S0-AYQ-285

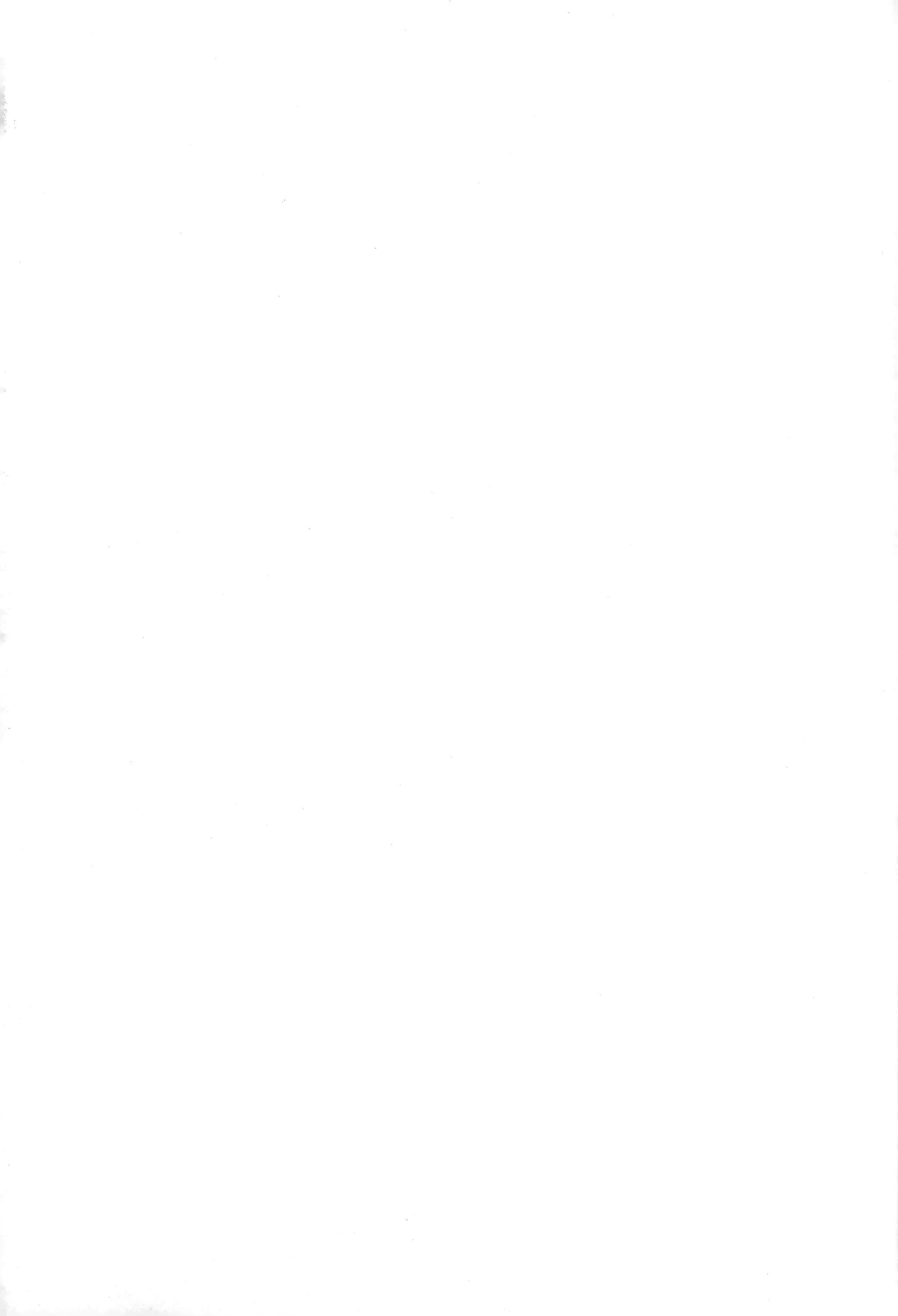

PATHOLOGY
OF THE
PLACENTA

PATHOLOGY
OF THE
PLACENTA

Second Edition

Edited by

Steven H. Lewis, MD
Clinical Associate Professor of Obstetrics, Gynecology, and Pathology
University of South Florida School of Medicine
Tampa, Florida

Director of Anatomic Pathology, Obstetrics and Gynecology
The Florida Women's Center
Department of Obstetrics, Gynecology, and Pathology
Indian River Memorial Hospital
Vero Beach, Florida

Eugene Perrin, MD
Department of Pathology
Wayne State University School of Medicine
Detroit, Michigan

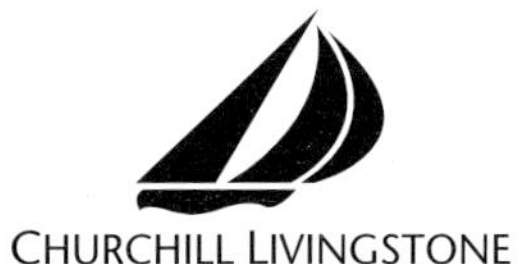

CHURCHILL LIVINGSTONE

New York, Edinburgh, London, Madrid, Melbourne, San Francisco, Tokyo

CHURCHILL LIVINGSTONE

A Division of Harcourt Brace & Company

The Curtis Center
Independence Square West
Philadelphia, Pennsylvania 19106

Library of Congress Cataloging-in-Publication Data

Pathology of the placenta / [edited by] Steven H. Lewis, Eugene
Perrin. — 2nd ed.
p. cm.
Includes bibliographical references and index.
ISBN 0-443-07586-7
1. Placenta—Diseases. I. Lewis, Steven H. II. Perrin, Eugene
V. D. K.
[DNLM: 1. Placenta—pathology. 2. Placenta Diseases—pathology.
WQ 212 P297 1999]
RG591.P37 1999
618.3'4—dc21
DNLM/DLC

98-23008

PATHOLOGY OF THE PLACENTA ISBN 0-443-07586-7

Printed in the United States of America

Last digit is the print number: 9 8 7 6 5 4 3 2 1

To
Heidi Dries Gorsuch
and
Makena Frances Natanella Lewis

In Memory of

Stephen A. Heifetz, MD

Contributors

Geoffrey Altshuler, MB, BS
Clinical Professor of Pathology and Pediatrics, University of Oklahoma Health Sciences Center; Pathologist, Children's Hospital of Oklahoma, Oklahoma City, Oklahoma
Infectious Disorders of the Placenta

Virginia J. Baldwin, MD, FRCP(C)
Associate Professor of Pathology, Faculty of Medicine, University of British Columbia; Consultant Pediatric Pathologist and Head, Autopsy and Embryopathology Service, Children's and Women's Health Center of British Columbia, Vancouver, British Columbia
Placental Pathology and Multiple Gestation

Robert W. Bendon, MD
Associate Clinical Professor of Pathology and Pediatrics, University of Louisville; Pathologist, Kosair Children's Hospital, Louisville, Kentucky
Examination of the Placenta

Kurt Benirschke, MD
Professor Emeritus of Pathology and Reproductive Medicine, University of California, San Diego, San Diego, California
Overview of Placental Pathology and Justification for Examination of the Placenta

Enid Gilbert-Barness, MD
Professor of Pathology, Pediatrics, and Obstetrics and Gynecology, University of South Florida School of Medicine, Tampa, Florida
Placental Membranes

Brendan Harrington, MA, MB, ChB, MRCP
Clinical Lecturer in Child Health, University of Manchester; Honorary Senior Registrar in Paediatrics, St. Mary's Hospital for Women and Children, Manchester, United Kingdom
Molecular Biology of the Placenta with Focus on Special Placental Studies of Infants with Intrauterine Growth Retardation

†Stephen A. Heifetz, MD
Professor of Pathology and Laboratory Medicine and Director of the Division of Pediatric Pathology, Indiana University Medical Center, Indianapolis, Indiana
Pathology of the Umbilical Cord

---

†Deceased.

Debra S. Heller, MD
Associate Professor of Clinical Pathology and Laboratory Medicine, New Jersey Medical School, University of Medicine and Dentistry of New Jersey, Newark, New Jersey
Gestational Trophoblastic Disease

Scott R. Hyde, PhD
Assistant Professor of Pathology, University of Oklahoma College of Medicine—Tulsa; Scientific Director of Perinatal Pathology and Molecular Diagnostic Laboratory, Saint Francis Hospital and South Tulsa Pathology, Inc., Tulsa, Oklahoma
Infectious Disorders of the Placenta

Eric Jauniaux, MD, PhD
Senior Lecturer, University College London; Consultant in Materno-Fetal Medicine, University College Hospitals, London, United Kingdom
Clinical Ultrasound and Pathologic Correlation of the Placenta

Dagmar K. Kalousek, MD
Professor, Department of Pathology, The University of British Columbia; Director, Cytogenetic Laboratory, British Columbia's Children's and Women's Hospital, Vancouver, British Columbia
Molecular Biology of the Placenta with Focus on Special Placental Studies of Infants with Intrauterine Growth Retardation

Cynthia G. Kaplan, MD
Associate Professor of Pathology, State University of New York, Stony Brook; Pediatric Pathologist, University Hospital, State University of New York, Stony Brook, Stony Brook, New York
Embryonic Pathology of the Placenta

John C. P. Kingdom, MD, MRCOG, MRCP, DCH
Associate Professor, Department of Obstetrics and Gynaecology, University of Toronto; Staff Obstetrician, Maternal-Fetal Medicine Division, Department of Obstetrics and Gynaecology, Mount Sinai Hospital, Toronto, Ontario
Clinical Ultrasound and Pathologic Correlation of the Placenta

Valia S. Lestou, PhD
Department of Pathology and Laboratory Medicine, University of British Columbia; British Columbia Research Institute for Children's and Women's Health, Vancouver, British Columbia
Molecular Biology of the Placenta with Focus on Special Placental Studies of Infants with Intrauterine Growth Retardation

Steven H. Lewis, MD
Clinical Associate Professor of Obstetrics, Gynecology, and Pathology, University of South Florida School of Medicine, Tampa, Florida; Director of Anatomic Pathology, Obstetrics and Gynecology, The Florida Women's Center; Department of Obstetrics, Gynecology, and Pathology, Indian River Memorial Hospital, Vero Beach, Florida
Overview of Placental Pathology and Justification for Examination of the Placenta; Placental Membranes

Richard L. Naeye, MD
Professor of Pathology, Pennsylvania State University College of Medicine, Hershey, Pennsylvania
The Placenta: Medicolegal Considerations

Robert Pijnenborg, MD
Associate Professor, Department of Obstetrics and Gynecology, University Hospital Gasthuisberg, Leuven, Belgium
Disorders of the Decidua and Maternal Vasculature

Edwina J. Popek, DO
Assistant Professor of Pathology and Pediatrics, Baylor College of Medicine; Pediatric Pathologist, Texas Children's Hospital, Houston, Texas
Normal Anatomy and Histology of the Placenta

Raymond W. Redline, MD
Associate Professor of Pathology and Reproductive Biology, Case Western Reserve University; Pediatric Pathologist, University Hospitals of Cleveland, Cleveland, Ohio
Disorders of the Placental Parenchyma

Wendy Robinson, PhD
Department of Medical Genetics, University of British Columbia, Vancouver, British Columbia
Molecular Biology of the Placenta with Focus on Special Placental Studies of Infants with Intrauterine Growth Retardation

Carolyn M. Salafia, MD
Associate Professor of Pathology, Albert Einstein College of Medicine of Yeshiva University and Montefiore Medical Center, Bronx, New York
Disorders of the Decidua and Maternal Vasculature

C. Maureen Sander, MD
Professor of Pathology and Director, Michigan Placental Tissue Registry, Michigan State University, East Lansing, Michigan
Examination of the Placenta

Douglas R. Shanklin, MD
Professor of Pathology and Obstetrics and Gynecology, University of Tennessee, Memphis, Memphis, Tennessee
Chorangiomas and Other Tumors

Aron E. Szulman, MB, ChB, FRCPath
Professor of Pathology Emeritus, University of Pittsburgh School of Medicine; Staff Pathologist (Consultant), Magee Women's Hospital, Pittsburgh, Pennsylvania
Trophoblastic Diseases: Complete and Partial Hydatidiform Moles

Contents

†Deceased.

Foreword

All physicians who care for the pregnant patient must have an appreciation of the pathologic basis of placental disease because this can have an important bearing on the health of the mother as well as on the development of the fetus. Similarly, scientists interested in obstetrical, prenatal, and neonatal disorders must have an understanding of the pathologic processes affecting the placenta to direct research endeavors. Yet in the past the pathology of the placenta has received relatively little attention, with most of the contributions to knowledge in this area coming from anatomists, physiologists, and endocrinologists. More recently, investigation of the placenta by pathologists has increased dramatically and provided a wealth of new information. Doctors Lewis and Perrin have assembled a highly talented group of individuals who have provided comprehensive treatises on all aspects of placental pathology.

The second edition of *Pathology of the Placenta* admirably fulfills its goal of providing a careful correlation of the clinical findings with the gross and microscopic features of the various diseases that can affect the placenta. The chapters on molecular biology, clinical ultrasound, and genetics enhance this even further. *Pathology of the Placenta* will be invaluable not only for pathologists but also for clinicians and basic scientists since its focus is not merely on morphology but on a correlation of morphology with function, thereby elucidating the clinical implications of the various pathologic alterations. This book will undoubtedly go a long way toward filling the lacuna in the understanding of placental pathology that has existed in the past, and it is a tribute to the vast breadth of knowledge of Doctors Lewis and Perrin and their special gifts as teachers that they have been able to present a large amount of complex material in a clear and concise fashion.

Robert J. Kurman, MD

Preface

The first edition of *Pathology of the Placenta* was used by pathologists, obstetricians, neonatologists, and students as an inclusive, easy-to-interpret text that served both as an introduction to the complexities of the placenta and as a diagnostic tool for those needing placental interpretation. In this regard, a complex subject with many ramifications was made available to a broad spectrum of physicians in a detailed yet simplified form.

Since its initial printing in 1984, much has transpired to update, clarify, and give added support to principles set forth in the first edition. It is the aim of this text to remain a resource both for those beginning a study of the placenta and for those who need a ready and inclusive reference for diagnosis—all in current context.

The contributors to this text are accepted experts in the field who have done much to illuminate the importance to clinical medicine of understanding the placenta. Their charge again has been to provide a guide to, as opposed to an encyclopedia of, their specific topics of evaluation. The all encompassing and definitive text on the placenta continues to be Benirschke and Kaufmann's *Pathology of the Human Placenta,* and the reader is referred there as well to the other excellent texts cited throughout this book for more in depth reviews on topics covered in this book.

I gratefully extend my appreciation to the contributors to this text and to those reviewers and staff who have provided excellent work, commentary, and production. I would also like to acknowledge Kurt Benirschke, who has patiently taught me much about the placenta and life, and my professors G. Barry Pierce and Ralph M. Richart, who have taught me much about the pursuit of quality in research and medicine.

Steven H. Lewis, MD

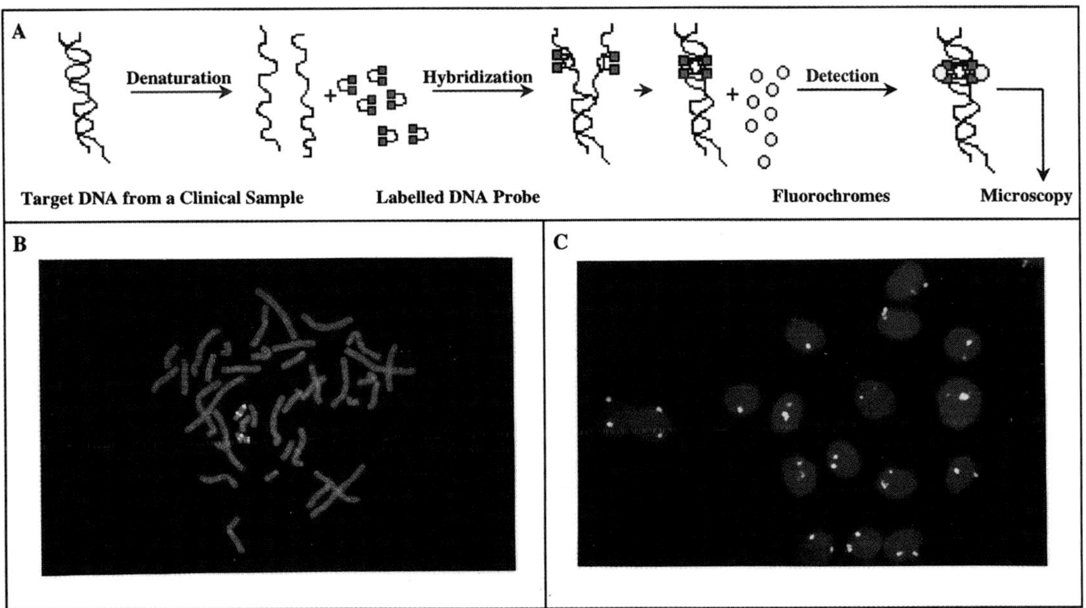

Figure 14–4. Fluorescence in situ hybridization (FISH) allows the direct localization of DNA sequences on chromosomes and within interphase nuclei. **A,** Labeled DNA probes are hybridized to complementary target DNA. The probes are detected with fluorochrome-marked specific antibodies. A fluorescence microscope is used for visualization, and both chromosomes and nuclei are counterstained with propidium iodide. **B,** Metaphase showing the Di-George chromosome region (DGCR) using the specific probe at 22q11 (D22S75-Oncor) and a control probe on chromosome 22 at band q13.1 (D22S39-Oncor). **C,** Interphase nuclei hybridized with chromosome 18 α-satellite probe (D18Z1-Oncor) showing disomy.

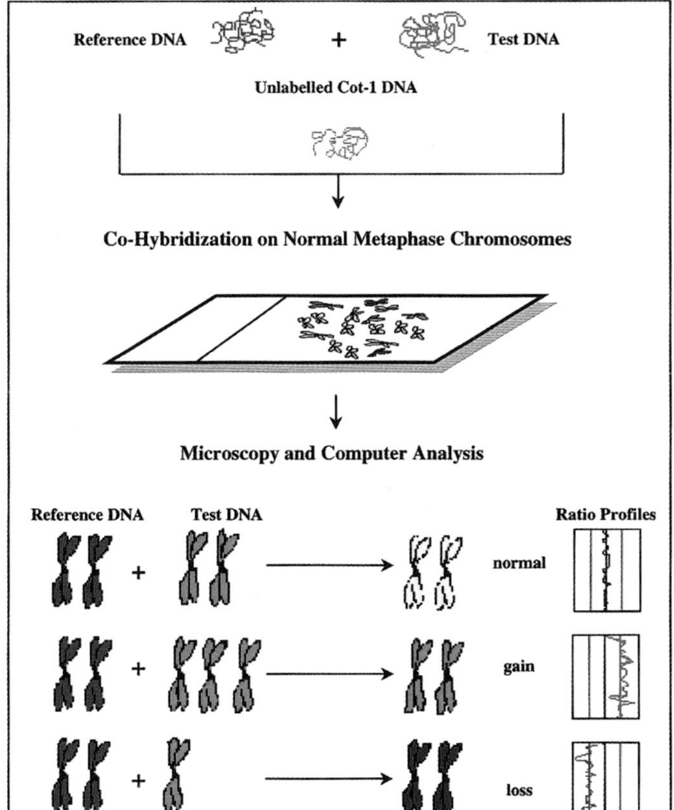

Figure 14–5. Comparative genomic hybridization (CGH). CGH permits a comprehensive analysis of the entire genome for gains or losses of chromosomal material. Test DNA, reference DNA, and Cot-1 DNA are hybridized to chromosome spreads obtained from a normal person (see text for details). Chromosomal imbalances are detected by fluorescence microscopy and computer analysis. Disomy is detected as a balanced ratio of green to red fluorescence and is indicated by the blue line. A gain is detected as a relative increase in the green fluorescence and is indicated by a shift to the right (green line). A loss is detected as a relative decrease in the green fluorescence and is indicated by a shift to the left (red line).

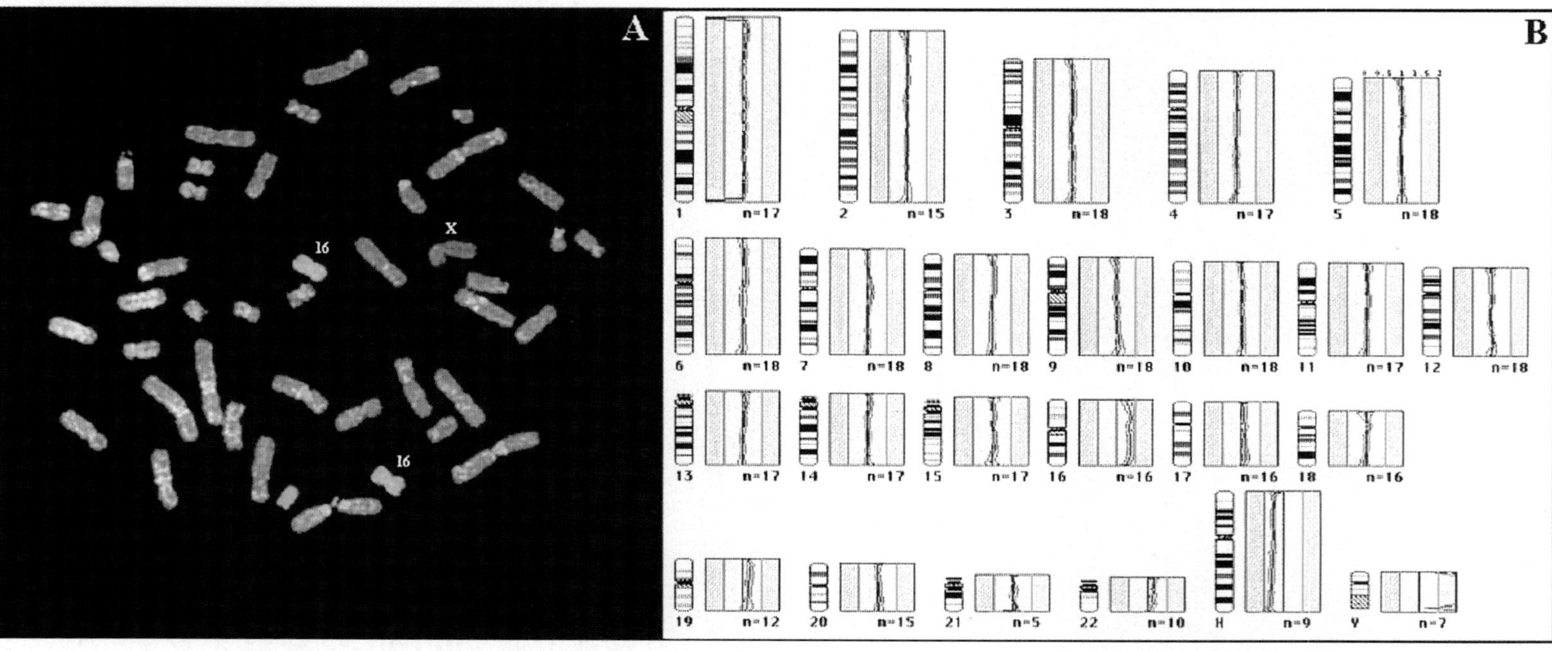

Figure 14–6. Detection of trisomy for chromosome 16 in placental tissues (47,XY, +16) by comparative genomic hybridization on a metaphase plate from a normal female. **A,** Greenish color indicates overrepresented chromosome 16 and reddish color underrepresented chromosome X, since the reference DNA originated from a female (XX) and the test DNA from a male (XY). **B,** The ratios are plotted along each single chromosome. The blue line represents the average green-to-red fluorescence profile ratio, and the gray lines represent the corresponding standard deviation. The profile for chromosome 16 demonstrates a shift to the right indicating a gain, while chromosome X demonstrates a shift to the left indicating a loss.

1

Overview of Placental Pathology and Justification for Examination of the Placenta

Steven H. Lewis and Kurt Benirschke

It is unfortunate that medicolegal concerns have been the impetus for an exponential growth of interest in the placenta. A well-managed placenta may be worth millions of dollars in a malpractice case, but its true value lies in its elegant depiction of in utero events. These events have enormous impact on gestational and neonatal care.

Despite the current fascination with the placenta, many impediments to commonplace expertise in and respect for the organ still exist. Although generally all specimens from a surgical suite are sent to pathology laboratories for evaluation, the delivery suite is not often considered an operating room. Placentas are usually left in limbo for someone to make a decision regarding their submission. (There is never any question whether a hernia sac should be "sent to pathology.") The uncertainty is compounded by the fact that not all placentas require examination. Most pregnancies are normal. Occasionally an adverse outcome is noted long after the mother and newborn have gone home, and no meaningful record of placental findings exists. A concise guide for handling and submission of all placentas is therefore required. A list of placental conditions necessitating submission should be present in all labor and delivery units (Table 1–1).[1]

Proper evaluation of the placenta is critical for establishing germane clinicopathologic correlates. Often gross and microscopic findings within the placenta indicate the presence of factors relating to adverse maternal and fetal outcome.

A coordinated approach to placental examination is required. Since not all placentas can be examined in a pathology laboratory, principally because of cost constraints, the obstetrician must decide whether submission is necessary based on clinical, neonatal, and placental observation. Inherent in this is that the obstetrician understand placentas. If the clinician sees no obvious need for submission, he or she is responsible for at least accurately recording a

Table 1–1. Indications for Placental Evaluation

Maternal	Fetus or Newborn	Placenta and Umbilical Cord
Diabetes mellitus	Stillborn	Infarcts
Pregnancy-induced hypertension (PIH)	Neonatal death	Abruptio placentae
Premature rupture of membranes (PROM)	Multiple gestation	Vasa previa
Preterm delivery before 36 weeks	Prematurity	Placenta previa
Postterm delivery at 42 weeks or later	Intrauterine growth retardation (IUGR)	Abnormal appearance of placenta or cord
Unexplained fever	Congenital anomalies	
Poor previous obstetric history	Erythroblastosis fetalis	
Oligohydramnios	Transfer to a neonatal intensive care unit	
History of drug abuse	Ominous fetal heart rate tracing	
	Presence of meconium	
	Apgar scores below 5 at 1 minute or below 7 at 5 minutes	

From College of American Pathology: The examination of the placenta: patient care and risk management. Arch Pathol Lab Med 115, 1991. Copyright 1991, American Medical Association.

gross description of the placenta. This takes only 2 or 3 minutes and should be a more salient observation than "The placenta was delivered intact." Noting the cord length and describing the membranes and the parenchyma requires a basic knowledge that the obstetrician probably can master with a single lecture and some limited practice. The obstetrician's note in the delivery record is commonly the only permanent record of placental findings. Therefore the obstetrician *must* have a core knowledge of placental pathology.

The coordinated approach continues further by recognizing that the placental pathology report is important not only to the obstetrician, but also to the pediatrician and neonatologist. Therefore pediatricians also require a fundamental base of knowledge to interpret and recognize the relevance of placental findings. Most pediatricians erroneously believe that the only important information to be derived from the placenta is whether infection is identified. It is dramatically helpful in this regard to have the pathologist make rounds with the pediatricians and neonatologists. In this way babies who are not doing well may benefit from information gleaned from the placenta, and pediatricians can be educated about the benefits and importance of a thorough placental examination.

The radiologist also plays an important role in a coordinated approach. As described in Chapter 15, many placental lesions may be identified antepartum through imaging performed by the radiologist and obstetrician. These should be confirmed post partum by the obstetrician or the pathologist.

The placenta's impact in medical care and legal concerns will be greatest if the obstetrician, pathologist, pediatrician, and imaging specialist interact in a manner that creates a synthesis of data. The director of the placental service in a hospital is best suited to effect this coordinated effort and can tremendously further the benefits of placental examinations.

Relationships between placental pathologic alter-

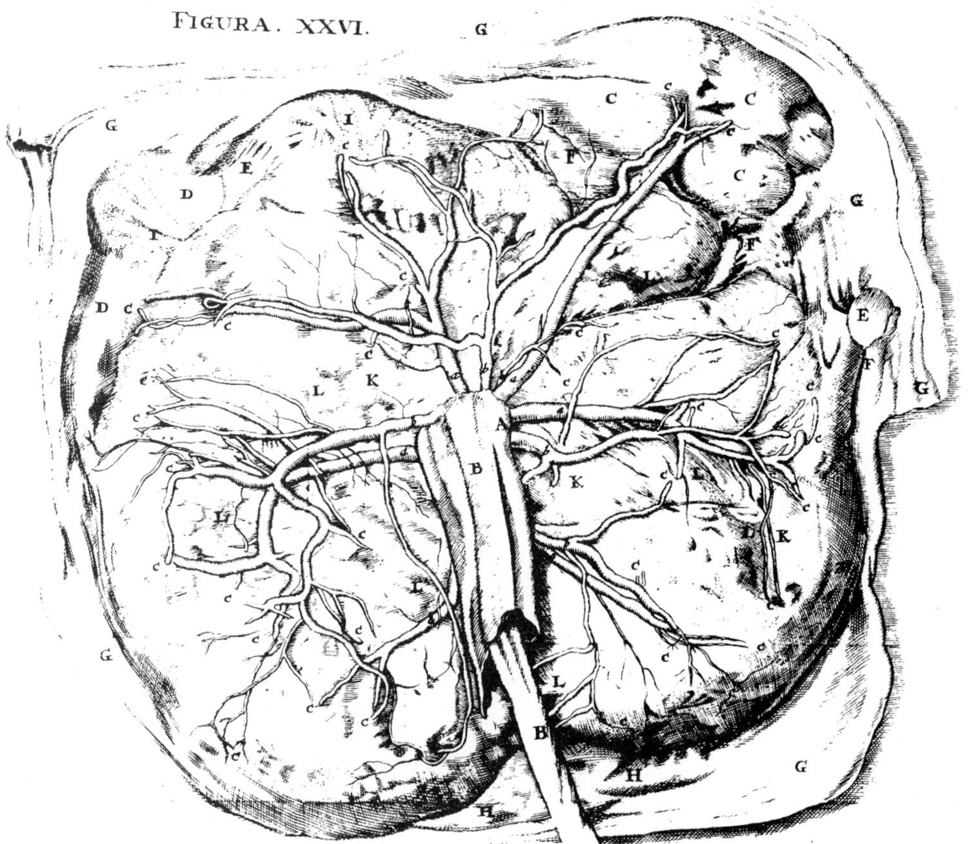

Figure 1–1. As early as 1669, Nicholas von Hoboken first described the accurate relations and compartments of the placenta as the cord, membranes, parenchyma, and decidua.

CLINICAL

Patient's Name ____________________ Med Record # ________________ Accession # ______________

Gestational Age ____________________

Medical Complications of Pregnancy (e.g., diabetes / hypertension / bleeding): 1st 2nd 3rd trimester / Infection (circle or add): ______________________________

Vaginal Delivery / Cesarean Section (circle)

Neonate: Wt ______ APGARS ______ CORD Ph______ NICU for ____________

Umbilical Cord Length in Total at Delivery ____________ cm

PLACENTA GROSS (circle choices)

Cord ______ cm × ______ cm Abnormalities

Membranes: In / Complete Clear Stained (color: __________) Opaque

Parenchyma: ______ cm × ______ cm × ______ cm
______ grams (trimed weight)
Red / Pale / Plethoric In / Complete
Infarcts _______% Central / Peripheral
Abruption ______%
Lesions: ______________________________
____

MICROSCOPIC AND FINAL DIAGNOSIS

Umbilical Cord:

Membranes:

Parenchyma:

Decidua:

Clinical Correlation:

________________________ Signed

Figure 1–2. User-friendly combination: clinical summary submission protocol, gross evaluation form, and microscopic reporting form—as a single document.

ations and clinical outcome take the form of identifying and supporting maternal and fetal diagnoses. Further, and not without minor benefit, is the role of placental diagnosis in medicolegal dispositions.

Placentas not submitted to the laboratory for immediate evaluation should be stored for at least 7 days at 4° C. This will allow later submission if warranted by maternal or neonatal conditions. The placenta is best examined fresh. Formalin fixation alters placental weight and renders some gross findings more difficult to interpret. The free membranes and cord should be trimmed from the placenta before it is weighed. The narrowest width of membranes should be assessed before membrane removal. The cord length is measured in toto (this is best accomplished in the delivery room). Abnormalities in the cord are identified (see below). The membranes are examined for their color and completeness. Abnormalities as reviewed below should be described. The chorionic vasculature is similarly studied, and notations regarding aberrance should be recorded. The parenchyma of the placenta is examined in breadloaf sections. Irregularities are identified, and both pathologic-appearing and normal-appearing regions are appropriately sampled for a full assessment of the pathologic features described below. The decidua is incompletely evaluated grossly. Microscopic sections are best appreciated from the "membrane roll," and one to three such sections may be submitted. At least three through-and-through sections of the parenchyma and one to three sections of umbilical cord should be included for microscopic diagnosis.

From the preceding it is clear that division of the placenta into the following compartments allows concise evaluation and diagnosis (Fig. 1–1):

- Umbilical cord
- Membranes (including the chorionic plate)
- Parenchyma (villi and intervillous space)
- Decidua

These compartments can serve as useful headings for reporting diagnoses in pathology reports (Fig. 1–2).

A majority of diagnoses relating to the placenta may be made during gross examination. Microscopic evaluation confirms these and enables diagnosis of specific histologic entities such as those that pertain to the decidua, as well as findings such as villitis.

The following is a compilation of pathologic processes that pertain to the placenta and have special clinical relevance. For a more detailed discussion and illustrations, the reader is referred to the appropriate sections of this text.

UMBILICAL CORD (see also Chapter 5)

The umbilical cord is formed as part of the development and maturation of the yolk stalk during embryogenesis. Functionally, the cord allows the transfer of nutrients and oxygen and the discard of waste and carbon dioxide. These occur through the cord's connection with the villous parenchymal capillaries by way of vessels of diminishing caliber that emanate from the chorionic vasculature. The cord is the main conduit of the vascular tree of the placenta, usually containing two arteries and a vein.

Abnormal Cord Length

The length of the umbilical cord varies according to gestational age. At term, short cords are those less than 32 to 35 cm and long cords are those greater than 70 cm. Short cords are associated with diminished fetal movement, abdominal wall defects, cord hemorrhage, and hematoma formation. Short cords have a statistically significant association with fetal growth retardation, increased perinatal mortality rate, and neurologic abnormalities. The association between short cords and fetal hypokinesia has been documented, but the etiology of this relationship is not well understood. Short cords are associated with a statistically significant increased relative risk of low intelligence quotient (IQ) and seizure disorders.

Long umbilical cords are prone to thrombosis and congestion. Knots, entanglements, and prolapse have been noted. Hyperactivity syndromes have been reported in neonates having long umbilical cords.

Accurate measurement of the umbilical cord is critical. Because umbilical cord gases are obtained and a section of umbilical cord often accompanies the neonate, it is crucial that the obstetrician measure the length of the cord in the delivery room. When the specimen arrives in the pathology department, sections may be missing and accuracy of cord length measurement is questionable. Having a sterilized paper tape measure in all delivery sets is simple and convenient. Cord length should be a part of the delivery report, especially when abnormal lengths are determined (see Table 3–1).[2–5]

Single Umbilical Artery

The absence of an umbilical artery may occur through agenesis or atrophy. Thrombosis is the presumed cause of the latter. The incidence overall is approximately 1%. Care must be taken to confirm the diagnosis by distal measurements, since two arteries may fuse close to the insertion on the placental disk. The association with congenital anomalies has been well documented. Major malformations occur twice as often in infants with a single artery as in those with three-vessel cords. Interestingly, the presence of a single umbilical artery is associated with short cords,

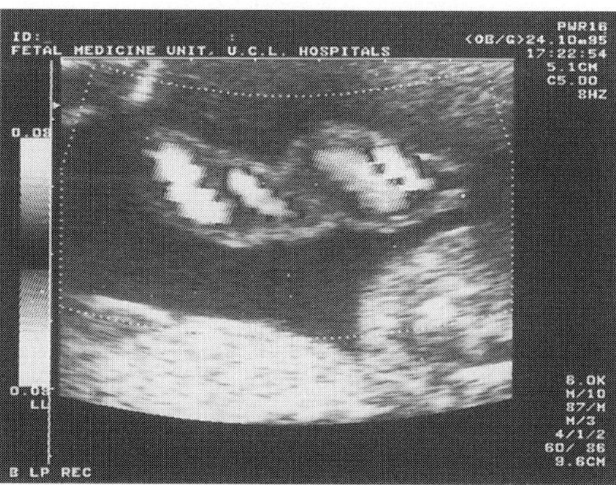

Figure 15–6. Color flow mapping at 22 weeks' gestation showing only one umbilical artery *(right)* next to the umbilical vein *(left)*. (See this figure enlarged in Chapter 15 by Eric Jauniaux and John C. P. Kingdom.)

marginal insertion of the cord, and small placentas. Stillbirth is four times as likely when a single umbilical artery is present. The risk of fetal growth retardation and preterm delivery is nearly doubled (Fig. 15–6).[2,6]

Abnormal Cord Insertions

The umbilical cord normally inserts centrally or paracentrally in the chorionic plate. Abnormal insertions take the form of marginal (at the periphery without membranous vessels) or velamentous insertions in which the umbilical cord inserts into the fetal membranes and is associated with membranous vessels that do not implant directly in the chorionic plate. These vessels course through the chorion of the fetal membranes before inserting into the disk proper.

The marginally inserted umbilical cord is associated with a slightly increased risk of fetal growth retardation and stillbirth.[2,4]

Certainly of pathologic significance is the velamentous (membranous) cord insertion. Statistically significant correlates include multiple gestations and congenital syndromes. Diabetes, advanced maternal age, and smoking are also correlates. Congenital syndromes carry an almost four-fold risk, as does diabetes. It is also found twice as frequently in patients with advanced maternal age. Adverse pregnancy outcomes have been studied, and preterm births in conjunction with velamentous insertions account for three per 1000 births. Neurologic abnormalities at 7 years of age carry a relative risk twice that of the normal population. Hyperactivity syndromes are also two to three times as likely.[2,4]

Catastrophic fetal blood loss with rupture, fetal distress, and vasa previa are noted complications of velamentous cords. Further, putative assessment regarding resultant nonhemorrhagic complications occurs from compression of unprotected vessels (without Wharton's jelly) and subsequent thrombosis (Fig. 5–9*A*).[2–4,7,8]

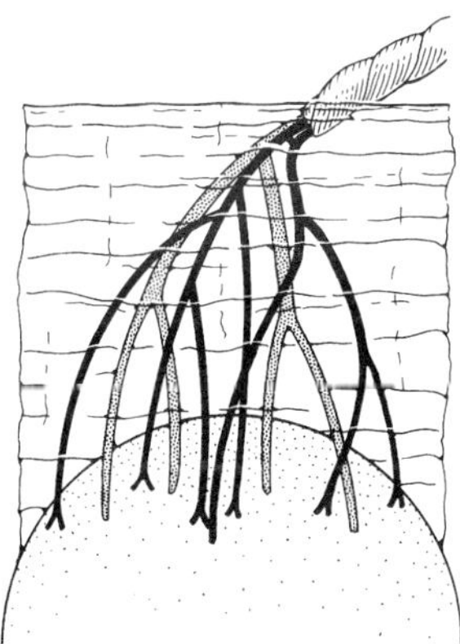

Figure 5–9. A, Velamentous insertion. The cord inserts into the membranes at some distance from the placental disk margin. Thereafter the three vessels branch while divested of and unprotected by Wharton's jelly as they course to the disk surface. When vessles branch and lose their jelly before their insertion but insert directly on the disk surface rather than into the membranes, the condition is termed a furcate cord insertion. (See this figure enlarged in Chapter 5 by Stephen A. Heifetz.)

Umbilical Vasculature Thrombosis

Umbilical vascular thrombosis can result from velamentous insertion, marked funisitis (cord inflammation), entangled cords, intravascular exchange transfusions, and fetal protein C deficiency. The occurrence has been calculated as seven per 1000 deliveries. Tight true knots and acute chorioamnionitis carry increased risks for thrombosis three and two times that of the normal population, respectively. Adverse associated pregnancy outcomes include preterm birth, stillbirth, and neonatal death. Stillbirth rates increase 300% with thrombosis. There is a high degree of association (and therefore it is medically probable) that thrombosis of the umbilical cord vasculature can be responsible for the causation of cerebral palsy (Fig. 5–16).[2,3,7]

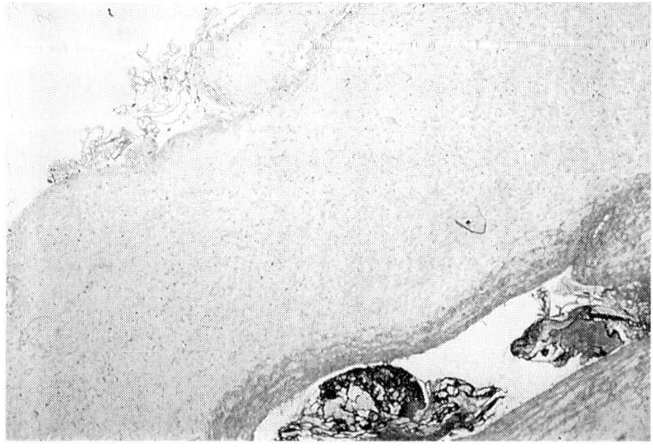

Figure 5–16. Umbilical vein thrombus at the site of cord strangulation by an amniotic band that is seen as the stringy material on the cord surface. (See this figure enlarged in Chapter 5 by Stephen A. Heifetz.)

Umbilical Cord Hematoma

Hemorrhage and hematoma formation in the umbilical cord are rare events. They occur in probably one per 1000 births. The antecedent event is usually considered to be an anomalous vessel in the cord. Such anomalous vessels may be vitelline remnants or tortuous varicosities of the umbilical vein. Stillbirth is a common result with a risk seven times that of the normal population. Associations include long umbilical cords and major congenital malformations, both of which occur approximately twice as often when this pathologic entity is present. It is important to differentiate true hematoma from the artifact of cord clamping in the delivered placenta. Serrated marks produced by a surgical or cord clamp at the site of hematoma distinguish this artifact (Fig. 5–15*A*).[2,3,7,9,10]

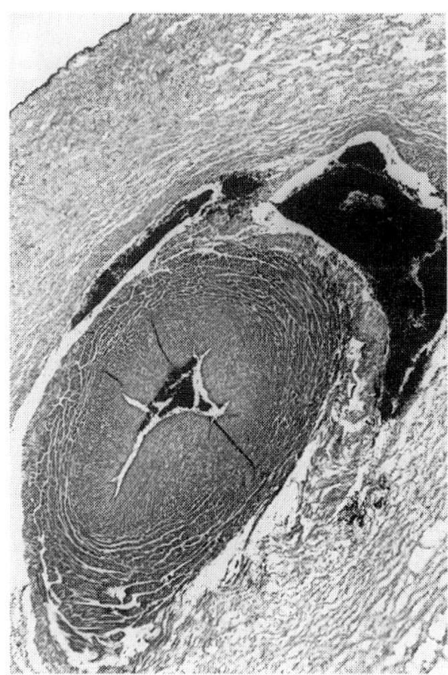

Figure 5–15. A, Periarterial intrafunicular hematoma forming a perivascular lake of extravasated blood. (See this figure enlarged in Chapter 5 by Stephen A. Heifetz.)

Umbilical Cord Stricture

Localized narrowing of the umbilical cord is associated with loss of Wharton's jelly and is most commonly seen close to the fetal body. Normal values for umbilical cord thickness have been determined. Narrow cords are three to four times as likely in patients who smoke and are also found in dysmature fetuses or those with major malformations. Small placentas and villi with unevenly accelerated maturation may be seen also three to four times as often in placentas with cord stricture.[2,3] Cord stricture is associated with both fetal growth retardation and fetal death (Fig. 5–13).[2,3]

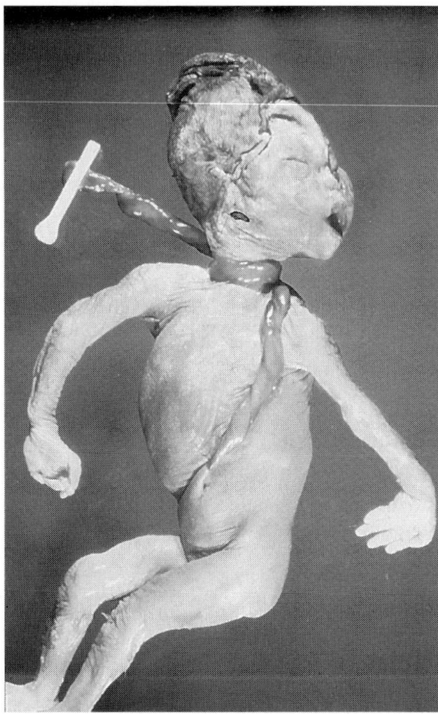

Figure 5–13. Severly macerated 27-week fetus with two nuchal coils that were deemed responsible for the fetal demise because of marked congestion of the cord distal to the entanglement and venous thrombi noted on microscopy. The cord "stricture" at the umbilicus showed no thrombi. The gradually diminishing quantity of Wharton's jelly as the cord approaches the abdomen was due to autolysis, which proceeds from the fetus toward the placenta. (See this figure enlarged in Chapter 5 by Stephen A. Heifetz.)

Umbilical Cord Torsion

Torsion is derived from excessive spiraling of the cord. Most often (7:1) a left-to-right twist occurs. This is probably because the right umbilical artery is usually larger than the left. Helix in the cord can be identified as early as 42 days' gestation. Increased fetal activity correlates with excessive spiraling. Excessive spiraling is seen more frequently in elongated umbilical cords. Statistically significant increases in fetal death from constriction and obstruction of vascular flow has been attributed to excessive spiraling.[2,7] Diminished

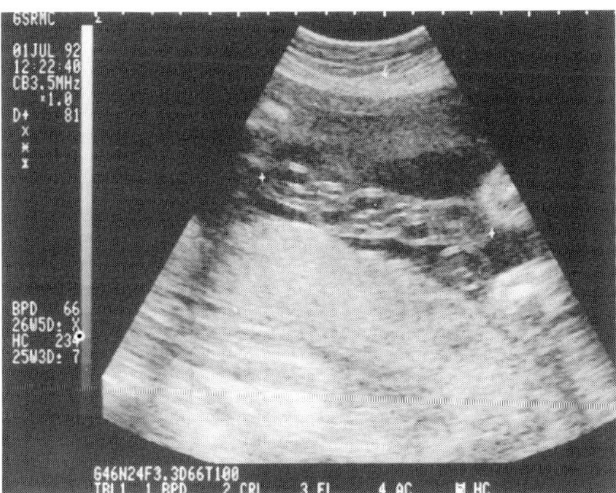

Figure 1–3. Excessive spiraling and torsion of the umbilical cord identified antepartum by ultrasonography. (Courtesy Thomas Strong, MD.)

spiraling may be associated with fetal distress and decreased fetal activity (Fig. 1–3).[11]

Edematous Umbilical Cord

Gross edema of the umbilical cord is seen in approximately 3% of deliveries. Hypertension with preeclampsia and eclampsia, uteroplacental insufficiency, chorioamnionitis, and increased subchorionic fibrin deposition are all frequently associated conditions. Preterm birth and stillbirth are twice as likely when cords are edematous. Normal gestational age-dependent values for cord thickness have been established (Fig. 5–7).[2,3,7]

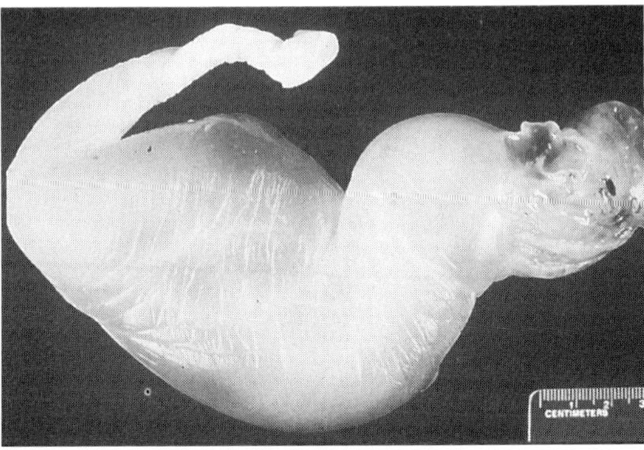

Figure 5–7. Localized edema of the umbilical cord (mucoid degeneration of Wharton's jelly). Cross sections commonly demonstrate a pseudocyst without an epithelial lining. If edema is located at the umbilicus, the cord should be transilluminated before ligation at delivery to search for a possible patent urachus, herniated portion of fetal intestinal tract, or hemangiomatous nodule. (See this figure enlarged in Chapter 5 by Stephen A. Heifetz.)

Cord Inflammation

The presence of polymorphonuclear leukocytes in the umbilical cord is a fetal response to intraamniotic infection. Circulating neutrophils permeate Wharton's jelly. The cord may appear opaque or even yellow. Distinct microabscesses caused by *Candida* can be identified on the cord surface as white plaques. One, two, or three vessels may be involved with acute inflammation. The vein usually demonstrates inflammation before the arteries. Subsequent inflammatory mechanisms promote luminal thrombosis. Preterm labor and distress from vascular spasm have been identified. Necrotizing funisitis is manifest as a severe inflammatory process that may create calcium deposition in the cord. Congenital infections such as syphilis and herpes are often reported causes of inflammation, but any severe infectious event may be etiologic (Fig. 13–2).[3,7,12,13]

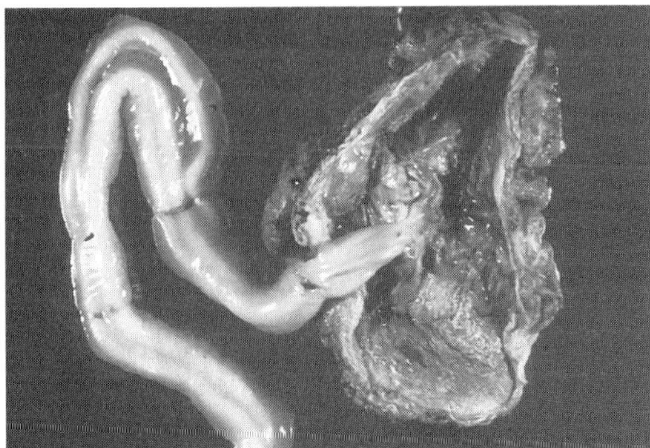

Figure 13–2. Necrotizing funisitis. Placenta with umbilical cord that manifests extensive edema and prominent blood vessels but not a so-called barber's pole appearance. On cut section the cord had chalky white linear streaks between the blood vessels and the amniotic surface of the umbilical cord. (See this figure enlarged in Chapter 13 by Scott R. Hyde and Geoffrey Altshuler.)

Meconium Changes

Chronic meconium exposure results in an opaque to green, mucoid-appearing umbilical cord. The Wharton's jelly of the cord becomes grossly stained only after the membranes are so affected. Meconium-laden macrophages are unusual in the cord. Long-standing exposure results in necrosis of vascular muscle ("meconium myonecrosis"). Spasm of umbilical vessels may result in fetal distress patterns. Meconium aspiration syndrome enhances the severity of these clinical effects (Fig. 5–18).[1,3,14]

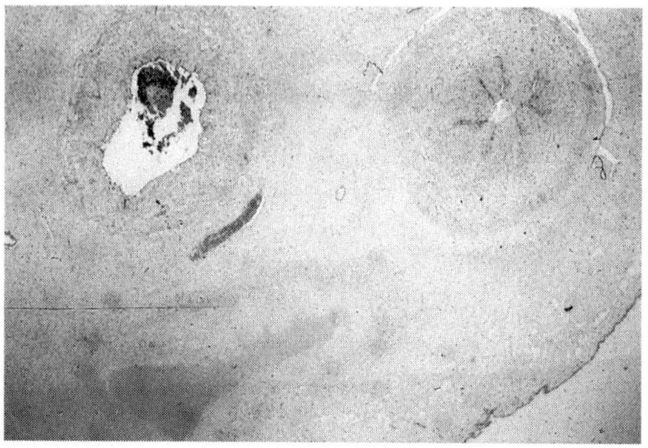

Figure 5–18. Meconium-induced necrosis of one umbilical artery. The portion of the arterial wall oriented toward the surface is most severely affected. (See this figure enlarged in Chapter 5 by Stephen A. Heifetz.)

Amniotic Web

The presence of amnion extending along the cord surface for several centimeters off the chorionic plate limits movement of the umbilical cord. The web is attributed to anomalous cord development. Circulatory compromise and decreased in utero movement are thought to be associated findings. Additional study is required to establish statistically significant clinical correlates.[1,3]

Embryologic Remnants

Embryologic remnants in the placenta are most commonly seen in the cord. The allantoic duct may persist and is identified between the two umbilical arteries. It has no clinical significance. The omphalomesenteric duct may persist and represents the connection between the developing gut and yolk sac through the yolk stalk. On occasion its prominence may be related to omphalocele formation, persistence of vitelline vessels, and unusual entrapped enteric mucosa that can ulcerate the cord when gastric epithelia are present. These embryologic associations account for the persistence of Meckel's diverticulum. A remnant of the yolk sac may be identified on the disk plate in some placentas and is a normal finding (Fig. 5–1).[3]

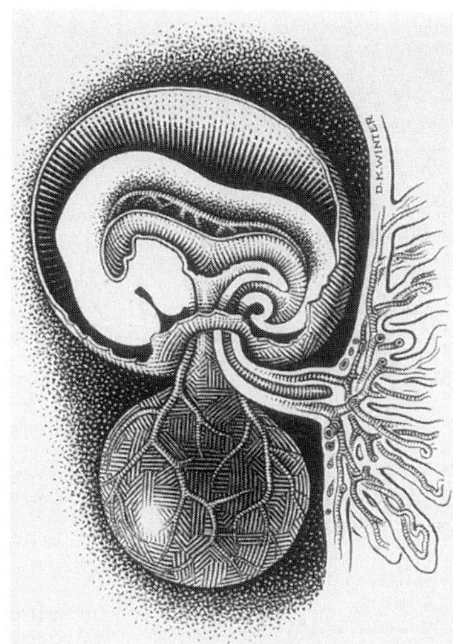

Figure 5–1. Formation of the umbilical cord. Between postconception days 18 and 40 the embryo rotates, so that the yolk sac turns toward the implantation site, and herniates into the enlarging amniotic cavity that compresses the connecting stalk, allantois, and the omphalomesenteric duct into a slender cord covered by amniotic epithelium. (See this figure enlarged in Chapter 5 by Stephen A. Heifetz.)

Tight Knots

Tight knots have marked clinical significance, and in the absence of other significant pathologic alterations they may cause fetal demise or significant compromise. The presence of "notching" and proximal dilatation is indicative of clinically significant tightness. Loose knots are often present in healthy infants.[7] True knots should be distinguished from false knots which are simply varicosities of the umbilical vein. On rare occasions such varicosities may be prone to thrombosis (Fig. 5–12*A*).

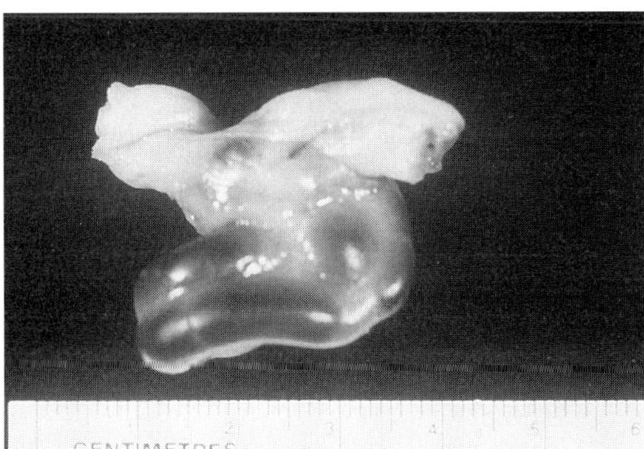

Figure 5–12. A, Thrombosis of redundant umbilical vein varix (false knot). (See this figure enlarged in Chapter 5 by Stephen A. Heifetz.)

MEMBRANES (see also Chapter 6)

The membranes of the placenta are composed of the "reflected" membranes and those of the chorionic plate on the placental disk. Embryologic concerns are germane because membrane development requires appropriate atrophy of villi that make up the chorion laeve during expansion of the amnionic cavity. The mesodermal investments from the embryo are responsible for vascular formation and associated mesenchymal tissue within the chorion. The remainder of the extravillous chorion is derived from trophoblast. The amnion develops from ectodermal layers of the fetus, and the amnion and chorion together form a distinct structural and functional unit. The following pathologic alterations are critical in examination of the delivered placental membranes.

Squamous Metaplasia of the Amnion

The most significant aspect of squamous metaplasia is distinguishing its normal appearance from the alterations consistent with amnion nodosum. Squamous metaplasia occurs with great frequency and reflects the ectodermal nature of the amnionic cell layer. Occasionally, large plaques of metaplastic epithelium caused by traumatic events are identified. Where large anomalous fetal formations rub chronically against the amnion (in the absence of oligohydramnios), large metaplastic lesions may occur. When immersed in water, these areas do not hydrate. This distinguishes them from amnion nodosum, which unlike metaplasia may be readily abraded from the amnionic surface (see below) (Fig. 6–4*B*).[3]

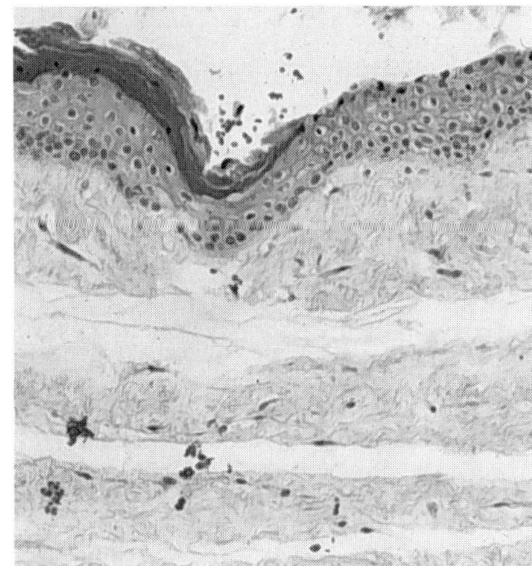

Figure 6–4. B, Microscopic squamous metaplasia. (See this figure enlarged in Chapter 6 by Steven H. Lewis and Enid Gilbert-Barness.)

Amnion Nodosum

Amnion nodosum is identified as innumerable nodules or plaques along the fetal surface of the placenta. It is pathognomonic of oligohydramnios. Exfoliated cells from the fetal epidermis, hair, and amnion aggregate with sebaceous material and fibrillar debris, forming the characteristic plaques. Long-standing oligohydramnios may result from renal agenesis and amniotic fluid leak-

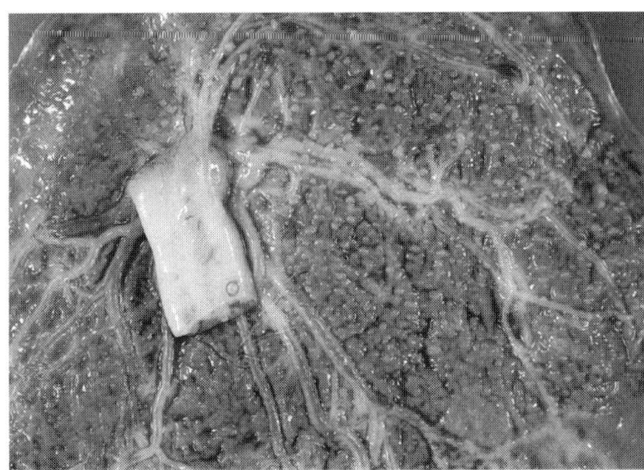

Figure 6–5. A, Innumerable papules of amnion nodosum. (Courtesy K. Benirschke, San Diego, California.) (See this figure enlarged in Chapter 6 by Steven H. Lewis and Enid Gilbert-Barness.)

age and cause pulmonary hypoplasia. Associated morbidity and mortality have been rigorously documented (Fig. 6–5*A*).[3,7]

MECONIUM CHANGES

Meconium pigment on the surface or within macrophages in deeper layers produces a characteristic amnionic epithelial degeneration with associated epithelial pseudostratification and necrosis of the amnion. Meconium passed into the amnionic fluid diffuses into membranes and may be phagocytosed by macrophages. Meconium staining is generally not seen before 32 to 34 weeks' estimated gestational age. Pigments identified before this period generally are indicative of hemosiderin and represent earlier hemorrhagic events. Other pigments such as lipofuscin, when not readily distinguishable microscopically, may be stained specially for confirmation purposes. Precise temporal relationships between meconium passage and staining have not been established, although estimations are available.[2,3,7]

Based on in vitro and retrospective data, meconium is a toxic agent that can cause fetal distress by producing vascular spasm and in severe cases vascular medial necrosis. In the Collaborative Perinatal Study, neurologic abnormalities at 7 years of age, including motor abnormalities and severe mental retardation, accounted for 230 per 1000 births in which meconium staining was noted. Motor abnormalities and severe retardation were also identified. Interestingly, statistically significant correlates include acute chorioamnionitis, advanced maternal age, and what has been termed birth asphyxial disorder in the Collaborative Perinatal Study. In this instance, 454 per 1000 births were so affected, six times more than in control subjects.[2,14]

Notably, meconium aspiration syndrome occurs in approximately 9 per 1000 births. Whether in utero aspiration results from gasping produced by physiologic responses to hypoxia or occurs through normal fetal breathing remains to be determined. Although aspiration syndrome has been hypothesized to be a function of direct toxicity to respiratory passages and alveoli, meconium instilled into experimental animals does not cause characteristic necrosis and inflammation. The high degree of association between chorioamnionitis and the presence of meconium (567 cases per 1000 births) has led to the speculation that infected amniotic fluid dramatically contributes to the pathophysiology of meconium aspiration syndrome (Fig. 6–10).[2,3,7,14]

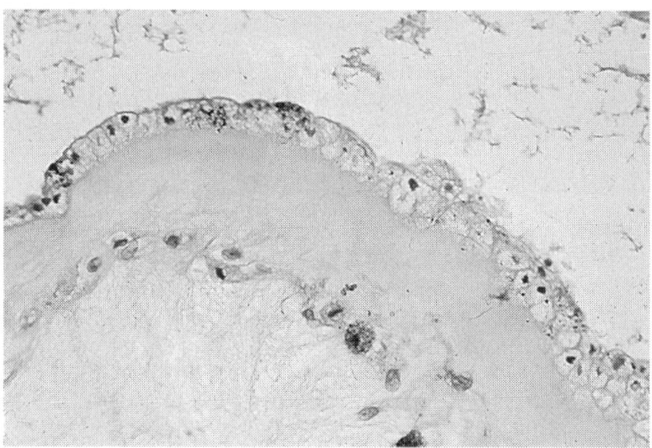

Figure 6–10. Membrane edema caused by meconium. Note vacuolated amnionic epithelial degeneration and marked edema of the compact and fibroblastic layers. Meconium is seen in macrophages. (See this figure enlarged in Chapter 6 by Steven H. Lewis and Enid Gilbert-Barness.)

ACUTE MEMBRANITIS (CHORIOAMNIONITIS) (see also Chapter 15)

Acute membranitis represents both maternal and fetal response to intraamniotic infection. The direction of polymorphonuclear leukocyte migration indicates the location of the antigen. This directionality may be confused insofar as funisitis appears to be a fetal response, whereas most chorioamnionitis represents maternal response. Initial maternal inflammation occurs in perivascular decidual layers. Inflammatory cells percolate to involve the chorion and subsequently the amnion. The degree of response does not correlate with clinically associated severity. Specifically, group B streptococcal sepsis is generally associated with small amounts of inflammatory infiltrate.[2,3,7,13]

Acute chorioamnionitis is identified in 160 of 1000 deliveries in which fetal membranes ruptured 1 to 12 hours before the onset of labor. In vitro weakening of fetal membranes results from staphylococcal and *Escherichia coli* infections, whereas group B streptococci are not associated with collagenase stimulation.[2]

The strong association of membranitis with preterm delivery and premature rupture of membranes has been noted. Associations with umbilical vascular spasm and thrombosis are described above. In such cases aberrant velocimetry may be identified. In severe inflammatory cases, extraplacental and placental membranes may appear white and purulent. In milder cases the membranes may demonstrate varying degrees of opacification and loss of normal sheen and translucency (Fig. 6–7*B*).[2,3,7,13]

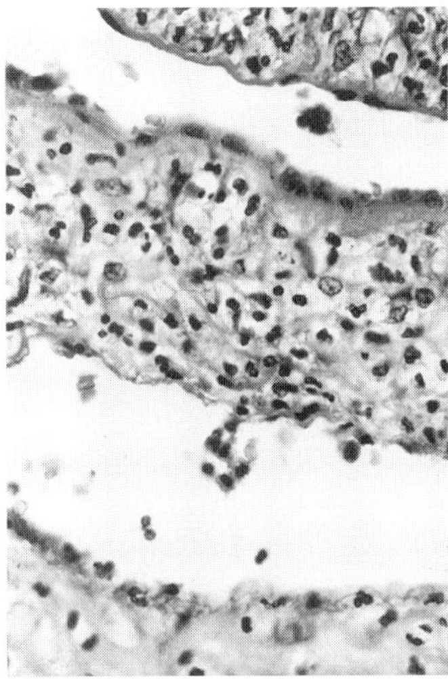

Figure 6–7. B, Acute chorioamnionitis involving the reflected membranes. (From Lewis SH, Benirschke K: The placenta. In Sternberg S [ed]: Histology for pathologists. New York, 1977, Raven Press.) (See this figure enlarged in Chapter 6 by Steven H. Lewis and Enid Gilbert-Barness.)

Amnionic Bands

The presence of amnionic bands is a result of former rupture of the amnion. This occurs for undetermined reasons. The characteristic appearance of the fetal surface of the chorionic plate is noteworthy for its lack of sheen. This is due to the absence of amnion above the remaining chorion. Strands or bands of residual amnion cross the fetal surface and attach directly to the umbilical cord. This attachment represents the firmest adherence of the amnion, and the bands cannot easily be stripped from this attachment site. Amputations, constrictions, disruptions, compression, and oligohydramnios may be identified. The temporal relationship between amnionic rupture and type of associated malformation may be presumed. Major anomalies occur with early rupture and include anencephaly and limb reduction (third week of gestation), with amputations occurring later (7 weeks and onward). Asymmetric disorders aid in ruling out chromosomal disorders and congenital syndromes. Thorough evaluation of the placenta generally establishes the diagnosis. Because of the heterogeneous nature of the condition, terminologic distinctions have been proposed, including "early amnion rupture sequence," "amnion disruption sequence," and "fetal disruption complex" (Fig. 6–11*C*).[2,7]

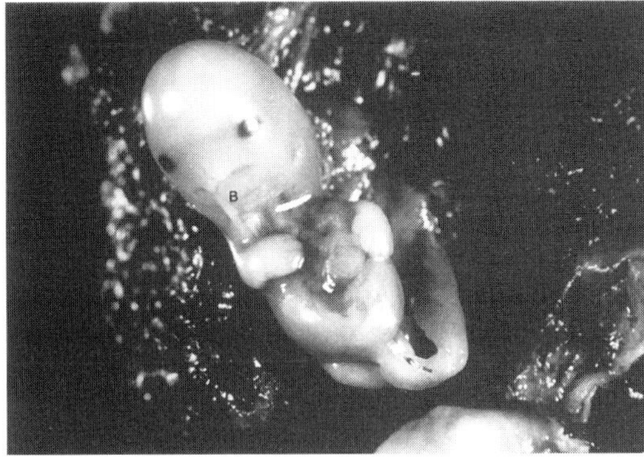

Figure 6–11. C, An unusual case of amniotic band *(B)* with facial deformity in the first trimester. (Courtesy Diane Spice.) (See this figure enlarged in Chapter 6 by Steven H. Lewis and Enid Gilbert-Barness.)

Gastroschisis-Associated Vacuolization

A peculiar vacuolization of the amnionic epithelium is pathognomonic and diagnostic of gastroschisis. Although clinical findings are generally sufficient without supportive diagnosis

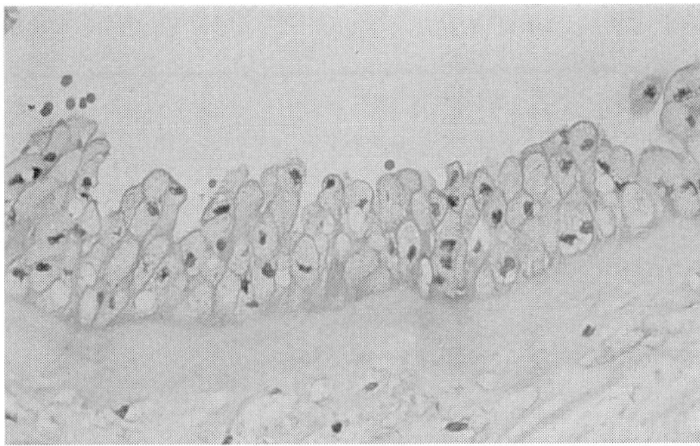

Figure 6–13. Gastroschisis amnionic vacuolization. Vacuolated epithelial cells are in turn filled with innumerable smaller vacuoles. (From Benirschke K, Kauffmann R: Pathology of the human placenta. New York, 1995, Springer-Verlag.) (See this figure enlarged in Chapter 6 by Steven H. Lewis and Enid Gilbert-Barness.)

through placental evaluation, it is interesting that this finding is seen only in this condition. The pathophysiology relates to deposition of vacuolar inclusions consisting of lipid, which can be confirmed by electron microscopy. The origin of this is not clear, especially since the fibrinous coating of the intestines seen in gastroschisis is without lipid (Fig. 6–13).[7]

Extrachorial Placentation

Extrachorial placentations are marked by *circumarginate* and *circumvallate* placentas. In the circumarginate placenta a rim of fibrin lies beneath the amnion and extends circumferentially medial to the disk margin. In circumvallation the amnion folds back onto itself, forming a distinct ridge, and remains loosely adherent to the peripheral chorion. The clinical significance of circumargination has been speculative, and distinct pathologic correlates remain obscure. There is an association with major fetal malformations and decidual necrosis. On the other hand, circumvallate placentas occur in approximately 6% of gestations, and associations with fetal growth retardation, preeclampsia, and decidual necrosis have been documented. The finding of associated bleeding disorders during gestation has long been known to coincide with circumvallate placentas. Such bleeding has been identified as maternal and may be either acute or chronic. Additional data are required to confirm the reported association between circumvallation and premature rupture of membranes, preterm delivery, and oligohydramnios (Fig. 6–12*A*).[2,3,7,15]

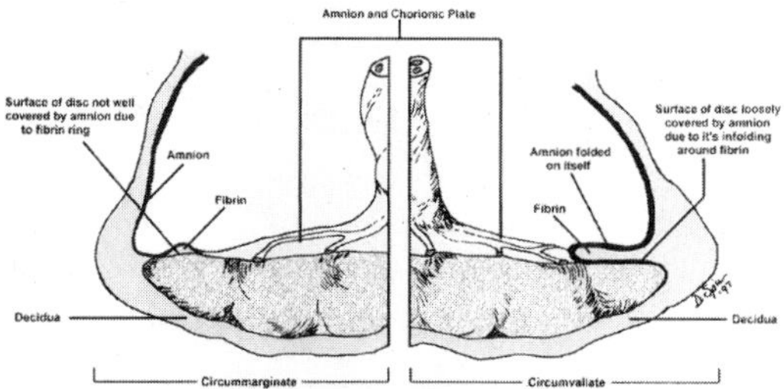

Figure 6–12. A, Cross-sectional diagram of circummargination and circumvallation. (See this figure enlarged in Chapter 6 by Steven H. Lewis and Enid Gilbert-Barness.)

Chorionic Vascular Thrombosis

Thrombosis of the chorionic vessels conceptually represents an extension of thrombosis of the umbilical vascular counterparts. Thrombosis results from compression, inflammation, immune mechanisms, factor deficiencies, congestion, and unknown causes.

Fetal compromise is a demonstrable correlate of thrombosis. The diagnosis is readily made by gross examination and can be accomplished in the delivery room. The observation of white to gray streaks running parallel to the periphery of luminal vascular structures is pathognomonic. Notation of such findings is critical, since adverse clinical outcome is a known consequence (see discussion of umbilical vascular thrombosis) (Fig. 6–14).[2,3,7,10,16]

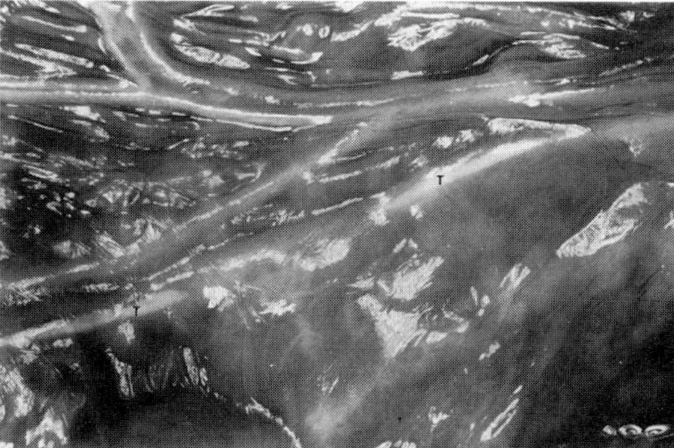

Figure 6–14. Chorionic vascular thrombi *(T)*. (From Benirschke K, Kauffmann R: Pathology of the human placenta. New York, 1995, Springer-Verlag.) (See this figure enlarged in Chapter 6 by Steven H. Lewis and Enid Gilbert-Barness.)

Multiple Gestations (see also Chapter 9)

Multiple gestations are conveniently discussed under the heading of membranes, since membranous relations are important and aid in establishing zygosity. In the evaluation of placentas from twin gestations, zygosity is a clinical concern. With the presence of a monochorionic placenta, diagnosis of monozygosity is certain. Approximately one third of monozygotic twins have dichorionic placentations, and therefore additional workup, including blood groupings, HLA marker studies, and "DNA fingerprinting," satisfies concerns regarding the nature of twinning. When monozygotic twins have dichorionic placentas, early splitting of the zygote (before 3 days of development) is likely. Late splitting results in monozygotic twinning with monochorionic and monoamnionic placentas. In such cases no intervening membrane is present and cord entanglements cause significant morbidity and mortality. Morbidity from monochorionic gestations with an intervening membrane is related to abnormal cord insertions, including increased incidence of velamentous cords (with their attendant associated complications; see above) and transfusion syndromes. Vein-to-vein, artery-to-artery, and artery-to-vein transfusions and shifts occur in decreasing order of frequency. Of greatest pathologic significance is the artery-to-vein transfusion (through a villous district), which may lead to the classic transfusion syndrome. Recent investigation of such syndromes has led to the conclusion that classic findings do not always occur. Complex vascular dynamics and flow patterns also involving artery-to-artery and vein-to-vein anastomosis account for discrepancies in the classic transfusion pattern (anemic donor and plethoric recipient). Injection studies are helpful in confirming the nature of anastomosis. Surface ablation of anastomotic vasculature via intrauterine surgery is of current interest.[2,3,7,17,18]

A convenient method of assessment for monochorionic twinning involves transillumination of the intervening membrane. The absence of velamentous vascular remnants establishes the diagnosis of monochorionicity. This is true because the amnion does not possess a vasculature and therefore the absence of a chorion between juxtaposed amnions coincides with diamnionic monochorionic placentation (Fig. 6–19*E*).[2,3,7,17,18]

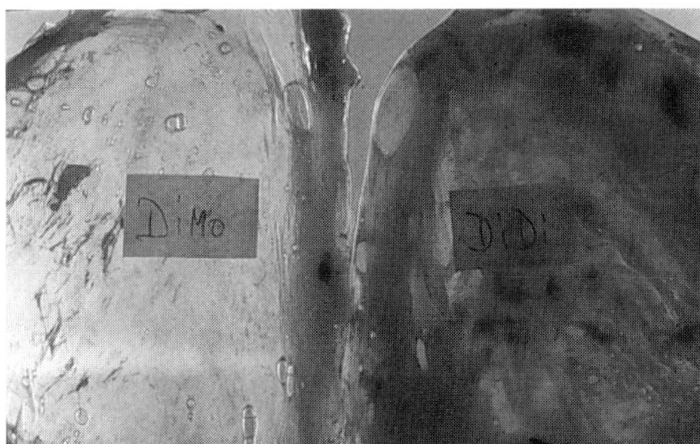

Figure 6–19. E, Transillumination of DiMo and DiDi intervening membranes. (Courtesy K. Benirschke, San Diego, California.) (See this figure enlarged in Chapter 6 by Steven H. Lewis and Enid Gilbert-Barness.)

PARENCHYMA (see also Chapter 7)

The placental parenchyma, for convenience designated as a "compartment," is composed of the villous ramifications of the disk. Taking off from the chorion, the vascular tree ramifies from stem to primary, then secondary, and finally tertiary villi. The intervillous space is also included. Developmentally, characteristic trophoblastic derivatives and their mesenchymal investments take on specific morphogenic appearances that are gestational age dependent. Pathologic entities germane to the parenchyma are described below.

Abnormal Placental Weight

Fetal placental weight ratios have been determined for normal ranges at different gestational ages. The ratio is 4 at 24 weeks and increases to 7 at term (see Table 3–1). Small placentas coexist with preeclampsia, low birth weight, and uniformly accelerated villous maturation. Small placentas are also associated with an increased incidence of stillbirth (400 per 1000). Neurologic abnormalities at 7 years and mental retardation without motor abnormalities are increased relative risks as well. Thin placentas coincide with small placentas; with placental thickness less than 2 cm this diagnosis can usually be established.[2,3,18,19]

Unusually large placentas are associated with villous edema, maternal diabetes, severe maternal anemia, fetal anemia, congenital syphilis, large intervillous thrombi, retained blood clot beneath the subchorionic layer, toxoplasmosis, congenital fetal nephrosis, idiopathic fetal hydrops, and multiple placental chorangiomas. In the Collaborative Perinatal Study, 9% of children with excessively large placentas showed neurologic aberrancies at 7 years of age. Most such cases are due to placental edema.[2,3,7,19]

Abnormal Color

The placental substance is ordinarily deep red. Pallor indicates anemia or infection in the villous

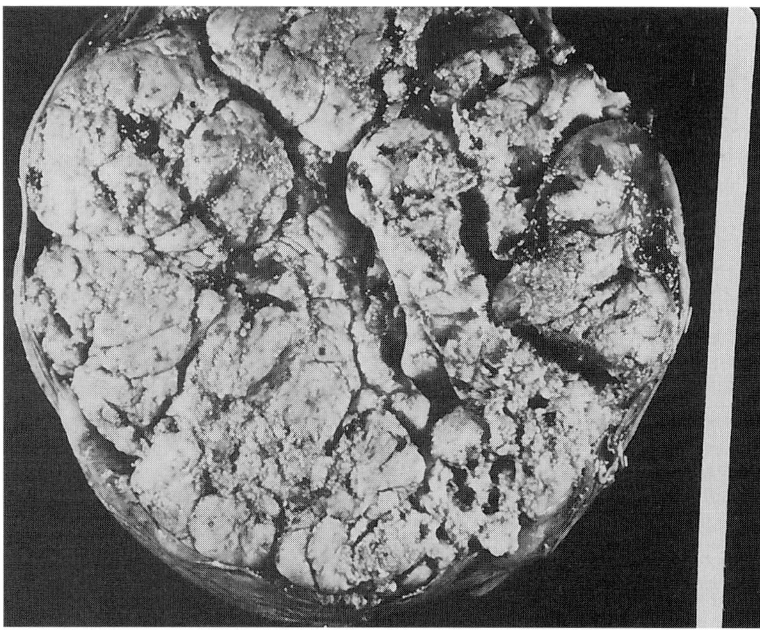

Figure 1–4. A large placenta in Rh incompatibility. It is hydropic, pale, and bulky and weighs 780 g.

parenchyma, whereas deeper hues of bright red in conjunction with increased weight are demonstrative of plethora and polycythemia. Other causes of deep, diffuse reddening of the placenta include placental congestion and chorangiosis (see below). Severe anemia is responsible for ischemia and neonatal organ system failure. Plethora may cause sludging and vascular thrombosis with attendant end organ damage (Fig. 1–4).[3,7,20]

ABNORMAL SHAPE

Irregular nonovoid shapes including multilobed placentas, reflect abnormalities of implantation, including failed involution of the chorion laeve. In addition, intracavitary uterine abnormalities (septa and leiomyomas) may result in accessory lobe formation. Important pathologic correlates include the presence of vasa previa from membranous vessels connecting lobes and retained placental tissue from unrecognized remaining lobules of placenta. Membranous vessels are also subject to compression and thromboses, as is the case with velamentous cord insertions. In approximately 1 in 40,000 pregnancies placenta membranacea occurs. In this condition an extensively thin placenta forms an entire sac and there is no distinct "membrane bag." Complete failure of involution of the chorion laeve is causal. This results in placenta previa and abnormal uterine bleeding both antepartum and postpartum. Postpartum bleeding reflects the high degree of association between placenta accreta and placenta membranacea (Fig. 6–15).[3,7,21]

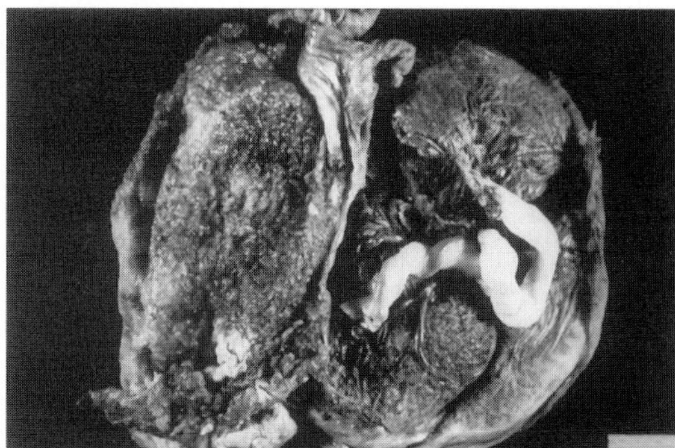

Figure 6–15. Placenta membranacea. No significant free membranes are present. (See this figure enlarged in Chapter 6 by Steven H. Lewis and Enid Gilbert-Barness.)

PLACENTA ACCRETA

Placenta accreta, placenta increta, and placenta percreta are complications that arise from the absence of intervening decidua between villous tissue and myometrium. Placenta accreta is a superficial process, whereas placenta increta penetrates the myometrium and placenta percreta progresses through the uterine serosa. A layer of intervening fibrin in the absence of decidua does not alter the diagnosis. An increased occurrence derives from previous cesarean section, uterine trauma, and low placental implantation. In unusual cases this diagnosis may be established by examination of the delivered placenta, which shows myometrial cells adherent to chorionic tissue in the absence of intervening decidua. Postpartum hemorrhage usually necessitates hysterectomy (Fig. 3–28).[3,7,22]

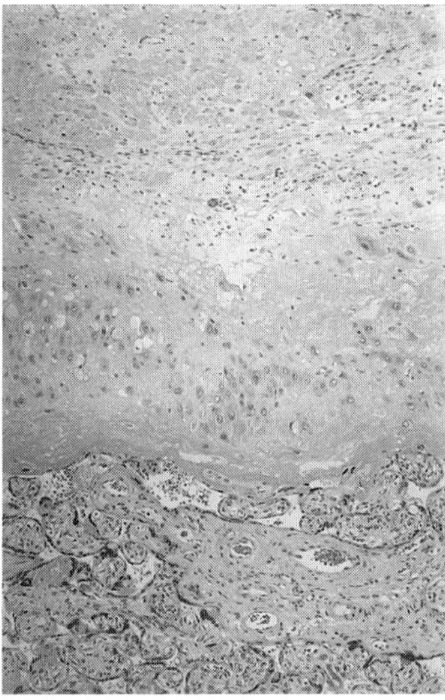

Figure 3–28. A large area of placenta accreta, which shows absence of decidua basalis. The mononuclear cells seen between the villi and the myometrial smooth muscle are invading intermediate trophoblast. The intact uteroplacental specimen is the result of a postpartum hysterectomy in a patient with known placenta accreta (×4). (See this figure enlarged in Chapter 3 by Edwina J. Popek.)

Placenta Previa

Low implantations of the placenta covering the cervical os carry increased relative risks of neonatal death and neurologic abnormalities at 7 years of age. Motor abnormalities, severe mental retardation, and cerebral palsy are all increased in incidence when placenta previa is present. Restriction of uterine blood flow to the endometrium resulting from uterine abnormalities and suboptimal implantation with subsequent diminution of placental blood flow in utero, as well as continued unabated bleeding, are presumed causes for these adverse outcomes. Preterm birth is an important correlate and occurs five times as often when placenta previa is present. Nineteen percent of patients with placenta previa have associated placental abruptions. The perinatal mortality rate is 320 per 1000 when abruption is present versus 99 per 1000 when no abruption is associated with placenta previa ($p < .001$). A positive correlation exists between cigarette smoking and the occurrence of placenta previa (Fig. 15–4*A*).[2,3,23,24]

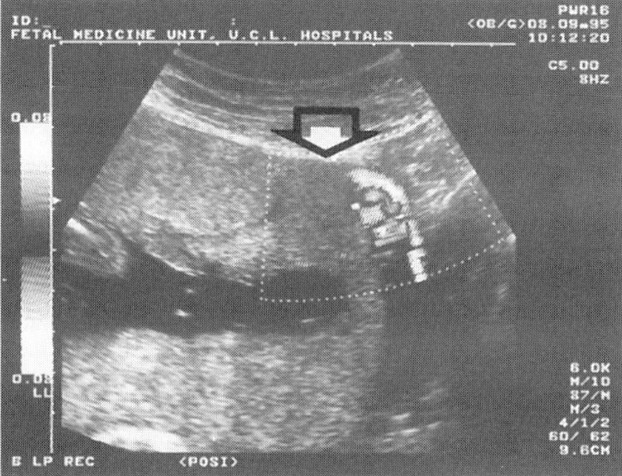

Figure 15–4. A, Longitudinal view of a complete placenta previa located partially under the scar of a previous cesarean section *(arrow).* Note the absence of decidual interface and an area of increased vascularity with dilated blood vessels. (See this figure enlarged in Chapter 15 by Eric Jauniaux and John C. P. Kingdom.)

Placental Abruption

Abruptio placentae is a clinical term. The histopathologic diagnosis is retroplacental hemorrhage. Such clotting, especially when chronic, deforms the base of the maternal surface. Chronicity is determined by coloration of the clot (darker collections and presence of brownish pigment are consistent with longer standing accumulations). Microscopic evaluation reveals compression of surrounding villi and in longer standing cases infarction. This may be present in degrees from acute to old (see below). Breakdown of decidual vasculature from either inflammation or hypertensive rupture is a known cause of abruptio placentae. Trauma is also a notable antecedent event. Associ-

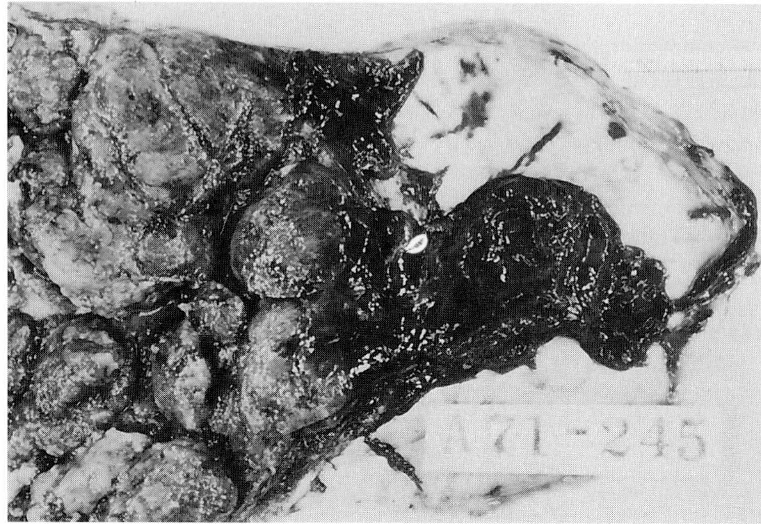

Figure 1–5. Abruptio placentae, marginal. The clot is densely attached to an infarct. Moderate bleeding occurred per vagina, and a 250 cc clot was found behind the placenta.

ations with long umbilical cord, acute chorioamnionitis, congenital malformations, preeclampsia, and smoking during pregnancy are also seen (Fig. 1–5).[2,3,7,25] The relative risks of stillbirth, neonatal death, and preterm delivery are increased.

Intervillous Hemorrhage (Intervillous Thrombus)

An intervillous thrombus is composed of a mixture of fetal and maternal blood. It is presumed that maternal blood percolating through the intervillous space mixes with fetal blood from villous capillary disruption. The incidence of fetal-maternal hemorrhage is prominent in such cases, and Kleihauer-Betke testing or other suitable maternal serum markers document this occurrence. Associated fetal-maternal hemorrhage may induce isoimmunization and subsequent erythroblastosis. The histologic appearance is characterized by a laminated thrombus, which may be recognized on gross examination with its "lines of Zahn." Long umbilical cord, fetal malformations, and immunization or infection in the first trimester are contributory events. The overall incidence has been reported as 6 per 1000 births, but the condition is probably much more common. Cases have also been seen in association with systemic lupus erythematosus and circulating antiphospholipid antibodies. Villous breakdown with capillary leakage is often considered to be trauma induced and may even result from vigorous fetal movements. This speculation correlates with the associated finding of long umbilical cords (Fig. 7–17*B*).[2,3]

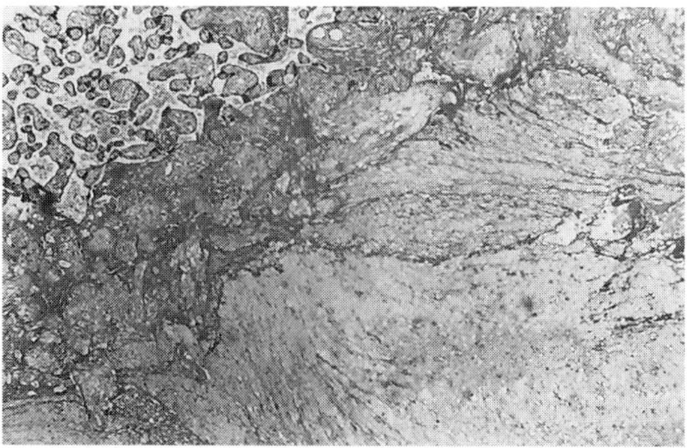

Figure 7–17. B, The blood products have become laminated (H&E, ×40). (See this figure enlarged in Chapter 7 by Raymond W. Redline.)

Subchorionic Fibrin Deposition

Laminated fibrin thrombi below the fetal surface (subchorionic) reflect eddying of maternal blood in the intervillous space. In some cases thromboses extend to the basal plate. This is termed Breus' mole and is seen in missed abortion; it occurs in live-born fetuses as well and can be documented ultrasonographically. Increased subchorionic fibrin deposition is associated statistically with tight cord knot, edematous umbilical cord, umbilical vascular thrombosis, cord hematoma, opaque fetal membranes, maternal floor infarction, and neurologic and behavioral abnormalities (Fig. 7–18).[2]

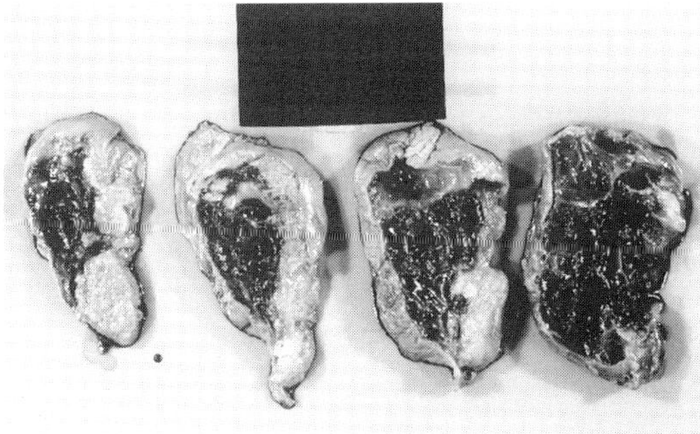

Figure 7–18. Subchorial thrombus. Laminated enlarging hematoma separating the villous parenchyma from the chorionic plate with substantial elevation of the latter structure. (See this figure enlarged in Chapter 7 by Raymond W. Redline.)

SUBCHORIONIC AND SEPTAL CYSTS

Cysts of the placenta generally have no pathologic significance. They are derived from intermediate trophoblastic cells (X cells). Yellow, serous, or even hemorrhagic fluid, often with gelatinous characteristics, is noted within these cysts. The gross appearance of the placenta may be distinctly aberrant with marked deformation from numerous cysts. No clinicopathologic correlation is concurrent unless massive fibrin deposition is also noted (see below) (Fig. 6–16).[1,3]

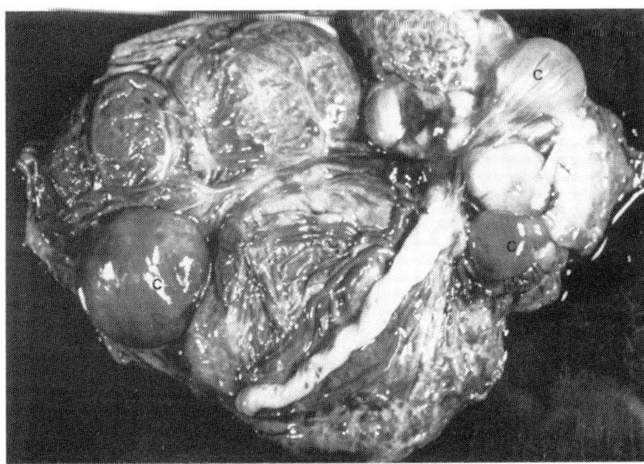

Figure 6–16. Subchorionic cysts *(C).* The two lower cysts are associated with increased fibrin deposition. (From Lewis SH, Benirschke K: The placenta. In Sternberg S [ed]: Histology for pathologists. New York, 1997, Raven Press.) (See this figure enlarged in Chapter 6 by Steven H. Lewis and Enid Gilbert-Barness.)

MATERNAL FLOOR INFARCTION (MATERNAL FLOOR FIBRIN DEPOSITION)

Maternal floor infarction is an improper term used to describe a serious placental pathologic alteration. Extensive deposition of fibrin (and not infarction) at the basal plate of the placenta is identified in such cases. This has been closely associated with intrauterine fetal demise and recurrence in subsequent gestations. The etiology has not been established, although immunologic considerations have been suspected. The condition is not a postmortem artifact. Associated decidual vasculopathy may be identified. In some cases maternal serum α-fetoprotein levels are elevated. "Major basic protein" has been identified as a secretory product and may become a marker for surveillance. Ultrasonography may also be used to identify this aberrancy, especially when the history indicates occurrence in a previous gestation. In addition to midtrimester loss of pregnancy, intrauterine growth retardation is noted. Stillbirth rates are 26 times normal when other factors are considered and excluded in multivariant analysis. Motor abnormalities and mental retardation are also increased relative risks. Long umbilical cords and diffuse subchorionic fibrin deposition are commonly seen as concomitants (Fig. 7–15*A*).[2,3,7,26]

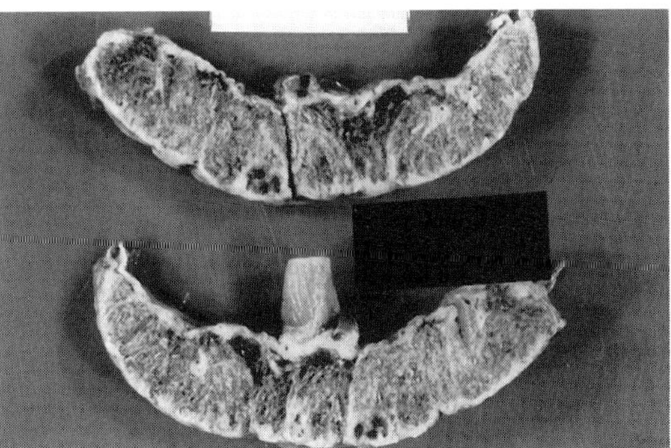

Figure 7–15. A, Maternal floor infarction (gross). Thickening of the basal plate, septal infoldings, and paraseptal villi secondary to diffuse deposition of extracellular matrix and fibrin. (See this figure enlarged in Chapter 7 by Raymond W. Redline.)

INFARCTION

Infarction in the placenta is a common occurrence. Size, degree, and location are important.

Findings in the gross examination are generally characteristic but may be documented histologically. Acute infarction involves villous crowding and congestion followed by necrotic changes and intervillous polymorphonuclear leukocyte infiltration. Later forms of infarction (old infarct) are characterized by ghost villi without villous stromal fibrosis. These findings can be discerned from perivillous fibrin deposition in that infarction is palpably granular and fibrin deposition is palpably smooth. With placental infarction of 10% to 15%, especially with central localization, growth retardation and uteroplacental insufficiency are seen. Extensive infarction can result in fetal distress and demise. Associations with preeclampsia, diabetes, and systemic lupus erythematosus are well established. Interruption or decrease in maternal blood supply is etiologic (Fig. 7–11*A*).[1,3,7]

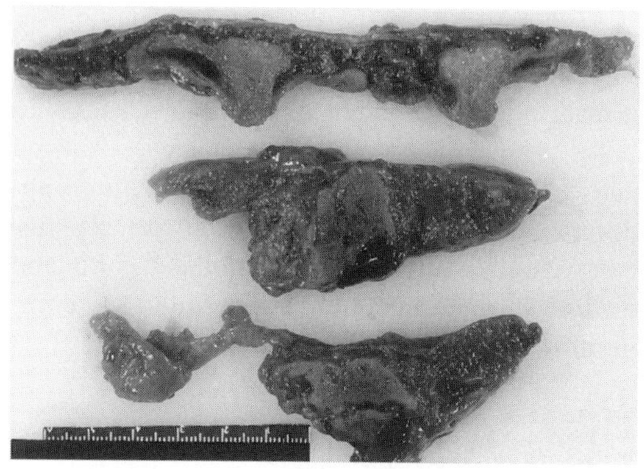

Figure 7–11. A, Gross pathology. Pale, firm, granular, wedge-shaped lesions with their broad base paralleling the basal plate reflect total occlusion of one or more decidual arterioles. (See this figure enlarged in Chapter 7 by Raymond W. Redline.)

Villous Edema (Nonhydropic)

Focal villous edema is identified microscopically. The diagnosis cannot be made on gross examination. The presence of individual swollen and edematous villi distinguished from neighboring normal-appearing villi establishes the diagnosis. It has been suggested that the insult producing such edema increases the thickness of the vasculosyncytial membrane, which diminishes oxygen and nutrient exchange capabilities. Villous edema is associated with fetal compromise, especially when chorioamnionitis is present. Much has been written about placental villous edema, which has been stated to be "the most frequent cause of stillbirth, neonatal death and neonatal morbidity in children born . . . before 28 weeks gestation."[2] Documented associations include acute chorioamnionitis, preterm birth, stillbirth, and neonatal death, all of which are three to six times more likely when focal villous edema is found. Neurologic abnormalities at 7 years of age and motor abnormalities with severe mental retardation are also associated findings (Fig. 7–12*B*).[2,27,28]

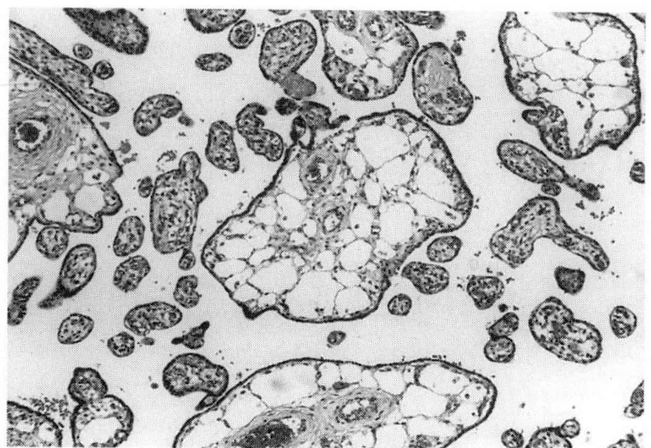

Figure 7–12. B, Villous edema (nonhydropic) is characterized by an exaggeration of the normal lacunae seen in immature intermediate tertiary stem villi of late second- and early third-trimester placentas. (See this figure enlarged in Chapter 7 by Raymond W. Redline.)

Nucleated Red Blood Cells in Fetal Vessels

Nucleated red blood cells should not be seen in the placental villous fetal circulation after 30 weeks of gestation. Abnormal release of hematopoietic elements stimulated by erythropoietin is considered etiologic. Conditions in which such a release occurs include erythroblastosis, fetal anemia, infection, intrauterine growth retardation, severe cases of fetal distress, hypoxia, and ischemia. A vigorous attempt to establish temporal correlations between cord blood erythropoietin levels and fetal hypoxemia has met with lack of success in experimental models. Recent evidence suggests that a temporal relationship exists between the identification of cord blood normoblasts and lymphocytes and hypoxic events (Fig. 7–14).[7,29]

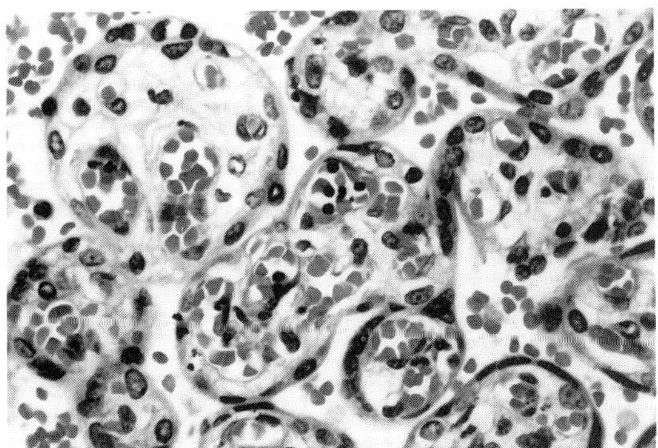

Figure 7–14. Increased nucleated red blood cells. Multiple villous capillaries in one low-power field showing normoblasts with perfectly round nuclei, featureless hyperchromatic chromatin, and glassy eosinophilic cytoplasm. (See this figure enlarged in Chapter 7 by Raymond W. Redline.)

CHORANGIOSIS

Increased numbers of villous capillaries (10 vessels per 10 villi per 10 10× fields) are associated with chronic hypoxia, maternal diabetes, villitis, and perinatal death. There is additionally the association of fetal malformation (Fig. 7–6).[7,15]

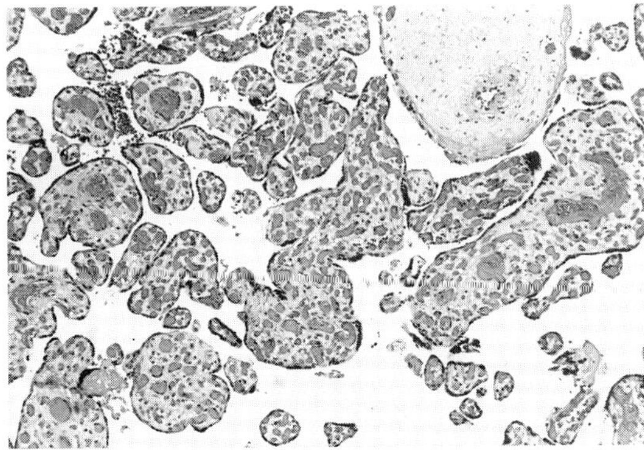

Figure 7–6. Villous chorangiosis defined as hypercapillarization of terminal and tertiary stem villi with greater than 10 capillaries per villous cross section. (See this figure enlarged in Chapter 7 by Raymond W. Redline.)

VILLITIS

Villitis is broken down into several distinct entities.

Acute villitis is associated with parenchymal microabscesses composed of polymorphonuclear leukocytes and is most commonly identified in listerial infection. Other bacteria occasionally are causal (Fig. 13–7).

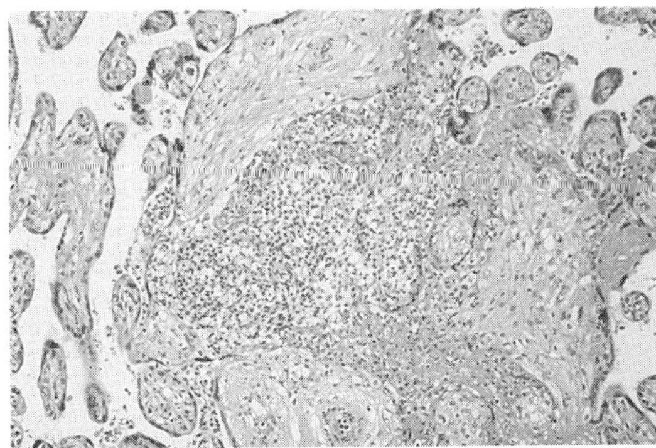

Figure 13–7. Placental tissue demonstrating focal intense acute intervillositis with perivillous fibrin deposition induced by congenital *Listeria* infection. There is also acute villitis (H&E, ×50). (See this figure enlarged in Chapter 13 by Scott R. Hyde and Geoffrey Altshuler.)

Chronic villitis is characterized by inflammatory infiltrates that range from mild processes with focal increase in villous Hofbauer cells (villous macrophages bearing leukocyte-specific macrophage antigen markers) to aggregates of lymphocytes and plasma cells. With microscopic search for specific morphologic characteristics or special studies using immunohistochemistry or in situ hybridization, such infiltrates may be seen in conjunction with cytomegalovirus, toxoplasmosis, rubella, and syphilis. Fetal infections are common in these cases (Fig. 13–9*B*).

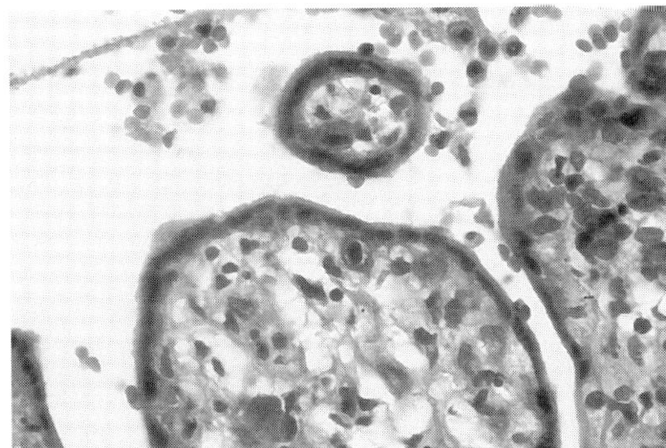

Figure 13–9. B, Villus containing pathognomonic intranuclear inclusions (H&E, ×50). (See this figure enlarged in Chapter 13 by Scott R. Hyde and Geoffrey Altshuler.)

Villitis of unknown etiology (VUE) produces a similar mononuclear leukocytic infiltrate, yet no pathogen can be identified. Such inflammatory events occur in 8% to 10% of normal deliveries. An association with adverse outcome, however, has been noted, and immunogenic localization has determined that the origin is fetal. From these data it is speculated that the putative relationship with maternal immunologic events is less likely and occult infection more probable (Fig. 13–8*A*).

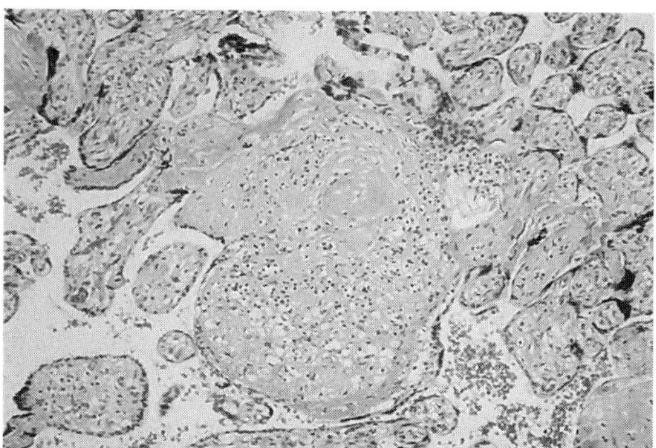

Figure 13–8. A, Lymphohistiocytic villitis of unknown etiology. Note the disruption of the normal villous cytoarchitecture, including fetal vascular obliteration (H&E, ×50). (See this figure enlarged in Chapter 13 by Scott R. Hyde and Geoffrey Altshuler.)

"Silent villitis" occurs in the absence of inflammatory infiltrate or characteristic inclusions. It is identified by the presence of viral antigens within villous tissue. This is the type that occurs in human immunodeficiency virus (HIV) infection (Fig. 1–6).[3,7,16,30]

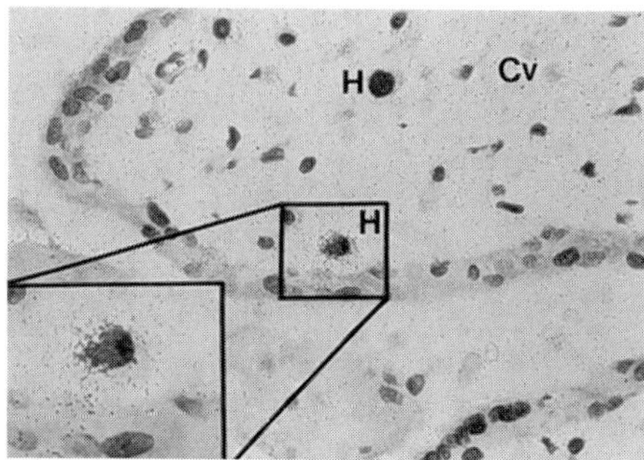

Figure 1–6. In situ hybridization of an S35 HIV probe to villous Hofbauer cells of the first-trimester placental tissue. (From Lewis SH, Reynolds-Kohler C, Fox HE, Nelson JA: Lancet 355:565, 1990.)

Abnormal Maturation

Abnormal maturation takes several forms. Accelerated maturation, retarded maturation, and irregular maturation are all notable.

Accelerated maturation is most commonly seen in hypertensive disorders. The characteristic increase in syncytial knots is considered to be a pathophysiologic response to hypoxemia and an aborted attempt to increase the surface area of villous syncytial vascular membrane to accommodate hypoxic surroundings. Fetal compromise, growth retardation, and intrauterine fetal demise are documented correlates (Fig. 7–10*B*).

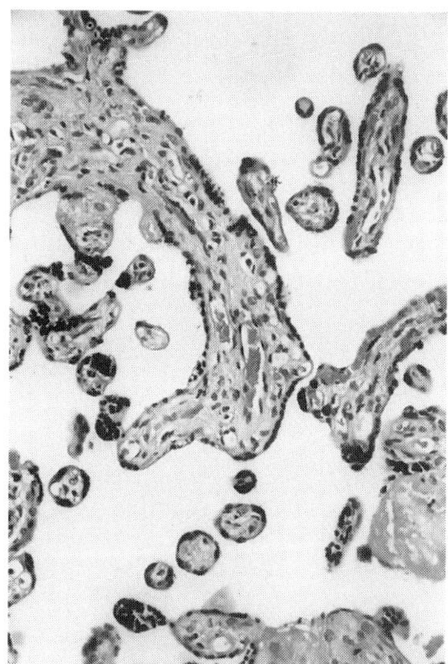

Figure 7–10. B, Accelerated maturation. Long, thin stem villi with stromal fibrosis give rise to tiny, sparse, terminal villous projections, many of which lack capillaries and others of which show increased syncytial knots. (See this figure enlarged in Chapter 7 by Raymond W. Redline.)

Retarded maturation is seen when the villous development is not appropriate for the gestational age and may be retarded. Hofbauer cells, nucleated red blood cells, and unexpected double-layer trophoblasts are found in excess. Maternal diabetes, fetal anemia, and fetal heart failure are known correlates. Both immune and nonimmune hydrops can also be present (Fig. 7–10*A*).

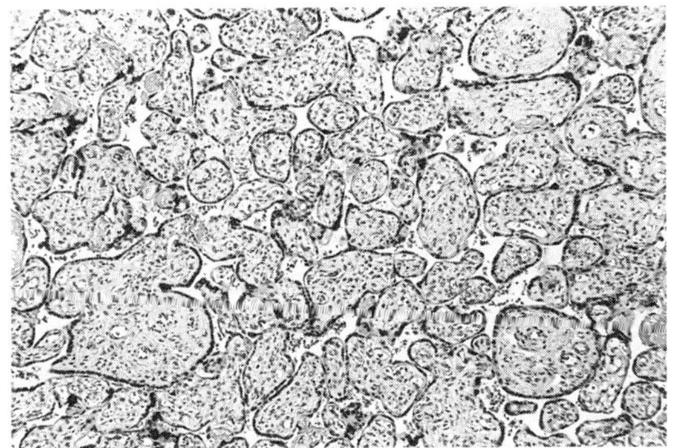

Figure 7–10. A, Delayed maturation. Terminal villi in a term placenta show characteristics of immature intermediate villi with loose edematous stroma, central capillaries, and cellular villous trophoblast. (See this figure enlarged in Chapter 7 by Raymond W. Redline.)

Irregular villous maturation is noteworthy in that villi of varying immature and advanced mature forms are seen for a given gestational age. Such findings correlate with genetic abnormalities including trisomy 18 and chronic villitis.[1]

Fetal Vascular Obliteration (Villous Fibrosis)

Distinct from maternally induced infarction is the phenomenon of villous fibrosis and obliteration that results from lack of fetal perfusion. Infarction, conversely, results from absence or diminution of maternal perfusion. Stillbirth risk rates are nine times higher when this condition is present. Relative risks of chronic villitis, preterm birth, neonatal death, and preeclampsia are also increased. Diffuse fibrosis is a common finding in intrauterine fetal demise. Hemorrhagic endovasculitis may be a part of the disease spectrum, but this finding has been met with debate and is viewed by some as a postmortem artifact (Fig. 7–1*B*).[7]

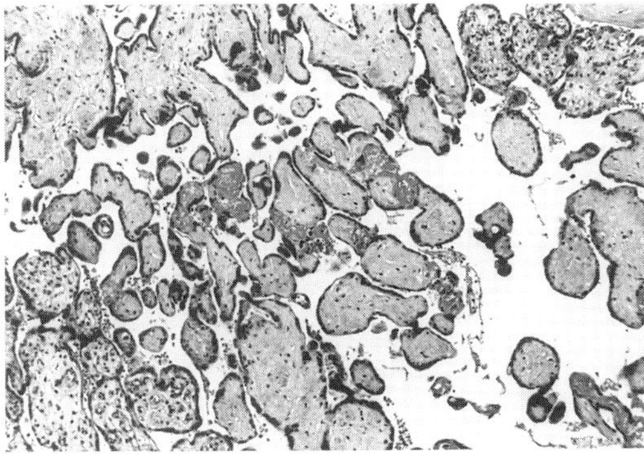

Figure 7–1. B, Focally avascular villi related to upstream arterial occlusion show bland homogeneous collagenized stroma and interdigitate with normally vascularized villi. (See this figure enlarged in Chapter 7 by Raymond W. Redline.)

Chorangioma

Anomalous vascular development within the placental parenchyma takes the form of chorangiomas. A variety of terms have been applied to distinguish degrees of components, but there is no differentiation in clinical significance. Small lesions have no clinical impact; large lesions may result in microangiopathic anemia with associated disseminated intravascular coagulation and high-output failure resulting in fetal cardiac decompensation. The gross appearance may be confused with infarcts or thrombi, but the histologic appearance is pathognomonic (Fig. 15–5*A*).[3,7]

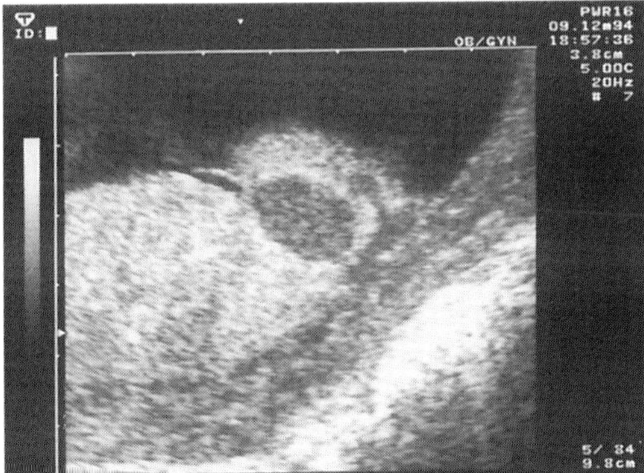

Figure 15–5. A, Longitudinal sonogram of the placenta at 20 weeks' gestation showing a hypoechoic mass corresponding to a chorioangioma. Polyhydramnios had been noted. (See this figure enlarged in Chapter 15 by Eric Jauniaux and John C. P. Kingdom.)

Intervillous Fibrin Deposition

On gross examination, intervillous fibrin deposition is somewhat similar to chronic infarction; however, the glistening and smooth surface distinguishes this entity from the granular surface of infarction as discerned by palpation. Fibrin deposition is distinguished from intervillous thrombi through the recognition of laminated lines of Zahn in thrombi.

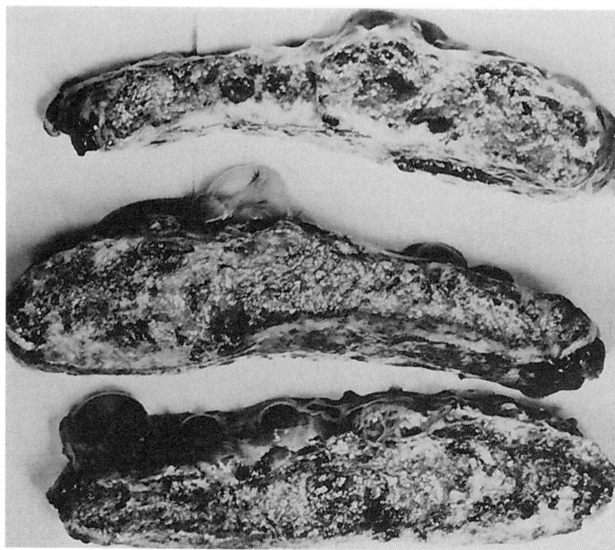

Figure 1–7. Extensive intervillous fibrin deposition ("Gitterinfarkt").

Histologic examination shows trapped trophoblastic cells of either cytotrophoblast or intermediate trophoblastic derivatives. No particular adverse outcome is identified except when large areas are involved. When greater than 30% of the placental disk is involved with intervillous fibrin deposition, there is a strong association between fetal growth retardation and intrauterine fetal demise (Fig. 1–7).[3,7]

HISTOLOGIC REPRESENTATION OF ABNORMAL CELLS IN THE INTERVILLOUS SPACE

The histologic identification of aberrant cells in the intervillous space may identify a maternal pathologic condition. The presence of sickle cells may document sickle cell anemia in the mother. It should be noted that storage of placentas causes low oxygen tension in remaining intervillous erythrocytes, and in patients with sickle trait or sickle cell anemia the presence of sickling in the placenta does not necessarily denote that sickling was present at delivery. Additional findings may include metastatic lesions such as breast carcinoma and melanoma, which, although rare in the placenta, have great clinical import for future care and management of the mother (Fig. 12–8*B*).[7]

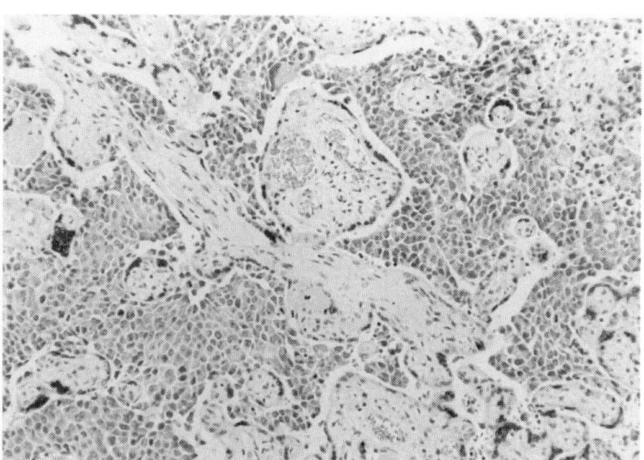

Figure 12–8. B, Extensive infiltration of intervillous space by poorly differentiated epidermoid carcinoma from lung. The tumor conforms to the villous outline. No sites of direct infiltration of villi are apparent in this field (H&E, ×100). (See this figure enlarged in Chapter 12 by Douglas R. Shanklin.)

DECIDUA (see also Chapter 8)

The maternal decidua is gestational endometrium. Spiral arterioles that terminate and leave openings in the decidual surface permit maternal blood to bathe the placental villi, effecting transfer of nutrients and waste. This highly specialized tissue is best examined histologically on the surface of the reflected membranes or from endometrial biopsies at delivery. There is often little decidua associated with the base of the placental disk at delivery. Important pathologic conditions include the following.

DECIDUAL INFLAMMATION

The presence of decidual inflammation correlates with acute and chronic infections. Acute inflammation is commonly the earliest form of maternal response to intraamniotic bacterial infection. Associated decidual necrosis is not uncommon, especially in moderate to severe cases. Resultant breakdown of decidual vasculature may lead to hemorrhage and retroplacental bleeding. The presence of plasma cells and lymphocytic infiltrates should signal the possibility of conditions such as cytomegalovirus and syphilis (Fig. 7–9).[1,3,7]

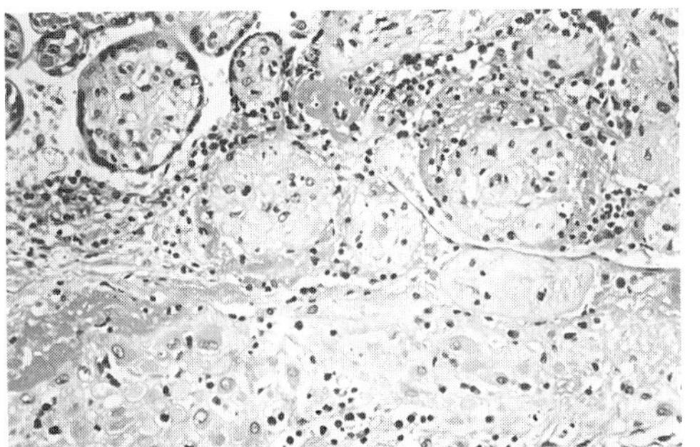

Figure 7–9. Basal villitis with basal lymphoplasmacytic deciduitis. A plasma cell–rich decidual infiltrate spills over into anchoring villi but fails to extend into so-called floating villi. (See this figure enlarged in Chapter 7 by Raymond W. Redline.)

Decidual Vasculopathy

Aberrancies of decidual vessels have been noted for many years. Several forms are identified, among which are atherosis and muscular hyperplasia. Such conditions are identified in hypertensive disorders or in immune conditions. These vascular abnormalities alter perfusion and can lead to growth retardation and fetal demise (Fig. 8–5*A*).[3]

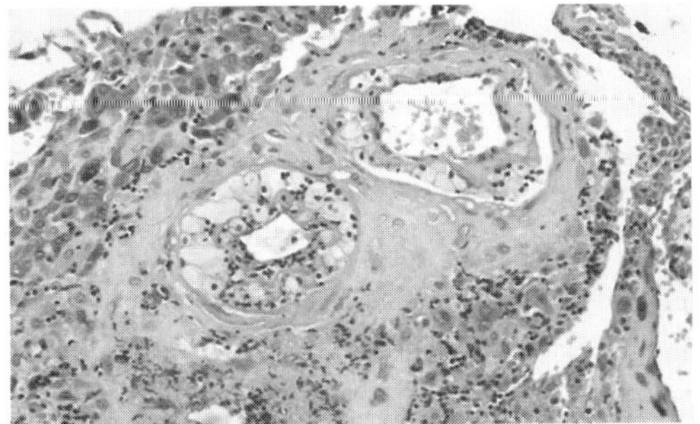

Figure 8–5. A, Basal plate of delivered placenta, uteroplacental artery with fibrinoid necrosis and atherosis. Note numerous foamy macrophages ("atherosis," *arrows*) within the homogeneous eosinophilic wall of the vessel. Dense chronic vasculitis is associated with the foamy macrophages. The infant was growth restricted at term, the mother was normotensive, and there were no clinical risk factors (H&E, ×40). (See this figure enlarged in Chapter 8 by Carolyn M. Salafia and Robert Pijnenborg.)

GESTATIONAL TROPHOBLASTIC DISEASE (see also Chapters 10 and 11)

The potential for causation of neoplasia should be kept in mind when considering potential pathologic alterations of the placenta. Accurate pathologic diagnosis is essential so that appropriate clinical management can be undertaken. A detailed discussion of the subject is beyond the scope of this chapter. The following is a brief description of entities encountered.

Hydropic Degeneration

Hydropic degenerative change is seen in villi from early gestations that have undergone demise. No cytologic atypia or abnormal proliferation of trophoblasts is present to aid in the diagnosis. Fetal parts or villous vasculature may be obscure, confounding the interpretation. Careful attention to criteria for diagnosis of complete and incomplete mole allows the pathologist to establish this benign finding (Fig. 10–3).

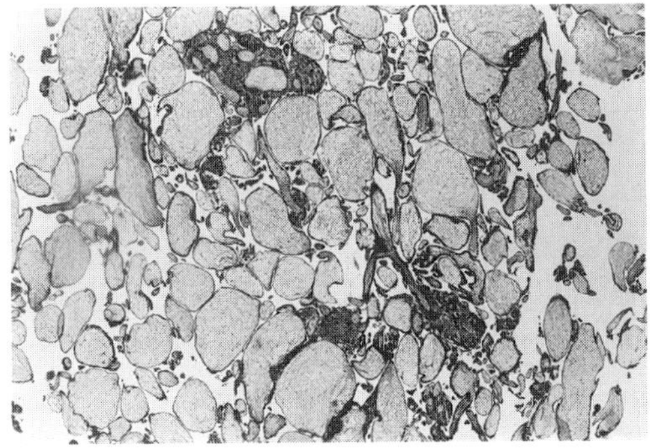

Figure 10–3. Hydropic abortus, placenta; "blighted ovum," 10 weeks MA. Uniform villous edema, without trophoblastic hyperplasia and without cistern formation. An occasional trophoblastic column must not be misinterpreted as expressing hyperplasia. (See this figure enlarged in Chapter 10 by Aron E. Szulman.)

Complete Mole

Complete mole is a neoplasia that is usually derived from paternal XX chromosomes. On histologic examination, villi are hydropic and devoid of fetal vasculature and exhibit trophoblastic hyperplasia and atypia. No fetal parts are present. The potential for invasion, persistence, and development of choriocarcinoma is well known (Fig. 10–2*F*).[7]

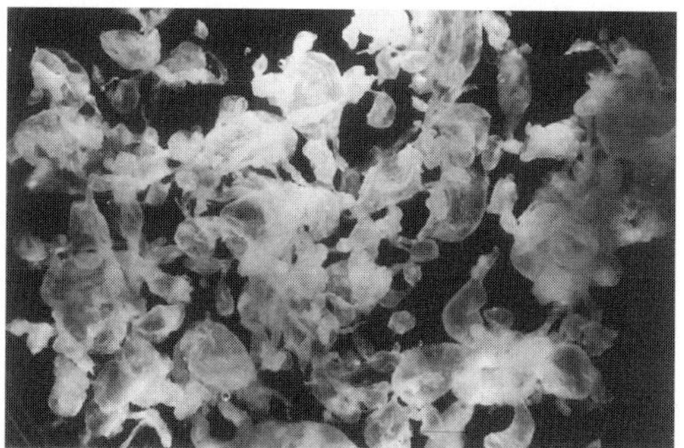

Figure 10–2. F, CHM, 15 weeks MA. "Bunch of grapes" group of hydatidiform villi floated on saline solution and photographed in a transillumination setup. Note the translucent vesicles (maximum 15 mm in this specimen). Most of the vesicles represent end-station cisterns. (See this figure enlarged in Chapter 10 by Aron E. Szulman.)

Partial Mole

Partial moles are usually derived from triploid gestations and have associated fetal development.

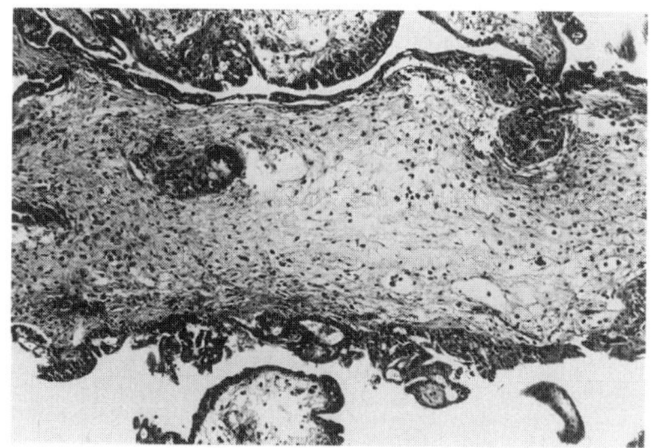

Figure 10–4. E, PHM, 10 weeks MA. A villus showing two inclusions, formed by incursions of both layers of surface trophoblast into the subjacent stroma. (The one on the right seems to have just started on its journey from the surface.) The inclusions are lumenless; the lucent areas in the center are produced by syncytial cytoplasmic vacuolation. (See this figure enlarged in Chapter 10 by Aron E. Szulman.)

Their propensity to form persistent or invasive disease is limited, and such disease is rare. Histologic examination shows hydropic villi with characteristic scalloped borders, which when sectioned tangentially appear as villous inclusions or islands (Fig. 10–4*E*).

Syncytial Endometritis

This misnomer (in that there is no associated infection or inflammation) refers to an exaggerated implantation site forming a nidus of abundant trophoblastic derivatives. More serious diagnoses (see below) are excluded by the absence of atypia (Fig. 11–5*B*).

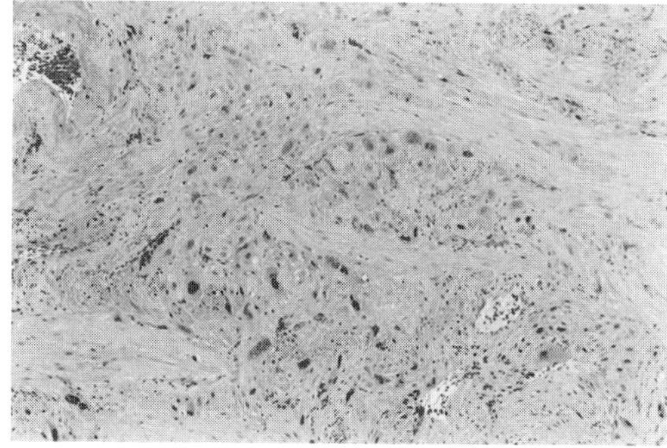

Figure 11–5. B, Numerous intermediate trophoblastic cells are seen infiltrating myometrium. (See this figure enlarged in Chapter 11 by Debra S. Heller.)

Choriocarcinoma

Choriocarcinoma is a malignancy derived from trophoblastic tissue, usually from a former gestation and most commonly from complete moles. The

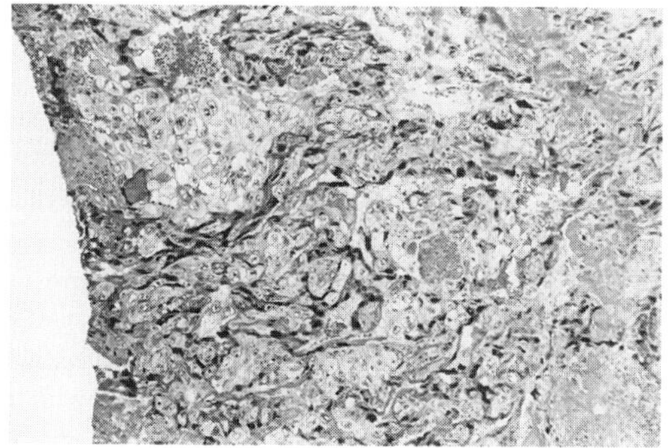

Figure 11–3. C, The tumor is biphasic, and no chorionic villi are present. (See this figure enlarged in Chapter 11 by Debra S. Heller.)

marked proliferation and pronounced atypia are characteristic. No coexisting villi are present. Although choriocarcinoma is curable in early stages, advanced disease requires aggressive treatment and may not respond satisfactorily (Fig. 11–3*C*).

Placental Site Trophoblastic Tumor

Placental site trophoblastic tumor is an unusual neoplasm characterized by a uterine proliferation of trophoblastic X cells (intermediate trophoblast) usually diagnosed through curettage. Locally aggressive lesions necessitate hysterectomy (Fig. 11–4*A*).

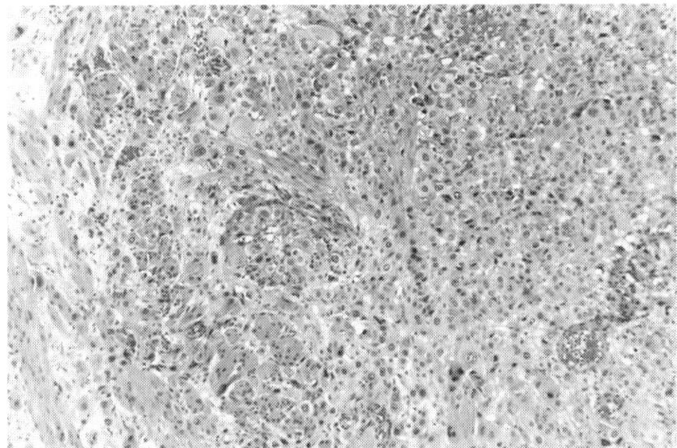

Figure 11–4. A, Intermediate trophoblastic cells splaying myometrial bundles. (See this figure enlarged in Chapter 11 by Debra S. Heller.)

CONCLUSION

Scientifically based correlation distinguishes the causes of morbidity and mortality resulting from pathologic conditions of the placenta. That these conditions exist is not debated. The problem with providing relevant data for patient care lies in the common misunderstanding that the placenta is not valuable for diagnosis. Pathologists and clinicians must become better informed about the causes of perinatal and maternal morbidity and mortality associated with placental pathologic conditions. When they do, the placenta may become more widely used to enhance the understanding of adverse outcomes and improve the quality of patient care. This chapter is a synopsis of placental conditions that underscore this premise and validate the importance of the placental examination.

REFERENCES

1. College of American Pathology: The examination of the placenta: patient care and risk management. Arch Pathol Lab Med 115, 1991.
2. Naeye RL: Disorders of the placenta, fetus and neonate. St. Louis, 1992, Mosby.
3. Lewis SH, Benirschke K: The placenta, histology for pathologists, 2nd ed. New York, 1997, Raven Press.
4. Naeye RL: Umbilical cord length significance. J Pediatr 107:278, 1985.
5. Rayburn WF, Beynen A, Brinkman DL: Umbilical cord length and intrapartum complications. Obstet Gynecol 57:450, 1981.
6. Froehlich LA, Fujikura J: Significant of a single umbilical artery: report for the collaborative study of cerebral palsy. Am J Obstet Gynecol 94:274, 1966.
7. Benirschke K, Kaufmann R: Pathology of the human placenta. New York, 1995, Springer-Verlag.
8. Uyanwah-Akporm P, Fox H: The clinical significance of marginal and velamentous insertion of the cord. Br J Obstet Gynaecol 84:941, 1977.
9. DeSa DJ: Diseases of the umbilical cord. In Perrin EVDK (ed): Pathology of the placenta. New York, 1984, Churchill Livingstone.
10. Fox H: Thrombosis of foetal arteries in the human placenta. Br J Obstet Gynaecol 73:961, 1966.
11. Strong TH: Factors that provide optimal umbilical protection during gestation. Contemp OB Gyn March, 1997.
12. Gersell DJ, Kraus RF, Reffle M: Diseases of the placenta. In Kurman R (ed): Blaustein's pathology of the female genital tract, 3rd ed. New York, 1987, Springer-Verlag.
13. Blanc WA: Pathology of the placenta, membranes, and umbilical cord in bacterial, fungal and viral infections in man. In Naeye RI, Caisson JM, Kaufmann N (eds): Perinatal disease. Baltimore, 1981, Williams & Wilkins
14. Altshuler G, Hyde S: Meconium induced vasoconstriction: a potential cause of cerebral and other fetal hypoperfusion and of poor pregnancy outcome. J Child Neurol 4:137, 1989.
15. Fox H, Sen DK: Placenta extrachorialis: a clinicopathologic study. J Obstet Gynaecol Br Commonw 79:32, 1972.
16. Altshuler G, Herman A: The medicolegal imperative: placental pathology and epidemiology. In Stevenson DK, Sunshine P (eds): Fetal and neonatal brain injury. Mechanisms, management, and the risks of practice. Philadelphia, 1989, BC Decker.
17. Baldwin VJ: Pathology of multiple pregnancy. In Dimmick JE, Kalousek DK (eds): Developmental pathology of the embryo and fetus. Philadelphia, 1992, Lippincott.

18. Baldwin VJ: Pathology of multiple gestation. New York, 1993, Springer-Verlag.
19. Molteni RA, Stys SJ, Battaglia FC: Relationship of fetal and placental weight in human beings: fetal/placental weight ratios at various gestational ages and birth weight distributions. J Reprod Med 21:327, 1978.
20. Kaplan CG: Color atlas of gross placental pathology. New York, 1994, Igaku-Shoin.
21. Fujikura T, Benson RC, Driscoll SG: The bipartite placenta and its clinical features. Am J Obstet Gynecol 107:1013, 1970.
22. Fox H: Placenta accreta, 1945–1969. Obstet Gynecol Surg 27:475, 1972.
23. McShane PM, Heyl PS, Epstein MF: Maternal and perinatal morbidity resulting from placenta previa. Obstet Gynecol 65:176, 1985.
24. Naeye RL: Placenta previa, predisposing factors and effects on the fetus and surviving infants. Obstet Gynecol 52:521, 1978.
25. Paterson MEL: The etiology and outcome of abruptio placentae. Acta Obstet Gynecol Scand 58: 31, 1979.
26. Benirschke K, Kaufmann P: The pathology of maternal floor infarction. In Pathology of the human placenta. New York, 1990, Springer-Verlag.
27. Shen-Schwarz S, Ruchelli E, Brown D: Villous edema of the placenta: a clinicopathological study. Placenta 10:297, 1989.
28. Naeye RL, Maisels J, Lorenz RP, Botti JJ: The clinical significance of placental villous edema. Pediatrics 71:588, 1983.
29. Naeye RL, Localio AR: Determining the time before birth when ischemia and hypoxemia initiated cerebral palsy. Obstet Gynecol 86:5, 713, 1996.
30. Lewis SH, Reynolds-Kohler C, Fox HE, Nelson JA: HIV-1 in trophoblast, Hofbauer cells and hematologic precursors in 8-week fetuses. Lancet 355:565, 1990.

2

Examination of the Placenta

Robert W. Bendon and C. Maureen Sander

The full pathologic examination of the placenta is a time-consuming process that requires specialized skill and knowledge. To achieve a high-quality examination, the pathologist must understand the significance of the obstetric history and of the gross placental lesions. An inexperienced pathologist attempting to preserve a record by random sections will miss important observations. Such samples can be used only to evaluate diffuse disease or provide DNA analysis. The pathologist undertaking the placental examination must learn much that is foreign to surgical pathology.

This chapter guides the pathologist systematically through a complete examination of the placenta. The basics of the clinical history, gross findings, microscopic sampling, and reporting are considered. Gross pathologic lesions are listed here in the context of a systematic examination; their pathologic description is found in subsequent chapters.

CLINICAL HISTORY

The following section lists and discusses the clinical information needed to interpret the placental examination. Knowing this information before the gross examination can focus observations and detect inconsistencies, such as labeling errors, that might occur. Experience is needed to use the information fully, but with a rational and alert approach, starting the examination with a known history should increase efficiency and quality.

Information to be Gathered

Identification of Mother and Infant

The mother and infant may be linked by the hospital computer system, but if not, both identifications should be obtained, and the report sent to both charts.

Gestational Age and Weight

The infant's gestational age and weight help to identify that the correct placenta is being processed. In addition, a small for gestation placenta and baby prompt a differential diagnosis that may include more directed sampling of maternal vessels, looking for maternal floor infarction and other conditions. A large baby and placenta again prompt a differential diagnosis that may influence sampling or other testing and alert the prosector to look for hydrops.

Type of Delivery

Knowing whether a delivery was vaginal or a cesarean section may be useful. Completeness of the maternal surface is a lesser concern with direct removal. If the placenta is anterior in the uterus, the chorionic or membranous vessels may be cut during the cesarean incision. Such cut vessels are not significant, but had they occurred from amniotomy with a vaginal delivery, they would have been a site of fetal hemorrhage.

Apgar Scores

A 5-minute Apgar score of 7 or above is good evidence against fetal asphyxia. A low score has poor specificity for asphyxia but is still a useful estimate of fetal well-being. For example, a fresh blood clot on the maternal surface is more likely to be from abruption if the Apgar scores are low and if the history is supportive.

Indication for the Placental Examination

A good practice to focus the placental examination for both obstetrician and pathologist is to require that an indication for the examination be specified. Such focusing decreases missed diagnoses and wasted effort. For example, knowing that the examination is because of fetal anemia will prompt a search for any gross placental site of blood loss such as ruptured velamentous vessels that might otherwise have been overlooked. Keeping a list of indications for pathologic examination of the placenta in the obstetric suite facilitates this goal (see Table 1–1).

Matching of Twin to Placenta

The umbilical cords should be identified as belonging to twin A (firstborn) or B (or more in higher multigestation). Unless there is an accepted hospital standard, the pathologist cannot assign A and B if there has been no designation. In such cases it is reasonable to assign the cords as twin X or Y. The pathologist should be aware that the designation at birth may not match the designation of twins on prenatal ultrasound.

Information Needed to Interpret the Placenta

Ideally, all the clinical information is available at the time of gross placental examination. It is possible to complete the placental examination on the basis of the minimal history suggested above. However, the more complete the information available to and understood by the pathologist, the more likely that the placental report will have clinical utility. For example, if a placenta is more mature than the stated gestation, is this the result of utero-placental ischemia, or is the gestational age wrong? If the dates are based on an early ultrasound (and hence accurate), the advanced maturity of the placenta is the result of uteroplacental ischemia. If a placenta is sent for examination because of fever and abdominal tenderness and no chorioamnionitis is found, the possibility of another abdominal problem such as appendicitis must be considered.

Means of Obtaining the Needed Clinical Information

Requisition for Pathologic Examination of the Placenta

The requisition is the time-honored way to obtain information. However, the requisition may not be completed if it requires labor-intensive reentering of information. Below are three solutions that have been effective in different circumstances:

1. Hospitals generally have a single-sheet labor and delivery (L&D) record that records all the essential information about the labor and delivery. By addition of a line to request placental examination, the L&D sheet can become the pathology requisition. A carbon copy or photocopy then must accompany the placenta to the laboratory.
2. For outside hospitals a copy of the physician and nursing notes for the current labor and delivery and a copy of the prenatal record if available at delivery are required parts of the requisition. Having this additional information is important because the chart cannot be directly examined if needed, as it can at the base hospital.
3. A specific placental pathology requisition can be produced. The information to be completed should be kept simple and focused. One approach is to provide on the requisition form a checklist of indicators for the placental examination or a list of questions about the case that the physician hopes to have answered. Requisitions should be available in the nurseries as well as the labor and delivery suite. An example of a requisition accompanying specimens referred to the Michigan Placental Registry is shown in Figure 2–1.

Other Information

Prior pathology reports are important and are available without requiring a request in most laboratories. Looking at past material may help confirm a diagnosis; for example, previous growth retarda-

FOR REGISTRY USE ONLY

PR# ________________

RC'D ________________

TOTAL WGT. __________

TRIMMED WGT. _______

PLACENTAL TISSUE REGISTRY

MICHIGAN STATE UNIVERSITY
Dept. of Pathology
A-203 Clinical Ctr.
E. Lansing, MI 48824-1313

(517) 432-1012: Dr. Sander
(517) 432-1011: Placental Lab
(517) 353-4365: Clin. Secretary
(517) 432-1053: Fax

MOTHER

Last Name: ______________________ First: ______________________ Initial: _______

Soc. Sec. #: _______-_______-_______ Hospital Record ______________________

Date of Birth: ______________ Age: __________ Race: __________ Marital Status: __________

Parity: G __________ P __________ Still __________ Abortions __________ Live births __________
(Including this pregnancy)

Abnormalities in past pregnancies: ______________________________________

THIS PREGNANCY: EDC: ______________ DATE DELIVERED ______________

Please circle: (**Y** = yes/**N** =no)

Y N	Toxemia/Pre-eclampsia	Y N	Gestational diabetes	Y N	Alcohol abuse
Y N	Hypertension of pregnancy	Y N	Diabetes mellitus	Y N	Drug abuse
Y N	Pre-existing hypertension	Y N	Seizure disorder	Y N	Herpes
Y N	Cigarette smoking (>5 cig/day)	Y N	Anemia	Y N	CMV

Other: ______________________ Infections: ______________________

Medications during pregnancy: ______________________________________

INFANT: Live _______ Apgar 1 _______ Apgar 5 _______ **Sex:** Male Female

Still _______ Birth Wgt (gm) _______ Fetal Distress Yes No

TWIN: Indicate placental sectors A/B: Stillbirth: A / B Live: A / B Apgars 1 & 5: A _______ B _______

PLACENTA: (gross) **Normal:** Yes No If no, describe: ______________________

CORD: (gross) **Normal:** Yes No If no, describe: ______________________

AMNIONIC FLUID: **Normal** _________ **Excessive** _________ **Oligo** _________ **Color** _________

Reason for sending specimen:
____

Name of physician who will be following child: ______________________

Attending Physician: ______________________ Phone: ______________________

Hospital: ______________________ Address: ______________________

City: ______________________ Zip Code: ______________________

INSTRUCTIONS: Specimen must be thoroughly fixed in formalin for three or four days, then mailed in a tightly sealed container thoroughly cushioned and taped to retain formalin. A tightly sealed plastic bag containing formalin also may be used. The history form should be put in a separate plastic envelope. Mail to the above address. Physician's report will be sent to Department of Pathology, unless otherwise requested.

NOTE: ALL PLACENTAS WILL BE RETURNED IF NOT LABELED CLEARLY WITH PATIENT'S NAME Rev 7/94

Figure 2–1. Michigan Placental Tissue Registry clinical information and mailing form.

tion in an infant is consistent with a current diagnosis of massive perivillous fibrin and maternal floor infarction (a lesion with an approximately 50% recurrence rate). Access to laboratory test results can also save time. In one example, funisitis with smooth muscle necrosis and cellular hydrops of the villi were seen in a placenta from a stillbirth. Looking up a Veneral Disease Research Laboratory (VDRL) test done in the delivery room provided support for the diagnosis of syphilis. The physician was called and ordered penicillin before the patient left the hospital. Positive umbilical staining for spirochetes was obtained subsequently.

Electronic Information

Computerized office and hospital records offer new possibilities for quickly obtaining patient information. In the pathology department, old pathology records and laboratory results are most likely to be available electronically. The full potential of this information revolution should benefit placental pathology by forever linking the placental findings to the infant. Some placental observations that did not correlate with disease in the infant, such as single umbilical artery or fetal vascular thrombi, may prove predictive of disease in the future.

Interpretation of the Obstetric Chart

The pathologist must grasp the basic vocabulary of obstetrics and neonatology and understand the common diseases, complications, and procedures. Interpretation of placental pathology requires the same type of understanding the pathologist brings to other specimens such as a lymphoma or renal biopsy. Residents interested in perinatal pathology would benefit from clinical rotations in obstetrics, rounds in the neonatal intensive care unit (NICU), and a formal fellowship in pediatric and perinatal pathology. For pathologists without special training the following is a brief introduction to the field, but it is not a substitute for reading basic texts in perinatal medicine and maintaining communication with clinical colleagues.

The obstetric record cannot be deciphered without knowing the common abbreviations. Some of these are relatively standard, such as P (para), G (gravida), LMP (last menstrual period), and EDC (expected date of confinement). However, the alphabet soup is often regional and needs to be learned at each institution. A labor record is likely to state, "US: IUGR with oligo, FHR: Loss LTV and late decels, PIH, IDDM, with MSF." This translates as, "The baby was known to have intrauterine growth retardation and oligohydramnios by prenatal ultrasound. During the labor the fetal heart rate monitor showed a loss of long-term variability (an ominous finding) and late decelerations (the fetal heart rate bradycardia following a contraction often associated with fetal acidosis). The mother had pregnancy-induced hypertension (preeclampsia) and was an insulin-dependent diabetic. At some point meconium stained the amniotic fluid." There are many other common abbreviations, such as PROM (premature rupture of membranes—before the onset of detectable labor) and VBAC (vaginal delivery after cesarean section). The pathologist should never assume that an unknown abbreviation is unimportant but rather should speak with the obstetrician when in doubt.

Two practical devices are useful when submitting placental pathology specimens. One is an obstetrician's wheel (usually provided by a drug company) that converts LMP or EDC to gestational age. The other is a table of birth weight distributions by gestation with percentiles. A method for converting pounds and ounces to grams may also be needed (2.2 lb/kg). An algorithm is necessary to select the best gestational age estimation.

As a general rule an ultrasound in the first trimester is the most accurate of dating tools. Here the estimated gestational age (EGA) is plus or minus (±) 1 week. Early in the second trimester the EGA begins to span ± 1 to 2 weeks by ultrasound. With progression to the third trimester, EGA by ultrasound begins to vary ± 2 to 3 weeks. Here, in later gestations, symmetric IUGR may occur, and this further confounds dating parameters by ultrasound. A known LMP, an early quantitative β-human chorionic gonadotropin, and an early first examination by the obstetrician are also helpful in establishing EGA.

When examining a placenta the pathologist should keep in mind a variety of maternal-, fetal-, and labor-specific processes, all of which may confer greater importance on placental findings.

Specific clinical parameters should thus direct the pathologist to look for specific and therefore supportive findings in the placenta. Several such entities that may be brought to the pathologist's attention by the accession form or through personal communication are discussed below, together with the attendant placental findings. For more in-depth discussions regarding these pathologic entities, the reader is directed to the appropriate chapters throughout the text. Following this brief description of "what to watch out for" is a discussion of the necessary systematic approach for placental evaluation.

Maternal Disorders

Pregnancy-induced hypertension is often associated with infarction (both early and old), retroplacental bleeding (clinically termed abruption), decidual vasculopathy, and increased villous syncytial knotting. Rarely, partial molar change may be seen.[1–5] *Maternal diabetes* may be gestational or type I with the potential for attendant maternal systemic (e.g., renal, hypertensive, retinal) disorders. In suboptimally controlled gestational diabetes usually, infants and placenta are increased in size and weight. In type I diabetes, placentas tend to be small and fetuses may be growth restricted. In these cases villous dysmaturity may be identified.[6,7] *Vaginal bleeding* throughout gestation may be associated with retroplacental hematoma, circumvallate placentation, marginal placenta or placenta previa, and decidual hemosiderin deposition. *Elevated maternal serum α-fetoprotein* may be associated with fetal maternal hemorrhage, and large intervillous thrombi can be identified. *Preterm PROM* is associated with the risk of chorioamnionitis (which may either cause or result from PROM). *Viral and other infectious illness* in the mother can be confirmed by specific findings in the placenta. In severe bacterial infection the membranes may appear white with diffuse polymorphonuclear leukocytes. Other characteristic histologic findings herald a variety of pathogens. A history of *preterm labor* can be associated with infection, abruption, and uterine anomalies. In the last mentioned, depression and infarction may be present in the placenta, which, for example, may have been situated over a submucous myoma.

Fetal and Neonatal Disorders

Fetal hydrops may have a variety of etiologies. Commonly these are considered immune and nonimmune in origin. Evaluation of the placenta may help to establish the diagnosis, especially when infection (such as parvovirus B19, cytomegalovirus [CMV], or syphilis) is present.[8] Large chorangiomas and acardiac twins are other potential causes of hydrops delineated by examining the placenta. Large, often anemic (pale) placentas are common in such cases. On microscopic examination, increased erythropoiesis is marked by the finding of nucleated erythroid precursors and villous stromal edema. *Intrauterine growth retardation* (IUGR) in many cases may be accounted for by specific placental findings. Notable among these causes are excessive perivillous fibrinoid deposition (maternal floor infarction),[9,10] excessive parenchymal infarction, and infection. Other contributing factors include amnion nodosum, seen in oligohydramnios, and fetal anomalies, which may be heralded by a cord with a single umbilical artery. *Oligohydramnios* caused by long-standing rupture of membranes or Potter's syndrome may be confirmed by the identification of amnion nodosum on the fetal membranes.[11,12] *Macrosomic or large for gestational age* (LGA) infants may be further evaluated through findings specific to the placenta. In such cases villous hydrops may be noted. Abnormal villous maturation may signal diabetic effects. *Fetal malformations and anomalies* may be elucidated by the identification of amnionic bands, villous abnormalities suggesting chromosomal defects, single umbilical artery, and lysosomal storage phenomenon.[13] Twins and multiple gestations carry a many-fold increase in perinatal morbidity and mortality. The placenta is often instrumental in establishing the cause of problems, with findings including vascular anastomoses causing twin-twin transfusion syndrome (and its typical and atypical constellation of effects in the placenta and fetus), malformations with associated single umbilical artery, and another characteristic cord lesion seen in twins (such as velamentous insertion).[14–16] *Intrauterine fetal demise* (IUFD) and *stillbirth* are devastating events that often require a diligent search for the antecedent causative events. In all cases the pathologist should be attuned to the pathologic conditions of the placenta that can be cited as contributory. Such placental findings with their attendant associations include hydrops, ischemic lesions (including infarction, excessive perivillous fibrin, and maternal floor infarction), infection (both chorioamnionitis and villitis), cord anomalies, vascular thrombosis, and cord accidents and lesions. These are but a few of the potential etiologic factors that should be sought during placental evaluation in IUFD.[17]

Complications of Labor and Delivery

A variety of processes notable during the labor and delivery process should be considered when evaluating the placenta. *Vaginal bleeding* should signal a need to assess for abruption, placenta previa, intervillous thrombi, and ruptured vascular anomalies. *Meconium-stained fluid* during labor requires an evaluation of the placenta to discern the extent of involvement. This can be accomplished by observing the staining characteristics of the placenta. The amnion, then the chorion, and lastly the cord become grossly green. Identification of macrophages in the chorion, amnion, and decidua can also be helpful in distinguishing between meconium and hemosiderin from bleeding. *Fetal heat rate tracing abnormalities* should be considered by the pathologist. Late decelerations are seen with uteroplacental insufficiency and its associated placental lesions (including infarction, edema, infection, abruption, excessive fibrin, and decidual vascular disease). Severe variable decelerations reflect cord compression. Compression is usually secondary to oligohydramnios, but cord lesions such as stricture, knots, velamentous insertion, and entanglements may also be related. Fetal acidemia and fetal distress may be documented during labor by an abnormal scalp pH or an ominous fetal heart rate tracing. In the latter, loss of variability in conjunction with late and moderate to severe variable decelerations, a rising baseline (associated also with infection), a sinusoidal pattern (seen with anemia and narcotics), or bradycardia may all be significant enough to be diagnostic of fetal distress.[18] Here again, placental lesions noted to be related to uteroplacental insufficiency should be documented. Abnormal fetal heart rate patterns that would have little significance at term (such as mild to moderate variables) may take on increased significance in the preterm gestation.

Clinical Follow-up of Abnormal Placentas

The placental examination has a role in diagnosis and quality review. The proof of that statement requires studies of correlation with clinical outcome and eventually trials of intervention based on the placental findings. In practice, however, if the placental findings are unusual or uncertain or do not make sense in terms of the clinical history, the pathologist can initiate the follow-up. A call to the clinician or request for the maternal or neonatal chart may be enough. The call to the pediatrician becomes an obligation for diagnoses that have a direct impact on treatment, such as CMV or parvovirus inclusions or lysosomal storage cells.

HANDLING AND STORAGE OF THE PLACENTA

Transportation and Storage Before Pathologic Examination

The placenta should be in a container that will not leak or lose its label. As long as the placenta is kept cold, but not frozen, the pathologic examination is satisfactory for days after delivery. If unfixed placentas are kept in refrigerated storage, a simple system is a set of bins for the number of days of storage. Emptying and filling the bins sequentially prevents the placentas from accumulating. The longer the storage, the greater the ability to reexamine the placenta when an infant is transferred from the well baby nursery to the NICU.

Handling of the Pathology Specimen

The placenta, like any other fresh specimen, is a potential source of contamination. Thus the pathologist may decide to fix the placenta before transport from the labor and delivery room or on receipt in the pathology department.

Fixed Placenta System

Fixation reduces contamination with blood and may be the safest way to transport placentas from outside the hospital. Ten percent neutral buffered formalin is the most practical all-around fixative. Proper penetration of the fixative is necessary for appropriate demonstration of structural detail. The placenta should be allowed to lie flat in a round bottom container of adequate size. Rolled or compressed edges hamper penetration of the fixative. The specimen should be covered with fresh fixative at least three times the volume of the sample. Proper penetration requires a minimum of 24 hours before sectioning. Compete fixation of the core of the placenta may require several days even with adequate formalin volume. If specimens have been mailed from outside hospitals, old fixative should be replaced with fresh fixative. It is important to wash the specimen under water for at least several hours before gross examination, which should be performed under a well-ventilated hood to avoid atmospheric contamination. Fixation characteristically increases the placental weight by 10%.

Fresh Placenta System

The fresh placenta has the advantage of permitting accurate color description, of easy palpation of focal lesions, of fixing the membranes in a compact jelly roll, and of microbiologic or chromosomal culture. For safety, however, adequate universal precautions and clean-up procedures must be followed. There is also the potential for contaminating injury while cutting the placenta. The use of scissors and a long, sharp knife with a blunt end is safer than scalpels and knives with pointed ends.

The placenta is one of the bloodiest pathologic specimens. The refrigerated storage area becomes contaminated with blood and must be kept clean. A large work area that can be cleaned with running water is needed. The space must be easily protected from contaminating blood splashes and spills and easily cleaned and decontaminated. The morgue may be a better choice than the surgical cutting area. With the fresh placenta, blocks of tissue can be fixed in formalin. (Bouin's fixative can decrease the time necessary for fixation and makes fixed tissues firmer, enhancing the ability to section the tissue before placing it into the cassettes.) The specimen can then be trimmed and submitted later in the day or next day. Far less formalin and storage space are needed with this method.

GROSS EXAMINATION

If a gross lesion is not observed, it may not be rediscoverable by the histologic examination. To avoid such errors the pathologist should be aware of the implications of the clinical history before examining the placenta, examine the placenta systematically with a checklist for each region, and examine as many placentas as possible to gain experience. The following section describes a systematic approach to the gross examination and provides a brief list of lesions. The reader is referred to other chapters for clinical significance and pathologic description of the lesions.

The College of American Pathology consensus conference on the placenta in 1990, reissued and reproduced in the current guidelines,[19] resolved that a gross description of the placenta is the responsibility of the physician delivering the infant. The condition of the placenta should be noted in the chart. A strong knowledge of gross placental pathology is therefore essential for the obstetrician. This knowledge will also aid in determining which grossly abnormal placentas should be sent for pathologic examination. The delivering physician is also best able to obtain an accurate umbilical cord length.

Procedure for Examining the Placenta

The intervillous blood has usually drained from the fresh placenta into its container. Any discolorations (sections in the air are redder than those in the blood) or distortions from the position in the container should be noted to avoid confusion during the examination. After the placenta is removed, it often needs a brief rinse to restore the natural color. The container, commonly filled with bloody fluid, should be searched for any unattached specimen. Fresh clot, which is usually not significant, may develop behind the placenta after delivery of the infant. Older clot (drier, brown, or more friable) is significant. The size of such clots can be estimated and recorded. The container may have other biologic components, such as vernix or meconium, and occasionally an additional specimen, such as pieces of cord or a fragment of endometrial tissue or myoma. The odor should be noted as evidence of bacterial overgrowth.

The gross examination and sampling should proceed systematically to avoid unintentional omissions. This section describes the basic approach to each anatomic area of the placenta. Increasing the number of samples increases the chance of identifying lesions that are not seen macroscopically, either because they are easy to overlook (e.g., *Candida* plaques) or because they are not necessarily visible (e.g., acute atherosis of maternal spiral arteries or villitis). In other instances increased sampling aids diagnosis because of inherent variability between samples, for example, evaluating villous adaption to uteroplacental ischemia. The benefits of more samples must be balanced against cost, both for the processing and for the pathologic reading. With exceptions, such as multiple infarctions, distinctly pathologic areas of the placenta should be sampled. The following should be considered a minimum for histologic processing of the placenta: two or three cross sections of umbilical cord, one or two cross sections of the membrane roll, three through-and-through sections of normal-appearing parenchyma, and representative sections of all grossly identified lesions that might require histologic confirmation.[19]

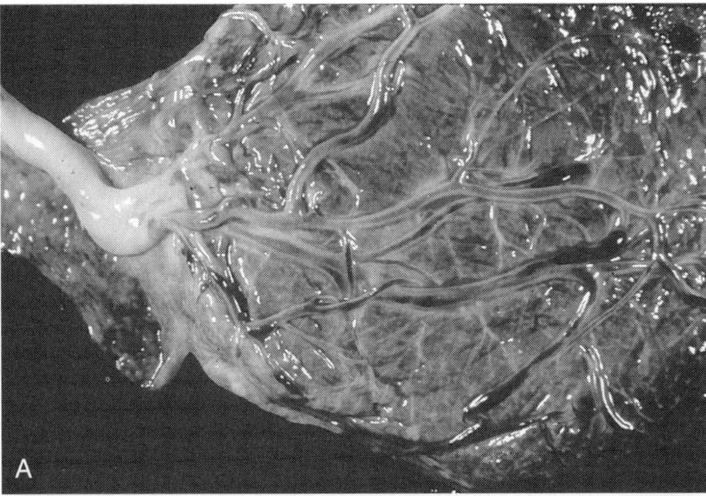

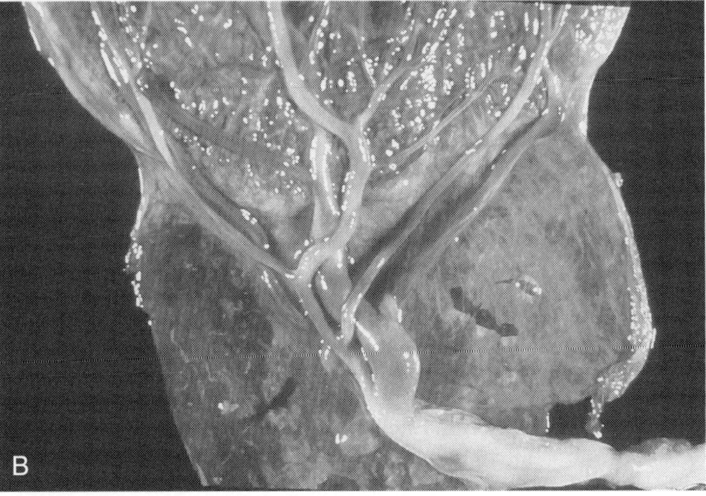

Figure 2–2. A, Marginal cord insertion. (Note small abnormal membranous vessel located on the membranes adjacent to the cord insertion site, indicating partial velamentous insertion.) **B,** Velamentous cord insertion.

Umbilical Cord

Since not all of the cord may be sent to the pathology laboratory, the true length should be obtained by the obstetrician in the delivery room. However, the pathologist should measure all segments of the cord available, since this may document that the cord was at least not abnormally short. At term any cord less than 30 cm or more than 70 cm may be abnormal. Normal values have been published (see Table 3–1).[20] Cord length is probably a function of fetal activity.[21,22] The umbilical cord insertion is noted. The cord may insert onto the placental surface (may be described as central or eccentric), at the margin (battledore insertion) (Fig. 2–2*A*), or in the membranes (velamentous insertion) (Fig. 2–2*B*). If Wharton's jelly ends before the cord vessels reach the placental surface, the insertion is called furcata ("like a fork"). Next the cord is cut from the placenta. All pieces of the cord are measured, and a mean diameter can be estimated. The diameter of the mature cord is between 0.8 and 1.5 cm.[23] A cross section of the middle umbilical cord permits counting of the vessels. Because the two arteries constrict and the vein is flaccid, the appearance with the normal three vessels often resembles two eyes and a mouth. The portion of the cord near the fetus is likely to contain remnants of the allantoic and omphalomesenteric ducts. The portion near the placenta may reflect abnormal insertion or the fetal arterial anastomosis (which is normal) (Fig. 2–2*C*). The color of the cord is helpful to classify. White to cream is normal; green or yellow green

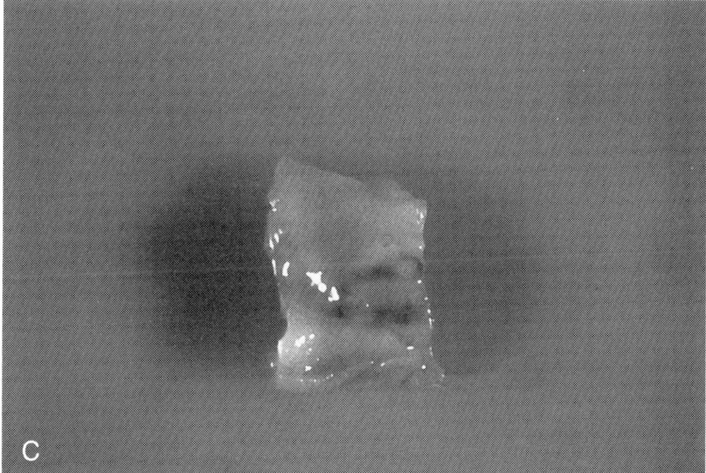

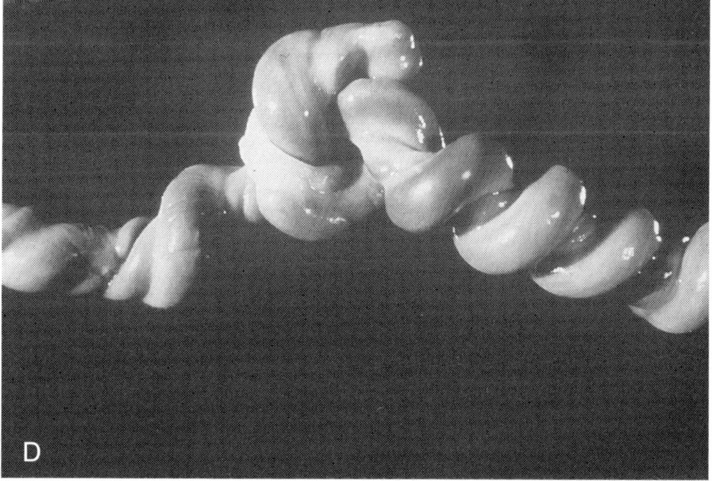

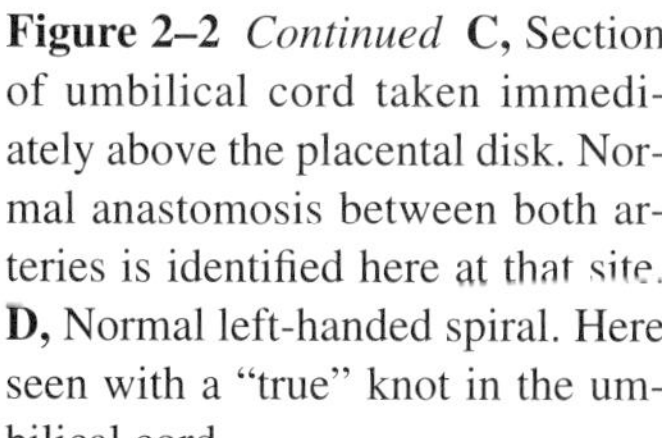

Figure 2–2 *Continued* **C,** Section of umbilical cord taken immediately above the placental disk. Normal anastomosis between both arteries is identified here at that site. **D,** Normal left-handed spiral. Here seen with a "true" knot in the umbilical cord.

indicates meconium, red or brown means hemoglobin, and transparent suggests immaturity, edema, or necrotizing funisitis. The red color may be generalized after fetal death. If the cord is red in a live-born infant, especially if the red follows only one arterial spiral, umbilical arterial thrombus may be present.[24] The normal umbilical cord has a helical spiral of the blood vessels, usually left handed (Fig. 2–2*D*). The spiral may be decreased or accentuated from the usual.

The most common anomaly is a single umbilical artery. An extra umbilical vein is rare. Vascular looping (pseudoknots), or false knots (Fig. 2–3*A*), may give the illusion of more than three vessels in cross section, but this potential error can be identified. Other vascular abnormalities include aneurysms (Fig. 2–3*B*) and thrombus (Fig. 2–3*C* and *D*). Venous aneurysms with nonocclusive thrombus may occur at the insertion. A barber pole spiral of white bands adjacent to the vessels that appears as a white crescent in cross section is often due to subacute necrotizing funisitis (Fig. 2–3*E*). Surface lesions often follow the vascular spiral and include the fine yellowish nodules of *Candida* (Fig. 2–3*F*), and the ulcerations associated with bowel atresia.[25] Hematomas are often massive, sausagelike swellings of the cord starting at the fetal end. Small hematomas, often with clamp marks or needle punctures, are created post partum. Hemorrhages from percutaneous umbilical blood sampling are difficult to find. True overhand knots of the umbilical cord occur in utero. They may retain flattened areas after untieing if they are "tight." If a knot causes venous obstruc-

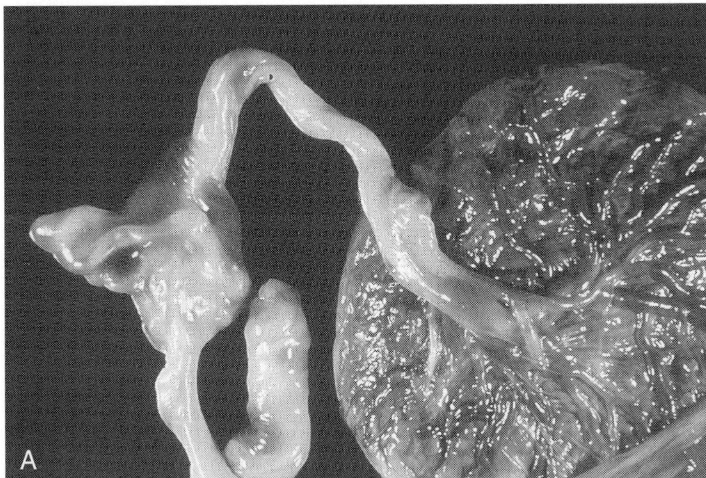

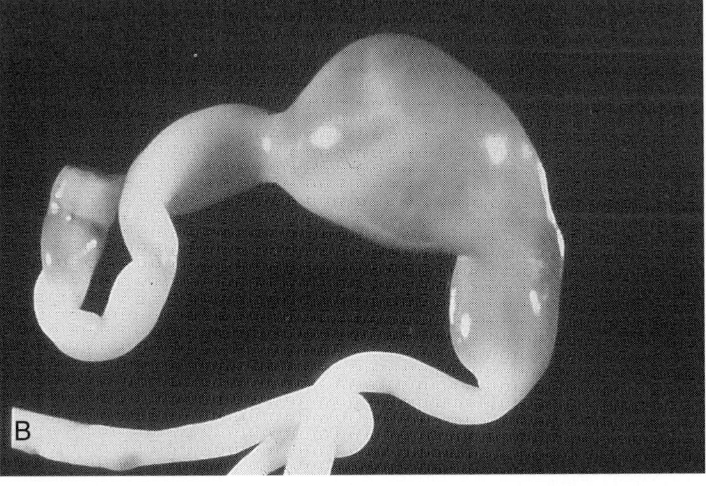

Figure 2–3. A, False knot of the umbilical cord. **B,** Cord aneurysm.

tion, the vein should be dilated on the placental side. Tumors, cysts, hemangiomas, and teratomas may also be seen.

Placental Membranes

The membranes include the reflected membranes of the fetal sac and the membranes of the chorionic plate or "fetal surface" of the placenta. Both are composed of amnion and chorion. The chorionic vessels reside in the chorion of the fetal surface (chorionic plate). Maternal decidua is found at the deep surface of the chorion on the reflected membranes. The fetal sac is usually still attached to the rim of the placenta. All of it or fragments may also be separate, having been removed during delivery. The membrane sac may have inverted over the maternal surface with delivery but can be flipped back to the in situ position. If the sac is not shredded, pulling the membranes up can reproduce a rough image of the sac in utero. The location of the opening and the size of the sac can be reconstructed. The sac had to open to deliver the infant, but the point of rupture that usually overlies the os may be eccentric to the actual tear in the sac. In some cases the sac is opened at the time of cesarean section and thus the opening is not related to the location of the os. When possible the membrane sample should include the sac opening because this may demonstrate distinct pathologic effects of rupture.

The color and any focal lesions of the membranes should be noted. The amnion is a thin

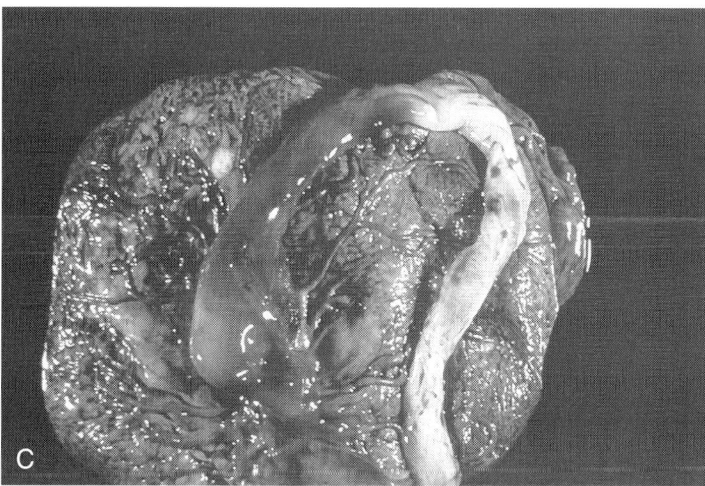

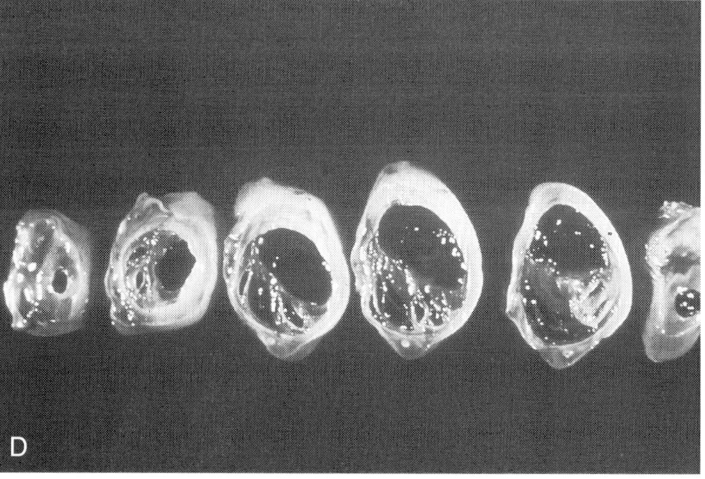

Figure 2–3 *Continued* **C,** Umbilical vascular thrombosis. **D,** Thrombosis identified in cross-sectional study of the umbilical cord.

Illustration continued on following page

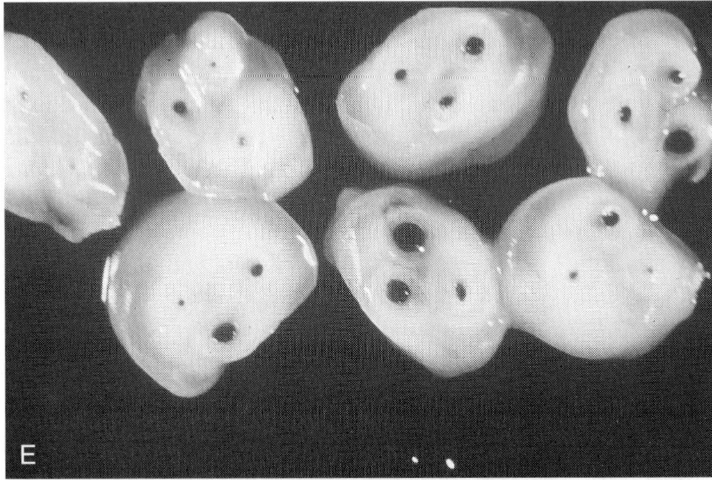

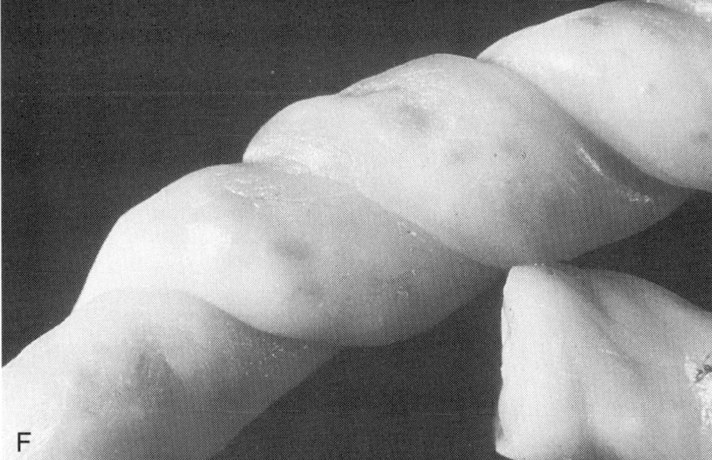

Figure 2–3 *Continued* **E,** Necrotizing funisitis. **F,** *Candida* plaques of the umbilical cord.

membrane, resembling plastic wrap, that can be peeled from the fused chorion and decidual membranes. The decidua (endometrium) may separate at different depths, appearing translucent if just below the chorion but as a spongy tissue with maternal vessels if nearer the basal layer. To sample maternal vessels, the pathologist should choose an area that demonstrates gross vessels. Pathologic lesions may also be included in the sample roll (see below). In twin pregnancy, in addition to the samples of the membranes that line the uterine wall, a sample of the septal membrane (intervening) should also be taken if present. A diamnionic septum is clear, whereas a dichorionic membrane is thicker with opaque markings.

The technique for sampling the membranes has many variations, but most texts recommend creating a roll of membranes and cutting it transversely, like a jelly roll, for the histologic sample (Fig. 2–4). One procedure is to make two parallel cuts with scissors from the margin of rupture to the placental attachment, approximately 2 to 3 cm apart. This strip is grasped approximately 1 cm from the

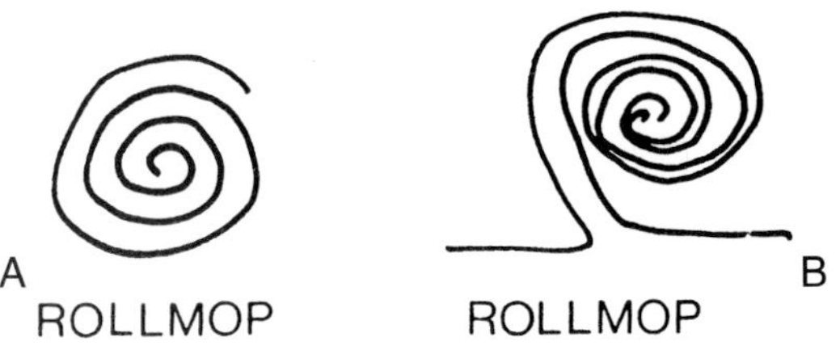

Figure 2–4. **A,** Roll of free membranes for cross-sectional study. **B,** Roll of intervening membrane from twin gestation.

margin by placing and closing a hemostat completely across it. The free 1 cm of membrane is then placed flat against the fixed end, and the whole is rolled around the hemostat until the edge is reached. The membrane is cut from the edge, and a single tie with string is made around the middle and lightly tightened. The hemostat is released and carefully removed. The tie is tightened, and the specimen is fixed in formalin until firm. The pathologist then submits one or two cross sections, depending on how many fit in the processing cassette. Some pathologists are content simply to stuff a random sample of membranes into the cassette. This can be used to produce a diagnostic slide but lacks the orientation and adequate surface area that make the membrane roll easier to read and interpret.

The following is a list of items for recording membrane findings and some examples of lesions: The completeness of the sac should be assessed. The site of rupture and its shortest distance from the parenchymal disk should be recorded. Velamentous or membranous vessels crossing within the membranes should be described. Any abnormal-appearing vessels should be noted and sampled for inflammation or thrombus. The membranes are usually white with a faint bluish sheen. As in the cord, blood stains red to brown, and meconium yellow to green. Purulent inflammation may show pus or a dull cream to pale green hue (Fig. 2–5*A*). The nodules of amnion nodosum vary in size from barely perceptible with the correct angle of illumination to several millimeters in diameter (Fig. 2–5*B*). They need to be distinguished

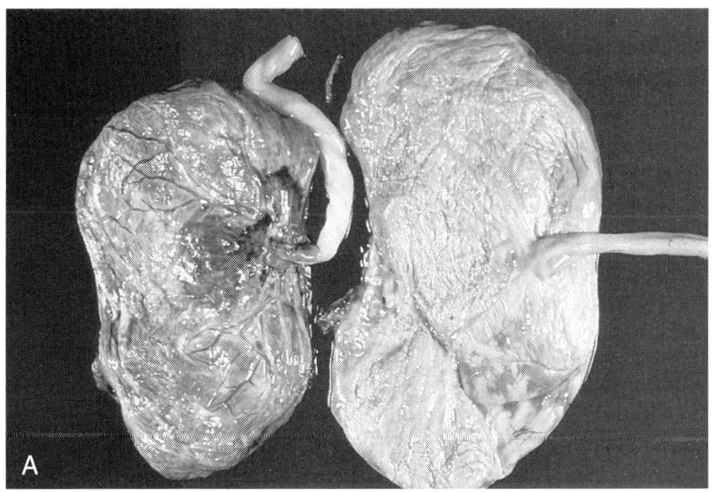

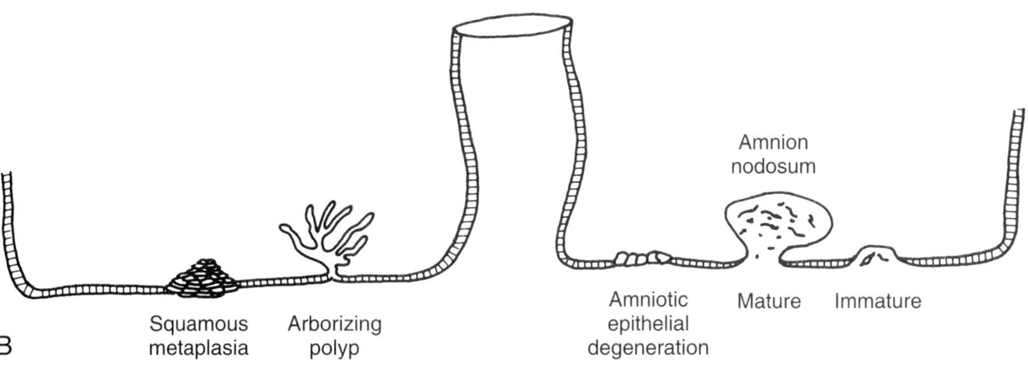

Figure 2–5. A, Chorioamnionitis with gross identification of "pus" in the affected larger placenta. **B,** Abnormalities of the fetal or amniotic sac. *Illustration continued on next page*

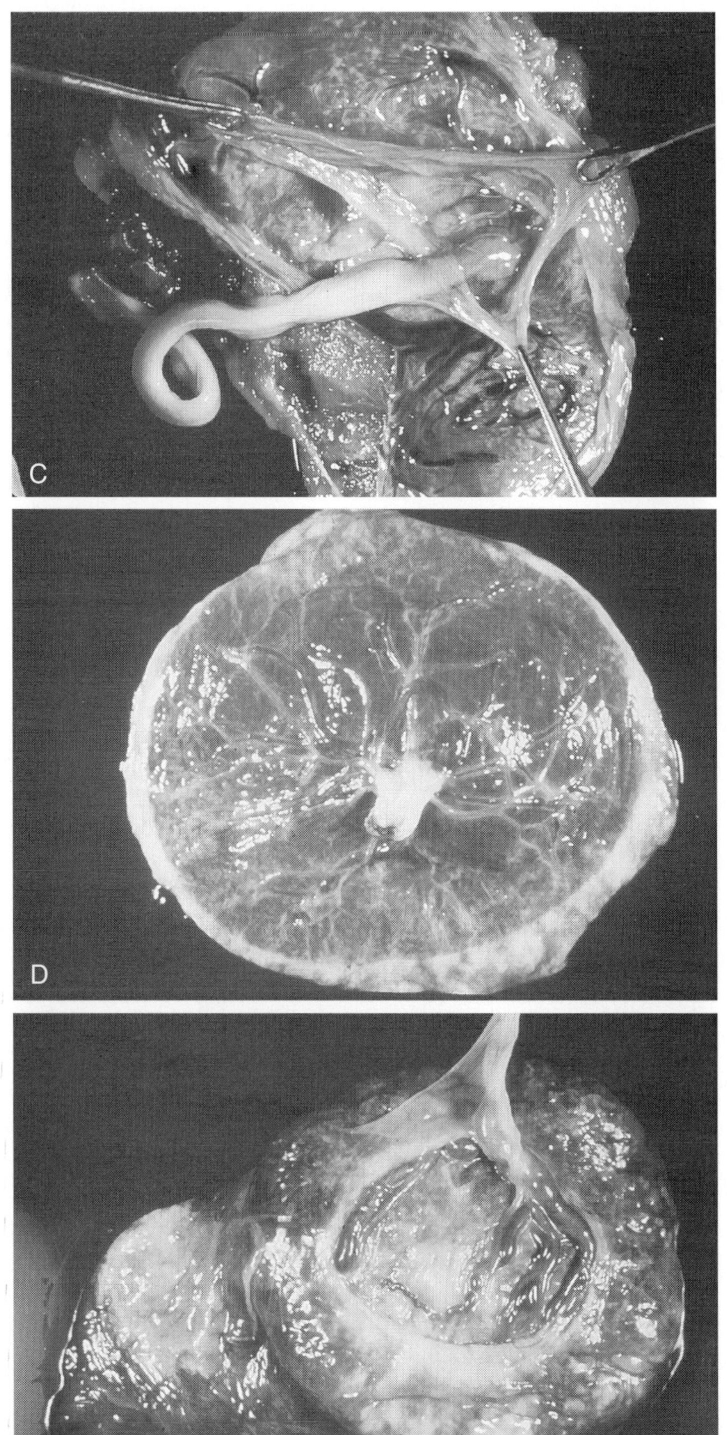

Figure 2–5 *Continued* **C,** Amniotic band or sheet. **D,** Circummarginate placenta. **E,** Circumvallate placenta.

from squamous metaplasia. The yolk sac is seen as a small, white nodule and need not be sampled. A fetus papyraceus may be found in the membranes, but often the residua of a "vanished" twin appears amorphous. A radiograph may demonstrate skeletal remains. Amnionic bands (Fig. 2–5*C*) are composed of strands of tissue attached to the fetus and have two distinct morphologies. One appears to be residua of the shredded amnion, often attached to the umbilical insertion. The placenta surface appears dull, and amputated fetal parts may rarely be present. A sample of the surface membranes does not demonstrate amnion. In the other variety the chorion still has an intact amnion lining, but there are bands between the fetus and amnion analogous to scars or adhesions.[26–28] Foci of yellow necrosis or tan hematoma may be recognized on the decidua, reflecting older hemorrhage. The percentage of circummarginate (Fig. 2–5*D*) or circumvallate membrane (Fig. 2–5*E*) insertion should be noted, the chorionic surface vessels described, and samples taken of any thrombi, aneurysms, surface vascular tumors (chorangiomas), or angiomatous malformations.

Placental Parenchyma

The membranes should be trimmed from the placenta, and the trimmed, drained weight of the placenta obtained (see Table 3–1). The shape is described: discoid, bilobed (Fig. 2–6*A*), elongated, or multilobed (Fig. 2–6*B*). This weight is considerably lighter than the weight obtained fresh in the

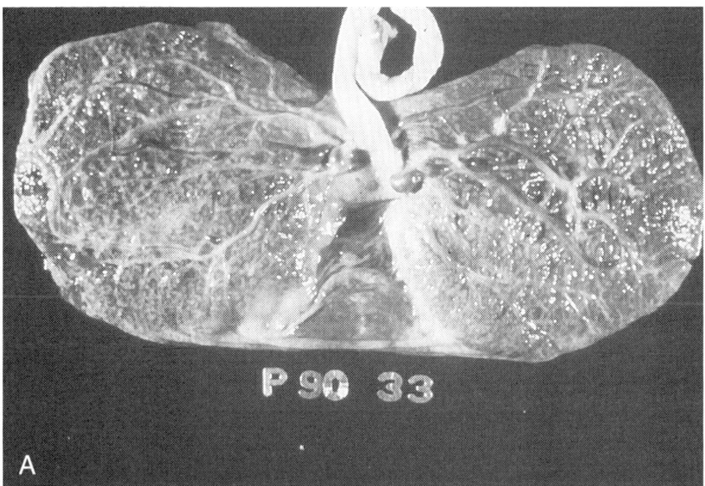

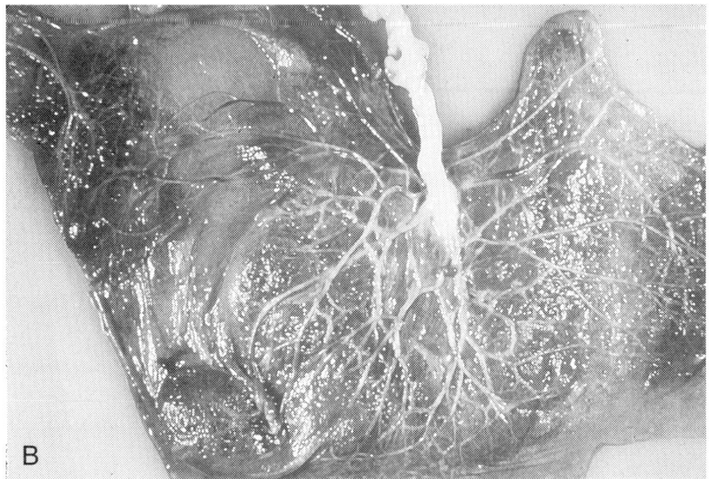

Figure 2–6. A, Bilobed placenta. **B,** Multilobed placenta (succenturiate lobes).

delivery room, which usually includes the intervillous maternal blood. An infant more than 36 weeks' gestational age typically weighs six to eight times the placenta; thus a 3000 g infant typically has a 375 to 500 g placenta. The weight can be a useful reference point; for example, a histologically mature-appearing placenta weighing 180 g is abnormal. If multigestation placentas are fused and cannot be weighed separately, the percentage associated with each infant can be estimated from the surface. In monochorionic twins the vascular relationships should be noted. The placenta should be inspected on both surfaces. As described for the membranes, on the fetal surface the vessels should be systematically inspected, especially for thrombi, which are often calcified. If hemorrhage is present, its location, subamnionic or subchorionic, should be noted. There is a distinct maternal surface (the side without the umbilical cord) composed, starting from the uterine side, of adherent decidua, a trophoblastic layer, and a fibrinoid layer. A lobular organization exists, with septa that appear related to the maternal circulation but not the fetal cotyledons. The placenta separates at the decidualized endometrium similar to menstruation. If most of the placenta fails to separate, this is placenta accreta and usually results in severe postpartum hemorrhage and hysterectomy. However, smaller portions of adherent placenta leave a gap on the maternal surface with evidence of a torn villus. This must be distinguished from insignificant tearing of the surface.

The placental dimensions can be measured as the longest axis, its perpendicular surface axis, and an

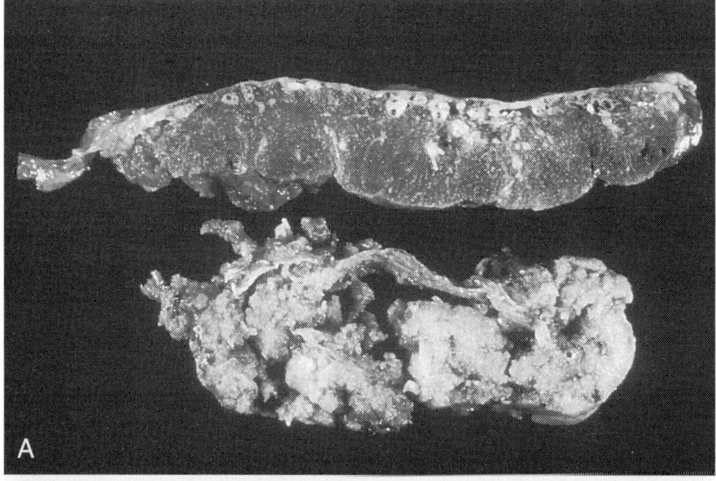

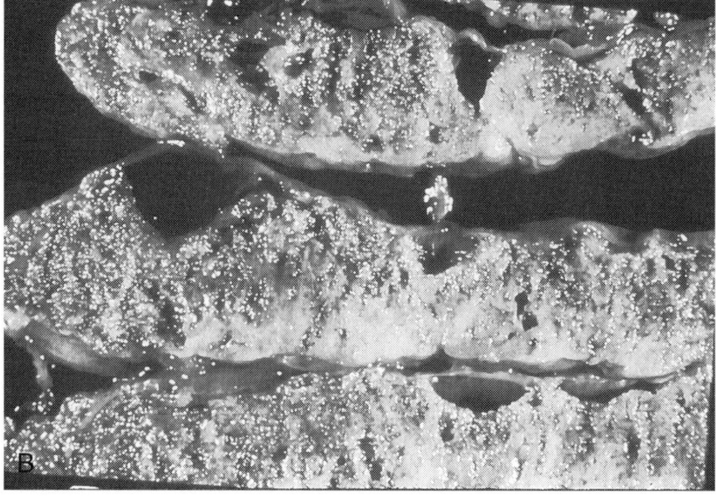

Figure 2–7. A, Hydrops identified in the placental cross section viewed below. **B,** Maternal floor infarction.

estimated mean thickness. In some cases the placenta has been removed manually or by curettage with such disruption that it can only be weighed. Any photographs of unusual features should be taken at this point before further processing. If cytogenetic studies are desired, they are best performed at this point. The placenta is next palpated to localize any parenchymal lesion and then is cut in full thickness (breadloafing) across the entire placenta at 1 cm intervals. A blunt-tipped large knife makes the cuts simple and safe. If small abscesses are seen, these should have microbial culture. Lesions should be sampled, although documentation of every infarction or laminated intervillous thrombus is unnecessary. Often there is no need to document small areas of marginal perivillous fibrinoid or normal variations in subchorionic fibrin. Normal placenta should be sampled both to look for microscopic lesions that cannot be detected macroscopically and to document physiologic villous changes. In a mature placenta the cut surface frequently has an area overlying the spiral artery inflow, which has an open "cystic" appearance (so-called jet lesions) with a more compacted periphery. This is a normal finding. There is also a variation of architecture from the maternal to the fetal surface of the placenta. Thus sections should be taken from the fetal surface to the maternal surface. If necessary, these may be divided to fit in the sampling cassette. To obtain good sections, a large full-thickness block (1 cm thick) can be fixed, then a thinner sample submitted for processing. If the placentas are put into fixation in the morning, the section can be trimmed in the late afternoon and submitted for histologic

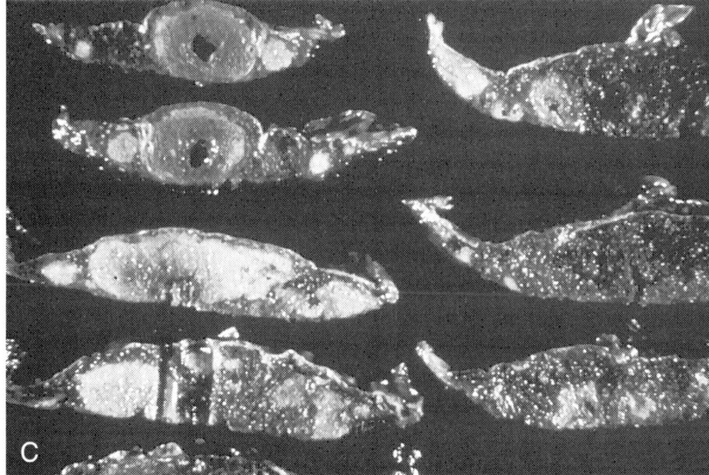

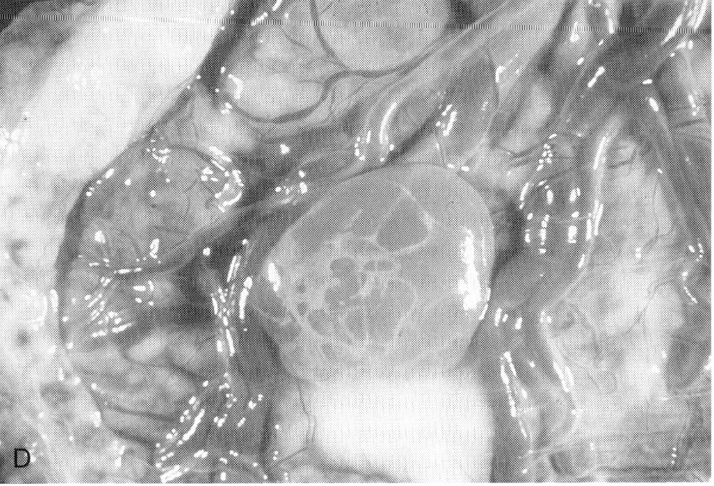

Figure 2–7 *Continued* **C,** Multiple, principally old infarcts. **D,** Chorionic cyst of the placenta.

examination the same day. Three normal sections, not involving the margin, are usually sufficient to give a representative sample of the villi.

In addition to the placental weight, shape, and dimensions, the following should be identified and documented. The completeness of the parenchyma should be assessed, since absence of fragments may indicate portions left in utero. The color is usually normal red. Paleness is indicative of anemia, and a deep red color denotes plethora. A "boggy" appearance or texture reflects immaturity or hydrops (Fig. 2–7*A*). Excessive fibrin (throughout the parenchymal substance known as "gitter-infarct" or along the basal plate indicative of the misnomer "maternal floor infarction" [Fig. 2–7*B*]), infarction (firm granular areas that are red when early and yellow to white as they age [Fig. 2–7*C*]), and thrombi (noted as dark collections of blood when "fresh" that become laminated as they age) should be noted and described by location and percentage of the placenta affected. Retroplacental hematomas should be measured and described as a percentage of the maternal surface affected. Subchorionic fibrin collections reflect maternal eddying of blood and are normal findings. A large subchorionic hematoma is, however, abnormal and representative of a Breus' mole. Subchorionic (Fig. 2–7*D*) and septal cysts are lined by intermediate trophoblasts, contain clear fluid, and generally are of no pathologic significance other than sometimes being associated with maternal floor infarction.

Decidua

The decidua is difficult to assess by gross examination. As described previously, it is best examined with the reflected membranes because it most commonly adheres to them. Finding significant amounts of decidua attached to the basal plate of the placenta is unusual, since this is mostly sheared from the base of the maternal surface and remains in utero until being shed with maternal lochia. The decidua associated with the chorion laeve may show evidence of old blood that should not be confused with meconium (which is more diffuse). Decidual spiral vessels may be examined microscopically for atherosis.

MICROSCOPIC EXAMINATION

Stains

A well-done hematoxylin and eosin preparation is still the best all-around stain for most purposes. As with other staining procedures, care must be taken with preparation of the stain. Freshness of the stain and tincture of staining are extremely important. Overstaining of slides with either hematoxylin or eosin may obscure important histologic detail. Likewise, freshness of dehydrating solutions and purity of embedding media are essential for clarity of microscopic detail.

Old stains and solutions result in as much distortion of the tissue and are as great a hindrance to histologic and eventual clinical interpretation as poorly handled fixation.[29] Other stains may be used, mostly for the identification of infectious agents. Periodic acid–Schiff (PAS) or methenamine-silver stains are useful for identifying fungal hyphae or spores. In addition to Gram's stain for bacteria, silver impregnation methods may be helpful in detecting organisms such as *Listeria,* spirochetes, or fusobacteria.

Assessment of Extent and Severity of Microscopic Placental Lesions

The extent and severity of placental alterations may have important clinical implications.[30] The

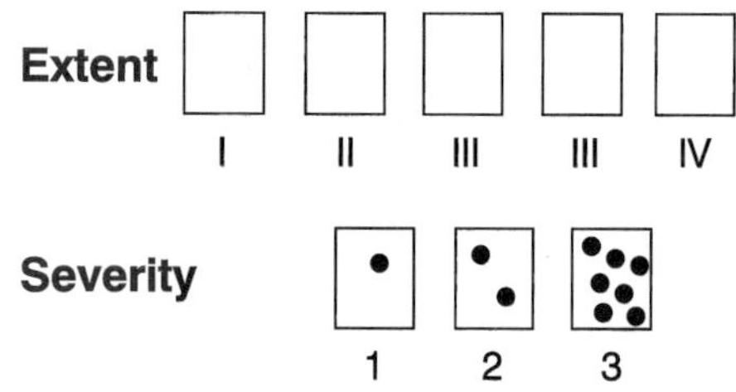

Figure 2–8. Method for evaluating the extent and severity of microscopic placental lesions. Extent equals number of histologic sections exhibiting the lesion (I to IV). Severity equals number of affected areas per section (I to III). I equals focal; II equals at least two; III equals multiple or diffuse. Extent/severity index equals extent number times average severity number. Example, extent of II × average severity of 2.5 equals 5.

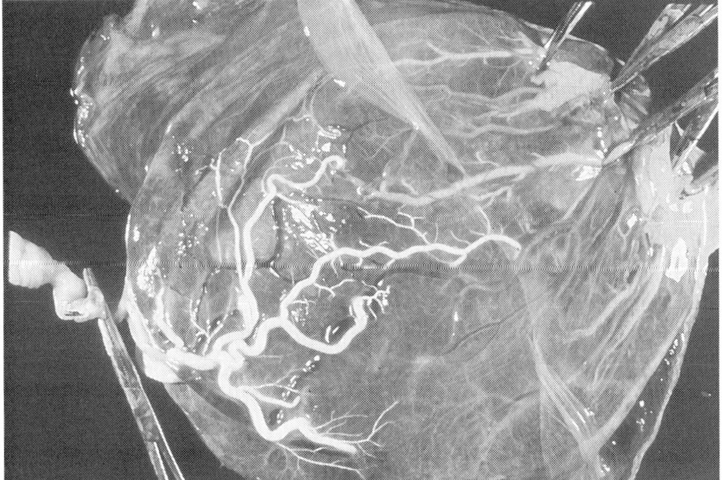

Figure 2–9. Assessment of vascular anastomoses in diamniotic monochorionic twin placenta (artery at left anastomosis with vein at right; note: invariably, chorionic arteries pass over chorionic veins as viewed from the fetal surface).

extent of gross lesions such as primary infarcts or massive perivillous fibrin deposition can be estimated at the time of gross examination, and a statement made about the percentage of placental volume involved. One method for assessing the extent of microscopic lesions is to count the histologic slides exhibiting the lesion in question. In this scheme severity is reflected by the number of affected areas per slide. Multiplying the extent number by the average severity number enables calculation of an extent/severity index or score for parenchymal lesions, such as chronic villitis, hemorrhagic endovasculitis, or fetal placental vessel thrombi (Fig. 2–8).

Special Techniques

Vascular Injection

The simplest vascular injection technique is to insert a needle into a superficial vein or artery (Fig. 2–9). More complicated injection into the umbilical cord or into vessels with catheters is also possible. Many injection media can be used, among which are air, milk, and water. The advantage of low-viscosity solutions is that they pass through the villous circulation. The advantage of oral barium solution with colored dye added is that at least the most viscous preparation stays in the surface vessels, facilitating photography of the vascular relationships. With this technique, blood clots in the vessels may have to be massaged through. The needle site and umbilical cords must be clamped. The use of a short intravascular catheter instead of a needle facilitates removing the syringe to refill it. Injection studies are not required for diagnostic examination of twins, since most artery-to-artery and vein-to-vein anastomoses can be visualized and confirmed by pushing blood with a finger to verify continuity in suspect areas. Artery-to-vein shunts require more patience, but if each arterial branch is followed out, a vein should accompany it. If there is no vein, or clearly a vein from the other placenta, a shunt is presumed to be present in the underlying fetal cotyledon.

Once mastered, the barium technique is not intimidating and can be performed routinely by a pathology assistant using viscous oral barium from the radiology department mixed with standard tissue marker paint in a specimen container. The barium is drawn into a 50 ml syringe, and an 18-gauge needle is attached. The injection is made into a large surface vessel, which is clamped with a hemostat after the needle is withdrawn. Multiple colors can be used, for example, for artery versus vein or for twin A versus twin B. Excess barium can be washed off the surface for photography. Some leakage may occur from the parenchyma, but high-viscosity barium does not leak easily through the capillary bed.

Cytogenetics

Placental villi uncontaminated with maternal blood or decidua are fetal tissue. With aseptic technique the placental surface can be removed to avoid bacteria and a portion of clean villi can be sampled. A sterile scalpel blade and a suture removal kit are adequate tools. Placental karyotyping is often performed on stillborn infants because no other viable tissue is available (unless amnionic fluid was collected). The villi remain perfused by maternal blood, while the umbilical cord and amnion fibroblasts often fare less well.

Microbial Culture

Vaginal delivery may lead to contamination of the placenta. A technique for avoiding this is to lift the amnion off the chorion and swab the inner membrane area. One study of fetal morbidity using this technique recovered *Mycoplasma* and *Ureaplasma.*[31] Whether the technique is valid for recovering all types of organisms and truly reduces contamination is unknown. However, placental culture may be the only way to demonstrate the origin of an infection. In one unpublished case of pneumococcal pneumonitis in a newborn the refrigerated placental specimen was cultured and grew *Streptococcus pneumoniae.* In subacute funisitis, direct culture of Wharton's jelly has been successful.[32]

REPORTING AND DATA MANAGEMENT

A practical report format for the placental diagnosis is to use three headings: gross diagnoses, microscopic diagnoses, and clinical correlation (when appropriate). The first two present the clearly diagnostic features such as single umbilical artery or meconium macrophages to the level of the decidua. The clinical correlation relates these preceding diagnoses to the clinical history and presents the known clinical implications. The nondiagnostic observations, gross and microscopic, are retained in a descriptive database portion of the report. A computer database modeled on the examples of clinical history and gross findings presented above, and coupled with a record of microscopic findings, can simplify retrieval, summation, and follow-up of cases for research and quality reports. A convenient format that details gross findings and microscopic diagnoses is shown in Figure 1–1.

Working with a Pathology Assistant

With a large number of placentas, training an assistant may be a cost-effective investment. However, delegating responsibility for gross examination and sampling of the placenta is controversial. There are two prerequisites. One, the use of an assistant presupposes that the pathologist is competent in placental gross examination. Two, the pathologist must be certain that the assistant is competent to perform the examination. The assistant needs to perform an adequate number of examinations with a pathologist experienced in placental pathology. There is no formula for an adequate number, but seeing enough of the gross pathology discussed in this chapter requires several hundred supervised examinations at the minimum. The outline of clinical findings and of gross lesions will aid in training the assistant and provide a format for dictation. The assistant must also know his or her limitations and be able to consult the pathologist about any unfamiliar finding or history. A list of specific case types that must be done with the pathologist is useful: stillbirth, low Apgar scores, suspected abruption, and discordant or monochorionic twins, for example. The training of an assistant should be complemented by good Kodachrome slides and saved sample cases. In some cases microscopic comparison to the gross findings is essential for diagnosis, and in such cases the pathologist should perform the gross examination.

REFERENCES

1. Bendon RW, Siddiqi T, Soukup S, Srivastava A: Prenatal detection of triploidy. J Pediatr 112:149, 1988.
2. Szulman A, Surti U: The clinicopathologic profile of the partial hydatidiform mole. Obstet Gynecol 59:597, 1982.
3. Bartholomew RA, Colvin ED, William H, et al: Criteria by which toxemia of pregnancy may be di-

agnosed from unlabeled formalin-fixed placentas. Am J Obstet Gynecol 82:277, 1961.

4. Salafia CM, Pessullo JC, Lopez-Zeno JA, et al: Placental pathologic features of preterm preeclampsia. Am J Obstet Gynecol 173:1097, 1995.
5. Redman C: Pre-eclampsia and the placenta. Placenta 12:301, 1991.
6. Singer DB: The placenta in pregnancies complicated by diabetes mellitus. Perspect Pediatr Pathol 8:199, 1984.
7. Clarson C, Tevaarwerk GJM, Harding PGR, et al: Placental weight in diabetic pregnancies. Placenta 10:275, 1989.
8. Machin G: Hydrops revisited: literature review of 1414 cases published in the 1980s. Am J Med Genet 34:366, 1989.
9. Andres R, Kupyer W, Resnik R, et al: The association of maternal floor infarction of the placenta with adverse perinatal outcome. Am J Obstet Gynecol 163:935, 1990.
10. Mandsager NT, Bendon R, Mostello D, et al: Maternal floor infarction of the placenta: prenatal diagnosis and clinical significance. Obstet Gynecol 83:750, 1994.
11. Bendon RW, Ray MB: The pathologic findings of the fetal membranes in very prolonged amniotic fluid leakage. Arch Pathol Lab Med 11:47, 1986.
12. Bourne G: Amnion nodosum. In The human amnion and chorion. Chicago, 1962, Year Book, pp 196–213.
13. Rapola J, Aula P: Morphology of the placenta in fetal I-cell disease. Clin Genet 11:107, 1977.
14. Bajoria R, Wigglesworth J, Fisk N: Angioarchitecture of monochorionic placentas in relation to the twin-twin transfusion syndrome. Am J Obstet Gynecol 172:856, 1995.
15. Machin G, Still K, Lalami T: Correlations of placental vascular anatomy and clinical outcomes in 69 monochorionic twin pregnancies. Am J Med Genet 61:229, 1996.
16. Bendon RW: Twin transfusion: pathological studies of the monochorionic placenta in liveborn twins and of the perinatal autopsy in monochorionic twin pairs. Pediatr Pathol 15:363, 1995.
17. Rayburn W, Sander C, Barr M Jr, Rygiel R: The stillborn fetus: placental histologic examination in determining a cause. Obstet Gynecol 65:637, 1985.
18. Clark S, Miller F: Sinusoidal fetal heart rate pattern associated with massive fetomaternal transfusion. Am J Obstet Gynecol 149:97, 1984.
19. Langston C, Kaplan C, Macpherson T, et al: Practice guidelines for examination of the placenta. Arch Pathol Lab Med 121:449, 1997.
20. Naeye R: Umbilical cord length: clinical significance. J Pediatr 107:278, 1985.
21. Moessinger A: Fetal akinesia deformation sequence. Pediatrics 72:857, 1983.
22. Miller M, Higginbottom M, Smith D: Short umbilical cord: its orgin and relevance. Pediatrics 67:618, 1981.
23. Boyd JD, Hamilton WJ: The human placenta. Cambridge, UK, 1970, W Heffer & Sons, p 209.
24. Cook V, Weeks J, Brown J, Bendon R: Umbilical artery occlusion and fetoplacental thromboembolism. Obstet Gynecol 85:870, 1995.
25. Bendon RW, Tyson RW, Baldwin VA, et al: Umbilical cord ulceration and intestinal atresia: a new association? Am J Obstet Gynecol 164:582, 1991.
26. Higginbottom M, Jones K, Hall B, Smith D: The amniotic band disruption complex: timing of amniotic rupture and variable spectra of consequent defects. J Pediatr 95:544, 1979.
27. Lockwood C, Ghidini A, Romero R, Hobbins J: Amniotic band syndrome: reevaluation of its pathogenesis. Am J Obstet Gynecol 160:1030, 1989.
28. Torpin R, Miller G, Culpepper B: Amniogenic fetal digital amputations associated with clubfoot. Obstet Gynecol 24:379, 1964.
29. Sander CH: The surgical pathologist examines the placenta. Pathol Annu 20:235, 1985.
30. Sander CM, Gilliland D, Flynn MA, Swart-Hills LA: Risk factors for recurrence of hemorrhagic endovasculitis of the placenta. Obstet Gynecol 89:569, 1997.
31. Knudsin RB, Driscoll SG, Pelletier PA: *Ureaplasma urealyticum* incriminated in perinatal morbidity and mortality. Science 213:474, 1981.
32. Wright J, Stinson D, Wade A, et al: Necrotizing funisitis associated with *Actinomyces meyeri* infection: a case report. Pediatr Pathol 14:927, 1994.

3

Normal Anatomy and Histology of the Placenta

Edwina J. Popek

Because many complications of the later stages of pregnancy have their origin in the first months of placental development, those early stages require evaluation. The embryo cannot develop without a placenta, and genomic imprinting is important in implantation, with paternally derived genes linked to placental proliferation and maternal genes necessary for the development of a fetus.[1] The complexity of implantation in the mammalian placenta is reviewed elsewhere.[2–5] The placenta has been said to "die" when the fetus is born, but the concept of a finite placental life span is controversial.[5] Most placental pathologists believe that age-related changes reflect maturation and not senescence, although a plateau of growth and maturation is reached during the later stages of gestation.[5–7]

The age of early pregnancy is often referred to by the fertilization or conceptional age, which is the time from union of sperm and egg which occurs a few days after ovulation to 55 or 56 days after ovulation and is also the period of embryogenesis. The menstrual age, estimated from the first day of the last menstrual period, is usually 14 days greater than ovulatory age, spans 10 to 40 weeks, and is the age most often used when referring to fetal and placental pathology. This difference between ovulatory and menstrual age can be confusing; dates in this chapter are postmenstrual unless specifically identified as postovulatory or postfertilization.

NORMAL PLACENTAL WEIGHTS AND MEASUREMENTS

Normal placental weights and measurements for specific gestational ages have been established in numerous studies. Table 3–1 is a compilation of many of these studies, which have similar findings.[5,8–13] In recent years studies of selected gestational ages have measured moderately different expected weights for both fetus and placenta, resulting in significantly different fetal/placental ratios.[14–17] These newer studies addressed some of the objections to the earlier studies, correcting for gestational age and eliminating small and large for gestational age fetuses. Despite these alterations, the figures from the older studies seem to have stood the test of time.[18] These standard weight measurements have also been made after removal of the umbilical cord and free membranes and after blood has been allowed to drain from the maternal intervillous space. At term the umbilical cord weighs approximately 1 g/cm and the membranes weigh approximately 50 g. Placental weight is affected by formalin fixation, with an increase in weight of 5% to 10%.[5,19,20] Twin placentas have been found to weigh 1.69 to 1.94 times the expected weight of a singleton for a given gestational age.[10,18] There is no significant difference between monochorionic and dichorionic placentas.[18]

The length of the umbilical cord has also been studied at various gestational ages and is shown in Table 3–1.[11,21,22] Incomplete umbilical cord tissue is commonly received in the pathology laboratory, frequently because portions have been retained for blood gas studies or are attached to the fetus. It is therefore important for the obstetrician to measure cord lengh in the delivery room.

IMPLANTATION

Implantation is the process by which the blastocyst adheres to and invades the receptive en-

Table 3–1. Fetal and Placental Weights and Measurements

Weeks' Gestation, Postmenstrual	Fetal Crown-Rump Length (cm)	Fetal Weight (g)	Placental Weight (g)	Placental Diameter (cm)	Placental Thickness (cm)	Fetal/ Placental Ratio	Cord Length (cm)*
8	1.4	1.7	5	3.0	0.75	0.34	7
10	4.0	5	14	5.0		0.36	10
12	6.0	14	26	6.0	1.20	0.65	6–13
14	8.7	45	42	6.5		0.71	16
16	12.0	110	65	7.5	1.60	0.90	15–19
18	14.0	200	90	8.0		1.67	23
20	16.0	320	123	9.0	2.00	2.60	22–32
22	19.0	460	150	10.0		3.10	36
24	21.0	630	182	12.5	2.40	3.40	28–40
26	23.2	820	210	13.5		3.90	43
28	25.2	1045	250	15.0	2.80	4.20	28–45
30	26.5	1323	285	16.0		4.60	48
32	28.0	1700	323	17.0	2.80	5.20	42–50
34	30.0	2100	362	18.0		5.80	53
36	32.0	2478	404	20.0	3.00	6.10	46–56
38	34.0	2900	443	21.0		6.50	57
40	36.0	3400	482	22.0	3.00	7.00	35–60
42	37.2	3513	487			7.20	61
>42	39.1	4077	738		5.84	5.50	

*Shorter cord lengths are from Boyd and Hamilton.[11]
Data from references 5, 8 to 13, 17, 18, 22, and 54.

dometrium. In humans implantation is interstitial, which means that the blastocyst is completely surrounded by maternal tissues. The human placenta is hemochorial; that is, the placental trophoblast comes into direct contact with the maternal blood. This results in extensive interdigitation of fetal and maternal tissues. Other types of placentation have been reviewed elsewhere.[5]

The fourth day after fertilization the multicell morula becomes a blastocyst with the formation of a central cavity. The outer cell layer will become the trophoblast, while the inner cell mass becomes the embryo and the extraembryonic tissue. At 6 to 8 days after fertilization the blastocyst is ready to implant. The human blastocyst normally implants in the body of the uterus, most frequently on the upper part of the posterior wall near the midsagittal plane. At this stage of incomplete implantation some degeneration of endometrial glandular epithelium and a slight infiltration of lymphocytes and macrophages are noted but rarely are neutrophils found. Cytotrophoblast can already be distinguished at this time at the periphery of the blastocyst forming the trophoblast shell.[4]

Days 8 to 12 after ovulation constitute the lacunar stage (Fig. 3–1*A*). The trophoblast farther away from the embryo differentiates into a peripherally located syncytium, while the cells closer to the embryo continue to proliferate as mononuclear cytotrophoblast. Lacunar spaces that appear in the trophoblast are initially filled with fluid derived from maternal glandular secretions but will perforate the outer syncytium and establish communication between the endometrial vessels and the lacunae by postovulatory day 11 or 12. At this time the ovum is situated in the upper portion of the endometrium, just beneath the surface epithelium. On the summit of the implantation site is a defect in the uterine epithelium that is closed by a fibrin clot (Fig. 3–1*A*). Interstitial implantation is complete around 12 days after ovulation, with the formation of the decidua capsularis, endometrial tissue that completely covers the blastocyst. There is mostly cytotrophoblast and very little syncytium on the uterine luminal side of the implantation site, while on the myometrial side of the implantation, extensive cytotrophoblast and syncytium formation has occurred.[4]

The embryo and placenta now consist of the embryonic disk, with a small attached amniotic cavity (Fig. 3–1*B*). The peripheral portion of the chorionic cavity contains a weblike arrangement of primitive tissue, referred to as trophoblast mesoblast. This gives origin to some of the defin-

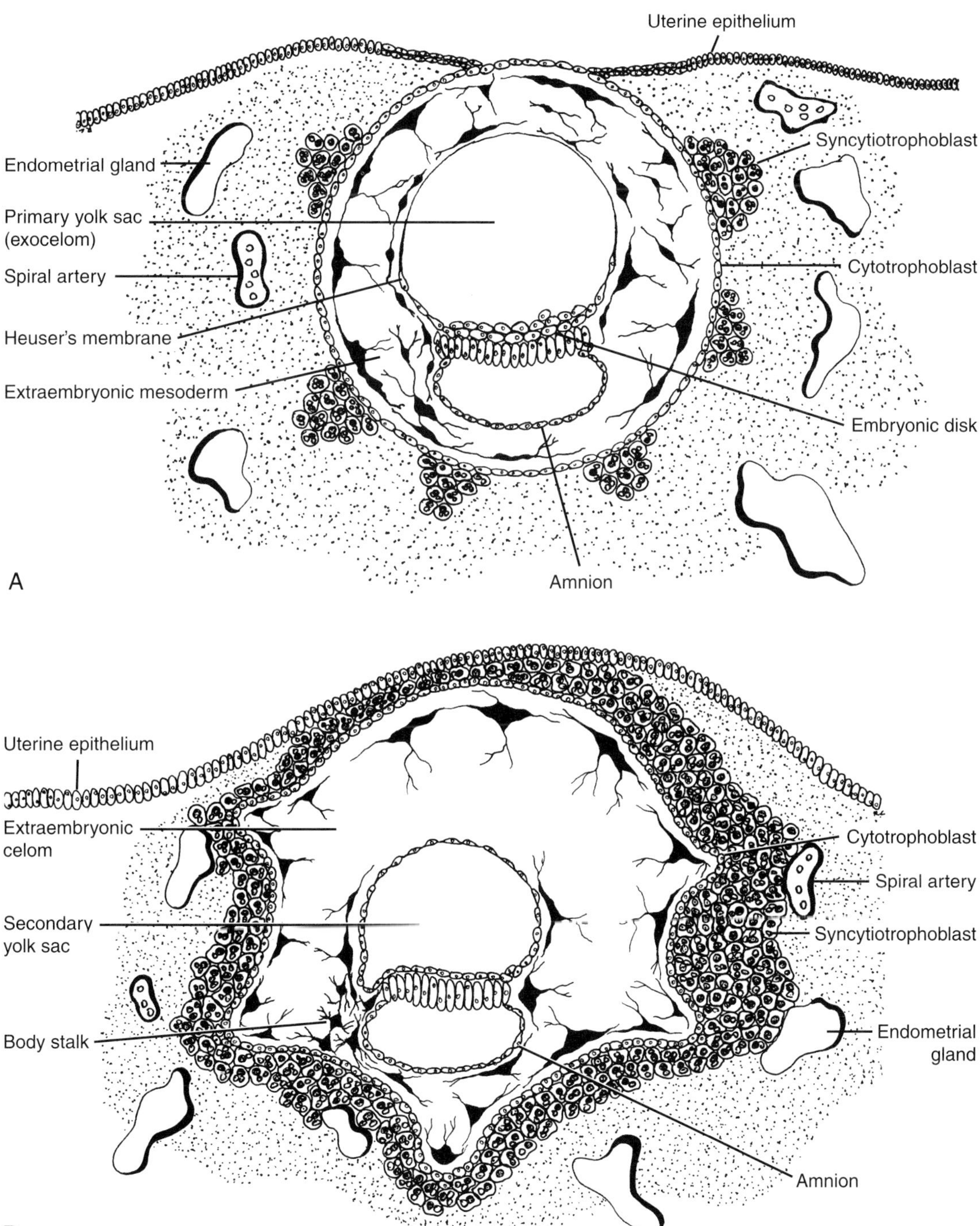

Figure 3–1. A, Interstitial implantation of the blastocyst 9 to 10 days after ovulation. **B,** Implantation is complete 12 days after ovulation with reepithelialization of the endometrium.

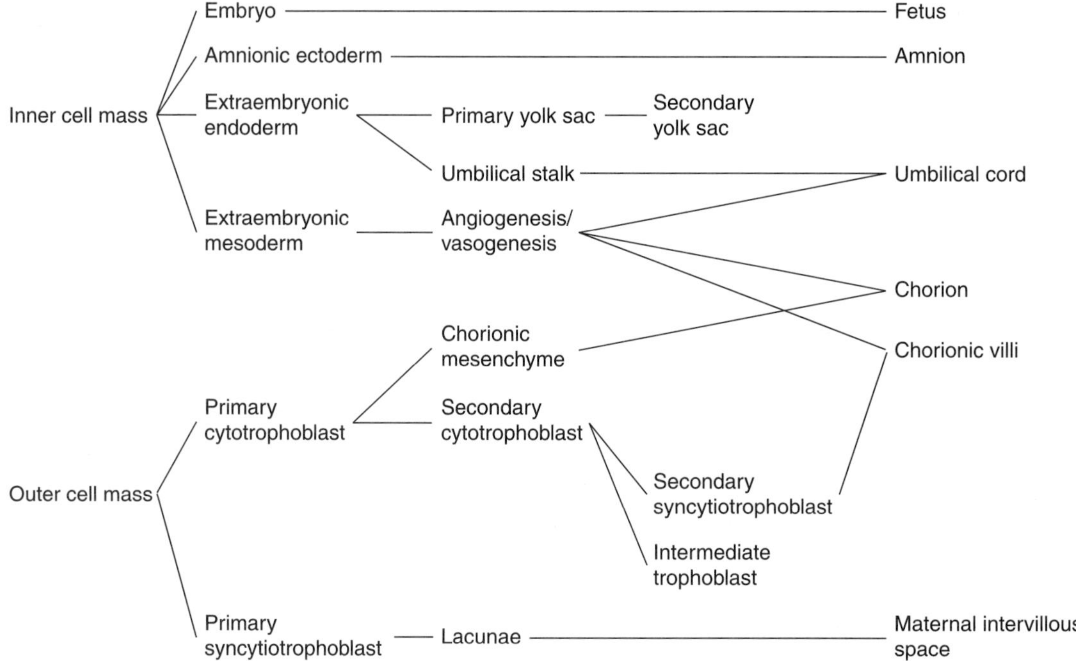

Figure 3–2. Diagrammatic representation of the origin of the various parts of the placenta from the inner and outer cell mass. The definitive structure is shown at the far right.

itive mesoderm and tissue of the chorion and villi. The space enclosed by the trophoblast mesoblast has been called the exocoelom or primary yolk sac. This structure should not be confused with the true or secondary yolk sac and the extraembryonic coelom, which is ultimately obliterated with fusion of the amnion and chorion. Development of the secondary yolk sac is discussed later in this chapter. The contributions from the various regions of the blastocyst to the fetus and placenta are shown in Figure 3–2.

In early pregnancy both cytotrophoblast and syncytiotrophoblast produce human chorionic gonadotropin (hCG), which later in pregnancy is produced only by the syncytiotrophoblast.[11] Serum hCG is measurable 12 to 24 hours after implantation, or 3 weeks after the last menstrual period, and peaks at 9 postmenstrual weeks. Levels of hCG double every 48 hours through 8 to 10 postmenstrual weeks and directly reflect the cytotrophoblast proliferation and differentiation into syncytium. If less than a 66% increase occurs in 48 hours, ectopic or nonviable pregnancy should be suspected. Serum hCG should become nondetectable by 6 to 8 weeks after evacuation of the uterine contents.

YOLK SAC

By postovulatory day 9 (Fig. 3–1*A*) a thin exocoelomic membrane (Heuser's membrane) extends around the blastocyst cavity enclosing a second cavity, the primitive yolk sac. The inner surface is a squamouslike endoderm, the outer is the cytotrophoblast shell, and an accumulation of primary mesodermal spindle cells is located between the primary yolk sac and trophoblast. The primary yolk sac degenerates by as yet an unknown mechanism that coincides with the formation of the secondary yolk sac.[23]

The secondary yolk sac lies between the amnion and chorion in the extraembryonic coelom, is connected to the embryo by a stalk containing blood vessels, and is present at the end of the fifth postmenstrual week during the previllous, postimplantation phase (Fig. 3–1*B*). How the secondary yolk sac develops is not clear, but it probably forms as follows: extraembryonic endodermal cells extend along the inside of the primitive yolk sac and then migrate medially to form the secondary yolk sac, as the primitive yolk sac degenerates.[23] Some refer to this structure as the umbilical vesicle, since in humans no yolk is involved.

The secondary yolk sac grows through the first 9 postmenstrual weeks, measuring 0.02 cm at 28 days, 0.5 cm at 9 postmenstrual weeks, and a maximum of 0.6 to 0.65 cm by the end of the tenth postmenstrual week. The early yolk sac does have a subtle yellow color and a transparent wall. It initially is located near the umbilical cord insertion, attached by a vascular stalk (Fig. 3–3*A*). The secondary yolk sac begins to degenerate at 9 to 10 postmenstrual weeks as the wall becomes cloudy.[23] By 12 weeks the secondary yolk sac can be seen as a flattened, yellow-white, calcified disk between the amnion and chorion, commonly near the placental margin or on the free membranes (Fig. 3–3*B*).

The yolk sac comprises three layers, an external mesothelial layer composed of a single layer of flattened cells, a vascular mesenchyme, and a thick endodermal layer facing the yolk sac cavity (Fig. 3–4*A*). The endoderm, which is the thickest layer, is α-fetoprotein positive and is where the red blood cells initially form. Large cells within this endoderm are considered to be the pluripotent cells.[24] Degeneration occurs by total necrosis and calcification or partial necrosis with fibrosis (Fig. 3–4*B*). An absent or small yolk sac is associated with spontaneous abortion.[25]

Biologic activity of the yolk sac is multifold. It possibly serves as a nutrient source and mediates transfer of nutrients and waste during the first 2 to 3 postovulatory weeks of embryogenesis. The fluid in the extraembryonic coelom is also probably a source of nutrients (vitamin B_{12} and folate) during the first trimester.[25] The yolk sac is the initial source of hematopoietic elements and primary germ cells.

Hematopoietic elements are mesenchymal in origin, initially forming in the secondary yolk sac

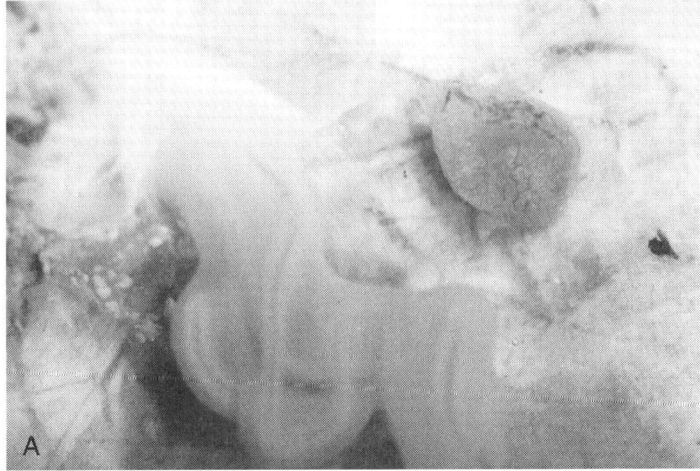

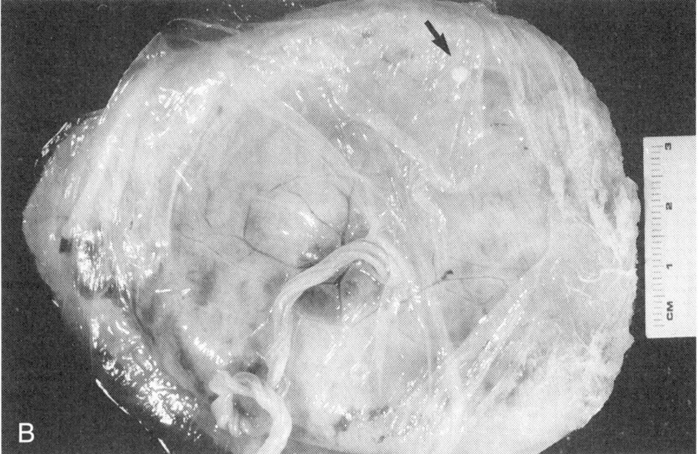

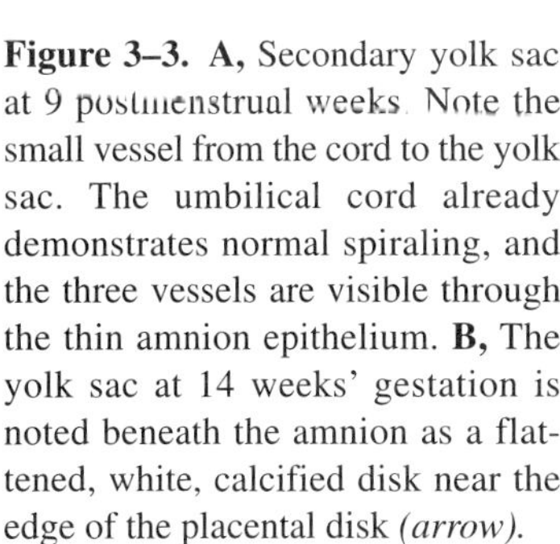

Figure 3–3. A, Secondary yolk sac at 9 postmenstrual weeks. Note the small vessel from the cord to the yolk sac. The umbilical cord already demonstrates normal spiraling, and the three vessels are visible through the thin amnion epithelium. **B,** The yolk sac at 14 weeks' gestation is noted beneath the amnion as a flattened, white, calcified disk near the edge of the placental disk *(arrow).*

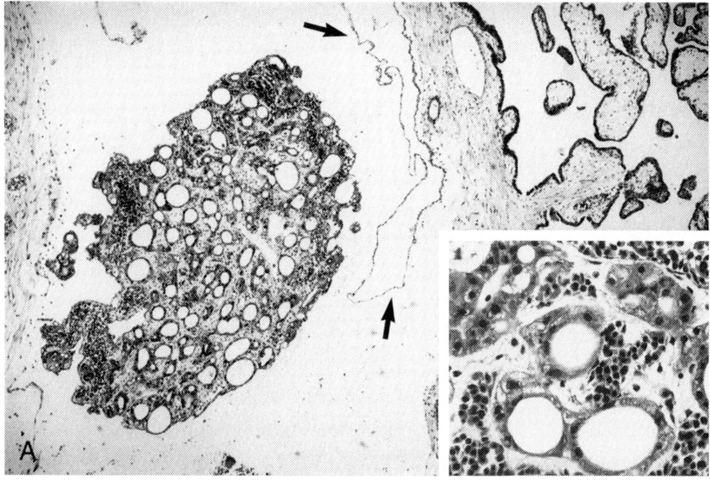

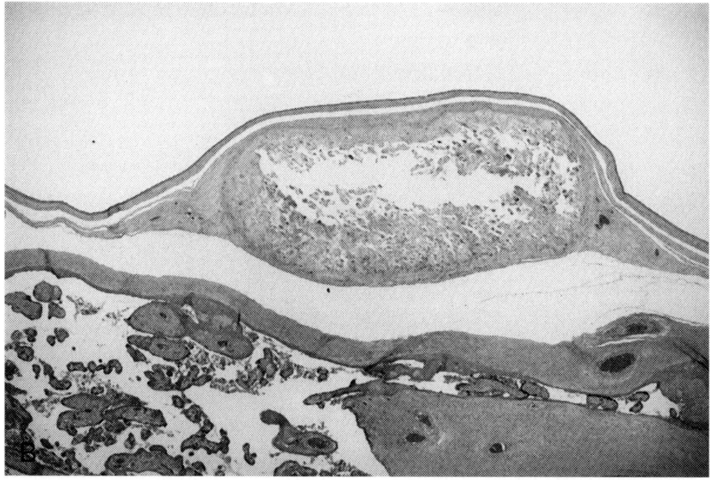

Figure 3–4. A, Early development of the placenta with the yolk sac (×4). Stem villi can be seen arising from the chorionic plate. The amnion is thin *(arrows),* almost a single cell thick, and is loosely associated with the chorion. The largest structure is the yolk sac, with its epithelium and vascular channels containing nucleated red blood cells. **B,** A calcified yolk sac from a term placenta is within the extraembryonic mesoderm of the amnion. Note that this remnant is similar in size to the earlier yolk sac, since both photographs are taken at ×4.

and in the chorionic plate vessels between 4 and 14 postmenstrual weeks until the fetal liver takes over at 8 to 18 postmenstrual weeks, ultimately to be replaced by the bone marrow at 16 postmenstrual weeks.[26] The hematopoietic elements include erythroid, granulated, megakaryocytic, and macrophages, which are found in the mesenchymal layer.[27] No lymphocytic, mononuclear, or granulocytic precursors are present.[28]

The yolk sac is the site of origin of primitive germ cells, which appear during the third postovulatory week in the posterior dorsal wall of the yolk sac near the allantois. They are large, have large nuclei and abundant pale cytoplasm, and are periodic acid–Schiff (PAS) and placental alkaline phosphatase positive. They migrate through the hindgut and mesentery into the genital ridge.

At the fourth postmenstrual week a part of the yolk sac becomes the primitive gut. The midgut is temporarily connected to the secondary yolk by the omphalomesenteric (vitelline) duct, which also contains a vitelline artery and vein. Occasionally these vitelline vessels are identified within the umbilical cord, near the amnion surface at its placental insertion, or on the chorionic plate itself. Remnants of the omphalomesenteric duct are also commonly seen near the cord surface. Other remnant structures are discussed in Chapter 5.

TROPHOBLAST

Trophoblast is used as a general term for the ectodermal covering of the conceptus and is the first epithelium. Initially referred to as trophectoderm, after implantation of the blastocyst it is called trophoblast.[29] Although there are several types of trophoblast, most investigators agree that they are all derived from the cytotrophoblast. Immunohistochemistry studies may be helpful in distinguishing the various types of placental trophoblast (Table 3–2).[30–34]

Cytotrophoblast

The villous cytotrophoblastic cells (Langhans' cells) are mononuclear with large nuclei, frequently with clumped chromatin and abundant pale, PAS-positive cytoplasm (Fig. 3–5*A*). They are frequently seen in mitosis during early gestation and stain with various proliferation markers.[31] During the latter half of pregnancy, rare cytotrophoblast mitoses can be seen. Cytotrophoblast forms an uninterrupted layer around the villus in the first trimester and is also found as a continuous layer at the chorionic plate and the chorion laeve. Cytotrophoblast covers only 50% of the villus circumference in the second trimester and 20% at term.[5] The cytotrophoblastic cells are frequently difficult to identify because they are flattened and often indistinguishable from other spindled stromal cells. Their location within the trophoblast basement membrane identifies them as cytotrophoblastic cells.

Ultrastructurally the cytotrophoblast is undifferentiated with few organelles and rare microvilli. Well-developed desmosomes join the lateral margins of adjacent cytotrophoblast as well as the overlying syncytiotrophoblast. A distinct reticular basement membrane separates the cytotrophoblast from the villous stroma. The cytotrophoblast in early gestation has abundant glycogen, which becomes less apparent as the placenta matures but does not completely disappear. Small amounts of lipid may be also seen. In the so-called postmature placenta, cytotrophoblastic cells are scarce and some show features of degeneration (vacuolation).[35,36] Prominence of the cytotrophoblast is considered a nonspecific indication of syncytiotrophoblast damage, possibly from ischemia, and is seen in preeclampsia, essential hypertension, preterm and prolonged pregnancy, diabetes mellitus, and Rh disease.[7] Whether this represents proliferation and hyperplasia or simply persistence of the cytotrophoblast is unclear.

Specialized forms of cytotrophoblast, cell columns, are seen at the tips of the anchoring villi at the end of 14 postovulatory days.[37] The cytotrophoblast of these cell columns is frequently polymorphic and enlarged (Fig. 3–5*B*). They have frequent mitoses and widespread persistence of large amounts of glycogen.

Cytotrophoblast of the chorion laeve divides maternal from fetal tissues and is residua from the uterine luminal portion of the cytotrophoblast shell. These cytotrophoblastic cells are frequently large and vacuolated and contain a large amount

Table 3–2. Immunohistochemistry Staining of Placental and Endometrial Components

	Keratin	EMA	hCG	HPL	PLAP	PCNA
Trimester	1 2 3	1 2 3	1 2 3	1 2 3	1 2 3	1 2 3
CT	4+ 4+ 4+	− − −	− − −	− − −	− − −	1+ 1+ 1+
ST	4+ 4+ 4+	− 1+ 1+	4+ 2+ 1+	2+ 3+ 4+	1+ 3+ 4+	− − −
IT	4+ 4+ 4+	1+ 3+ 2+	2+ 1+ −	3+ 3+ 3+	− 1+ 1+	1+ 1+ 1+
X cells	4+ 4+ 4+	− − −	1+ 1+ −	1+ 2+ 1+	1+ 3+ 3+	X + +
Amnion	4+ 4+ 4+	− 3+ 3+	− − −	− − −	± − −	X X X
Chorion	− − −	− − −	− − −	− − −	± − −	X X X
Villous stroma	− − −	− − −	− − −	− − −	− − −	± X −
Hofbauer cells	− − −	− − −	± − −	− − −	− − −	+ ± ±
Decidual stroma	− − −	− − ±	− − −	− − −	− − −	± − −
Endometrial glands	+ + +	+ + +	− − −	− − −	− − −	X X X

−, All cell negative; 1+, 1% to 24% cells positive; 2+, 25% to 49% cells positive; 3+, 50% to 74% cells positive; 4+, 75% to 100% cells positive; X, not reported; ±, not all specimens stained positive.

EMA, Epithelial membrane antigen; *hCG,* human chorionic gonadotropin; *HPL,* human placental lactogen; *PLAP,* placental alkaline phosphatase; *PCNA,* proliferating cell nuclear antigen; *CT,* cytotrophoblast; *ST,* syncytiotrophoblast; *IT,* intermediate trophoblast.

Data from references 5 and 30 to 34.

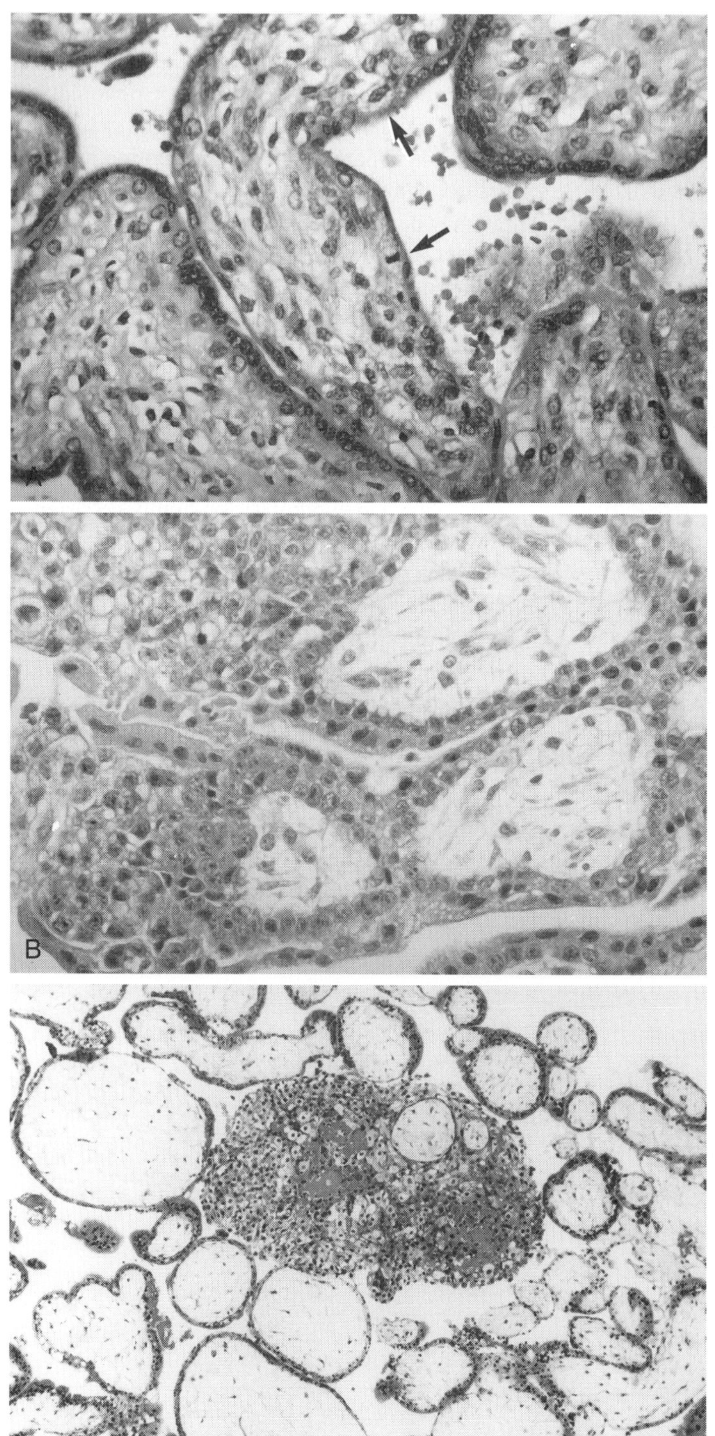

Figure 3–5. A, Cytotrophoblasts in the second trimester are plump with abundant clear cytoplasm and are occasionally seen in mitosis *(arrows)* (×40). **B,** Cytotrophoblast columns are only partially covered by syncytiotrophoblast, while the tips are composed of cytotrophoblast only. The vessels of these tertiary villi are inconspicuous in this photograph (×4). **C,** A cytotrophoblast island is a normal developmental structure composed of one or more villi surrounded by cytotrophoblast, syncytiotrophoblast, and intermediate trophoblast (×10). Such islands should not be mistaken for trophoblast proliferation of molar gestations.

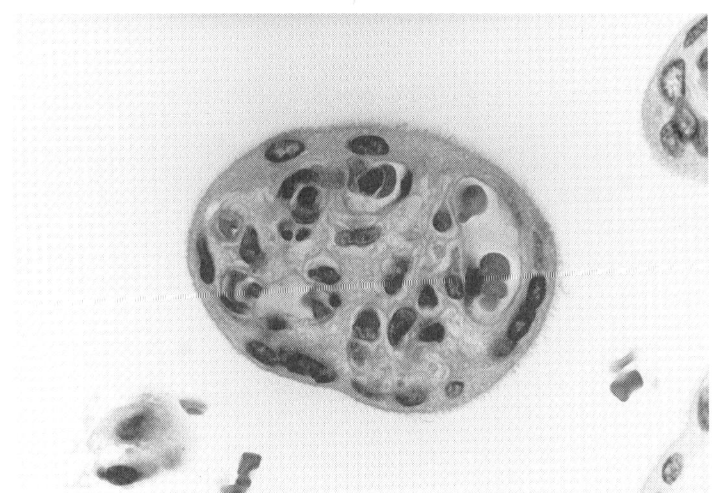

Figure 3–6. Syncytiotrophoblast near term with easily identified microvilli (×100).

of glycogen that persists throughout gestation. The chorion laeve is discussed in more detail later in this chapter.

Cytotrophoblast islands form at the tips of chorionic villi, especially in areas of poor blood supply (Fig. 3–5*C*). Seen initially late in the first month of gestation, they are most prominent during the third to sixth months but are also found in term placentas. Many are attached to anchoring villi or to placental septa and project into the maternal intervillous space. The islands are composed of cells of varying shape, frequently lack a syncytiotrophoblast covering, and measure approximately 1 mm in diameter.

Syncytiotrophoblast

The syncytiotrophoblast forms the outermost part of the trophoblast shell. It is also the outer covering of all villi, except the tips of the anchoring villi, and therefore acts as an endothelium within the intervillous space (Fig. 3–6). A specific basement membrane does not separate the syncytiotrophoblast from the cytotrophoblast. Syncytiotrophoblast initially have a large number of large, uniformly distributed, nuclei that tend to aggregate away from the intervillous space. Later in gestation the syncytiotrophoblast nuclei are smaller and irregularly shaped and have more evenly distributed chromatin. During the first trimester the syncytium is markedly vacuolated. These vacuoles may be so large as to distort the nucleus into crescentic shapes. Vacuolation becomes less pronounced with increasing gestation. The cytoplasm of the syncytium is more basophilic than that of the cytotrophoblast. The syncytiotrophoblast undergoes both apoptosis and necrosis. Apoptotic cells have margination and condensation of the nuclear chromatin and nuclear membrane blebbing, with loss of microvilli resulting in discontinuities of the syncytiotrophoblast surface.[38] Discontinuities begin to form in the syncytiotrophoblast layer at 9 to 12 postmenstrual weeks. Fibrin is deposited on the basement membrane, which is thought to permit reepithelialization of the denuded surface.[38] True necrosis of the syncytiotrophoblast is also seen adjacent to fibrin, with clumping of nuclear chromatin and swelling of cytoplasmic organelles. X cell proliferation may be present within these fibrinoid deposits.

The syncytiotrophoblast layer has a well-developed brush border of microvilli that can be seen even by light microscopy and are focally present throughout gestation (Fig. 3–6). Ultrastructurally there is a high concentration of endoplasmic reticulum suggesting protein or steroid synthesis, which is not surprising because syncytiotrophoblast produces the majority of hCG. Lysosomes are present and may contain storage product in some cases of inborn errors of metabolism.

The mechanism of formation of the syncytium has been controversial. The syncytiotrophoblast

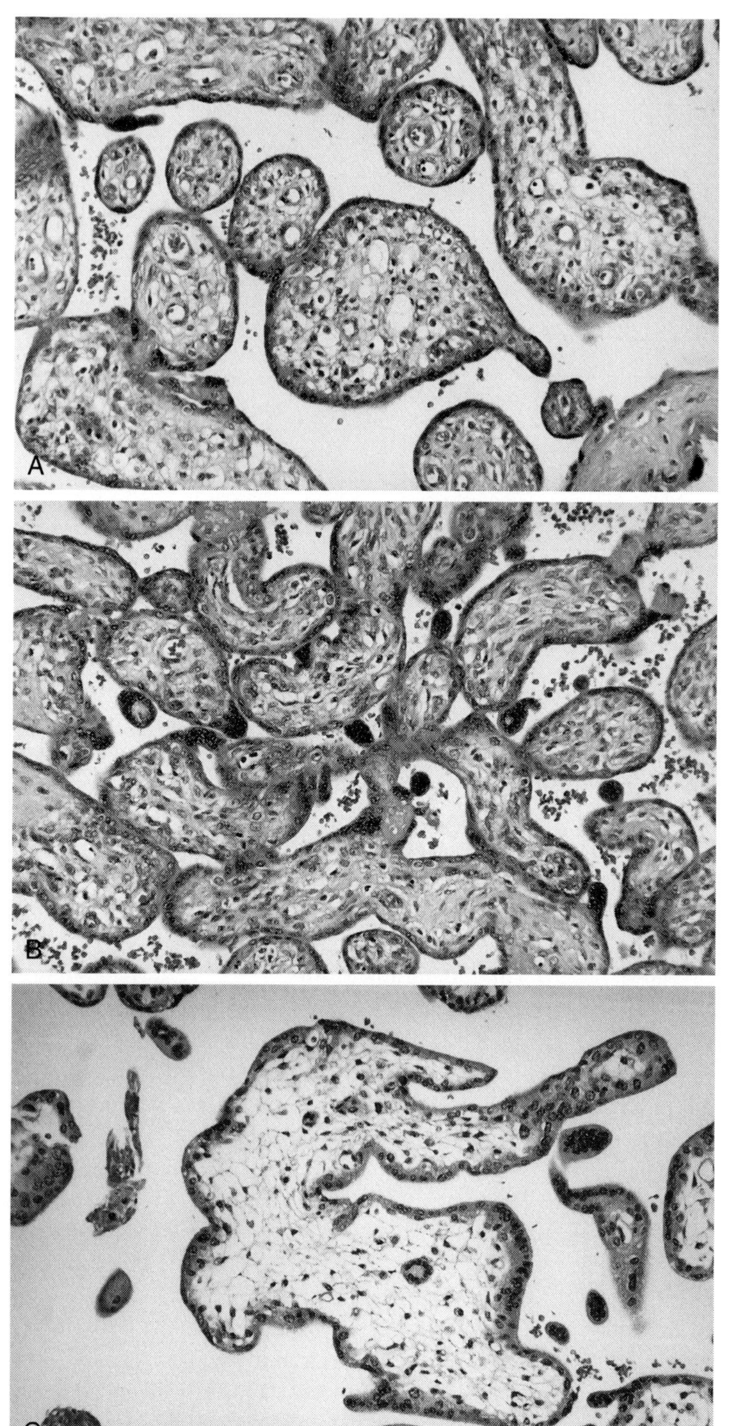

Figure 3–7. **A** and **B,** Second-trimester placenta with active villous production. **A,** A syncytiotrophoblast sprout with accompanying stroma will develop into another villus (×20). **B,** These syncytiotrophoblast sprouts, which are devoid of mesenchyme, are destined to become free floating within the intervillous space and maternal peripheral circulation (×20). **C,** Syncytiotrophoblast "buds," better known as trophoblast pseudoinclusions, are the result of sectioning of an irregular villus. This is a feature associated with chromosomal abnormalities (×20).

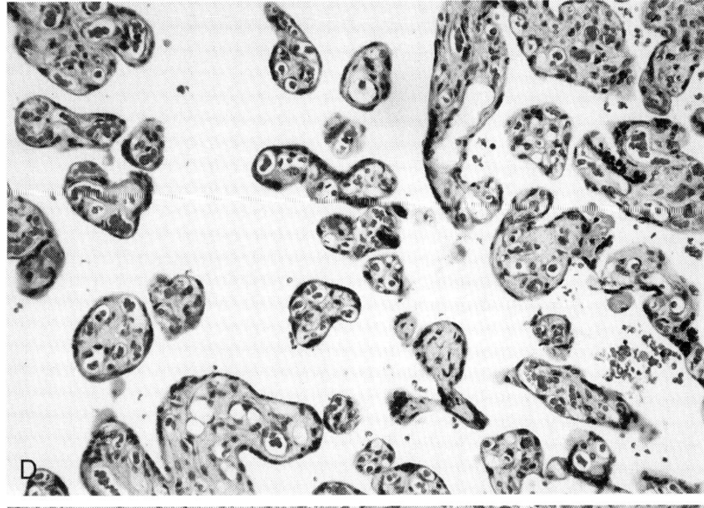

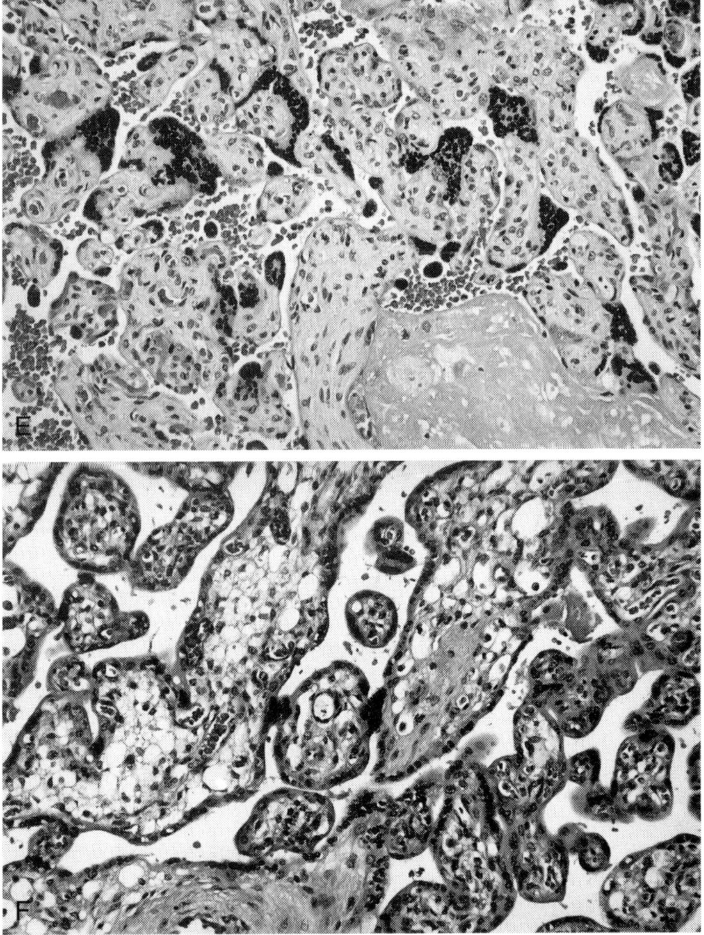

Figure 3–7 *Continued* **D,** Normal syncytial knots do not extend above the general outline of the villus (×20). **E,** In contrast, the exaggerated syncytial knots (Tenney-Parker sign) are composed of large numbers of very dense nuclei that extend well above the normal outline of the villus (×20). **F,** Syncytiotrophoblast bridges are shown connecting adjacent villi. They may provide internal structure of the mature placenta (×20).

arises from the progenitor cytotrophoblast. Syncytiotrophoblasts never show mitotic activity and only rarely stain positively with proliferating cell nuclear antigen (PCNA) in very early gestation. These cells stop proliferating, but DNA synthesis continues by endoreplication.[29] Most of the nuclei, however, are diploid. The presence of fragments of degenerated cell membranes within the cytoplasm supports the cell fusion theory with formation of a true syncytium.

A number of syncytiotrophoblast variants have been recognized. Recent scanning electron microscopic examination, however, suggests that many of these are only artifacts of sectioning.[39] Syncytial sprouts are surface elevations projecting into the intervillous space and attached to their parent villus by a constricted stalk. These sprouts may possess a central concentration of stroma and represent the initial phase of development of new villi (Fig. 3–7*A*). They eventually acquire cytotrophoblasts along with stroma of the villous stem. Vascularization of this core completes the process. Formation occurs throughout gestation but later produces more slender and delicate villi. Some sprouts never acquire a mesenchymal core, and the stalk of attachment becomes increasingly attenuated and eventually ruptures. This results in a freely floating syncytium in the intervillous space, which can be deported to the endometrial and myometrial veins and the maternal lungs throughout gestation (Fig. 3–7*B*).

Syncytial buds were originally described as projections of small masses of trophoblast into the villous stroma (Fig. 3–7*C*).[35,40] Another term that has been used is syncytial globules, but we now refer to these as trophoblastic pseudoinclusions and they are most pronounced early in gestation and in the stroma of chromosomally abnormal placentas, especially triploid, partial hydatidiform moles.

Syncytial knots are nuclear clumps whose formation and function have been reported as retrogressive, maturational, or functional. Syncytial knots are multilayered but extend only slightly above the villous contour (Fig. 3–7*D*). Their formation coincides with the formation of the vasculosyncytial membrane, which increases throughout the third trimester. Exaggerated knots, referred to as the Tenney-Parker sign, and are seen in so-called postmature placentas, preeclampsia, and ischemic areas such as the margins of infarcts (Fig. 3–7*E*).[41] Syncytial bridges are formed by the fusion of adjacent syncytial knots between villi and may act as an internal strut system to protect villous capillaries (Fig 3–7*F*).

Intermediate or Invasive Trophoblast

The intermediate trophoblast (considered by many as X cells[5]) based on light and electron microscopy and immunohistochemistry studies has intermediate differentiation between cytotrophoblast and syncytiotrophoblast.[34] Early in the first trimester, at the tips for cytotrophoblast columns the syncytiotrophoblast layer is penetrated by solid masses of intermediate trophoblast sprouting from the underlying cytotrophoblast. The mechanism of formation appears to be the stimulus of contact of the cytotrophoblast column with the maternal decidua.[2] Intermediate trophoblast is highly invasive into uterine epithelium, decidua, and the inner third of the myometrium (Fig. 3–8). Intermediate trophoblast also invades the maternal spiral arteries and is responsible for adapting them for pregnancy. The presence of intermediate trophoblast in the decidua is confirmation of an intrauterine pregnancy, even in the absence of chorionic villi.[42] Intermediate trophoblastic cells have larger nuclei and more abundant cytoplasm than decidual cells, but special stains may be necessary for definitive identification (Table 3–2). The intermediate trophoblast also expresses a nonclassic major histocompatibility antigen, HLA-G, which is trophoblast specific and prevents destruction by natural killer cells.[43,44]

Intermediate trophoblastic cells in the decidua are initially mononucleated but progressively become multinucleated through the first 6 months of gestation. Multinucleated trophoblasts are seen in the maternal decidua basalis and adjacent myometrium and are infrequently found in the decidua away from the implantation site (Fig. 3–8). They are often enmeshed in Rohr's and Nitabuch's fibrinoid and may be related to sclerosed and avascular anchoring villi of the decidua basalis. These multinucleated intermediate trophoblastic cells appear to have lost the ability to invade maternal arteries or veins. The immunohistochemistry staining characteristics of these cells are more similar to intermediate trophoblast than syncytiotrophoblast.[34]

Figure 3–8. Large numbers of intermediate trophoblastic cells from this anchoring villus are still visible within the maternal decidua (×4). The inset shows that most are mononucleated but some of those distant from the villus are multinucleated (×20).

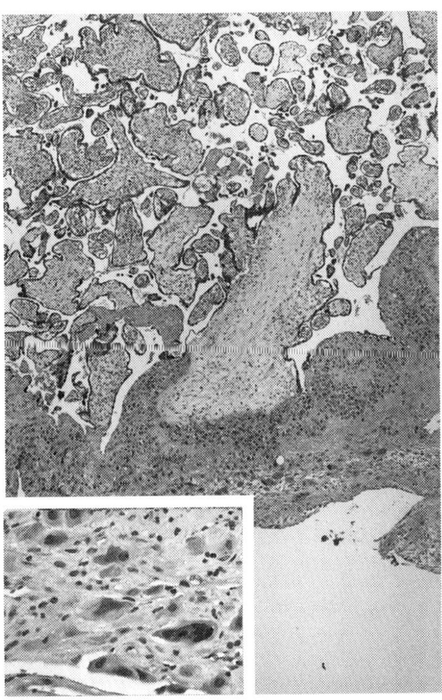

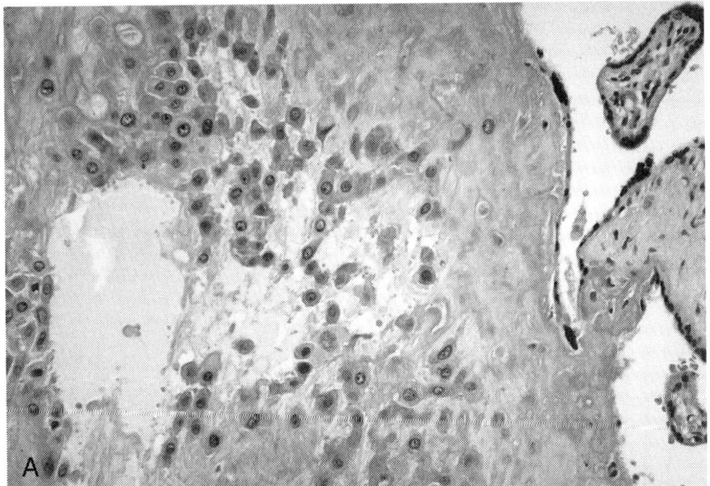

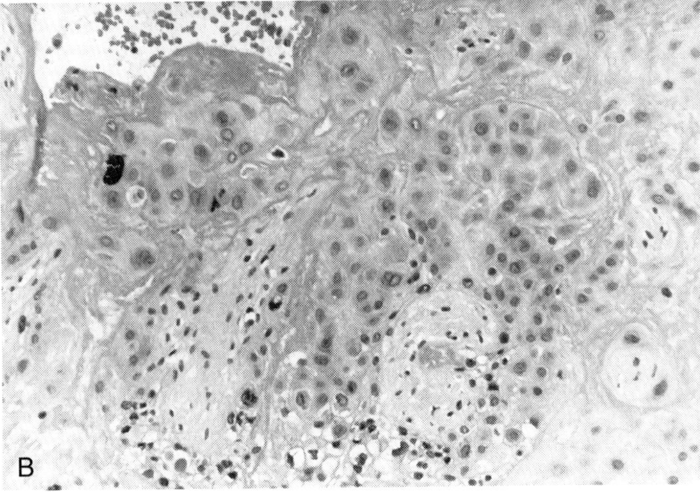

Figure 3–9. A, Septal cyst lined by X cells containing amorphous, homogeneous, rarely granular or hemorrhagic material (×20). **B,** Perivillous fibrinoid within which are numerous X cells (×20). Note the presence of avascular, atrophic but not necrotic villi at the center of the proliferation.

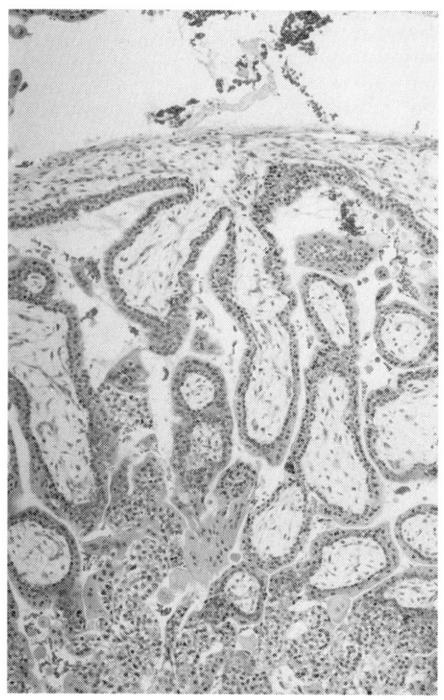

Figure 3–10. Tertiary villi with loose stroma and few blood vessels. At the periphery are almost solid nests of cytotrophoblast, which form the inner layer of the trophoblast shell (×10).

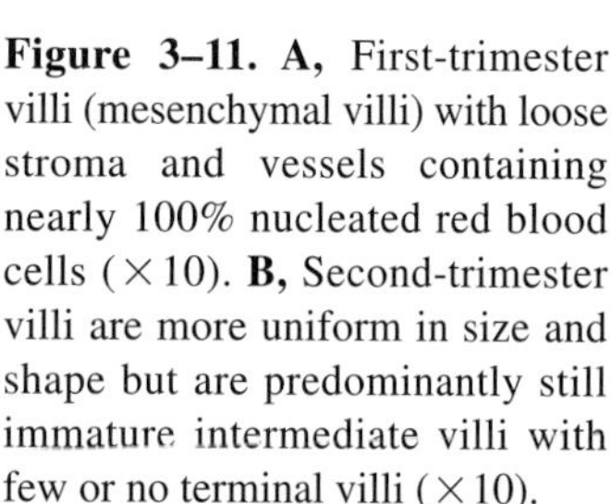

Figure 3–11. A, First-trimester villi (mesenchymal villi) with loose stroma and vessels containing nearly 100% nucleated red blood cells (×10). **B,** Second-trimester villi are more uniform in size and shape but are predominantly still immature intermediate villi with few or no terminal villi (×10).

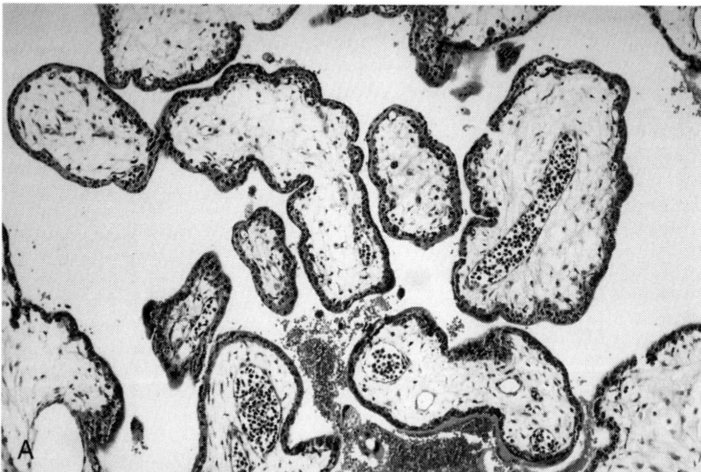

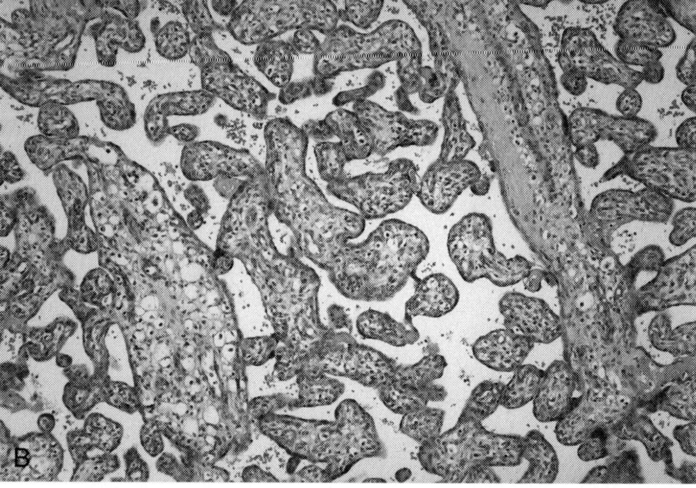

Extravillous Trophoblast

Extravillous intermediate trophoblastic or X cells are part of the placental septa, where they are found in solid nests or line cystlike spaces that may contain amorphous material (Fig. 3–9*A*). X cells are also located in areas of perivillous fibrinoid, where they may be an indicator of remote syncytiotrophoblast injury (Fig. 3–9*B*). X cells have large vesicular nuclei and abundant cytoplasm. Extravillous trophoblastic cells stain immunohistochemically like intermediate trophoblastic cells and are proliferative as demonstrated by stains for proliferation, such as PCNA.

The terminology pertaining to intermediate and extravillous trophoblast is nearly unparalleled in its nonuniform usage among various authors. For a comprehensive review of this topic the reader is referred to a more in-depth discussion.[5]

VILLI

Villous development has been thoroughly addressed elsewhere.[5] Primary villi are cytotrophoblast cores covered by syncytiotrophoblast that form late in the third postmenstrual week. Primary chorionic villi divide the chorion into radially oriented trabeculae that eventually fuse at the periphery of the implantation site to form the cytotrophoblast shell, becoming the first anchoring villi. Secondary villi are formed with the production of mesenchymal cores from the extraembryonic mesoderm during the fourth postmenstrual

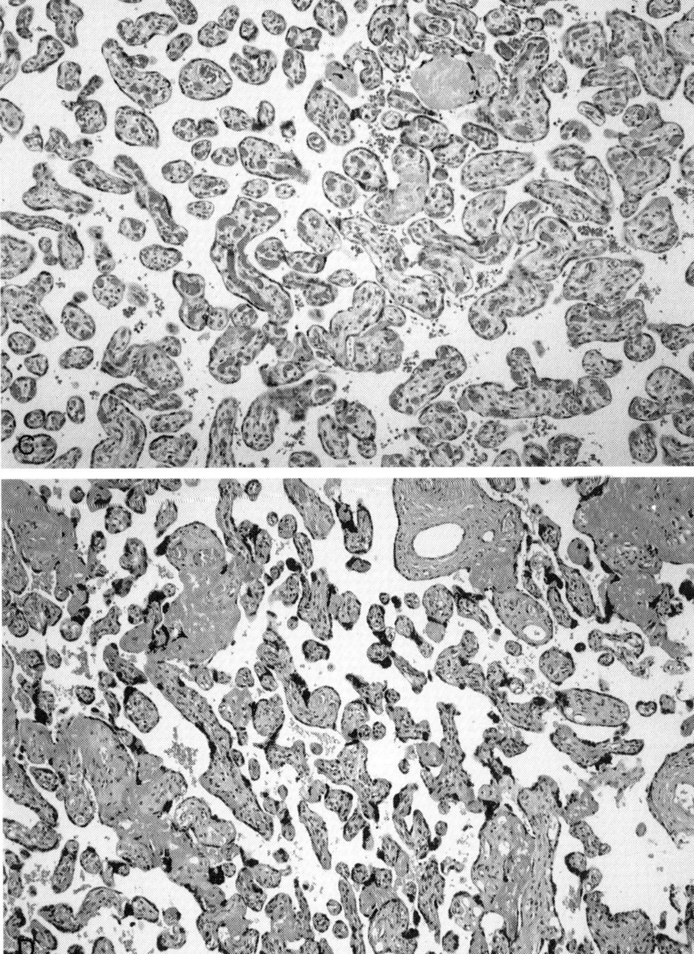

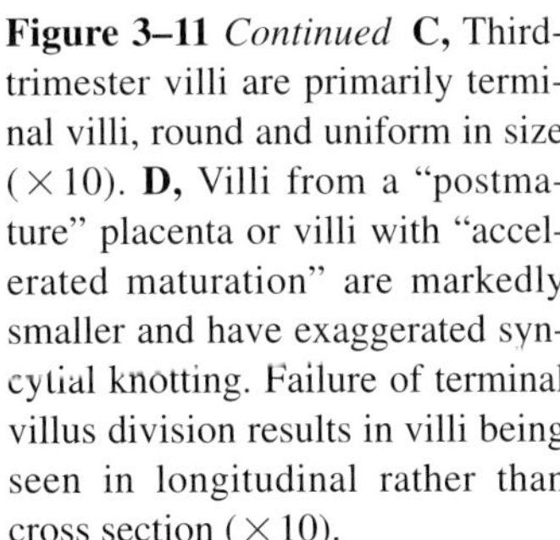

Figure 3–11 *Continued* **C,** Third-trimester villi are primarily terminal villi, round and uniform in size (×10). **D,** Villi from a "postmature" placenta or villi with "accelerated maturation" are markedly smaller and have exaggerated syncytial knotting. Failure of terminal villus division results in villi being seen in longitudinal rather than cross section (×10).

week. By the end of the fifth postmenstrual week, tertiary villi are formed with the appearance of embryonic blood vessels (Fig. 3–10).[11,14,45] Further villous development includes the formation of mesenchymal, stem, immature intermediate, mature intermediate, and terminal villi that represent the various levels of branching of the mature vascularized villous system. During normal development all forms of villi decrease in diameter except stem villi, which increase in diameter. The mean villous diameter is 200 μm in the first trimester because of the large variation in size and shape among immature villous types (Fig. 3–11*A*).[5,46] Terminal villous diameter is 70 μm during the second trimester (Fig. 3–11*B*) and 40 μm in the third trimester (Fig. 3–11*C*). The so-called postmature villus or villi with accelerated maturation may be considerably smaller (Fig. 3–11*D*).

During the third postmenstrual week, anchoring villi arise from the cytotrophoblast columns. They have tips formed of solid columns of cytotrophoblast that do not have a peripheral layer of syncytiotrophoblast (Fig. 3–10). The tips of the anchoring villi never acquire mesenchyme or fetal circulation. This is probably designed so that the fetal circulation will not come into direct contact with the maternal circulation or decidua. Anchoring villi may be identified at the basal plate even at term, although they are often embedded in fibrinoid and sometimes are associated with chronic inflammation (Fig. 3–8).

Mesenchymal villi are the most primitive and

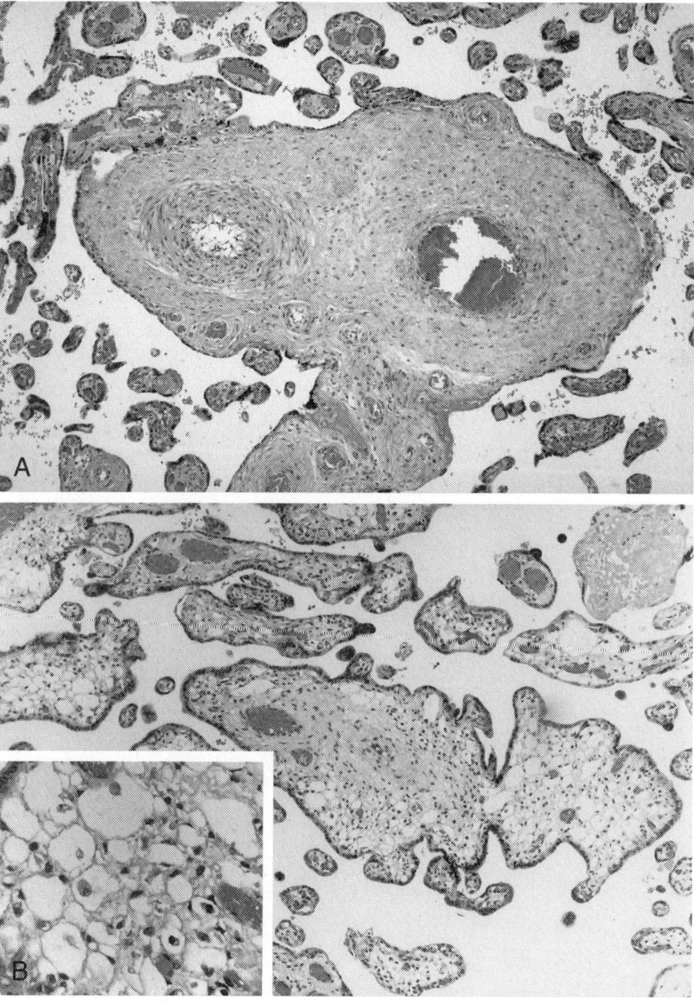

Figure 3–12. A, Intermediate-size stem villus with easily discernible artery and vein, each with muscular media and connective tissue adventitia. Smaller vessels at the periphery are similar to vasa vasorum and become more prominent in cases of obliteration of the stem vessels (×10). **B,** Immature intermediate villus with large abundant loose mesenchyme (×10). *Inset,* The prominent stromal channels, many of which contain Hofbauer cells (×20).

are present from 6 to 40 postmenstrual weeks. They form as the tertiary villi elongate and develop a loose mesenchyme with centrally placed, nondilated fetal capillaries (Fig. 3–11*A*).[5] Mesenchymal villi may develop along one of two routes. The larger mesenchymal villi form fibrous connective tissue surrounding the fetal vessels and are then called stem villi, and others become intermediate villi.

Stem villi range from 80 to 3000 μm in diameter, progressively increasing in size throughout gestation.[5] They have one to several large muscular vessels surrounded by a condensed fibrous adventitia that contains superficially located paravascular capillaries, similar to vasa vasorum. Within normal stem villi both arteries and veins are usually present. Early in gestation the stem villus is covered by a continuous trophoblast covering that at term is nearly totally replaced by fibrinoid (Fig. 3–12*A*). Anchoring villi are a form of primitive stem villus that branches numerous times, becoming progressively smaller.

Immature intermediate villi can be initially identified around the eighth postmenstrual week and persist in large numbers until the end of the second trimester (Fig. 3–12*B*). Even at term, immature intermediate villi can be seen in small clusters, often around a central cavity (Fig. 3–12*C*). Their large size, poor vascularity, and decreased stromal cellularity with sparse collagen often make them appear prominent and bulbous. The villous stroma contains reticulin and fibroblasts

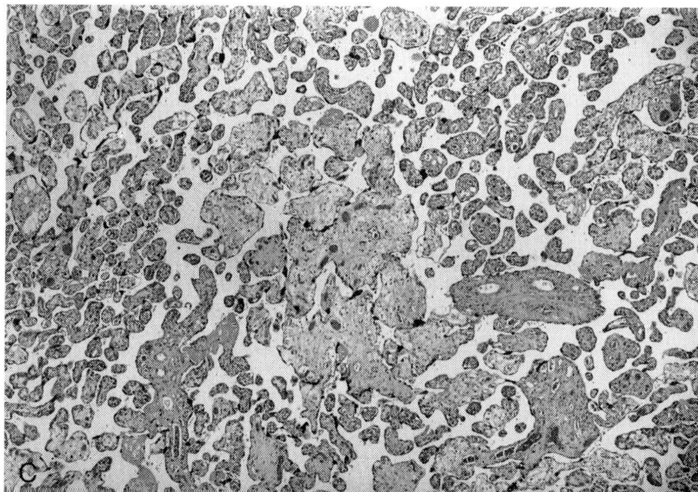

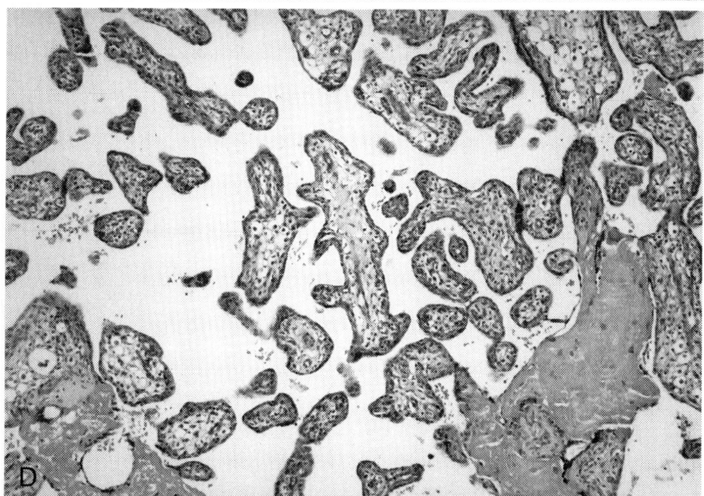

Figure 3–12 *Continued* **C,** A cluster of immature intermediate villi in an otherwise normal term placenta is an indication of continued villous production (× 10). **D,** Mature intermediate villus with prominent branching into terminal villi (× 10).

that form villous stromal channels. Hofbauer cells are prominent within the stromal channels, which may result in the mistaken impression that these villi are edematous. The fetal vessels do not have muscular walls, and arteries are difficult to distinguish from veins.

At the beginning of the third trimester some mesenchymal villi are transformed into mature intermediate villi. Mature intermediate villi measure 60 to 150 μm and are usually seen in longitudinal section. They have stroma composed of loose bundles of connective tissue and are poorly vascularized (Fig. 3–12*D*).

Terminal villi are the functional unit of the placenta. Initially forming at 21 to 24 weeks' gestation, they become the predominate villous structure at 33 to 36 weeks' gestation. They branch from mature intermediate villi, organized somewhat like clusters of grapes (Fig. 3–21).[37] Terminal villi have loose stroma and are well vascularized. Each terminal villus has two to six sinusoidally dilated and coiled capillaries (Fig. 3–11*B* and *C*).

Vasculosyncytial membranes (VSMs), also referred to as epithelial plates, begin forming at 18 to 20 weeks' gestation and are complete by 28 weeks. They increase in size only slightly until 37 weeks' gestation. The percentage of villous surface occupied by the VSMs varies from none at 12 weeks' gestation to 8% at 24 weeks and 24% at 28 to 40 weeks according to Stoz[46] or 11% to 30% at term according to Fox.[7] The VSM constitutes the effective metabolic barrier between the fetal and maternal circulations. The VSM is composed of syncytiotrophoblast cytoplasm, trophoblast basement membrane, stromal connective tissue, vascular basement membrane, and capillary endothelium. Formation of the VSM is also enhanced by the discontinuous layer of cytotrophoblast after the first trimester and the nonnucleated stretches of syncytial cytoplasm that result from clumping of the syncytial nuclei into the syncytial knots. The VSM becomes progressively thinner, measuring 1 to 3 μm at term. The capillary basement membrane and trophoblast basement membrane may come into such close proximity that they fuse (Fig. 3–13).[5]

The terminal villus has reached its final size and degree of differentiation by 28 weeks' gestation according to Stoz[46] or much later (36 weeks) according to Teasdale.[6] The total surface area of the placenta increases after 28 weeks' gestation by continued production of terminal villi, which reach a maximum number of 33,625 cm^2 at 36 weeks' gestation.[6,47] Villous maturation also involves a growth in number and relative volume of capillaries, which increases from 2.7% at 8 weeks' gestation to 4% at 12 weeks, 9% at 28 weeks, and 40% at 37 to 40 weeks.[5,46] Biochemical analysis of the placenta suggests a cellular growth phase, lasting until 36 weeks' gestation, that is followed by a hypertrophic phase continuing until term.[48] The increased placental weight noted from 36 weeks to term is due primarily to increased nonvillous connective tissue.[6]

Maturation of villi may be affected by their location within the placenta.[7] Villi near the chorionic plate and those at the margin of the placenta are smaller, with more collagenous stroma, thicker

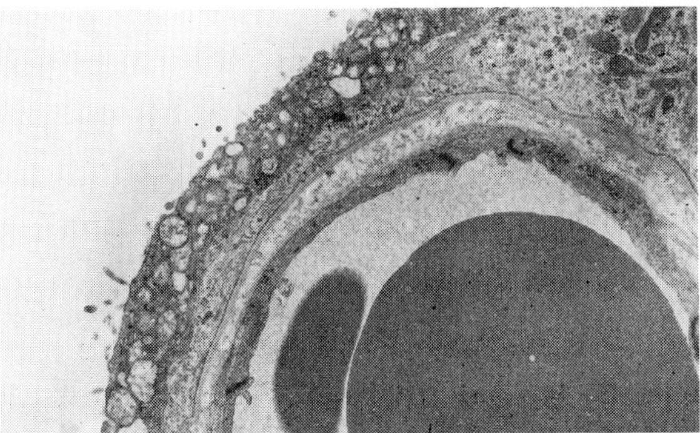

Figure 3–13. Electron microscopic study of a term villus showing the vasculosyncytial membrane formed by the thinned, anucleate syncytiotrophoblast cytoplasm, the cytotrophoblast cytoplasm, trophoblast basement membrane, a small amount of extracellular substance, and the capillary endothelium.

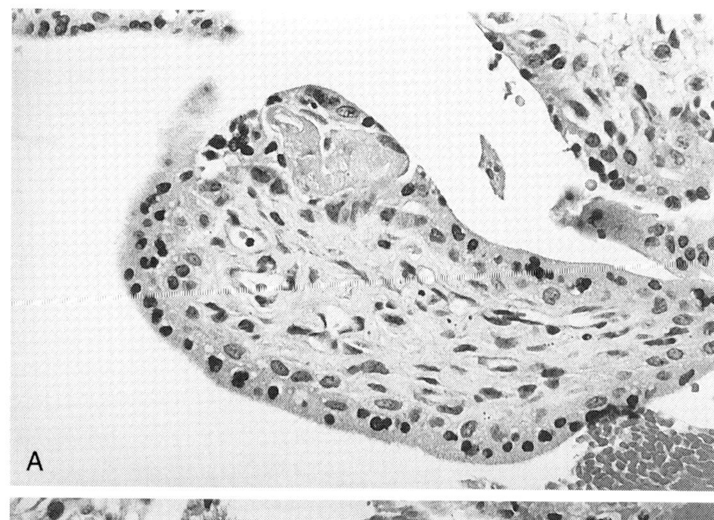

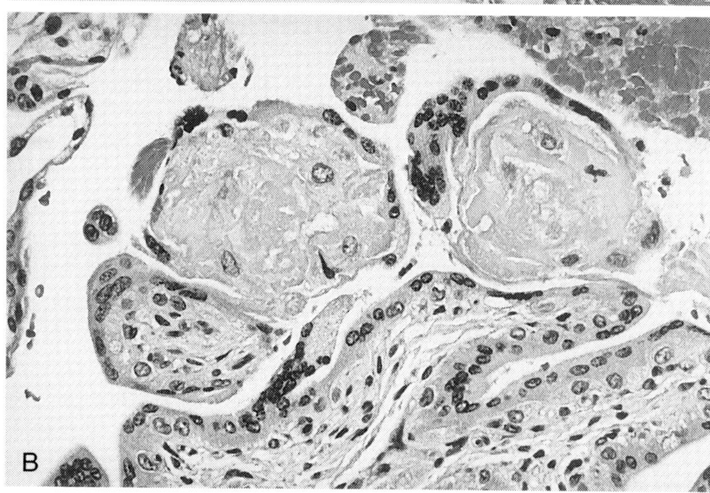

Figure 3–14. A, Fibrinoid necrosis of a villus begins with deposition of periodic acid–Schiff–positive material between the syncytiotrophoblast and cytotrophoblast (×40). The trophoblast basement membrane is intact. **B,** The mature lesion results in complete replacement of the villous stroma, while the villus is still covered by syncytiotrophoblast (×40).

trophoblast basement membranes, fewer vasculosyncytial membranes, and increased amounts of cytotrophoblast. These areas also have a tendency for increased perivillous fibrinoid, probably because of previous ischemic injury to syncytiotrophoblast. Care must be used in interpreting the maturation of the villi from sections of uncertain location. A more subtle effect may be noted with each lobule of the placenta. The question of "postmature" or accelerated maturation is controversial (Fig. 3–11*D*). The margins of the placenta and the periphery of infarcts frequently have some of these "ischemic" changes.

Villous fibrinoid necrosis (intravillous fibrinoid) results from degenerative changes in the cytotrophoblast of the villi thought to be an immunologic reaction, not merely the result of aging or villous ischemia, and similar to senile amyloid.[5,49] Fibrinoid necrosis begins external to the trophoblast basement membrane, between the cytotrophoblast and syncytiotrophoblast (Fig. 3–14*A*). The amorphous, PAS-positive material expands inward and gradually involves the entire villus (Fig. 3–14*B*). The syncytiotrophoblast covering is initially normal but slowly degenerates and later disappears. The fibrinoid then comes in direct contact with maternal blood. At term, fibrinoid necrosis in 3% of villi is considered normal.[50] Increased amounts in placentas may be seen in cases of maternal diabetes mellitus, Rh alloimmunization, pregnancy-induced hypertension, and premature onset of labor.

VILLOUS STROMA

The villous stroma first appears as a loose mesenchyme, derived from extraembryonic mesoderm during formation of secondary villi. It develops into connective tissue, the density of which depends on the age and the degree of differentiation of the particular type of villus investigated. Besides the blood vessels, the villous stroma has only two major components, fibroblasts and Hofbauer cells.

Fibroblasts are elongated and produce reticulin and collagen that are seen initially around the blood vessels. No elastic fibers have been identified within the villous stroma, although some have found elastin in the arterioles. Smooth muscle is a component of the blood vessels within stem villi only and is not found within the stroma. These mesenchymal-derived stromal components stain with vimentin, actin, and desmin.[5,51]

HOFBAUER CELLS

Hofbauer cells are special phagocytic cells of mesenchymal origin, found in the stroma of human villi, chorion, and amnion. They are present in the villi from the fourth postovulatory week, before the development of bone marrow. Hofbauer cells maintain their ability to undergo mitosis and self-replicate, a property that bone marrow–derived macrophages do not possess. Hofbauer cells are round or oval, are rarely irregular, and may show cytoplasmic projections. The nucleus is round or rarely crescentric and may be eccentric (Fig. 3–15). The cytoplasm is vacuolated, abundant, and eosinophilic. The vacuoles may contain lipid and PAS-positive, diastase-resistant material. Hofbauer cells are phagocytic, but less so than bone marrow–derived macrophages. The Hofbauer cell population is relatively constant throughout gestation, comprising about 40% of the stromal cells.[52] These cells are more easily seen in premature placentas, since they become more spindled and fibroblast like later in gestation, possibly because of compression by villous stroma. Hofbauer cells have cytoplasmic lysosomes and are therefore a target for storage product in some inborn errors of metabolism. Immunohistochemistry shows expression of T4 cell (CD4), leukocyte common antigen (CD26), KP-1 (CD68), and CD1a.[5,51] Hofbauer cells express some class II major histocompatibility complex determinants in the first trimester. Expression becomes stronger in the third trimester. This may suggest progressive functional maturation of the Hofbauer cell as regards cell adhesion and antigen presentation capacity. Villous stroma contains a sprinkling of mast cells; their function is uncertain, but they probably help to prevent intervillous thrombosis.

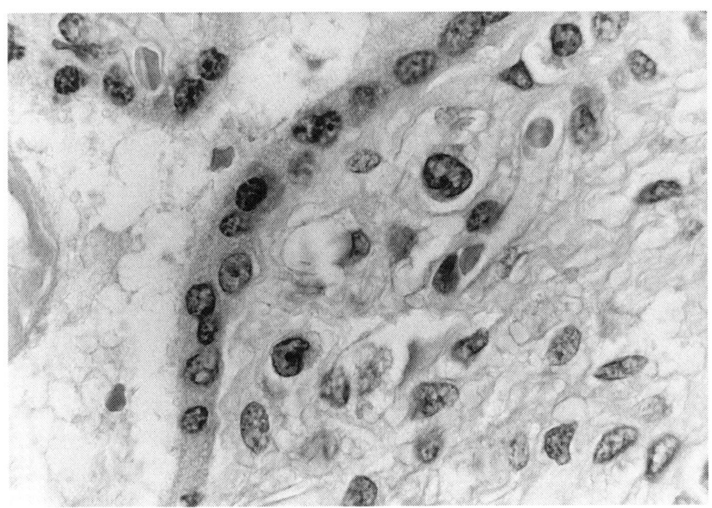

Figure 3–15. Hofbauer cell may resemble spindle cells or may appear more like macrophages, as they do here *(arrows)* (×100).

FETAL BLOOD VESSELS

UMBILICAL CORD

The umbilical stalk connects the embryo to the cytotrophoblastic shell. It is composed of the allantoic diverticulum, omphalomesenteric duct, and umbilical vessels and is sheathed by amnion. This stalk becomes the umbilical cord by the seventh postmenstrual week. The umbilicus, the skin-covered portion of the cord on the fetal abdomen, varies in length from about 1 to 3 cm. The omphalus or funis is the amnion-covered portion of the cord.

The umbilical cord varies considerably in length (Table 3–1).[11,21] The cord of female infants is on average 1.5 cm shorter than that of males.[53] The cord from a vertex delivery is approximately 4.5 cm longer than the cord from a breech delivery.[53] The umbilical cords of twins are approximately 10 cm shorter than those of singletons, probably related to decreased room for fetal movement.[21] Cord length does not increase much after 28 weeks' gestation, also probably because of decreased space within the amniotic cavity.[54]

The cord insertion onto the placental surface is a strong one, supported by sizeable amounts of connective tissue surrounding large muscular vessels and extending onto the chorionic plate for a short distance. This is probably a protective mechanism against cord avulsion. Most cords are inserted centrally (3% to 28%) or nearly centrally (62% to 91%).[5,11] Abnormal primary implantation (the polarity theory of the embryonic pole of the blastocyst) and trophism (placental wandering) may be responsible for some abnormal insertions.[5] During the early formation of the umbilical cord the embryo must rotate so that the umbilical stalk is toward the chorionic plate. If this rotation does not occur, the cord will seek its insertion on the chorion laeve, which will become the free membranes. Placental trophism is supported by ultrasound evidence of eccentric expansion of the placenta during gestation and the high percentage of abnormal cord insertions in twin gestations. Marginal insertion occurs in 5% to 20%, and velamentous or membranous insertion in only 0.5% to 1%.[5] The higher numbers are seen in stillbirths and multiple gestations.[5]

Spiraling of the umbilical cord is well established by the ninth postmenstrual week (Fig. 3–3*A*). Rather than a spiral, the form is actually a cylindric helix, with each vessel equidistant from a central axis and each spiral uniform in curvature. The spiraling is leftward (counterclockwise) in 83% and rightward (clockwise) in 12%; 5% have no spiraling.[54] "The spirality of an umbilical cord is the same, whether it be oriented with respect to the fetal or placental end or whether it be regarded as an independent object."[22] The number of cord spirals at term averages up to 40 with a maximum of 380.[55] Absent, decreased, or increased spiraling of the cord is currently thought to increase the risk of cord compression.[55]

In 99% of cords one vein and two arteries are present. Initially there are two arteries and two veins, but the right umbilical vein regresses at about 10 postmenstrual weeks. The caliber of the umbilical vessels increases from the fetal to the placental end. Anastomosis between the umbilical arteries (Hyrtl anastomosis) near their insertion onto the placental surface occurs in the majority of cords and is believed to indicate advanced development.[5]

The umbilical arteries are usually half the diameter of the vein because contraction of the umbilical artery results in the formation of "cushions" on the internal lumen (Fig. 3–16*A*). Plump endothelium often projects into the vascular lumen. In contrast to all other large muscle arteries, the umbilical artery does not have an internal elastin lamina, but does have delicate elastin fibers within the muscular wall, which has 50 to 60 layers of smooth muscle. The inner third are longitudinally oriented, but the outer layers have variable orientation (Fig. 3–16*B*).[56]

The umbilical vein has a thinner muscular wall, only 30 to 40 layers thick. The inner layer is discontinuous and longitudinally oriented, while the outer layers have variable orientation (Fig. 3–17*A*).[56] The vein has a well-developed internal elastic lamina that is usually single but may have up to four layers (Fig. 3–17*B*). No adventitia or vasa vasorum are associated with the umbilical vessels.

The umbilical cord stroma is derived from embryonic mesenchyme. Stellate cells within the cord stroma are myofibroblasts, with more myocyte differentiation near the vessels and more fibroblastic differentiation near the basement mem-

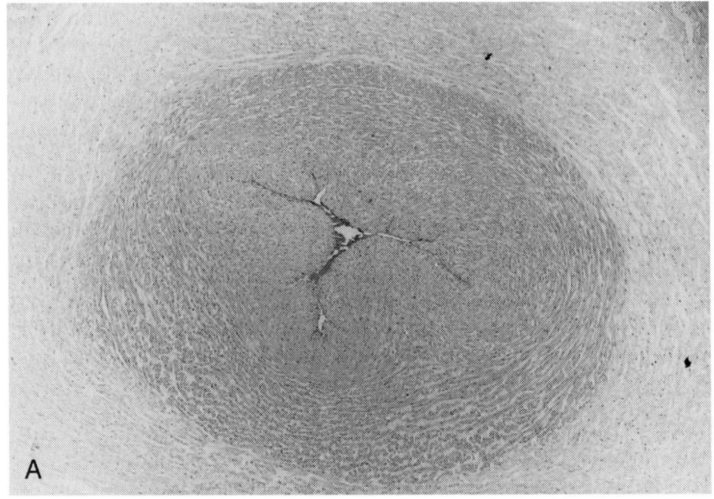

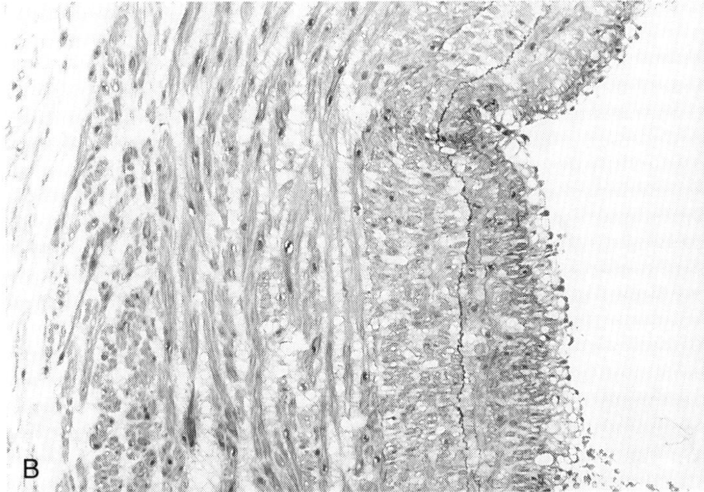

Figure 3–16. A, Constricted umbilical artery with small lumen and "cushions" (×4). **B,** An elastin stain shows the presence of thin elastic fibers only within the muscular wall (×20).

brane of the amnion.[57] Wharton's jelly forms first around the umbilical arteries and is an extracellular ground substance, rich in hyaluronic acid, chondroitin sulfate, and collagen. The cord substance is nourished by diffusion from the fetal vessels, primarily the thinner vein, and the amniotic fluid. Fluid balance of the cord and possibly the amniotic fluid may be influenced by movement of fluids from fetal blood through the vein wall. Mast cells within the cord stroma produce a heparin-like substance that may help to prevent thrombosis of the umbilical vessels. Macrophages are sparse but present within the cord stroma or can be recruited when needed. They may contain hemosiderin or meconium.

Chorionic Plate Vessels

The chorionic plate vessels at the insertion site have thicker connetive tissue, more fibers and cells, and less extracellular substance then the umbilical cord vessels, but it is not uncommon to see some Wharton's jelly substance within the larger chorionic plate vessels. The distribution of the chorionic plate vessels depends in part on the location of the umbilical cord insertion. A dispersed type of chorionic vasculature occurs with near central insertion of the cord; the two arteries divide dichotomously several times into a number of smaller vessels, rapidly diminishing in caliber (Fig. 3–18*A*). The magistral type of chorionic vasculature occurs most often with marginal or velamentous insertion of the cord, and the vessels extend almost to the margin of the placenta before diminishing in caliber; therefore there are longer undivided branches (Fig. 3–18*B*). Mixed forms may also occur. Arteries and veins are paired structures and most often found within close proximity. Arteries almost always cross over veins on the placental surface, 97% of the time according to Hamilton and Boyd.[11]

Each umbilical artery can produce eight or more terminal chorionic plate arteries. During division these perforating arteries form the basis for and determine the number of the cotyledons of the placenta (Fig. 3–19).[58] The magistral type of chorionic vasculature is associated with fewer penetrating arteries, fewer cotyledons, and abnormal umbilical artery blood flow.[58] The musculature in the perforating arteries decreases markedly as they enter the major stem vessels from the chorionic plate, and consequently the arterial caliber is increased. During the first 60 days of gestation before the chorion laeve is established, the entire chorion is vascularized from the umbilical cord vessels. Eventually only the chorionic plate possesses significant branches of the umbilical arteries, although a few straggling vessels to the membranous chorion may persist, resulting in intramembranous vessels. Each fetal cotyledon is supplied and drained by one and rarely two arteries and veins in variable arrangement.

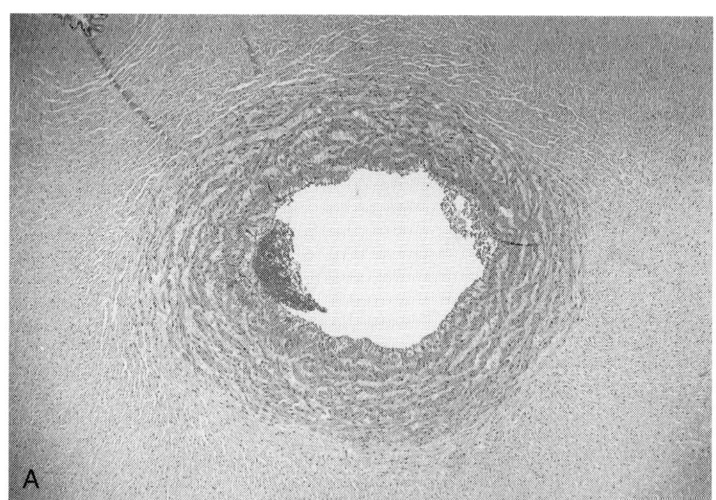

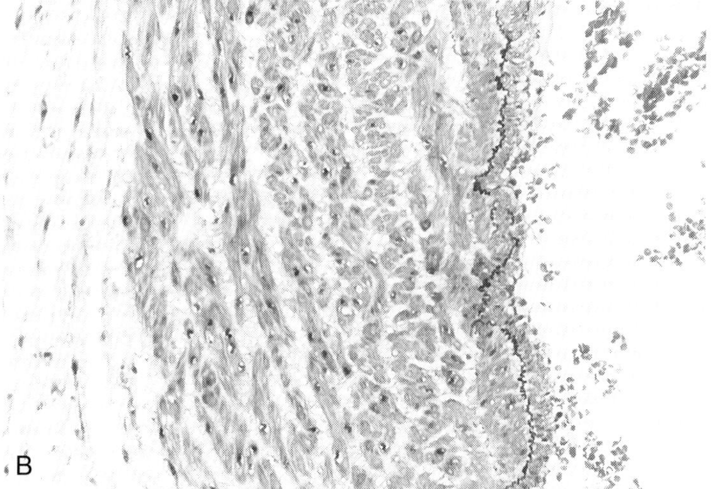

Figure 3–17. A, The umbilical vein is usually quite dilated (×4). **B,** Elastic stain highlights the internal elastic lamina (×20).

Villous Vessels

Blood vessels initially form from mesenchymal cells (vasculogenesis), which transform into cell cords that are forerunners of the capillary endothelium and hematopoietic stem cells. The lumina develop by dehiscence of intercellular clefts, forming the basis for vascularity from 5 to 26 postmenstrual weeks.[59] True angiogenesis occurs from 26 to 40 weeks' gestation and begins with proliferation of the endothelium, which sprouts from preexisting vessels, and formation of branches with longitudinal growth.[59] The vessels are composed of endothelium surrounded by pericytes, and a complete basal lamina is seen during the last 10 weeks of pregnancy. Only the vessels of the stem villi have muscular walls and peripherally placed capillaries that resemble vasa vasorum.

Nucleated Red Blood Cells

Red blood cells are first seen in the vascular lumen at 5 postmenstrual weeks. Before 6 weeks'

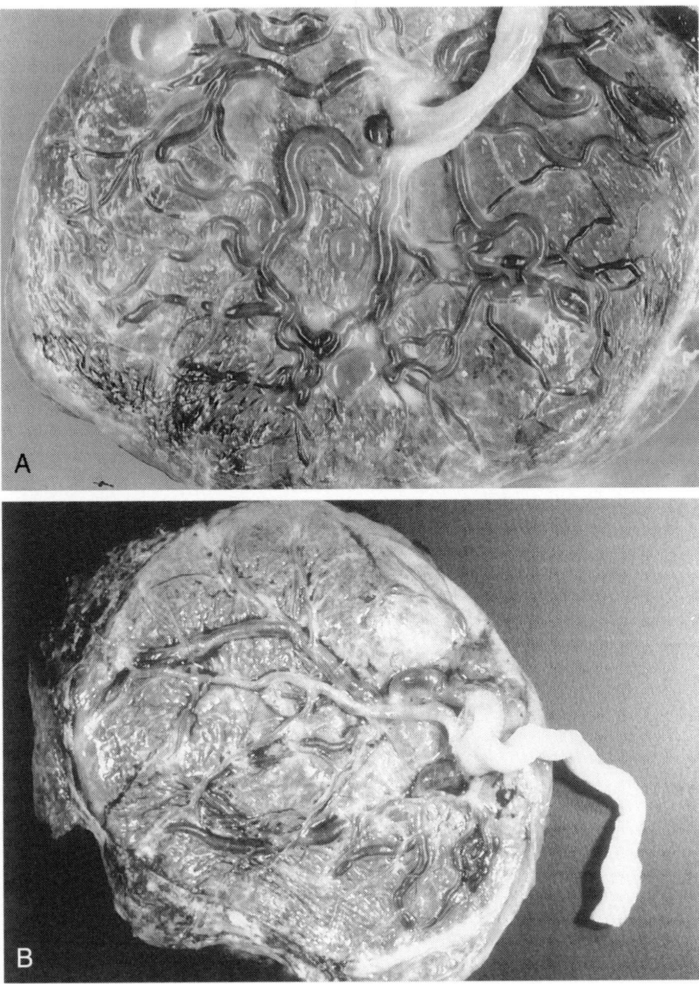

Figure 3–18. A, Near central insertion of the umbilical cord usually results in a dispersed type of chorionic plate vasculature. **B,** Insertion of the umbilical cord at the margin or within the membranes of the placenta results in the magistral type of chorionic plate vasculature. Note that the chorionic plate arteries nearly always cross over veins.

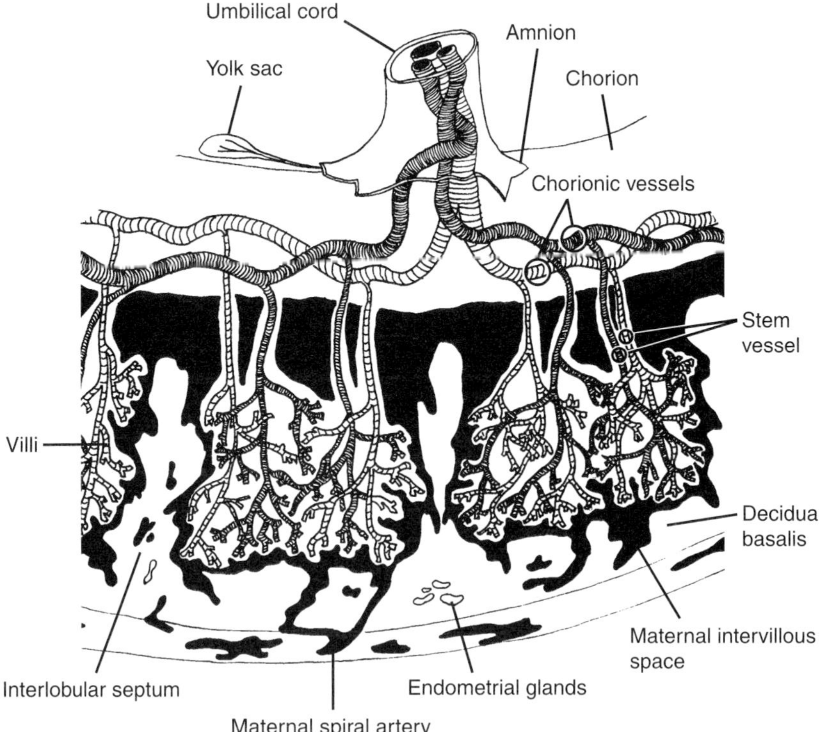

Figure 3–19. Diagrammatic representation of the structure of the placenta, with emphasis on the relationship between the placental lobule or cotyledon of fetal vascular origin and that created by the interlobular septa.

gestation 100% of fetal nucleated red blood cells are derived from the yolk sac and never become anucleate. At the end of the eighth postmenstrual week, hematopoiesis occurs in the sinusoids of the liver. From 12 postmenstrual weeks until term only 2% of red blood cells within the villi should have nuclei.[60] At term the identification of nucleated red blood cells within villous capillaries is frequently associated with increased circulating nucleated red blood cells,[61] an abnormal finding.

The color of the placental villi depends mainly on the amount of blood in the fetal capillaries; therefore the villi are pale in the first and second trimesters and darker thereafter. At term 10 ml of fetal blood exists for each 100 g of placenta if the cord is clamped immediately after delivery, and half that amount if cord pulsations cease before clamping.[5] This figure may be important in the calculation of massive fetal and maternal bleeding.

INTERLOBULAR SEPTA

The maternal surface of the placenta shows subdivisions into 10 to 38 lobes or lobules separated from one another by irregular and often indistinct grooves of variable depth occupied by tissue of the interlobular septa (Fig. 3–20). The lobes are often round but vary in shape and considerably in size. They are convex and covered by the decidua basalis, which has become detached during parturition. Hydropic placentas may lose this lobular appearance.

The septa first become apparent during postmenstrual weeks 8 to 12, beginning with focal incorporation of the innermost cytotrophoblast shell in the intervillous space.[11] Septum formation results from two main factors, differential growth in the system of villi and compression of the decidua in regions where the villous growth is more vigorous. Diminished growth rate in some of the anchoring villi results in a dragging of decidua and rarely maternal blood vessels into the intervillous space by the

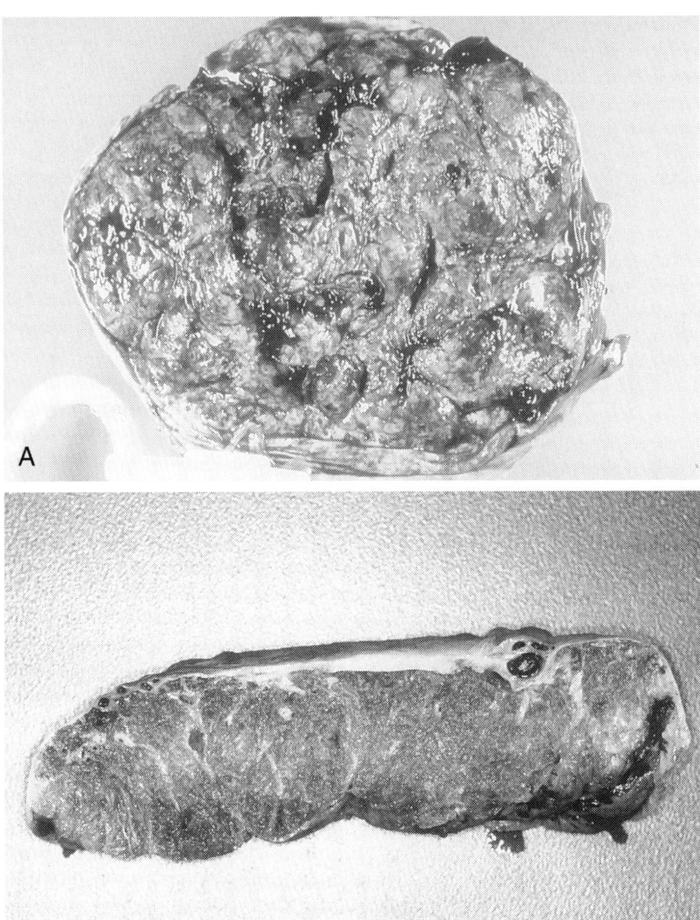

Figure 3–20. A, The maternal surface of the placenta may have a prominent lobular configuration because of the presence of irregularly spaced interlobular septa. **B,** The cross section of the placenta shows the interlobular septa as thin bands of connective tissue that do not extend to the chorionic plate but result in indentation of the maternal surface.

fourth month of gestation. These decidual elements are more centrally situated, but eventually the decidua degenerates and regressive changes in the accompanying maternal decidual vessels may be seen. This indentation of the decidual layer toward the chorion forms incompletely separated chambers within which the fetal vascular and villous systems project. The septa project from the basal plate toward the chorionic plate and are usually 1.2 to 1.5 cm long (Figs. 3–19 and 3–21).[33] The septa may become continuous with or abut septa projecting in other planes. When septa are first formed, the surfaces are covered by syncytiotrophoblast, but later in gestation this is replaced by fibrinoid. It is these septa that give the maternal surface its lobular appearance, which only loosely parallels the fetal vascular divisions of the placental parenchyma.

Degeneration of the central portion of the septa results in septal clefts or cysts lined with X cells that produce a clear fluid when warm and a firm colloidlike contents when cooled. They usually measure 0.5 to 1 cm and are found at the apex of a septum, although they may occur anywhere along the length of the septum, including the subchorionic plate (Figs. 3–22 and 3–9*A*). Septal cysts are seen in 11% to 20% of placentas and are more likely with hydrops.[5]

Calcifications are common in the interlobular septa, especially at the basal plate (Fig. 3–23). Calcification increases with gestational age, as much as 2.5 times during the last 4 weeks of pregnancy.[62] Calcification is especially common on the maternal surface, where it appears as small, irregular, hard yellow-white flecks that rarely penetrate the villous tissue. They may yield a gritty feel to the knife during sectioning. Macroscopic foci of dystrophic calcification are common at term but are rarely seen before 36 weeks. Calcification at term is not always

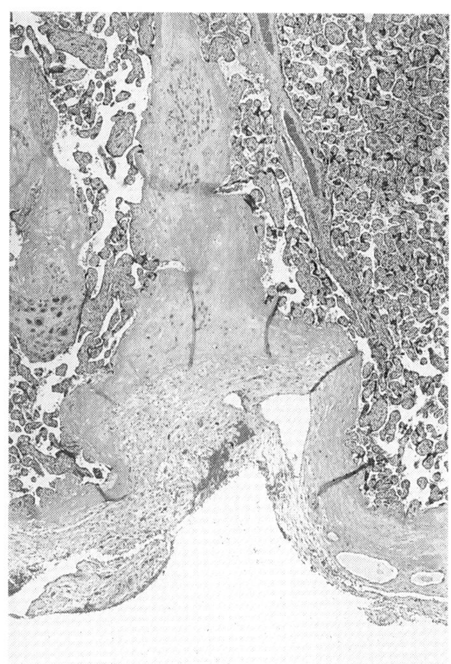

Figure 3–21. The interlobular septa are composed of connective tissue with variable amounts of maternal decidua and vessels that may be partially incorporated within the septum. This may cause disruption of the maternal decidual vessels, frequently resulting in thrombosis and secondary bland degeneration of the decidua basalis, which is more prominent during septal formation in early gestation.

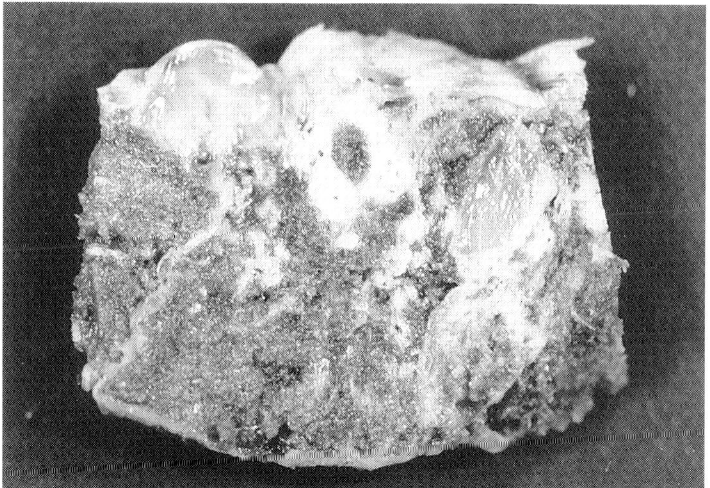

Figure 3–22. Septal cysts may be seen anywhere along the septum; an intraparenchymal and subchorionic cyst is shown here (×20).

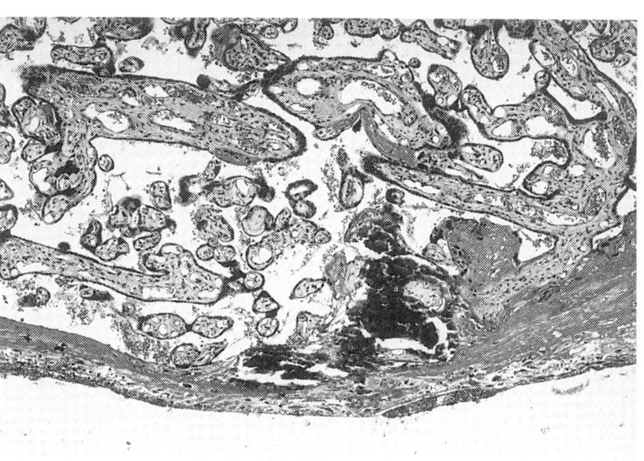

Figure 3–23. Calcifications of the maternal decidual tissue and connective tissues of the septa are normal findings near term (×10).

associated with tissue death. In preterm placentas, however, calcification is commonly associated with necrotic tissue. Staining these areas often reveals a combination of calcium and iron.

AMNION

Amnion arises from ectoderm immediately adjacent to the dorsal aspect of the embryonic disk at the end of the third menstrual week (Fig. 3–1). The amniotic cavity is formed by the fifth postmenstrual week. The amnion is continuous with the edges of the embryonic disk and the umbilical cord but is initially much smaller than the chorionic sac (Fig. 3–24*A*).

In early gestation the amnion epithelium is a flattened single layer and before fusion with the chorion is difficult to identify (Fig. 3–4*A*). Under normal circumstances, in the later stages of pregnancy the amnionic epithelium remains as a single layer with a variable distribution of microvilli (Fig. 3–25*A* and *B*). Late in gestation, squamous metaplasia occurs both on the amnion of the membranes near the cord insertion and on the umbilical cord itself, possibly as the result of minor trauma from fetal movement, but does not develop on the free membranes (Fig. 3–25*C*). The amnion of the umbilical cord is initially several layers thick, tightly adherent, and continuous with the amnion of the chorionic plate.

The amnion is considered to have five layers totaling 0.02 to 0.5 mm thick (Fig. 3–25*A*).[63] The amnion epithelium is flat, cuboidal, or columnar and appears to be an irregularly arranged mosaic if examined as a flat sheet. The amnion has a base-

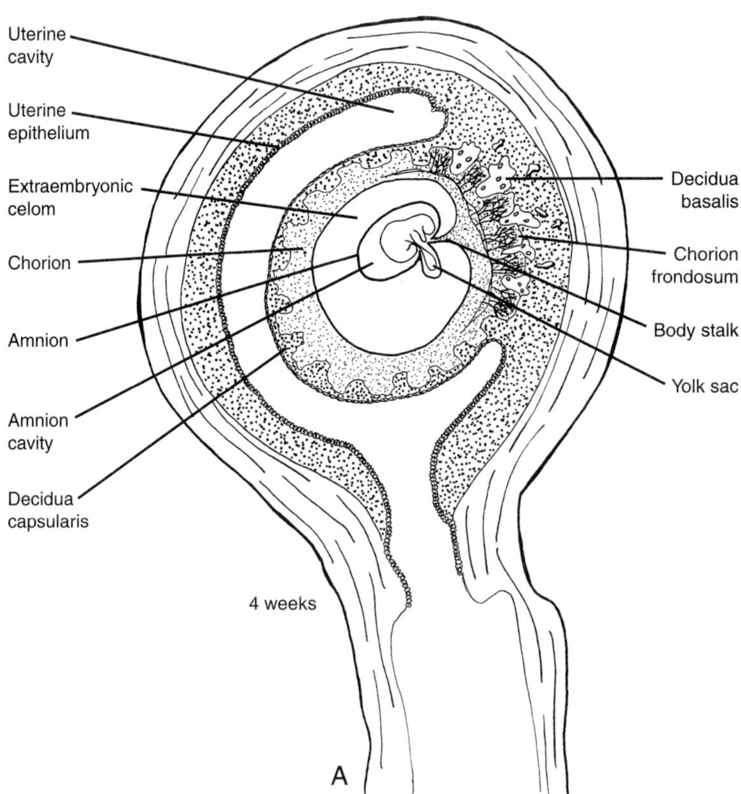

Figure 3–24. Diagrammatic representation of important developmental milestones in formation of the maternal-placental-fetal unit. **A,** At 4 weeks' gestation, implantation is complete and the decidua capsularis bulges into the uterine cavity. The chorion is completely covered by villi. The amniotic sac is still very small in comparison to the chorion.

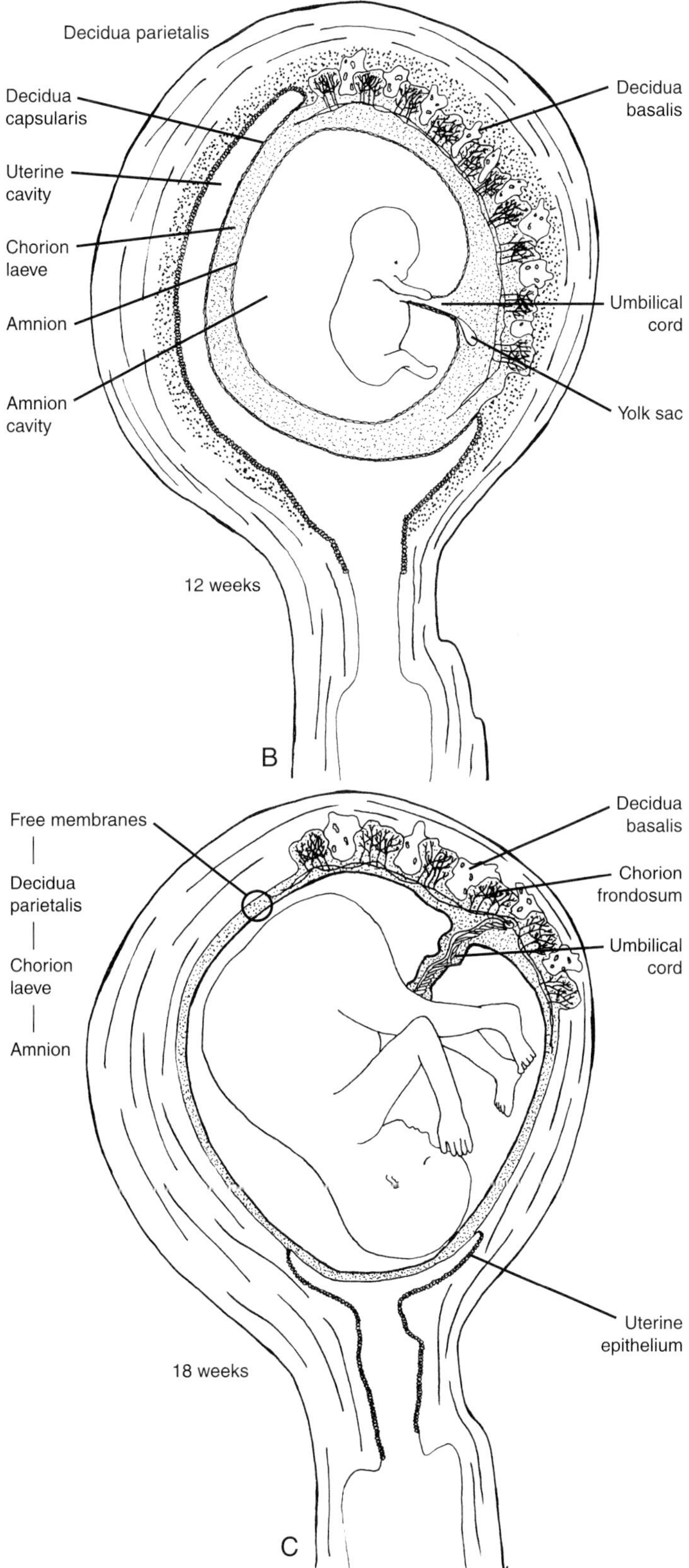

Figure 3–24 *Continued* **B,** At 12 weeks' gestation the amnion and chorion come into approximation, obliterating the extraembryonic coelom. Atrophy of the villi facing the uterine cavity forms the chorion laeve. **C,** At 18 weeks' gestation the maternal-placental-fetal unit is complete with obliteration of the uterine cavity, atrophy of the decidua capsularis, and fusion of the chorion with the decidualized endometrium, the decidua parietalis.

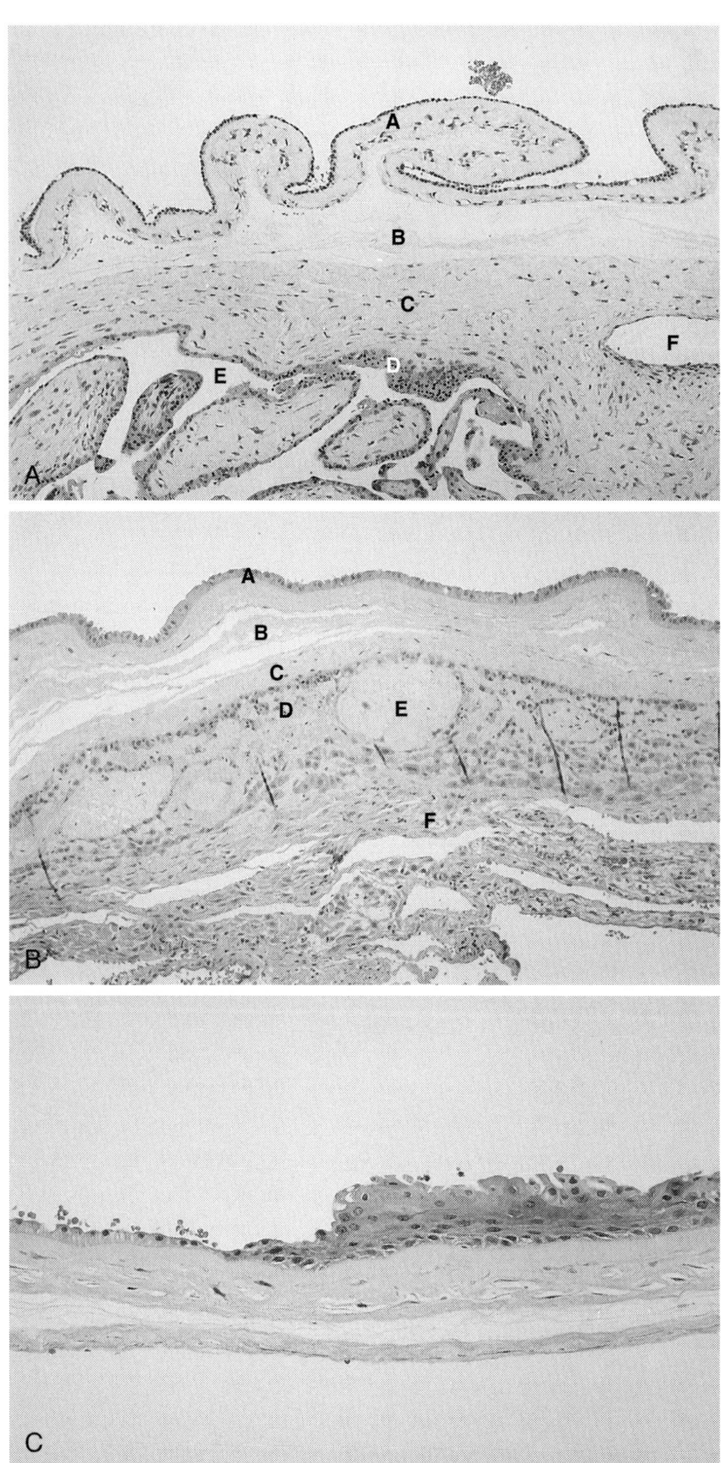

Figure 3–25. A, The attached membranes or chorionic plate from the second trimester is shown. The amnion epithelium *(a)* and the connective tissue of the extraembryonic coelom *(b)* are considered as the amnion. The chorion is formed primarily by fibrous connective tissue *(c)* and trophoblast *(d)* that covers the fetal chorion, separating it from the maternal intervillous space *(e)*. A large fetal chorionic plate vessel *(f)* is seen (×10). **B,** The free or reflected membranes in the third trimester are shown. The amnion epithelium *(a)* and the extraembryonic coelom *(b)* compose the amnion. The chorion has variable amounts of connective tissue *(c)* and a large amount of trophoblast *(d),* within which are atrophic villi of the chorion laeve *(e)*. The maternal decidua parietalis *(f)* is intimately associated with the fetal tissue (×10). **C,** Squamous metaplasia of the amnion occurs during the third trimester in response to minor injury. It is universally present on the amnion of the umbilical cord and commonly seen on the amnion of the chorionic plate at the cord insertion, often overlying large chorionic plate vessels (×20).

ment membrane. A compact layer that consists of reticulum and is devoid of cells is also resistant to edema and leukocytes is the next layer. The fibroblastic layer is the thickest and consists of a mass of reticulin and fibroblasts. This layer contains Hofbauer cells. The innermost layer is the spongy layer, which is tissue of the extraembryonic coelom. It contains mucin, wavy reticulin fibers, and Hofbauer cells and is the most susceptible to edema. This layer also frequently separates from the chorion, especially in cases of meconium, edema, or infection, and commonly results in sections of the "membrane roll" or chorionic plate that are devoid of amnion. If detached from the underlying chorion, the amnion of the free membranes is not usually distinguishable from the amnion of the chorionic plate, although frequently more prominent hyperplasia is seen on the amnion of the chorionic plate and squamous metaplasia is seen only on the amnion of the chorionic plate. In some cases vernix caseosa has dissected between the amnion and chorion.[64] Acute meconium, bacteria, and other debris are infrequently seen within the potential space of the extraembryonic coelom. The absence of reaction to the foreign material helps to identify this as an artifact, and its location distinguishes it from amnion nodosum. The amnion has no blood supply of its own.

Amniotic fluid volume varies with gestation; 200 ml at 16 weeks, 1000 ml at 28 weeks, 900 ml at 36 weeks, 800 ml at 40 weeks, and 350 ml at 42 weeks.[65,66] Early production of amniotic fluid is considered to be transmembranous, from the amnion, fetal lung secretions, and across fetal skin. Later in gestation the lungs secrete a large volume of fluid. Fetal urine production begins to comprise the greatest volume after 16 weeks' gestation. Amniotic fluid volume may be controlled by intramembranous absorption across the chorionic plate into the fetal vessels, as well as through fetal swallowing.[67] Polyhydramnios, defined as amniotic fluid volume greater than 2000 ml, can occur when fetal swallowing is absent, as with neuromuscular problems that prevent swallowing or with upper gastrointestinal tract obstruction that prevents reabsorption. Oligohydramnios, defined as less than 400 ml, usually occurs when urine production is deficient, as would occur with absence of kidneys, urinary outlet obstruction, and decreased fetal glomerular filtration rate. Premature rupture of membranes with loss of fluid and postdates pregnancy are also associated with oligohydramnios.

CHORION

The chorionic plate begins with the formation of the trophoblast shell and lacunae. Extraembryonic mesoderm spreads around the cytotrophoblast surface of the blastocyst cavity and thus forms the chorion (Fig. 3–24*A*). Because of the interstitial implantation, villi cover the entire surface of the membranes for the first 8 weeks of gestation, forming the chorion frondosum. The chorion frondosum becomes the chorionic plate or placental disk and is well defined by 12 postmenstrual weeks. The smooth area of villous regression is called chorion laeve, reflected chorion, or bald chorion. The villous atrophy is thought to result from deficient maternal vascularity of the abembryonic region. Ghostlike, atrophic villi can be identified even at term within the free membranes but are much more prominent during midgestation (Fig. 3–25*B*). The amnion and chorion fuse at about 12 menstrual weeks to produce the membrane we are most familiar with (Fig. 3–24*B*).

A failure of regression of the chorion laeve may result in abnormal placental shape. The most common abnormality is an accessory or succenturiate lobe, which occurs in 5% to 8% of placentas.[5] Multilobate placentas are seen much less frequently. The least common and most serious complication is placenta membranaceae, which is a thin, extremely large placenta, often measuring 30 cm or more with no or little free membrane. An abnormality of cord insertion is also common. The most frequent variation of placental shape, the bilobate placenta, is probably not related to abnormal regression of the chorion.

The chorion has four layers, all of which contain Hofbauer cells.[63] The cellular layer, an incomplete layer of interlacing fibroblasts, is closest to the amnion and is not seen at term. The reticular layer makes up the majority of thickness of the total membrane and is formed by parallel reticulin fibers. This is the area that contains the fetal blood vessels. Next is a pseudo–basement membrane formed by dense connective tissue. Closest to the maternal tissue is a trophoblast layer consisting of 2 to 10 layers of intermediate trophoblast in con-

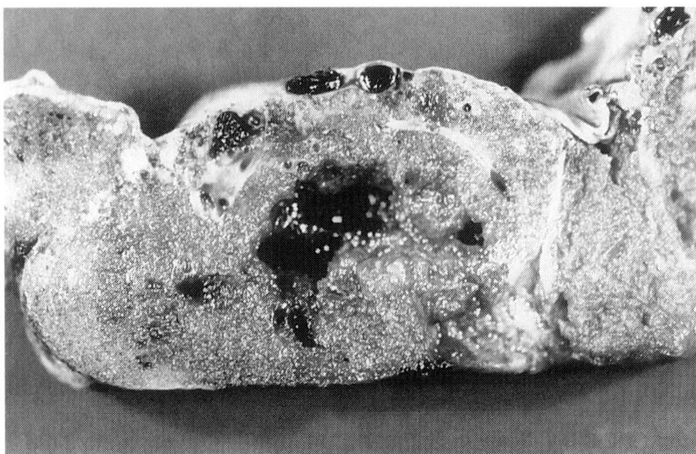

Figure 3–26. A "hole" within the placenta may be the result of the jet flow from a maternal spiral artery. No abnormalities of the surrounding villi are identified microscopically.

tact with maternal decidua of the free membranes or maternal intervillous space of the placental disk. This layer contains the atrophic villi of the chorion laeve of the free membranes (Fig. 3–25*B*). The trophoblast layer of the attached chorion is replaced at term by subchorionic or Langhans' fibrinoid, which varies in thickness from 0.1 to 1.5 cm (Fig. 3–25*A*). There is often evidence of true thrombosis with laminated fibrin, as well as glassy fibrinoid, in this location. Extreme cases, which are actually large subchorionic hematomas or thrombi, may be referred to as Breus' mole.

INTERVILLOUS SPACE

The intervillous space is an integral part of the hemochorial placenta. Initially the intervillous space is bathed by maternal plasma and uterine gland and decidual secretions. Controversy exists as to when this shifts to continuous maternal circulation.[68] At 8 weeks' gestation arteries open directly into the intervillous space but blood flow may be restricted by the presence of intraarterial intermediate trophoblastic plugs.[68] Ultrasound detects flow in all cases at about 12 weeks, but flow has been detected as early as 8 to 11 postmenstrual weeks with the use of more sensitive ultrasound instruments.[69–71] The blood within the space, although maternal, is outside the confines of an endothelium and in direct contact with fetal syncytiotrophoblast. Acoustic holes or cavitary spaces are noted on ultrasound.[72] These large gaps within intervillous space allow for or result from turbulence or blood "jets" from the maternal spiral arteries. Rarely, gross examination reveals such a cavitation within the center of the lobule (Fig. 3–26).

The placental venous sinus, marginal sinus, or circular vein of the placenta is a dilatation of the intervillous space at the placental margin and represents a functional rather than an anatomic structure. The subchorial lake is also an ultrasound finding based on pooling of blood in this relatively low-flow region, which results in increased fibrin deposition.

Intervillous fibrin, thrombus, or hematomas are seen in nearly half of term placentas. They are more common in hydropic placentas. They may be a mixture of fetal and maternal blood.[73] Large numbers of intervillous hematomas may be associated with intrauterine fetal demise and are suggestive of fetal-maternal bleeding.

Artifacts in the intervillous space can be caused by handling, fixation, and processing of the placental tissue. Adequate immersion fixation of the tissue before processing reduces the variation. Perfusion fixation through fetal vessels, maternal intervillous space, or both may yield superior preservation of the intervillous space but is not necessary for routine placental histologic examination.

Blood pressure in the uteroplacental arteries is 70 to 88 mm Hg, but within the intervillous space it has a mean value of about 10 mm Hg with the lowest pressures at the chorionic plate. This explains in part the variation in villous maturity and increased fibrin and fibrinoid at the subchorionic plate. Pressure within the uteroplacental veins is not more than 8 mm Hg. Blood flow to the intervillous space more than doubles during pregnancy. The mean volume of the intervillous space in the delivered placenta at term is 100 to 200 ml, but in vivo there is probably 400 to 500 ml, which contributes to the estimated blood loss during routine delivery.[5,6,47] Most of this blood is squeezed out of the intervillous space by uterine contractions during delivery of the placenta. Excessive blood noted either at delivery or within the placental bucket may be an indication of a recent abruption.

DECIDUA

Decidua is the term used to describe the endometrial stromal fibroblasts that under progestational influence become apparent by the twenty-eighth postmenstrual day. These stromal cells proliferate, become epithelioid, and accumulate glycogen and lipid (Fig. 3–27).[74] Because human implantation is interstitial, into the endometrium, decidua completely surrounds the blastocyst (Fig. 3–1*A*).

Decidua capsularis bulges into the uterine cavity. It is continuous with but always thinner than the basal decidua. Decidua capsularis atrophies because of a poor blood supply and can no longer be discerned by 22 weeks' gestation (Fig. 3–24). Decidua parietalis (decidua vera) lines the uterine cavity except at the implantation site. With growth of the gestational sac the decidua capsularis and decidua parietalis fuse, obliterating the uterine cavity as a fetomaternal tissue junction is established around the whole conceptus at 17 weeks' gestation (Fig. 3–24*C*).

The decidua basalis forms at the deep pole of the implanting blastocyst and is always thicker than that on the side of the uterine cavity but is rarely more than 0.1 cm thick at term. Immature placentas and those delivered by cesarean section often have a thicker decidua basalis. This is the area where fetal and maternal tissues become most intimately intermixed. It is through this region that the maternal vessels communicate with the intervillous space.

One function of the decidua basalis is presumably to limit excessive extension of the fetal trophoblast into the myometrium and thus prevent placenta accreta.[75] Placenta accreta may be partial (involving one or more lobes), focal (part of one lobe), or total (Fig. 3–28). The abnormal implantation may be onto the myometrium (accreta), into the myometrium (increta), or through the myometrium (percreta). Implantation in the lower uterine segment as in placenta previa is by definition accreta, because endometrium within this area or within the endocervix is insufficient for adequate decidualization. Cornual implantations are also associated with placenta accreta, as are prior surgical

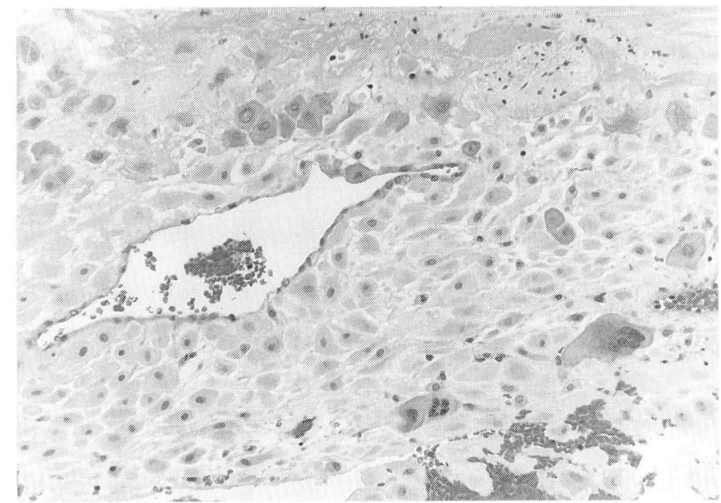

Figure 3–27. Maternal decidual cells have abundant but pale cytoplasm in contrast to the invading trophoblast with dense basophilic cytoplasm. Most of the trophoblastic cells are mononucleated, but a rare multinucleated form is seen *(arrows)*. A residual endometrial gland that contains displaced red blood cells is also present (×20).

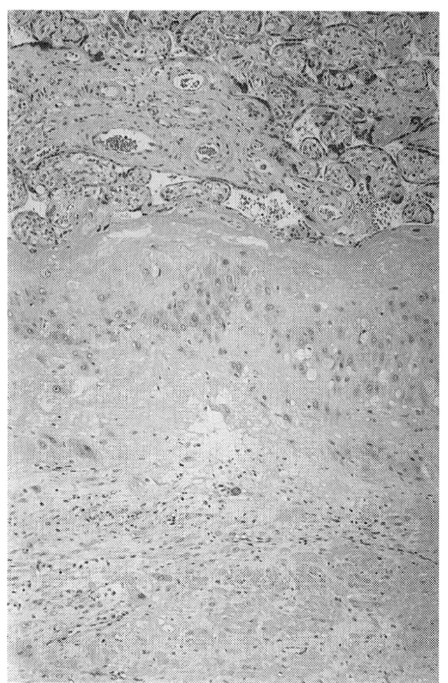

Figure 3–28. A large area of placenta accreta, which shows absence of decidua basalis. The mononuclear cells seen between the villi and the myometrial smooth muscle are invading intermediate trophoblast. The intact uteroplacental specimen is the result of a postpartum hysterectomy in a patient with known placenta accreta (×4).

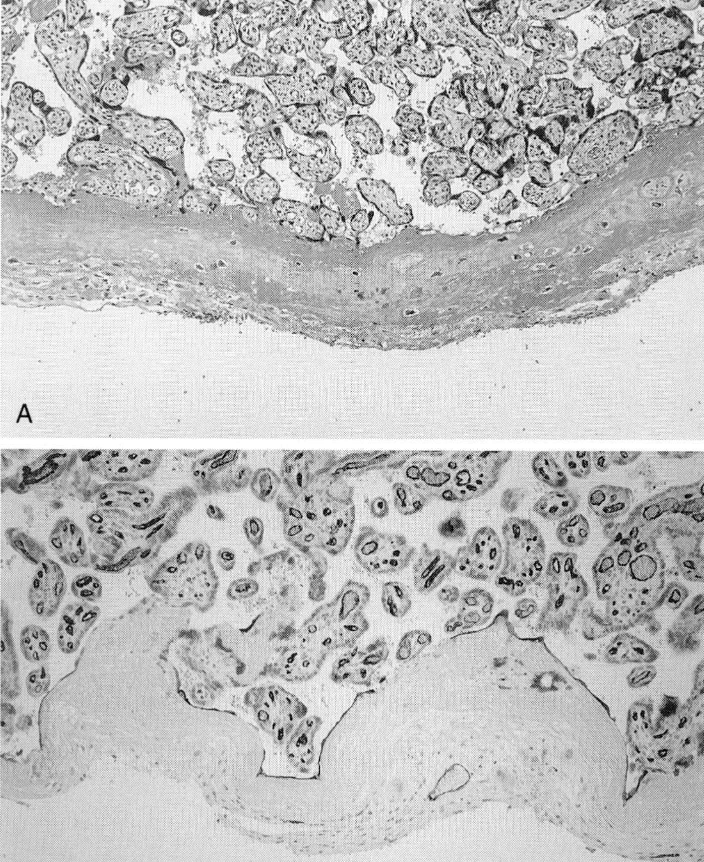

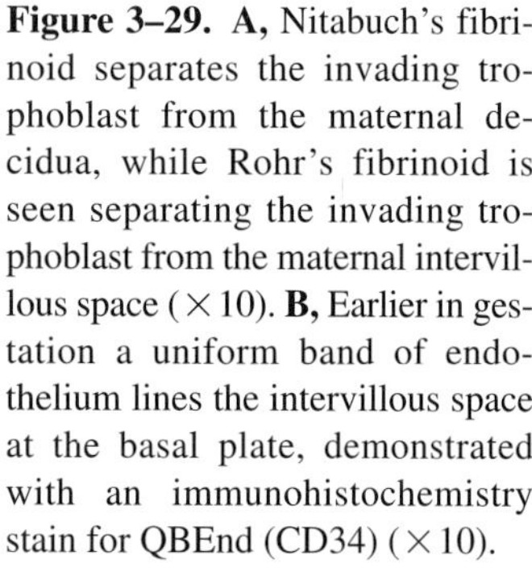

Figure 3–29. A, Nitabuch's fibrinoid separates the invading trophoblast from the maternal decidua, while Rohr's fibrinoid is seen separating the invading trophoblast from the maternal intervillous space (× 10). **B,** Earlier in gestation a uniform band of endothelium lines the intervillous space at the basal plate, demonstrated with an immunohistochemistry stain for QBEnd (CD34) (× 10).

procedures or manual placental extraction. Smooth muscle fibers are commonly found at the base of the placenta, especially in premature deliveries, manual extraction of the placenta, or cesarean sections.[76] Increased fibrosis and acute or chronic inflammation may also be seen within the implantation site, particularly within basal villi.[7]

Fibrinoid deposited at the boundary zone of the fetal trophoblast and the maternal decidua basalis is called Nitabuch's membrane or fibrinoid (Fig. 3–29*A*). Nitabuch's fibrinoid may extend diffusely out into the decidua. On the villous side of the implantation, initially the decidua basalis is separated from the intervillous space by endothelium (Fig. 3–29*B*), which is ultimately replaced by Rohr's fibrinoid (Fig. 3–29*A*). Rohr's fibrinoid is less uniformly present and frequently connects with Nitabuch's fibrinoid, making them difficult to distinguish as separate entities, especially at term.

Chronic inflammatory cells are a normal component of the decidua and are present in small numbers. They should be scattered diffusely throughout the decidua and not be localized around maternal or fetal structures within the decidua. Natural killer (NK) lymphocytes comprise 70%, macrophages 20%, and T lymphocytes 10% with few B lymphocytes.[44,77–80] The NK cells are a distinct form of lymphocyte that is positive for CD 56^{DIM} and CD16 and does not have granules. Many of the NK cells in the decidua are referred to as large granular lymphocytes. They have cytoplasmic granulation and are positive for $CD56^{BRIGHT}$ and negative for CD16, CD2, and CD3. When activated by cytokines they become lymphokine-activated killer (LAK) cells, which are capable of killing virally infected, malignant, or normal cells. The proportion of macrophages increases throughout gestation, and NK cells decrease steadily.

GLANDULAR EPITHELIUM

At the implantation site, early in gestation, some of the glandular epithelium disappears by apoptosis. During gestation the glandular epithelium undergoes changes referred to as the Arias-Stella reaction (Fig. 3–30*A*). The glandular epithelium is reportedly positive for S-100 protein.[81] The glandular epithelial cells may also have clear nuclei that are reminiscent of viral inclusions (Fig. 3–30*B*). This change is evident from 14 postmenstrual weeks to term and persists approximately 1 month post partum. It is caused by the intranuclear storage of biotin. This biotin may participate in gluconeogenesis, and it is metabolized during the first trimester but thereafter is stored. The presence of endogenous biotin interferes with the avidin-biotin-peroxidase method of immunohistochemistry, resulting in positive staining within both positive and negative controls.[82]

SPIRAL ARTERIES

During early implantation, on postovulatory days 14 to 18, necrosis of the maternal spiral artery wall is noted.[11] The endothelium becomes plump and hypertrophied and projects into the vessel lumen. An estimated 100 maternal arteries and 50 to 200 veins are present in the term placental implantation site.[4] Invasion and adaptation by intermediate trophoblast are discussed in Chapter 8. It is presumed that each placental lobule is fed by one or more spiral arteries and drained by one or more veins. On close inspection of the decidua basalis during gross examination the maternal spiral arteries may be identified as indentations or snail trail–like imprints (Fig. 3–31*A*). These spiral arteries on occasion can be identified as they enter the maternal intervillous space (Fig. 3–31*B*). Small muscular arteries, which are the basal branches of the spiral arteries, perfuse the endometrium and decidua. These basal branch vessels do not normally adapt for pregnancy and can be seen within both decidua basalis and decidua parietalis.

Maternal venous "sinusoids" in the implantation site are dilated and are filled with plasma and some maternal blood cells. The intervillous space communicates with these sinusoids by postovulatory day 14. When intermediate trophoblast invades the spiral arteries, a few intermediate trophoblastic cells can also be seen within decidual veins, but most often the veins are flattened, inconspicuous, thin-walled, endothelium-lined structures within the decidua.

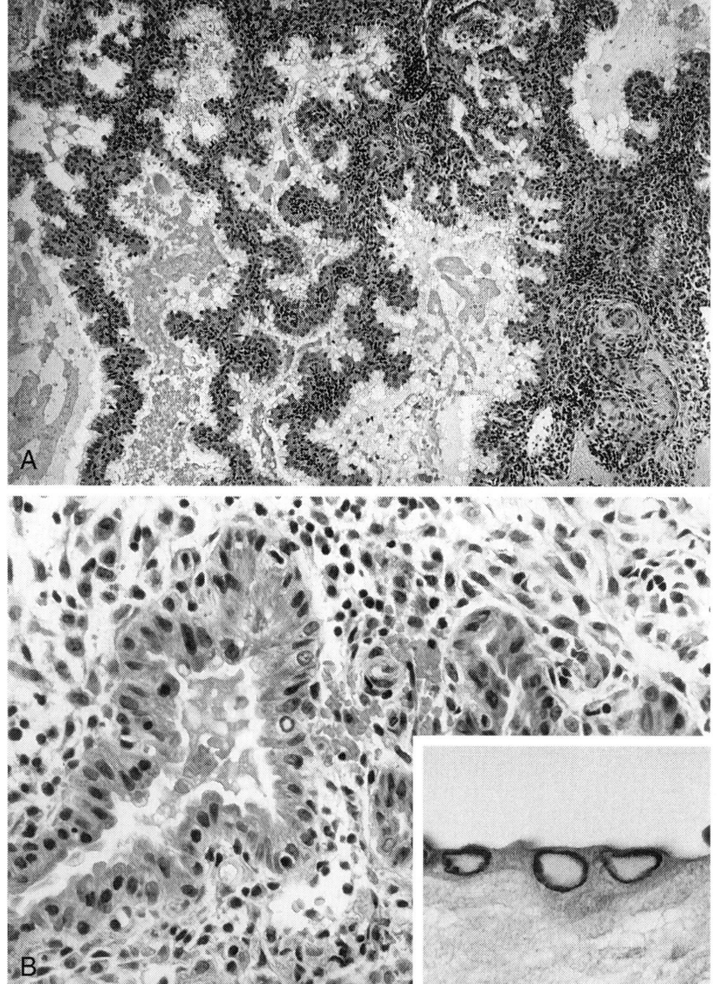

Figure 3–30. **A,** Arias-Stella reaction of the glands of the secretory endometrium in response to pregnancy during the first trimester (×10). **B,** At term the endometrial glands have lost the "hypersecretory" appearance of early gestation and have optically clear nuclei, which gives the appearance of intranuclear inclusions (×10; *insert,* ×100). These nuclei contain biotin, which results in nonspecific immunohistochemistry staining when the avidin-biotin method is used.

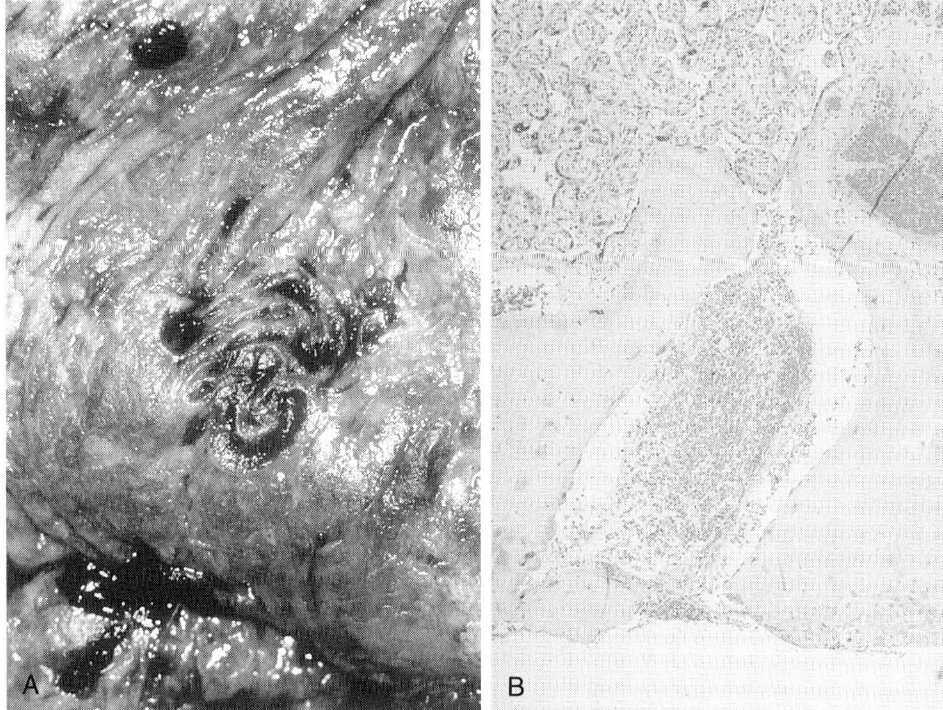

Figure 3–31. **A,** Spiral artery seen on the maternal surface of a term placenta, near the center of a lobule. **B,** Spiral artery shown cut longitudinally as it enters the maternal intervillous space (× 10).

REFERENCES

1. Franklin GC, Adam GIR, Ohlsson R: Genomic imprinting and mammalian development. Placenta 17:3, 1996.
2. Aplin JD: The cell biology of human implantation. Placenta 17:269, 1996.
3. Cross JC, Werb Z, Fisher SJ: Implantation and the placenta: key pieces of the development puzzle. Science 266:1508, 1994.
4. O'Rahilly R, Muller F: Human embryology and teratology, 2nd ed. New York, 1996, Wiley-Liss.
5. Benirschke K, Kaufmann P: Pathology of the human placenta, 3rd ed. New York, 1995, Springer-Verlag.
6. Teasdale F: Gestational changes in the functional structure of the human placenta in relation to fetal growth: a morphometric study. Am J Obstet Gynecol 137:560, 1980.
7. Fox H: Pathology of the placenta. Philadelphia, 1978, WB Saunders.
8. Molteni RA: Placental growth and fetal/placental weight (F/P) ratio throughout gestation—their relationship to patterns of fetal growth. Semin Perinatol 8:94, 1984.
9. Molteni RA, Stys SJ, Battaglia FC: Relationship of fetal and placental weight in human beings: fetal/placental weight ratios at various gestational ages and birth weight distributions. J Reprod Med 21:327, 1987.
10. Naeye RL: Do placental weights have clinical significance? Hum Pathol 18:387, 1987.
11. Boyd JD, Hamilton WJ: The human placenta. Cambridge, UK 1970, W Heffer & Sons.
12. Kalousek DK, Fitch N, Paradice BA: Pathology of the human embryo and previable fetus, an atlas. New York, 1990, Springer-Verlag.
13. Perrin EVDK, Sander CH: Introduction: how to examine the placenta and why. In Perrin EVDK (ed): Pathology of the placenta. New York, 1984, Churchill Livingstone, p 1.
14. Dombrowski MP, Berry SM, Hurd WW, et al: A gestational-age-independent model of birth weight based on placental size. Biol Neonate 66:560, 1994.
15. Alonso K, Portman E: Fetal weights and measurements as determined by postmortem examination and their correlation with ultrasound examination. Arch Pathol Lab Med 119:179, 1995.
16. McLean FH, Boyd ME, Usher RH, Kramer MS:

Postterm infants: too big or too small. Am J Obstet Gynecol 164:619, 1991.

17. Olofsson P, Saldeen P, Marsal K: Fetal and utero-placental circulatory changes in pregnancies proceeding beyond 43 weeks. Early Hum Develop 46:1, 1996.
18. Pinar H, Sung CJ, Oyer CE, Singer DB: Reference values for singleton and twin placental weights. Pediatr Pathol 16:901, 1996.
19. Jauniaux E, Moscoso JG, Vanesse M, et al: Perfusion fixation for placental morphologic investigation. Hum Pathol 22:442, 1991.
20. Fox GE, Van Wesep R, Resau JH, Sun C-CJ: The effect of immersion formaldehyde fixation on human placental weight. Arch Pathol Lab Med 115:726, 1991.
21. Naeye RL: Umbilical cord length: clinical significance. J Pediatr 107:278, 1985.
22. Edmonds HW: The spiral twist of the normal umbilical cord in twins and singletons. Am J Obstet Gynecol 67:102, 1954.
23. Enders AC, King BF: Development of the human yolk sac. In Nogales FF (ed): The human yolk sac and yolk sac tumors. Heidelberg, 1993, Springer-Verlag, p 33.
24. Jones CP, Jauniaux E: Ultrastructure of the materno-embryonic interface in the first trimester pregnancy. Micron 26:145, 1995.
25. Nogales FF, Beltran E, Gonzalez F: Morphologic changes of the secondary human yolk sac in early pregnancy wastage. In Nogales FF (ed): The human yolk sac and yolk sac tumors. Heidelberg, 1993, Springer-Verlag, p 174.
26. Takashina T: Histology of the human yolk sac and special reference to hematopoiesis. In Nogales FF (ed). The human yolk sac and yolk sac tumors. Heidelberg, 1993, Springer-Verlag, p 48.
27. Enzan H: Electron microscopic studies of macrophages in early human yolk sacs. Acta Pathol Jpn 36:49, 1986.
28. Fukuda T: Fetal hematopoiesis (1) electron microscopic studies on human yolk sac hemopoiesis. Virchows Arch B Cell Pathol 14:197, 1973.
29. Ilgren EB: Control of trophoblastic growth. Placenta 4:307, 1983.
30. Yeh I-T, O'Connor DM, Kurman RJ: Intermediate trophoblast: further immunocytochemical characterization. Mod Pathol 3:282, 1990.
31. Brescia RJ, Kurman RJ, Main CS, et al: Immunocytochemical localization of chorionic gonadotrophin, placental lactogen and placental alkaline phosphatase in the diagnosis of complete and partial hydatidiform moles. Internat J Gynecol Pathol 6:213, 1987.
32. Wolf HK, Michalopoulos GK: Proliferating cell nuclear antigen in human placenta and trophoblastic disease. Pediatr Pathol 12:147, 1992.
33. Sabet LM, Daya D, Stead R, et al: Significance and value of immunohistochemical localization of pregnancy specific proteins in feto-maternal tissue throughout pregnancy. Mod Pathol 2:227, 1989.
34. Kurman RJ, Main CS, Chen HC: Intermediate trophoblast; a distinctive form of trophoblast with specific morphologic, biochemical and functional features. Placenta 5:349, 1984.
35. Boyd JD, Hamilton WJ: Electron microscopic observations of the cytotrophoblast contribution to the syncytium in the human placenta. J Anat 100:535, 1966.
36. Boyd JD, Hamilton WJ: Development and structure of the human placenta from the end of the third month of gestation. J Obstet Gynaecol Br Cwlth 74:161,1967.
37. Vicovac L, Jones CJP, Aplin JD: Trophoblast differentiation during formation of anchoring villi in a model of the early human placenta in vitro. Placenta 16:41, 1995.
38. Nelson DM: Apoptotic changes occur in syncytiotrophoblast of human placental villi where fibrin type fibrinoid is deposited in discontinuities in the villous trophoblast. Placenta 17:387, 1996.
39. Kaufmann P, Luckhardt M, Schweikhart G, Cantle SJ: Cross-sectional features and three-dimensional structure of human placenta villi. Placenta 8:235, 1987.
40. Boyd JD, Hamilton WJ: Stromal trophoblastic buds. J Obstet Gynecol Br Cwlth 71:1, 1964.
41. Tenney B, Parker F: The placenta in toxemia of pregnancy. Am J Obstet Gynecol 39:1000, 1960.
42. Khong TY, Stewart CJR, Mott C, et al: The usefulness of human placental lactogen and keratin immunohistochemistry in the assessment of tissue from purported intrauterine pregnancies. Am J Clin Pathol 102:72, 1994.
43. Kovats S, Main EK, Librach C, et al: A Class I antigen, HLA-G, expressed in human trophoblasts. Science 248:220, 1990.
44. Deniz G, Christmas SE, Brew R, Johnson PM: Phenotype and functional cellular differences between human CD3- decidual and peripheral blood lymphocytes. J Immunol 152:4255, 1994.
45. Gilmour J: Normal haemopoiesis in intra-uterine and neonatal life. J Pathol 52:25, 1942.
46. Stoz F, Schuhmann RA, Schebesta B: The development of the placental villus during normal pregnancy: morphometric data base. Arch Gynecol Obstet 244:23, 1988.

47. Aherne W, Dunnill MS: Quantitative aspects of placental structure. J Pathol Bacteriol 91:123, 1966.
48. Winick M, Coscia A, Nobel A: Cellular growth in human placenta. I. Normal placental growth. Pediatrics 39:248, 1967.
49. Burnstein R, Frankel S, Soule SD, Blumenthal HT: Aging of the placenta: autoimmune theory of senescence. Am J Obstet Gynecol 116:271, 1973.
50. Fox H: Fibrinoid necrosis of the placental villi. J Obstet Gynaecol Br Cwlth 75:448, 1968.
51. Nakamura Y, Ohata Y: Immunohistochemical study of human placental stromal cells. Hum Pathol 21:936, 1990.
52. Goldstein J, Braverman M, Salafia C, Buckley P: The phenotype of human placental macrophages and its variation with gestational age. Am J Pathol 133:648, 1988.
53. Soernes T, Bakke T: The length of the human umbilical cord in vertex and breech presentations. Am J Obstet Gynecol 154:1086, 1986.
54. Walker CW, Pye BG: Length of the human umbilical cord. Br Med J 1:546, 1960.
55. Lacro RV, Jones KL, Benirschke K: The umbilical cord twist: origin, direction and relevance. Am J Obstet Gynecol 157:833, 1987.
56. Gebrane-Younes J, Mink HN, Orcel L: Ultrastructure of human umbilical vessels: a possible role in amniotic fluid formation? Placenta 7:173, 1986.
57. Nanaev AK, Kohnen G, Milovanov AP, et al: Stromal differentiation and architecture of the human umbilical cord. Placenta 18:53, 1997.
58. Nordenvall M, Ullberg U, Laurin J, et al: Placental morphology in relation to umbilical artery blood velocity waveforms. Eur J Obstet Gynecol Reprod Biol 40:179, 1991.
59. Demir R, Kaufmann P, Castellucci M, et al: Fetal vasogenesis and angiogenesis in human placental villi. Acta Anat 136:190, 1989.
60. Salafia CM, Weigl CA, Foye GJ: Correlation of placental erythrocyte morphology and gestational age. Pediatr Pathol 8:495, 1988.
61. Salafia CM, Minior VJ, Rosenkrantz TS, et al: Maternal, placental and neonatal associations with early germinal matrix/intraventricular hemorrhage in infants born at <32 weeks gestation. Am J Perinatol 12:427, 1995.
62. Jeacock MK, Scott J, Plester JA: Calcium content of the human placenta. Am J Obstet Gynecol 87:34, 1963.
63. Bourne GL: The microscopic anatomy of the human amnion and chorion. Am J Obstet Gynecol 79:1070, 1960.
64. Jacques SM, Qureshi F: Subamnionic vernix caseosa. Pediatr Pathol 14:585, 1994.
65. Elliott PM, Inman WH: Volume of liquor amnii in normal and abnormal pregnancy. Lancet 2:835, 1961.
66. Queenan JT: Polyhydramnios and oligohydramnios. Contemp Obstet Gynecol 36:60, 1991.
67. Brace RA: Current topic: progress towards understanding the regulation of amniotic fluid volume; water and solute fluxes in and through the fetal membranes. Placenta 16:1, 1995.
68. Carter AM. When is the maternal placental circulation established in man? Placenta 18:83, 1997.
69. Hustin J, Schaaps JP: Echographic and anatomic studies of the maternotrophoblastic border during the first trimester of pregnancy. Am J Obstet Gynecol 157:162, 1987.
70. Valentine L, Sladkevicius P, Laurini R, et al: Uteroplacental and leuteal circulation in normal first trimester pregnancies: Doppler ultrasonographic and morphologic study. Am J Obstet Gynecol 174:768, 1996.
71. Moll W: Absence of intervillous blood flow in the first trimester of human pregnancy. Placenta 16:333, 1995.
72. Crawford JM: Vascular anatomy of the human placenta. Am J Obstet Gynecol 84:1543, 1962.
73. Kaplan C, Blanc WA, Elias J: Identification of erythrocytes in intervillous thrombi: a study using immunoperoxidase identification of hemoglobins. Hum Pathol 13:554, 1982.
74. Dempsey EW, Wislocki GB: Observations on some histochemical reactions in the human placenta, with special reference to the significance of the lipoids, glycogen and iron. Endocrinology 35:409, 1944.
75. Fox H: Placenta accreta, 1945–1969. Obstet Gynecol Surv 27:475, 1972.
76. Sherer DM, Salafia CM, Minior VK, et al: Placental basal plate myometrial fibers: clinical correlations of abnormally deep trophoblast invasion. Obstet Gynecol 87:444, 1996.
77. Labarrere C, Faulk WP: Anchoring villi in human basal plate: lymphocytes, macrophages and coagulation. Placenta 12:173, 1991.
78. Starkey PM, Sargent IL, Redman CWG: Cell populations in human early pregnancy decidua: characterization and isolation of large granular lymphocytes by flow cytometry. Immunology 65:129, 1988.
79. Mincheva-Nilsson L, Hammarstrom S, Hammarstrom M-L: Human decidual leukocytes from early pregnancy contain high numbers of gamma delta+ cells and show selective downregulation of alloreactivity. J Immunol 149:2203, 1992.

80. Whitelaw PF, Croy BA: Granulated lymphocytes of pregnancy. Placenta 17:533, 1996.
81. Nakamura Y, Moritsuka Y, Ohta Y: S-100 protein in glands within decidua and cervical glands during early pregnancy. Hum Pathol 20:1204, 1989.
82. Yokoyama S, Kashima K, Inoue S: Biotin-containing intranuclear inclusions in endometrial glands during gestation and puerperium. Am J Clin Pathol 99:13, 1993.

4

Embryonic Pathology of the Placenta

Cynthia G. Kaplan

Spontaneous pregnancy loss is a common event, affecting about one in seven recognized pregnancies[1] and at least an equivalent number of earlier unrecognized ones.[2] The vast majority of gestational loss occurs in the first trimester, and "products of conception" (POC) is one of the most common specimens in most pathology laboratories. Many articles detail involved evaluation schemes for POC,[3–14] although the value of detailed examination of such material has been questioned.[14] Often the pathologist can gain much more information for the clinician and patient than just a determination of whether or not there was an intrauterine pregnancy or trophoblastic disease. However, a complete confirmation of cause and recurrence risk may not be apparent even with the most complete evaluation. Despite any limitations, in these days of infertility and valued pregnancy much potential benefit is gained for the parents in relieving guilt and reassuring them that a particular event in their lives did not cause loss of the pregnancy.[15]

When an embryo is present, its detailed evaluation is useful in classifying the spontaneous loss. This area is well covered elsewhere.[3–17] Often, however, the embryo is disrupted or has disintegrated, leaving only the placental tissues to examine. This chapter details the evaluation and implications of placental and implantation site morphology in the first trimester. The discussion includes the spontaneous losses in the embryonic period up to 10 menstrual weeks' development, as well as their time of intrauterine retention, which is frequently prolonged.

POCs are encountered daily by most surgical pathologists and are extremely variable specimens. The contents of these similarly labeled containers range from a blood clot with scant fragments of identifiable tissue to an intact sac with embryo. The questions to be answered regarding POCs range from simply whether there is evidence of intrauterine pregnancy to the etiology of recurrent loss, identification of specific syndromes, and prediction of malignant potential. The nature of the material received greatly influences the potential for diagnosis. Obviously, more complete and well-preserved specimens lend themselves to more detailed evaluation.

Certain techniques help in the gross examination of POCs and the selection of appropriate tissue for histologic examination. Ideally the specimen is received fresh so that material for special procedures (e.g., cytogenetics, flow cytometry) can be obtained. Choosing appropriate material for histologic sampling is also simpler in the fresh state, when the loose, usually abundant blood can be removed from the tissue. The finding of an embryo, gestational sac fragments, villi, or an implantation site is generally considered diagnostic of intrauterine pregnancy and should be documented. Histologic sectioning of large amounts of loose soft clot is rarely rewarding in finding evidence of intrauterine gestation. However, granular, degenerating blood often contains villi, or material from the implantation site. Intact gestational sacs are sometimes found,[3] particularly in spontaneously passed material (Fig. 4–1*A* and *B*). They may be encased in firmer blood clot or within a decidual cast (Fig. 4–1*C*). The fragmented tissue of a suction evacuation should be separated from the loose clot and roughly sorted into fetal and nonfetal components. Nonfetal tissue is usually more abundant. Clinicians at times separate components in their own examination. Typically, villous tissue is finely papillary. It may be held together by a smooth, shiny membrane constituting

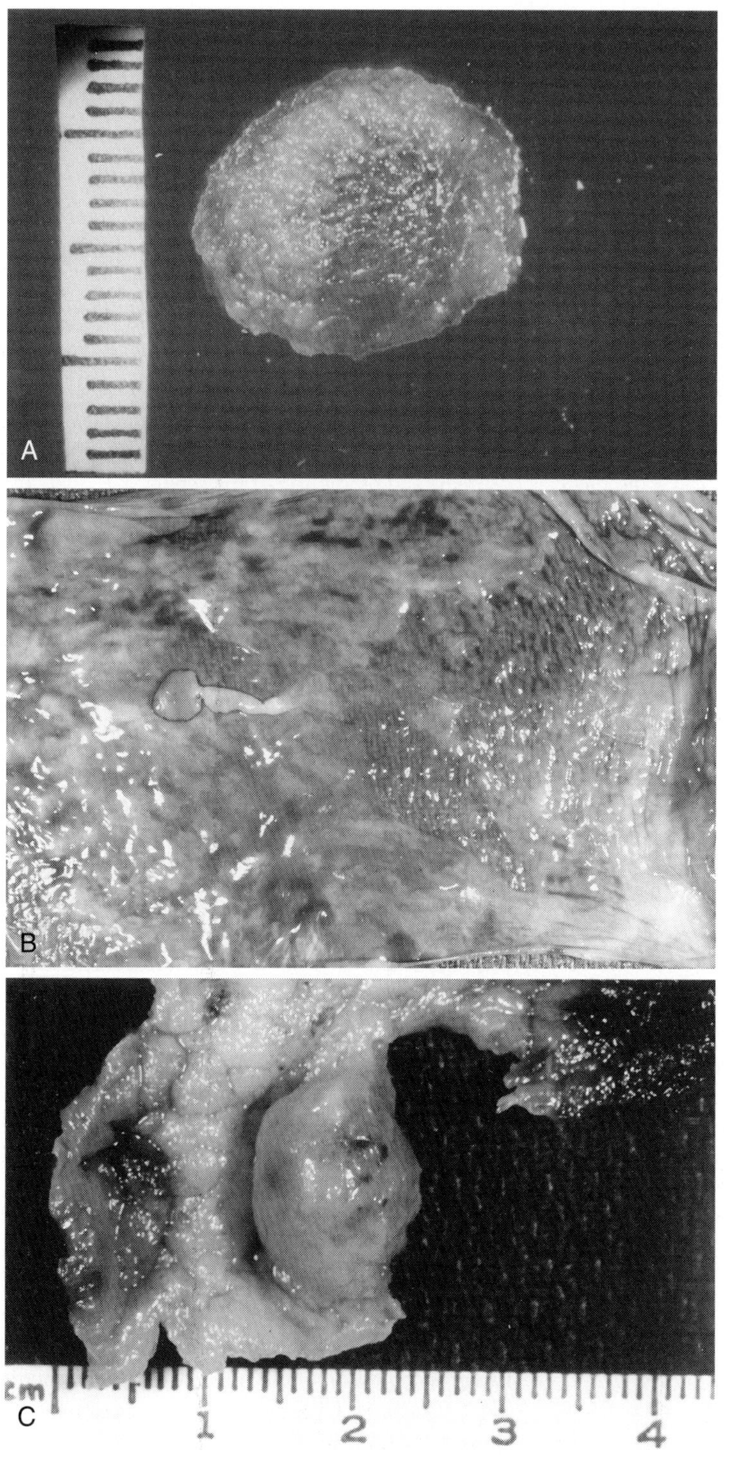

Figure 4–1. A, Intact gestational sac from a spontaneously passed abortion. The chorionic surface is completely covered by villi with early flattening in the capsular region. The sac contained a macerated growth-disorganized embryo. **B,** Opened inner surface of an intact gestational sac showing a degenerated embryonic remnant with a cord. This suggests long intrauterine retention of the specimen. Note the shiny amniotic surface and thin wall of the sac. Fragments of such when found have a similar appearance. **C,** Spontaneously passed decidual cast containing an intact embryonic sac. The decidua has a thick undulating appearance with hemorrhage at the edge. The enclosed embryo was not macerated, and an extraembryonic cause of spontaneous abortion is likely with such a specimen.

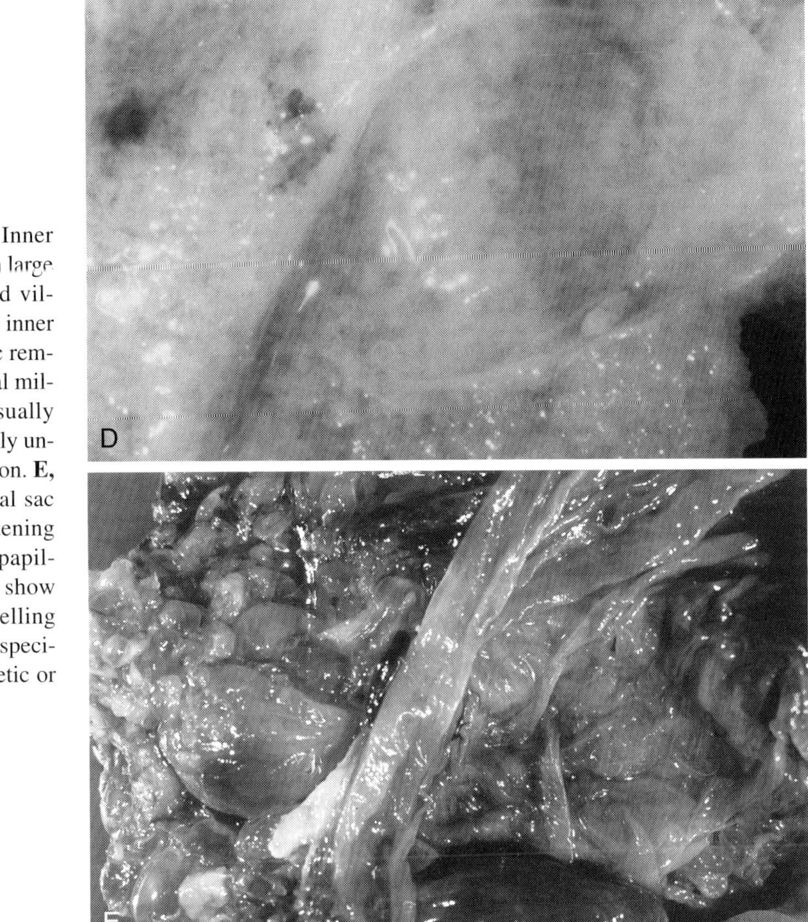

Figure 4–1 *Continued* **D,** Inner surface of gestational sac with large amount of papillary attached villous tissue. The nodule on the inner surface is probably a yolk sac remnant. Such nodules are several millimeters in diameter and usually yellow. They remain essentially unchanged for the rest of gestation. **E,** This fragment of a gestational sac shows both the smooth glistening amnion and some attached papillary villous tissue. The villi show some grossly abnormal swelling (hydrops), which makes this specimen a candidate for cytogenetic or ploidy analysis.

the remnants of the gestational sac (Fig. 4–1*D*). In both intrauterine and ectopic pregnancies a large volume of sheets of decidual and endometrial tissue is present. These tend to be smooth on one side and slightly undulating on the other, but never with the sheen of fetal membranes. They rarely contain the implantation site and do not require extensive sectioning. Fragments of gestational sac may be more visible if the specimen is suspended in saline solution. Examination under the dissecting microscope also reveals the villous character of the tissue. If cytogenetic examination is desired, villi or sac should be sent, attempting to eliminate maternal tissue. Embryonic tissue, even if present, will usually not grow. For specimens with grossly hydropic villi (Fig. 4–1*E*), flow cytometry for ploidy is most easily performed on fresh specimens. It should be recognized that although the finding of an intrauterine pregnancy markedly lessens the possibility of ectopic pregnancy, it does not eliminate it. Gross evaluation of embryos is usually much more valuable than histologic dissection.

Even in these times of cost containment, histologic examination has remained a necessary part of POC evaluation because even careful, experienced observers make errors in gross evaluation.[16] Furthermore, specimens containing only implantation site will be missed if only a gross examination is done. The number of histologic cassettes required varies with the specimen. If an obvious sac or complete or partial embryo is present, doc-

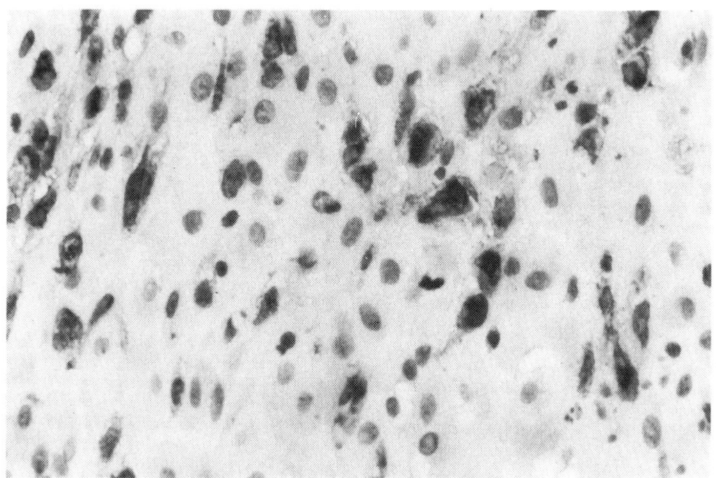

Figure 4–2. This histologic section of the implantation site has been stained for keratin. The trophoblastic cells have dark staining of the cytoplasm and can be distinguished from unstained decidual cells.

umentation of pregnancy requires only one block. However, more information about the potential etiology of pregnancy loss will be obtained if decidual tissue is also submitted to be examined for extraembryonic causes.

The presence of discrete chorionic villi is not necessary for the diagnosis of intrauterine pregnancy.[17] Identifying the region of trophoblastic implantation in the uterus is equally definitive. This consists of trophoblastic cells and typical alterations in blood vessels and stroma by the trophoblast. There is nearly always dense perivascular fibrin deposition containing the largely uninucleated and occasionally multinucleated intermediate trophoblastic cells. Vascular media are invaded and destroyed by the trophoblast, often with intraluminal mononuclear cells. At low-power magnification such areas generally stand out from bland decidual tissue and the loose fibrin of blood clot. If there is a question as to whether certain cells are trophoblastic, keratin staining can be performed. This stains the trophoblastic cells (and endometrial glandular cells as an internal control), but not decidual cells (Fig. 4–2). The pathologist should be cautious of an isolated multinucleated giant cell admixed with blood, since macrophages are frequently present from admixed cervical material. Even if a large cell was definitively trophoblastic, isolated cells (or possibly even a villus) might have been passed from an ectopic pregnancy, particularly one in the cornual region.

Pathologists have often felt compelled to search exhaustively for evidence to document intrauterine pregnancy, submitting and leveling blood clot and obvious decidual tissue in the usually futile attempt to find some implantation site or villi. Today's sensitive pregnancy tests and high-resolution ultrasound make this largely unnecessary, and discussions with the clinician before undertaking such extensive sectioning are appropriate.

DEVELOPMENTAL FEATURES

The detailed normal aspects of development of the placenta are considered elsewhere in this text. In evaluating a spontaneous abortion it is important to assess where the abortion fits in relation to normal development and the clinical history. This is done largely through histology, and even scant specimens containing a few villi may be quite informative. The presence of certain features gives the minimal time of development at the time of the loss (Table 4–1).

Trophoblastic cells have differentiated and begun endometrial invasion by the end of the first week of development, and syncytiotrophoblastic lacunar networks have formed by 12 developmental days. Primary placental villi and the secondary yolk sac have formed by 2 developmental weeks (4 menstrual weeks), with ingrowth of mesenchyme (secondary villi) early in week 3 (5 menstrual weeks). These villi cover the entire surface of the chorionic

Table 4–1. Morphologic Markers Useful for Dating Placental Tissue in First-Trimester Spontaneous Abortions

Developmental/Menstrual Age (Weeks)	Morphologic Feature
12 days/3½	Syncytiotrophoblastic lacunar network
2/4	Primary villi of cytotrophoblast and syncytiotrophoblast, secondary yolk sac
3/5 (early)	Secondary villi with mesenchymal cores
3/5 (late)	Tertiary villi with vasculature
3–4/5–6	Yolk sac hematopoiesis established
4½/6½	Yolk sac nucleated erythrocytes in placental capillaries
6–7/8–9	Nonnucleated erythrocytes from liver beginning to replace nucleated erythrocytes
9/11	Yolk sac present as remnant
10/12	Essentially all nonnucleated red blood cells circulating

Data from references 11 and 18 to 20.

sac. Some mesenchymal cells in the villi differentiate into vessels that fuse to form arteriocapillary networks during the third week of development (tertiary villi). Hematopoiesis and blood vessel development are seen in the yolk sac at the end of that week, and circulation begins.[17] Red blood cells derived from the yolk sac are all nucleated; only as the liver and other mesenchymal tissues in the embryo begin to take over this function in the fifth week (7 menstrual weeks) do nonnucleated red blood cells appear.[11,18,19] Thus the finding of remnants of blood vessels in villi indicates development to 5 menstrual weeks and the finding of nucleated red blood cells dates the development to 6½ weeks. By the percentage of nucleated red cells, the pathologist can estimate gestational age until essentially all red blood cells are nonnucleated at 12 menstrual weeks. The yolk sac becomes a well-delineated structure largely separate from the embryonic tissues at approximately 4 weeks (6 menstrual weeks). By 9 weeks (11 menstrual weeks) it has shrunk to a 3 to 5 mm remnant lying between the amnion and chorion.[17] Another temporally specific event is the apposition of the amnion and chorion, which occurs at about 10 weeks.[7]

Even though no embryo is found in many POCs, its existence can be postulated from the placental tissue. Villous stroma is derived from the extraembryonic mesenchyme, which in turn comes from the primary embryonic tissue.[11,17] Thus the presence of villous stroma indicates that embryonic tissue was once present but has disintegrated. More advanced embryonic development is often accompanied by stunted or disorganized remnants, but even these may disintegrate with time. The remnant of the secondary yolk sac is frequently identifiable without the embryo (Figs. 4–1*D* and 4–3).[20]

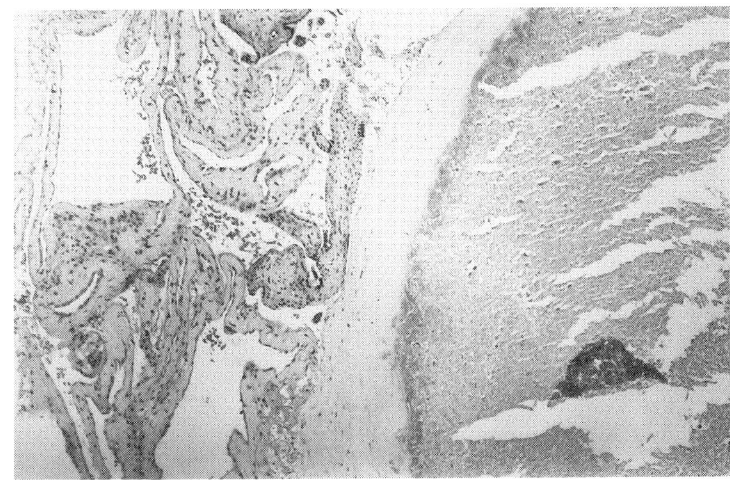

Figure 4–3. Yolk sac remnants are calcified debris lying between the amnion and chorion. Here such a nodule lies adjacent to loose fragments of amnion with a flattened surface layer.

MORPHOLOGIC CHANGES IN EMBRYONIC DEATH

Whether the gestation was viable at the time of the loss is a key feature to evaluate in POCs. Extraembryonic causes of early pregnancy loss (e.g., abnormal hormonal function of the corpus luteum, abnormal uterine form, abnormal endometrial function) tend to lead to nonmacerated specimens with well-developed embryos, while intrinsic embryonic causes are associated with intrauterine death and long retention, classically 3 to 4 weeks before spontaneous passage.[7,11] This natural time course is now frequently altered by the rapid ultrasound recognition of nonviability and immediate evacuation of the pregnancy, so that changes are often less striking.

Understanding the expected changes with intrauterine demise is an important part of the evaluation of any spontaneous abortion specimen. Degenerative changes occur rapidly in the embryo (Fig. 4–4). Placental changes occur more slowly and may show considerable variability with location. Rushton[10] and Szulman[11,12] have made important contributions in classification.

Rushton[10] divided specimens into three categories based largely on placental characteristics: blighted ova (group 1), macerated fetuses (group 2), and nonmacerated fetuses (group 3). The mean gestational age of group 1 was 11.4 menstrual weeks. These are typically intact or ruptured sacs, 1 cm or more in diameter and partially or totally covered by villi. Cystic villi are clearly present under the dissecting microscope and occasionally can be seen grossly. Histologic examination shows a variable proportion of hydropic villi and ones with stromal fibrosis and vascular obliteration. The difference between the two patterns is believed to relate to the time of the disturbance in development. Before the establishment of the extraembryonic circulation the villi become hydropic. The fibrous pattern results from problems after vascularization. Intermediate patterns exist with partial vascularization. The capsular villi generally do not become vascularized in any circumstance and thus always become hydropic eventually. To assess the developmental age at embryonic death, the pathologist needs to look for the most advanced region and recognize that incomplete specimens may give falsely low developmental ages, since the more central villi may not be represented.

Hydropic villi are characterized by loose, sometimes cystic stroma with rudimentary or absent blood vessels (Fig. 4–5*A*). The trophoblast is attenuated with loss of the inner cytotrophoblast, although occasional villi are still capped by trophoblast. This morphology is most commonly associated with an empty sac. The second pattern is smaller villi that may show two-layered trophoblast (Fig. 4–5*B*). Blood vessels are present and may contain nucleated red blood cells, but most often these are collapsed or undergoing obliteration (Fig. 4–5*C* to *E*).

Szulman[11,12] believes that the failure of fluid drainage from the villi leads to hydropic change.

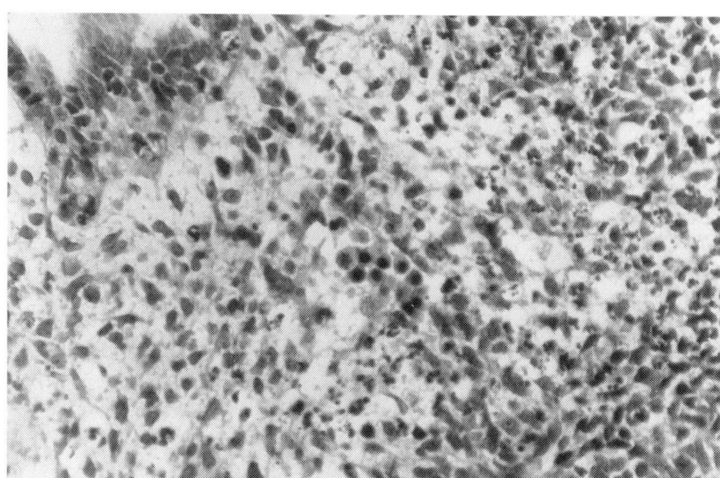

Figure 4–4. Although this pregnancy appeared nonmacerated on gross examination, intrauterine death had been diagnosed by ultrasound and nuclear fragmentation in the embryonic remnant is confirmatory.

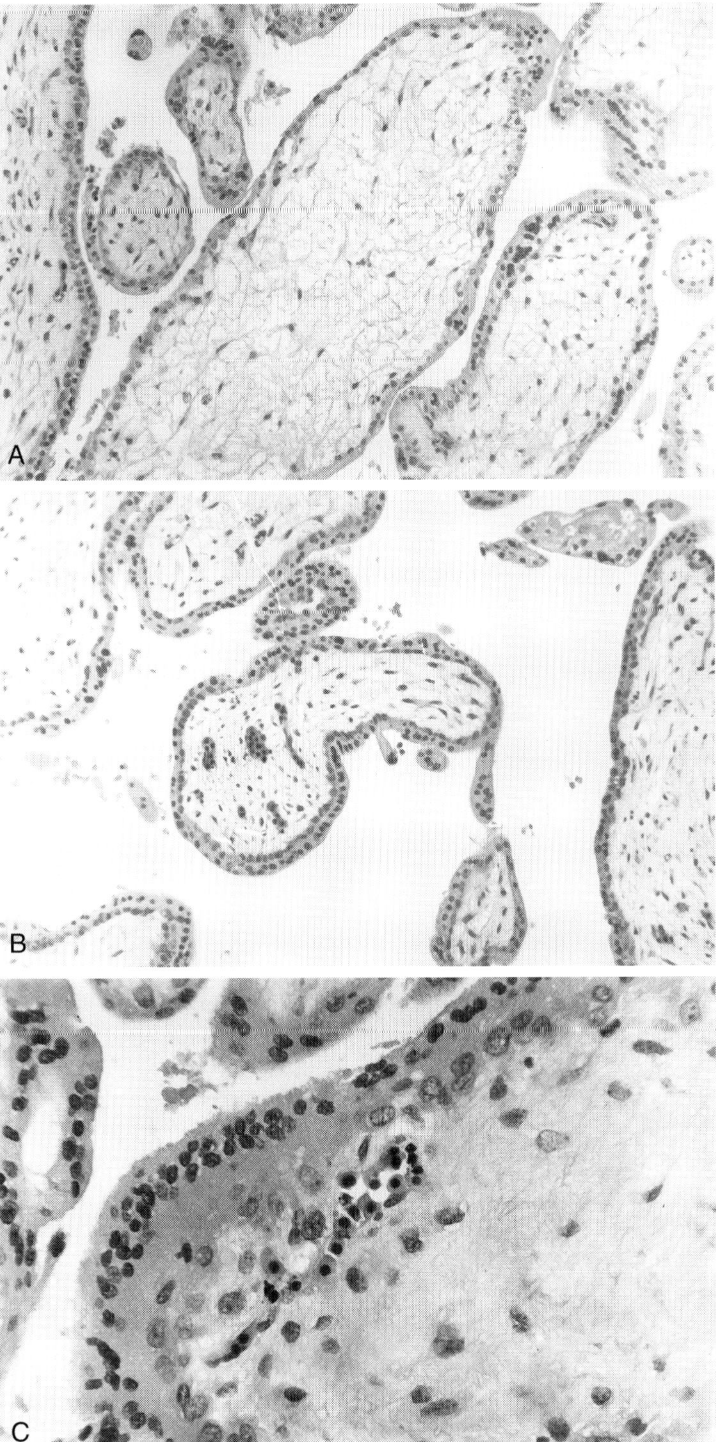

Figure 4–5. A, Typical hydrops and edema in a spontaneous abortion have led to the round, simple outlines. Macrophages with edema can be identified in the stroma. No vessels were noted in the majority of villi, although one villus at the far left does show a few collapsed, empty vessels. **B,** Low-power view of normal-appearing chorionic villi with all nucleated red blood cells and two-layered trophoblast with sprouts. Degenerative changes are minimal. **C,** Well-developed capillaries showing all nucleated red blood cells and surface cytotrophoblast and syncytiotrophoblast. Degenerative changes are minimal.
Illustration continued on following page

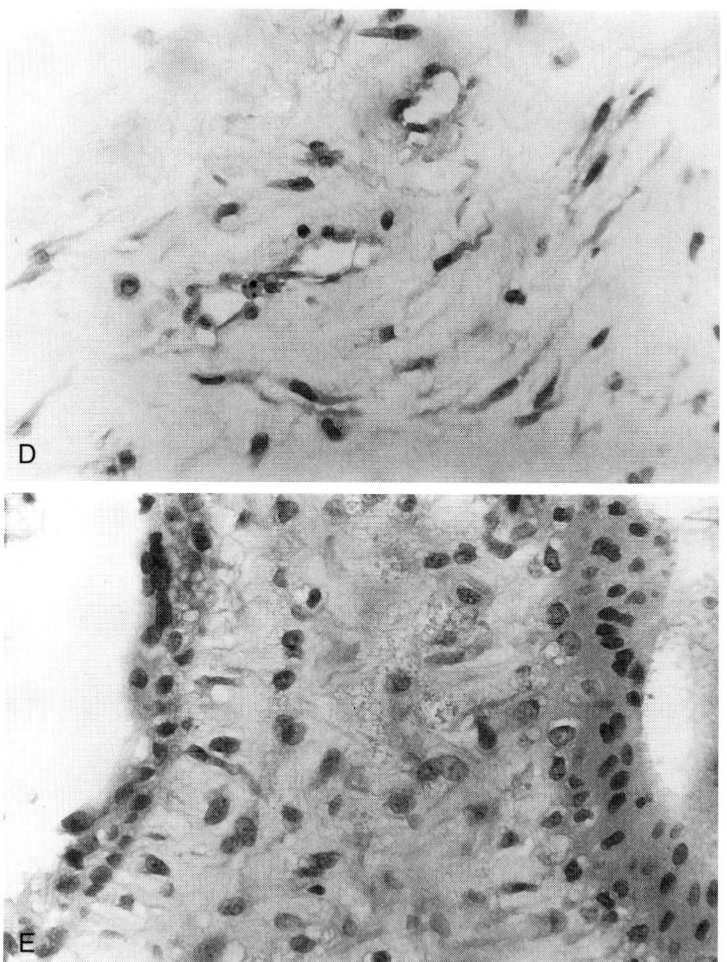

Figure 4–5 *Continued* **D,** Villous stroma showing remnant blood vessels with a single degenerating nucleated red blood cell. This indicates that development proceeded to at least 6½ weeks' menstrual age. **E,** The small fragments represent remnants of degenerated red blood cells and appeared eosinophilic. Note the relatively well-preserved trophoblast despite this change of long-standing death.

With embryonic death, drainage through capillaries ceases and the fluid pumped into the villus through the still viable trophoblast remains. The blood vessels recede rapidly in such cases. Hydropic spontaneous abortuses are usually empty sacs, with embryonic death having occurred before 6 to 7 menstrual weeks. Fibrosis of the villous mesenchyme develops when the embryo dies after 7 to 8 menstrual weeks. Erythrocytes are trapped within vessels and eventually degenerate. The time of development can be assessed by the proportion of cells with and without nuclei.

Developmental dating is particularly useful for recurrent abortions, in which timing of the loss may be important. It must be remembered that the degenerative changes in the capsular region and margin lead to variability in morphology (Fig. 4–5 *F* and *G*). Such varied villous appearance may also be explained by multiple gestations with varying time of death.

CYTOGENETIC ABNORMALITIES

Cytogenetic abnormalities are well recognized to occur in 50% of early spontaneous abortions. These are predominantly trisomy (27%), polyploidy (10%), and monosomy X (9%). Trisomy 16 is the most frequently occurring trisomy, about one third.[16] Taking into account the spontaneous abortion population consisting of empty sacs, growth-disordered embryos, and those with local defects, the incidence of abnormal karyotypes increases to 60% to 80% (Fig. 4–6).[6] Probably a

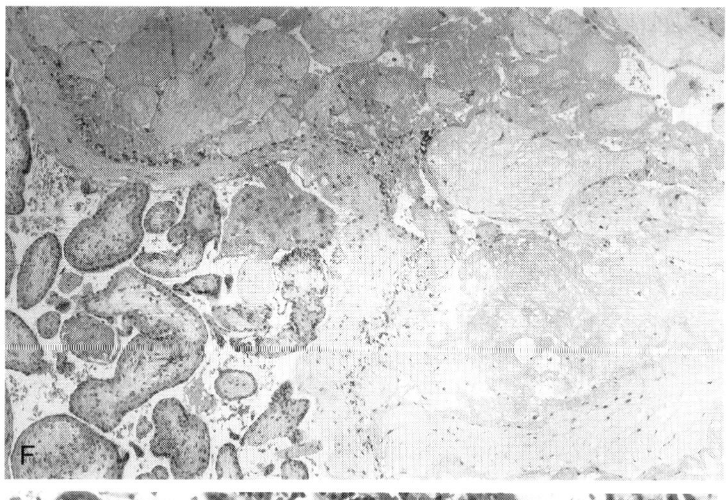

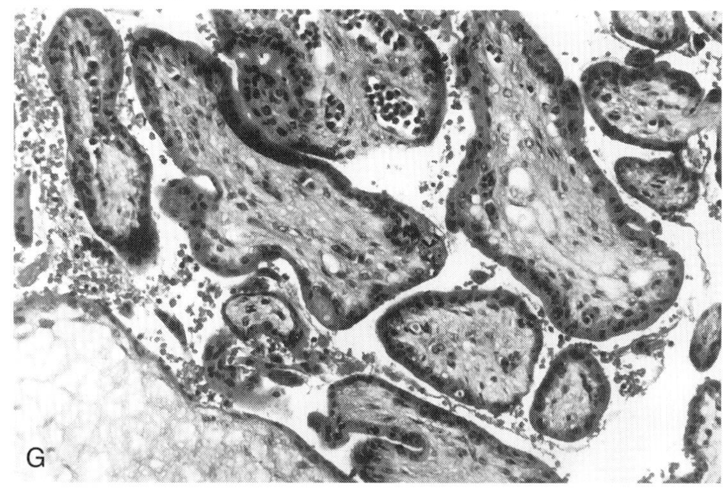

Figure 4–5 *Continued* **F,** Typical low-power view of a gestational sac fragment. The villi are quite variable. Some hydropic ones are ghosted and atrophic, while others have more cellular detail. As the early sac enlarges, the peripheral villi develop poorly and atrophy, leading to this appearance. The variability in the villous tissue makes wide sampling necessary. **G,** This specimen shows largely well-vascularized villi with all nucleated red blood cells. A portion of a typically hydropic villus is present in the lower left corner. This was thought to be related to capsular villi, not a second gestation.

substantial portion of the remaining specimens that have this gross morphology but are not obviously abnormal have other molecular abnormalities. Thus, finding a placental morphology associated with fetal death in a spontaneous abortion, the pathologist can predict with reasonable likelihood the presence of a chromosomal abnormality without actual karyotype. The incidence of such karyotypic abnormality in future pregnancies is either random or, for trisomies, related to maternal age.[21,22] Thus little true clinical value is gained from chromosomal analysis in an isolated spontaneous abortion, although information about what happened in the pregnancy may be important to the family and their grieving. As newer techniques become more widely available, they may simplify the analysis of karyotypes in spontaneous abortion. In situ studies in interphase nuclei for just the three chromosomes 16, X, and Y identify many trisomies, triploidy, and monosomy X.[7]

The issue of when the precise cytogenetic abnormality can be determined by the morphology of the placental tissue in a spontaneous abortion has long been debated in the literature.[8,9,23–30] A variety of features have been evaluated in an attempt to predict karyotype. These have included degree of hydropic change, fibrosis of villi, developmental arrest, intravillous cytotrophoblast, trophoblastic hyperplasia, villous profile and size, vascularization, erythrocytes, and regressive changes. The reliability of their identification by different observers has also been addressed, and poor correlation has been found in some cases.[29,30]

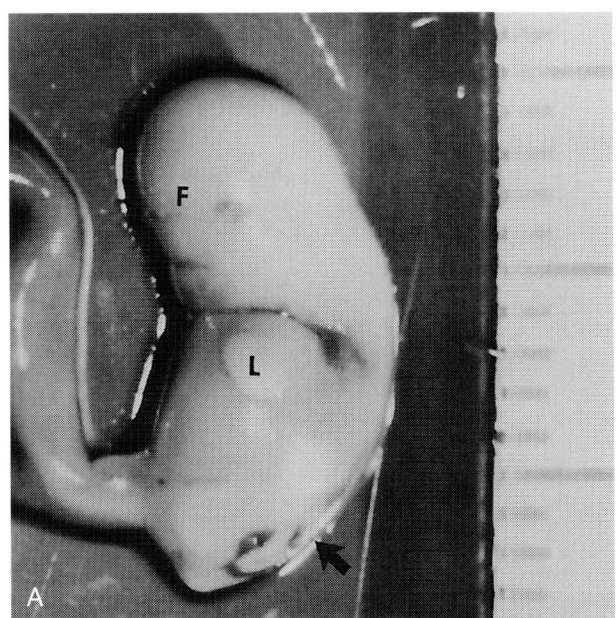

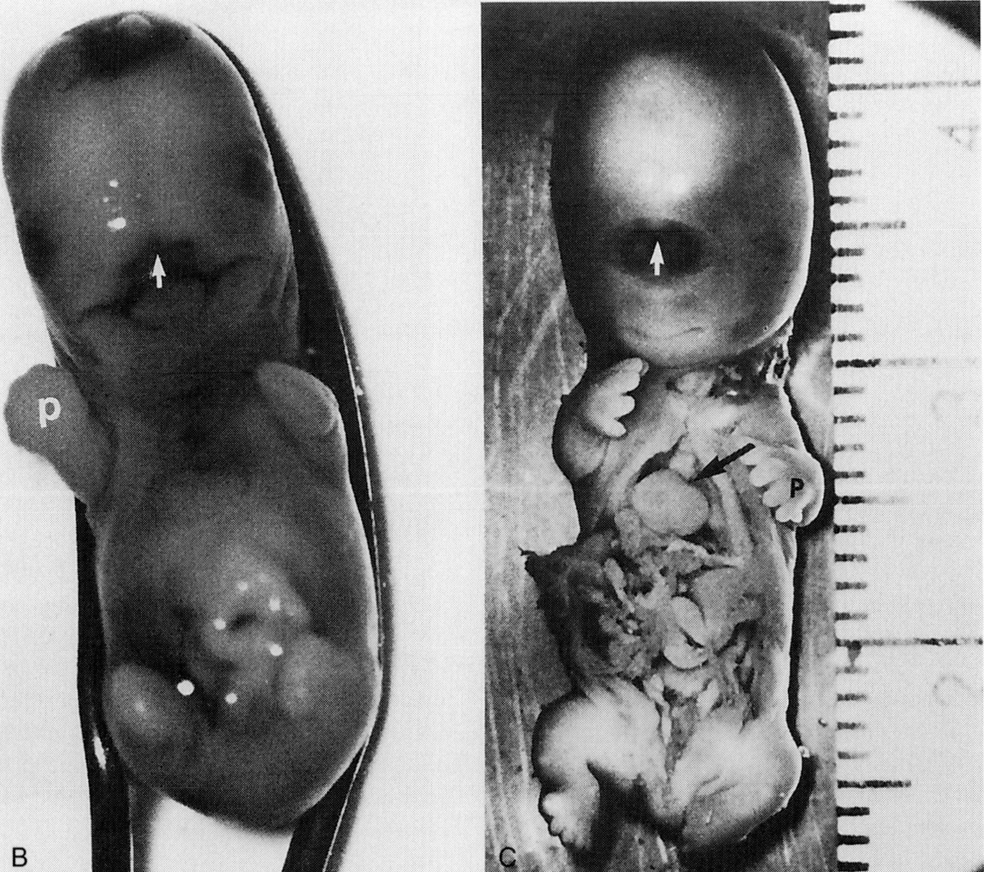

Figure 4–6. A, Triploid embryo showing retarded development of limbs *(L),* facial dysplasia *(F),* and lower spine neural tube defect *(arrow).* **B** and **C,** Trisomy D phenotype with facial clefting (*white arrow,* **B**), as well as polydactyly (*p,* **B** and **C**), cyclopia (*white arrow,* **C**), and abnormal heart development (*black arrow,* **C**).

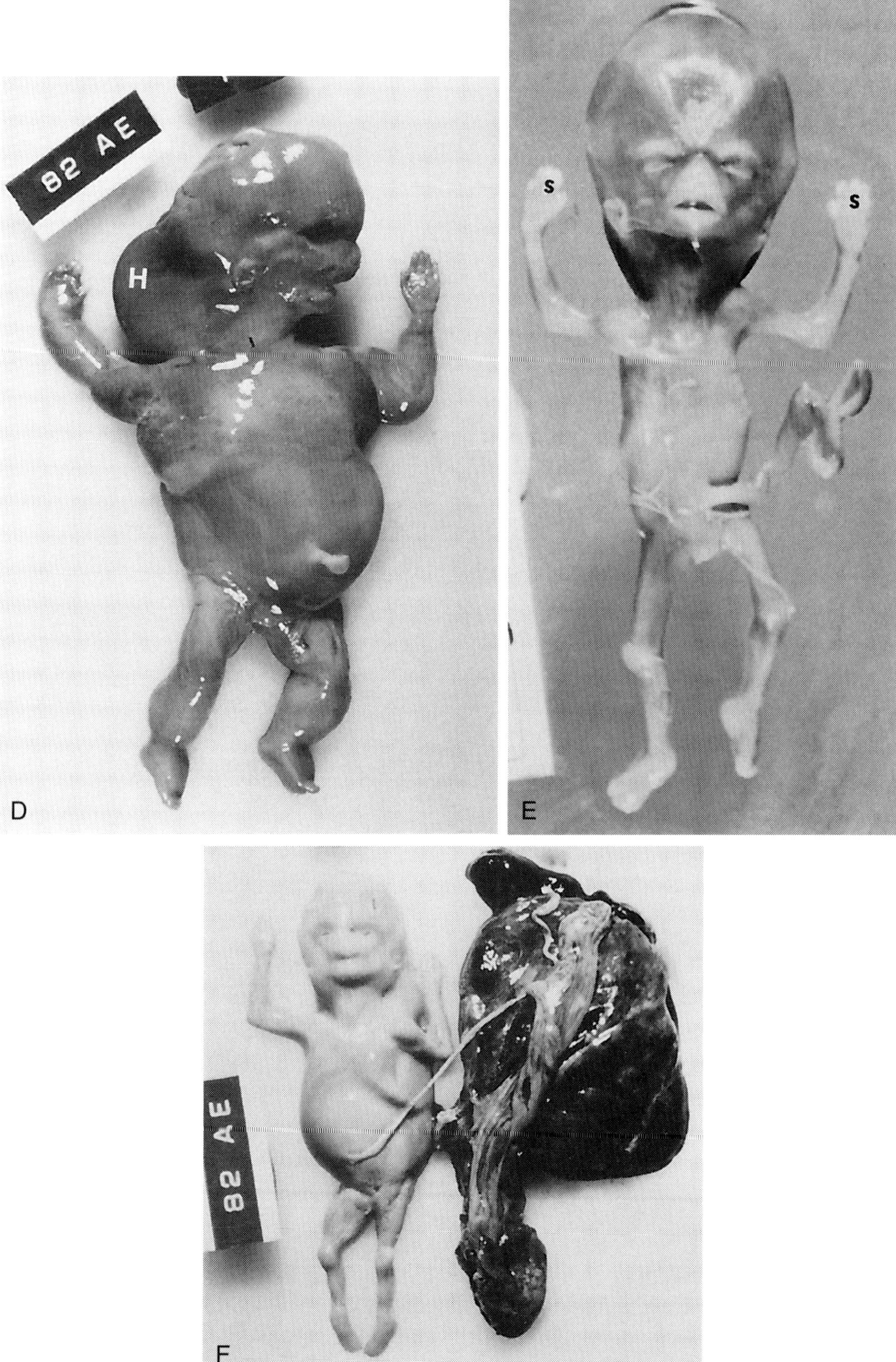

Figure 4–6 *Continued* **D,** Macerated female fetus of 14 developmental weeks showing generalized subcutaneous edema and posterior cervical hygroma *(H).* 45,X must be suspected. **E,** Macerated male fetus (69,XXY) of 12½ developmental weeks showing severe intrauterine growth retardation, a large head, and syndactyly *(S)* of the third and fourth fingers of both hands. **F,** Macerated female fetus of 12 developmental weeks with documented trisomy 18. Because of maceration, some typical features of trisomy 18 are missing, such as overlapping fingers (Courtesy Dagmar Kalousek, Vancouver, British Columbia.)

Most recent reports agree that except for triploidy, a specific abnormal karyotype cannot be predicted from the placental morphology,[23–30] and many spontaneous abortions that are found to be triploid do not show the distinctive features of cisterns and villous dysmorphism with scalloping. The other commonly identified villous changes are related merely to the time and duration of fetal demise. Since trisomies are so frequent in spontaneous abortions, it is not surprising that a nonspecific association exists.

The ability to predict a normal karyotype from morphology would also be a useful tool, since women who have had a spontaneous abortion may have subsequent reproductive problems.[28,29] Fetal anucleate erythrocytes, the presence of an umbilical cord, less villous hydrops, infarcts, and chronic inflammation have been associated with a normal karyotype. These relate to more advanced development in many karyotypically normal spontaneous abortions and continued circulation. However, some aneuploidies, particularly those considered more viable, share these histologic features. A study of spontaneous and induced trisomic abortions found similar differences, believed to be due largely to circulatory status at the time of the abortion.[31]

Confined placental mosaicism may occur when mitotic errors during early development lead to variations in karyotype between the fetus and the placenta.[32,33] If only placental tissue is cultured, this possibility must be kept in mind when evaluating the results. While confined placental mosaicism is clearly associated with intrauterine growth restriction and probably with late spontaneous abortions, its role in early losses is unclear.

OTHER CAUSES OF EARLY SPONTANEOUS ABORTION

Multiple Gestation

The rate of twinning in spontaneous abortions has been found to be three times that of liveborns. Spontaneously aborted twin embryos are virtually all monozygotic, and nearly all show abnormal development.[34] Many twin pregnancies are converted to singletons with early demise of one twin, as detected by ultrasound. Such very early losses may be undetectable at delivery or merely appear as a thickened plaque suggesting old hemorrhage on the membranes.

Infection

The role of infection is less well documented in first-trimester loss than in preterm delivery and second-trimester spontaneous abortion. Infection probably accounts for less than 5% of first-trimester losses.[35] Organisms such as *Ureaplasma* have been cultured with more frequency in patients with spontaneous abortion,[36] but specific histologic correlates have not been identified. Chronic and acute inflammatory patterns are commonly seen in patients with both positive and negative cultures (Fig. 4–7*A*). No serologic associations have been found with *Chlamydia*.[37] Plasma cell endometritis may reflect latent infection leading to spontaneous abortion.[38] HIV-positive patients were found to have an increased incidence of spontaneous abortion in one study.[39] Occasional specimens may show clear evidence of viral infection as with cytomegalovirus[40] (Fig. 4–7*B*) or bacteria such as *Listeria*[41] (Fig. 4–7*C*), but this is unusual.

Implantation Site and Endocrine Abnormalities

Proper functioning of the trophoblast is necessary for the maintenance of pregnancy. The trophoblast helps maintain the endocrine milieu, initiates implantation, and invades uterine vessels. Reduced trophoblastic penetration into decidua and spiral arteries has been found in the majority of spontaneously expelled spontaneous abortions.[42] The trophoblastic columns are thinner in such cases. Physiologic vascular changes may be absent[28] (Fig. 4–8). This is possibly related to maternal hypertensive disorders or genetic abnormalities in the embryo.

Aberrations in the maternal hormonal milieu in pregnancy are known to lead to spontaneous abortion, and the endometrial pathology related to luteal phase defects is well described.[43] Specific placental changes have not been noted. The association of stress with karyotypically normal gesta-

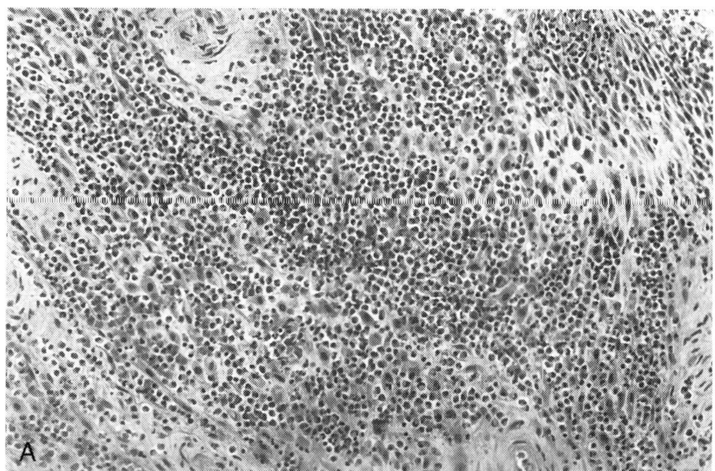

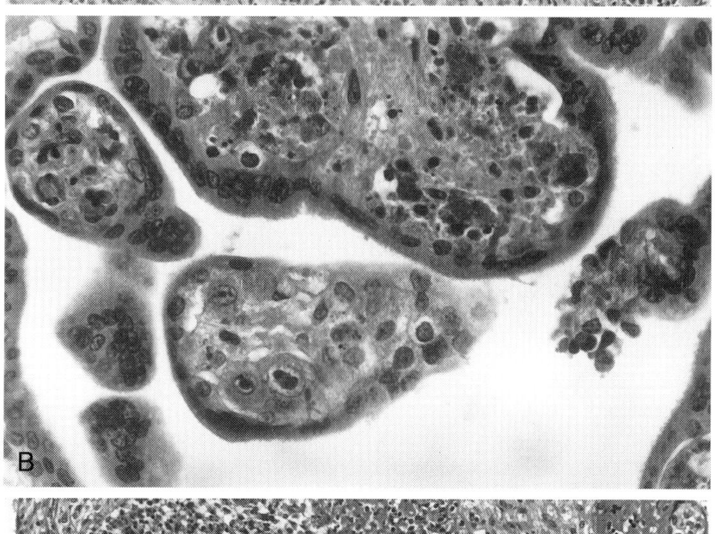

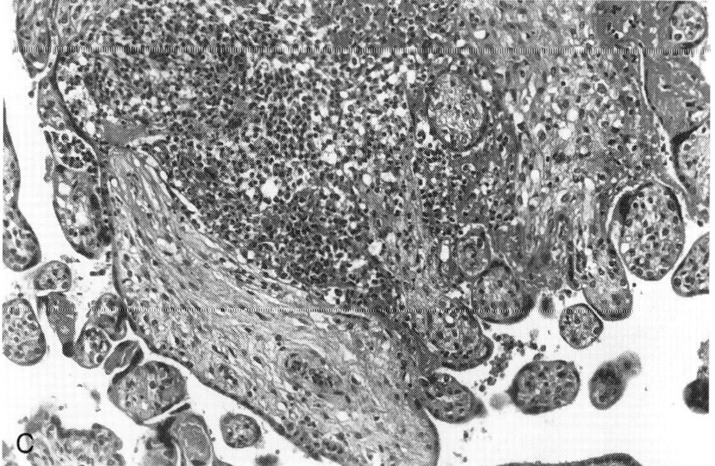

Figure 4–7. A, Portion of decidual tissue from a spontaneous abortion revealing a chronic inflammatory infiltrate. These changes are commonly found in such specimens and are not indicative of infection. **B,** Late first-trimester villi showing increased numbers of stromal cells and areas of necrosis. Typical cytomegalovirus inclusions are present. **C,** Villous microabscess showing necrosis and infiltration by numerous neutrophils. This pattern is typical of *Listeria* but may be seen with other maternal septicemic processes.

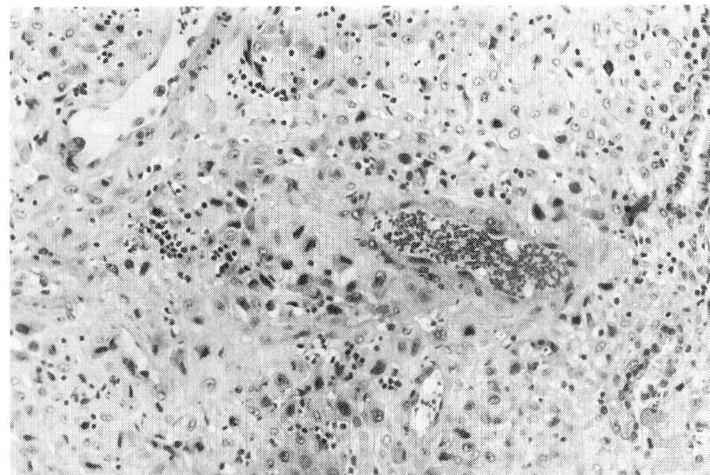

Figure 4–8. The decidual tissue from the implantation site is intermixed with numerous trophoblastic cells. The blood-filled vessel, however, still shows muscle in the wall and no trophoblastic invasion, an abnormal implantation site.

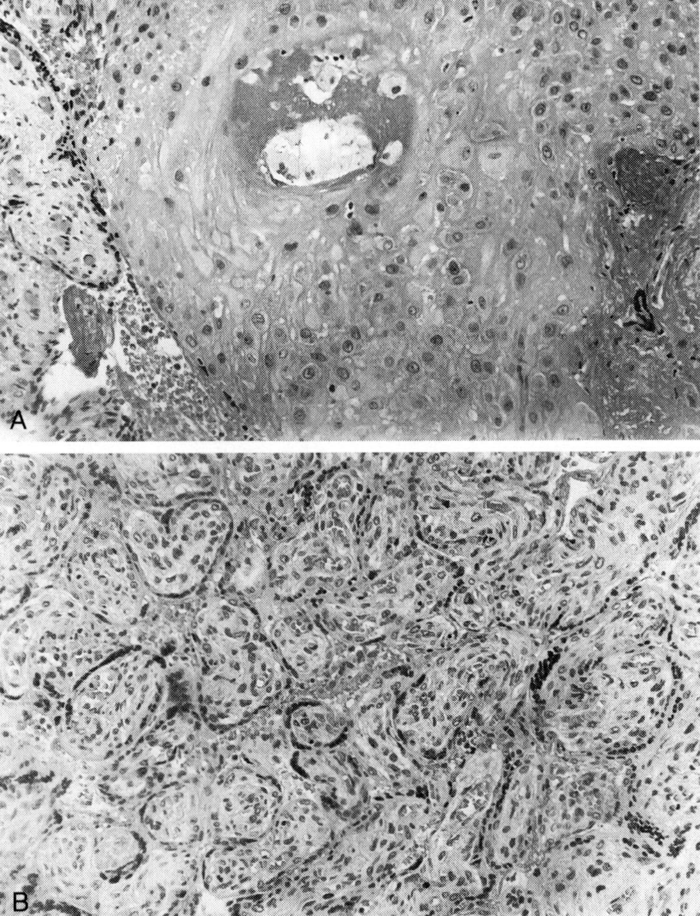

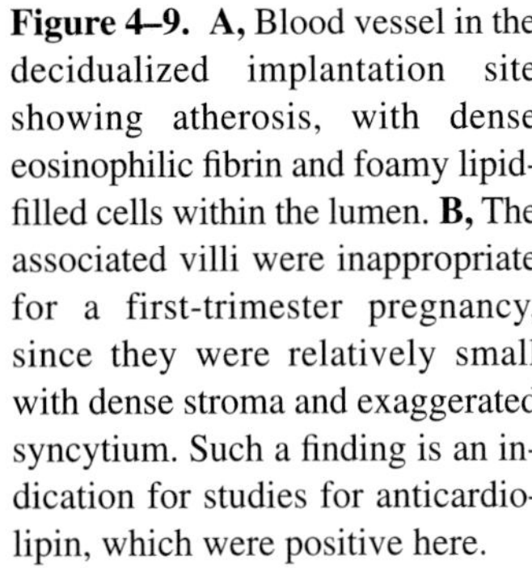

Figure 4–9. A, Blood vessel in the decidualized implantation site showing atherosis, with dense eosinophilic fibrin and foamy lipid-filled cells within the lumen. **B,** The associated villi were inappropriate for a first-trimester pregnancy, since they were relatively small with dense stroma and exaggerated syncytium. Such a finding is an indication for studies for anticardiolipin, which were positive here.

tions may indicate a hormonal role in these losses.[44]

Ectopic Pregnancy

Most ectopic pregnancies are lost in the first trimester, when the trophoblastic invasion of the abnormal site leads to symptoms. Some ectopic gestations are due to tubal structural abnormalities, but probably many are related to abnormal endocrine function of the mother or conceptus. The villous morphology depends largely on the state of the embryonic tissue at removal, since some are viable and others have died. Spontaneous abortion of ectopic pregnancies occurs for reasons similar to those in the uterus. Methotrexate treatment alters the morphology, limiting cytotrophoblastic proliferation with diminished trophoblastic spread, differentiation, and invasion.[45]

Immunologic Abnormalities

The literature contains considerable data relating to immunologic abnormalities associated with spontaneous abortion.[7,46] Information on pathologic changes in these areas is scant, dealing more with immunologic marking of cells in the decidua than placental morphology.[47] An exception is anticardiolipin antibodies. The vascular changes in the maternal decidual blood vessels and the ischemic villous morphology are well recognized.[41] While immunologic abnormalities are more often a problem after the first trimester, some early gestational loss has been recognized (Fig. 4–9). Heritable thrombotic disorders are currently being evaluated in their relationship to pregnancy loss. Again, much of this occurs after the first trimester.[48]

HABITUAL ABORTION

Habitual abortion is characterized by three or more consecutive spontaneous abortions. A variety of associated factors, including anatomic, structural genetic, hormonal, autoimmune, and infectious, can be identified currently in 60% of couples.[38]

Balanced translocations or other structural genetic defects in the parents cause less than 5% of cases. Even if the abortus is found to have an appropriate karyotypic abnormality, cytogenetic studies of the parents are still necessary to establish whether the translocation is related to them or occurred de novo. There is no increase in other karyotypic abnormalities in this population.[49,50]

A normal karyotype in the pregnancy (or inferred from parental karyotypes) suggests a hormonal, infectious, or immunologic problem or some other recurrent process known to be associated with spontaneous abortion. In abortions caused by teratogens or lethal microscopic genetic defects, karyotypes are also normal.

EARLY AND LATE FETAL LOSS

Spontaneous and induced fetal losses occurring from the late first through the early third trimester show a vast array of fetal and neonatal pathology. The fetus should be evaluated in the format of a mini-autopsy. The gestational age should be assessed (Table 4–2), the fetus should be evaluated for morphologic abnormalities (external and internal), and appropriate cytogenetic (as described above) and microbiologic studies should be performed. A description of the pathologic alterations affecting the fetus is beyond the scope of this text. For a more in-depth discussion the reader is referred elsewhere.[51]

The placentas usually demonstrate the pathologic findings found in later gestations, which are described throughout this text. The spectrum of findings can be summarized as follows: lesions affecting the umbilical cord (including abnormal length, inflammation, infection, spiraling and torsion, vascular rupture, thrombosis, and single umbilical artery) (see Chapter 5), the membranes (including inflammation, infection, amnion nodosum, chronic rupture, amnionic bands or complexes, and chorionic vascular thrombosis) (see Chapter 6), the villi (including infarction, intervillous thrombi, maternal floor infarction, partial molar change, edema, inflammation, infection, and fibrosis) (see Chapter 7), and the decidua (including inflammation, infection, retroplacental hemorrhage, and decidual vasculopathy) (see Chapter 8).

Table 4–2. Developmental Age of Fetus Estimated from Hand and Foot Lengths

Developmental Age (Weeks)	Hand Length (mm)	Foot Length (mm)
11	10 ± 2	12 ± 2
12	15 ± 2	17 ± 3
13	18 ± 1	19 ± 1
14	19 ± 1	22 ± 2
15	20 ± 3	25 ± 3
16	26 ± 2	28 ± 2
17	27 ± 3	29 ± 4
18	29 ± 2	33 ± 2
19	32 ± 2	36 ± 1

Modified from MacBride M, Baillie J, Poland B: Growth parameters in normal fetuses. Teratology 29:185, 1984.

CONCLUSION

Thorough gross and microscopic examination of early spontaneous abortions can be readily accomplished by the pathologist. Information gleaned includes confirmation of intrauterine pregnancy and precise time of embryonic death. Some assessment as to etiology can be made on morphologic grounds, based on knowledge of common events. Cytogenetic studies of the material yield additional information. This is most likely to have clinical utility in cases of recurrent loss. Early spontaneous abortion has many nonkaryotypic causes that are significantly less common.

REFERENCES

1. Warburton D, Fraser CF: Spontaneous abortion risks in man: data from reproductive histories collected in a medical genetics center. Am J Hum Genet 16:1, 1964.
2. Ellish NJ, Saboda K, O'Connor J, et al: A prospective study of early pregnancy loss. Human Reprod 11:406, 1996.
3. Poland BJ, Miller JR, Harris M, Livingston J: Spontaneous abortion: a study of 1961 women and their conceptuses. Acta Obstet Gynecol Scand Suppl 102:1, 1981.
4. Laurini RN: Abortion from a morphological viewpoint. In Huisjes HJ, Lind T (eds): Early pregnancy failure. New York, 1990, Churchill Livingston, p 79.
5. Novak RW, Malone JM, Robinson HB: The role of the pathologist in the evaluation of first trimester abortion. Pathol Annu 25:297, 1990.
6. Kalousek DK, Pantzar, Tsai M, Paradice B: Early spontaneous abortion: morphologic and karyotypic findings in 3912 cases. Birth Defects 29:53, 1993.
7. Kalousek DK: Pathology of abortion: the embryo and the previable fetus. In Gilbert-Barness E (ed): Potter's pathology of the fetus and infant. St. Louis, 1997, Mosby, p 106.
8. Philippe E, Boue J: Le placenta dans les aberrations chromosomiques lethales. Ann Anat Pathol 14:249, 1969.
9. Honore LH, Dill FJ, Poland BJ: Placental morphology in spontaneous human abortuses with normal and abnormal karyotypes. Teratology 14:151, 1976.
10. Rushton DI: The classification and mechanism of spontaneous abortion. Perspect Pediatr Pathol 8:269, 1984.
11. Szulman AE: Examination of the early conceptus. Arch Pathol Lab Med 115:696, 1991.
12. Szulman AE: Embryonic death: pathology and forensic implications. Perspect Pediatr Pathol 19:43, 1995.
13. Wolf GC, Horger EO: Indications for examination of spontaneous abortion specimens: a reassessment. Am J Obstet Gynecol 173:1364, 1995.
14. Fox H: Histologic classification of tissue from spontaneous abortions: a valueless exercise? Histopathology 22:599, 1993.
15. Frost M, Condon JT: The psychologic sequelae of miscarriage: a critical review of the literature. Aust NZ J Psychiatry 30:54, 1996.
16. Heatley MK, Clark J: The value of histopathologic examination of conceptual products. Br J Obstet Gynaecol 102:256, 1995.
17. O'Connor DM, Kurman RJ: Intermediate trophoblast in uterine curetting in the diagnosis of ectopic pregnancy. Obstet Gynecol 72:665, 1988.
18. Thompson EL: Time and rate of loss of nuclei by red blood cells of human embryos. Anat Rec 111:317, 1951.
19. Salafia CM, Weigl CA, Foye GJ: Correlation of placental erythrocyte morphology and gestational age. Pediatr Pathol 8:495, 1988.
20. Moore KL, Persaud TVN: The developing human, 5th ed. Philadelphia, 1993, WB Saunders.
21. Boue J, Boue A, Lazar P: Retrospective and prospective epidemiologic studies of 1500 karyotypes from spontaneous human abortions. Teratology 12:11, 1975.
22. Warburton D, Kline J, Stein Z, et al: Does the karyotype of a spontaneous abortion predict the karyotype of a subsequent abortus? Evidence from 271 women with 2 karyotyped spontaneous abortions. Am J Hum Genet 41:465, 1987.
23. Rehder H, Coerdt W, Eggers R, et al: Is there a correlation between morphologic and cytogenetic find-

ing in placental tissue from early missed abortions? Hum Genet 82:377, 1989.
24. Novak R, Agamanolis D, Dasu S, et al: Histologic analysis of placental tissue in first trimester abortions. Pediatr Pathol 8:477, 1988.
25. Van Lijnschoten G, Arends JW, Leffers P, et al: The value of histomorphological features of chorionic villi in early spontaneous abortion for the prediction of karyotype. Histopathology 22:557, 1993.
26. Van Lijnschoten G, Arends JW, Thunnissen FBJM, Geraedts JPM: A morphometric approach to the relation of karyotype, gestational age and histologic features in early spontaneous abortions. Placenta 15:189, 1994.
27. Minguillon C, Eiben B, Bahr-Porsch S, et al: The predictive value of chorionic villus histology for identifying chromosomally normal and abnormal spontaneous abortions. Hum Genet 82:373, 1989.
28. Salafia C, Maier D, Vogel C, et al: Placental and decidual histology in spontaneous abortions: detailed description and correlations with chromosome number. Obstet Gynecol 82:295, 1993.
29. Genest DR, Roberts D, Boyd T, Bieber F: Fetoplacental histology as a predictor of karyotype: a controlled study of spontaneous first trimester abortions. Hum Pathol 26:201, 1995.
30. Van Lijnschoten G, Arends JW, de la Fuente AA, et al: Intra- and inter- observer variation in interpretation of histological features suggesting chromosomal abnormality in early abortion specimens. Histopathology 22:25, 1993.
31. Van Lijnschoten G, Arends JW, Geraedts JPM: Comparison of histological features in early spontaneous and induced trisomic abortions. Placenta 15:765, 1994.
32. Kalousek DK: Confined placental mosaicism and intrauterine development. Pediatr Pathol 10:69, 1990.
33. Kalousek DK: The effect of confined placental mosaicism on the development of the human aneuploid conceptus. Birth Defects 29:39, 1993.
34. Livingston JE, Poland BJ: A study of spontaneously aborted twins. Teratology 21:139, 1980.
35. Simpson JL, Gray RH, Queenan JT, et al: Further evidence that infection is an infrequent cause of first trimester spontaneous abortion. Hum Reprod 11:2058, 1996.
36. Joste NE, Kundsin RB, Genest DR: Histology and *Ureaplasma urealyticum* culture in 63 cases of first trimester abortion. Am J Clin Pathol 102:729, 1994.
37. Osser S, Persson K: Chlamydial antibodies in women who suffer miscarriage. Br J Obstet Gynaecol 103:137, 1996.
38. Stephenson MD: Frequency of factors associated with habitual abortion in 197 couples. Fertil Steril 66:24, 1996.
39. Bakas C, Zarou DM, de Caprariis PJ: First trimester spontaneous abortions and the incidence of human immunodeficiency virus seropositivity. J Reprod Med 41:15, 1996.
40. Dehner LP, Askin FB: Cytomegalovirus endometritis: report of a case associated with spontaneous abortion. Obstet Gynecol 45:211, 1975.
41. Hustin J, Jauniaux E, Schapps JP: Histologic study of the materno-embryonic interface in spontaneous abortion. Placenta 11:477, 1990.
42. Hasegawa I, Tanaka K, Sanada H, et al: Studies on cytogenetic and endocrinologic background of spontaneous abortion. Fertil Steril 65:52, 1996.
43. Neugebauer R, Kline R, Stine J, et al: Association of stressful life events with chromosomally normal spontaneous abortions. Am J Epidemiol 143:588, 1996.
44. Floridon C, Nielsen O, Byrjalsen C, et al: Ectopic pregnancy: histopathology and assessment of cell proliferation with and without methotrexate treatment. Fertil Steril 65:730, 1996.
45. Houwer-de Jong MH, Bruinse HW, Termijtelen A: The immunology of normal pregnancy and recurrent abortion. In Huisjes HJ, Lind T (eds): Early pregnancy failure. New York, 1990, Churchill Livingston, p 27.
46. Lachapelle MD, Miron P, Hemmings R, Roy DC: Endometrial T, B, and NK cells in patients with recurrent SAB: altered profile and pregnancy outcome. J Immunol 156:4827, 1996.
47. Benirschke K, Kaufmann P: Pathology of the human placenta, 3rd ed. New York, 1995, Springer-Verlag.
48. Marzusch K, Dietl J, Klein R, et al: Recurrent first trimester spontaneous abortion associated with antiphospholipid antibodies: a pilot study of treatment with intravenous immunoglobulin. Acta Obstet Gynecol Scand 75:922, 1996.
49. Preston FE, Rosendaal FR, Walker ID, et al: Increased fetal loss in women with heritable thrombophilia. Lancet 348:913, 1996.
50. Stern JJ, Dorfmann AD, Gutierrez-Najar AJ, et al: Frequency of abnormal karyotypes among abortuses from women with and without a hisory of recurrent spontaneous abortion. Fertil Steril 65:250, 1996.
51. Gilbert-Barness E: Potter's pathology of the fetus and infant. St. Louis, 1997, Mosby.

5

Pathology of the Umbilical Cord

†*Stephen A. Heifetz*

The 1990 Professional Liability Survey by the American College of Obstetrics and Gynecology revealed that the majority of obstetricians have been sued at least once because of a poor obstetric outcome.[1] Rather than being prima facie evidence of substandard care or intrapartum negligence, tragedies such as perinatal death or severe neurologic impairment are increasingly being recognized as caused by pathologic conditions of the umbilical cord that frequently develop long before labor and delivery and cannot be prevented by the best of obstetric care.[2–6] Therefore informed examination of the umbilical cord, both in the delivery room and in the pathology laboratory, is a critical contribution to the investigation of failed pregnancies.

The umbilical cord is subject to a wide variety of lesions and untoward gestational events that are increasingly being diagnosed by prenatal ultrasonography.[7] Some lesions lead to indisputable cord failure that results from compromise of umbilical blood flow to a degree sufficient to prejudice the life or well-being of the fetus. Others may by themselves be innocuous, but herald more sinister associated conditions. Still others are of theoretical interest with unpredictable clinical significance. The mere presence of a cord lesion does not imply a causal relationship to poor pregnancy outcome, and the most conspicuous cord abnormalities may be harmless.

NORMAL DEVELOPMENT

The umbilical cord is formed between days 13 and 40 post conception.[8,9] By day 13 the implanted blastocystic cavity contains an embryo surrounded by a loose meshwork of extraembryonic mesoderm. The embryo is composed of two cavities (the amniotic cavity and the primary yolk sac) and the embryonic disk, which consists of two epithelial layers (the ectoderm and the entoderm) that form where the two cavities meet. The ectoderm is continuous with the amniotic epithelium, and the entoderm partially surrounds the primary yolk sac cavity.

By day 18 the extraembryonic mesoderm cavitates to form the exocoelom. Part of this mesoderm, the chorionic mesoderm, lines the inner surface of the trophoblastic shell, whereas the remainder covers the two embryonic cavities. As the exocoelom expands, these two portions of mesoderm remain connected in only one place, the connecting stalk, a mesenchymal bridge basal to the amniotic cavity. The allantois, the extraembryonic urinary bladder, forms as a fingerlike projection (duct) of the primary yolk sac into the connecting stalk at the presumptive caudal end of the embryonic disk and is surrounded by angiogenic mesenchyme.

Three developmental processes occur during the subsequent 3 weeks (Fig. 5–1): (1) The embryo rotates. The yolk sac, which originally faced away from the implantation site, turns toward the implantation site. (2) The amniotic cavity enlarges considerably, extends around the embryo, and compresses the exocoelom, which gradually is obliterated. (3) The originally flat embryonic disk bends in the anteroposterior direction and folds in the lateral direction toward the implantation site, herniating itself into the expanding amniotic cavity. By bending, the embryo subdivides the yolk sac into intraembryonic (primitive intestinal tract) and extraembryonic parts (the omphalomesenteric or vitelline duct with its accompanying angiogenic mesenchyme and its dilated peripheral portion, the

†Deceased.

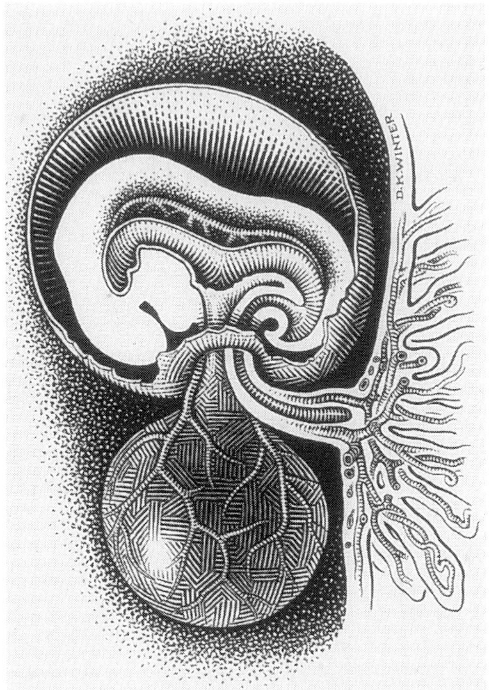

Figure 5–1. Formation of the umbilical cord. Between postconception days 18 and 40 the embryo rotates, so that the yolk sac turns toward the implantation site and herniates into the enlarging amniotic cavity that compresses the connecting stalk, allantois, and the omphalomesenteric duct into a slender cord covered by amniotic epithelium.

secondary yolk sac). As the amniotic cavity continues to expand, it compresses the connecting stalk, allantois, and omphalomesenteric duct into a slender cord covered by amniotic epithelium, thus forming the umbilical cord.

Meanwhile the angiogenic mesenchyme that accompanies the vitelline and allantoic ducts is forming arteries and veins destined to connect the developing fetal circulation with the capillaries developing in the placental villi. All mammals use either vitelline or allantoic vessels for fetal vascularization of the placental disk. In human beings the allantoic vessels become dominant. The two vitelline arteries and two veins involute by the end of pregnancy and may be seen as capillary channels in Wharton's jelly that may accompany a vestigial remnant of the omphalomesenteric duct (see below and Fig. 5–2). The two allantoic arteries originate from the internal iliac arteries to become the two umbilical arteries, and the left umbilical (allantoic) vein enters the hepatic vein. The right umbilical vein, originally present, disappears by the end of the second month.

NORMAL ANATOMY

The cord is covered by the amniotic epithelium, a mixed cuboidal-squamous epithelium that is continuous with the squamous epithelium of the umbilicus and the cuboidal-columnar epithelium of the placental-membranous amniotic surface. In contrast to the easily detached amnion of the placenta and membranes, the cord amnion adheres firmly to the underlying connective tissue, Wharton's jelly. Wharton's jelly is derived from the extraembryonic mesoderm and is mucoid, compressible, and thixotropic (liquefies under pressure), thereby protecting cord vessels.[10] It contains evenly distributed myofibroblasts or vascular smooth muscle–derived myofibroblast-like stromal cells within a ground

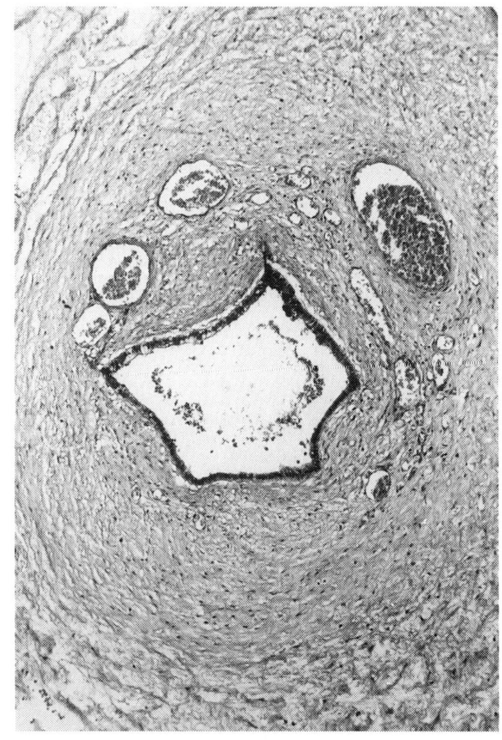

Figure 5–2. Cystic remnant of omphalomesenteric duct with angiomatous peripheral vascularity. Vitelline capillaries contain fetal erythrocytes with numerous nucleated forms.

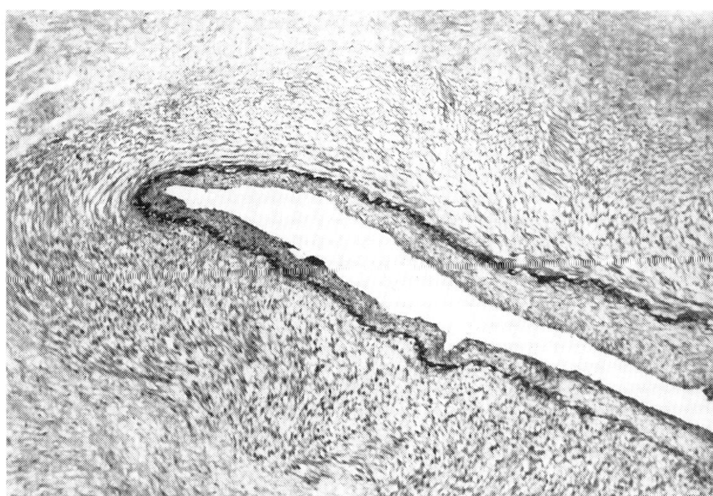

Figure 5–3. Elastic tissue stain of umbilical vein showing a well-developed lamina elastica interna.

substance rich in hyaluronic acid and chondroitin sulfate, similar to other avascular tissues nourished by diffusion (cornea and cartilage).[11–12] Numerous heparin-containing mast cells may facilitate diffusion and prevent intravascular thrombi in the long, tortuous course of the cord vessels.

The placenta has no neural supply, and no nerves traverse the umbilical cord from the fetus to the placenta.[13] Nerve fibers exist only in the immediate paraumbilical segment. No lymphatic vessels are present in the cord, and fixed macrophages are essentially absent. As a consequence, meconium-laden macrophages are rarely seen within Wharton's jelly (and only with prolonged exposure), hemosiderin tends not to be formed in situ after intrafunicular hemorrhage, and necrotic debris and spent neutrophils of a funisitis accumulate and are not cleared.

The extracorporeal human umbilical vessels differ from all other fetal vessels of comparable size. The vein, but not the arteries, has a well-developed lamina elastica interna (Fig. 5–3), although arteries have considerable elastic tissue within their media. The arterial media has no true circular or longitudinal layers but consists of decussating helicoid smooth muscle bundles that shorten to become more nearly circular with contraction.[14] The intraabdominal portion of the arteries has vasa vasorum from 20 weeks' gestation, but none are present beyond the paraumbilical cord segment. The cord's nutritional requirements are met by transmural diffusion, primarily across the thin-walled vein. Vascular tone is modulated by local prostaglandin production, which may be altered by maternal smoking, diabetes mellitus, and preeclampsia.[15–19] Preeclampsia also alters the collagen and ground substance content of Wharton's jelly and the walls of the arteries. These changes may be partly responsible for decreased umbilical blood flow in preeclamptic gestations by altering the compliance of the arterial walls and the contractile properties of the myofibroblasts in Wharton's jelly.[20]

Within 2 to 3 cm of the placental insertion of 95% of cords, segmental arterial fusion or macroscopic anastomosis equalizes the flow and pressure in the two arterial placental vascular territories (Fig. 5–4). The anastomosis is a safety valve comparable to the circle of Willis; in the event of luminal compression or occlusion of one artery the anastomosis is a source of blood to its deprived vascular territory from the other artery.

STRUCTURAL DEFECTS

Single Umbilical Artery and Supernumerary Vessels

The incidence of single umbilical artery (SUA) among prospective deliveries of white term infants is about 1%, slightly higher than among black or Asian infants.[21] The incidence rises throughout gestation, indicating that most cases result from progressive atrophy of a normally formed second artery. A markedly hypoplastic artery may be

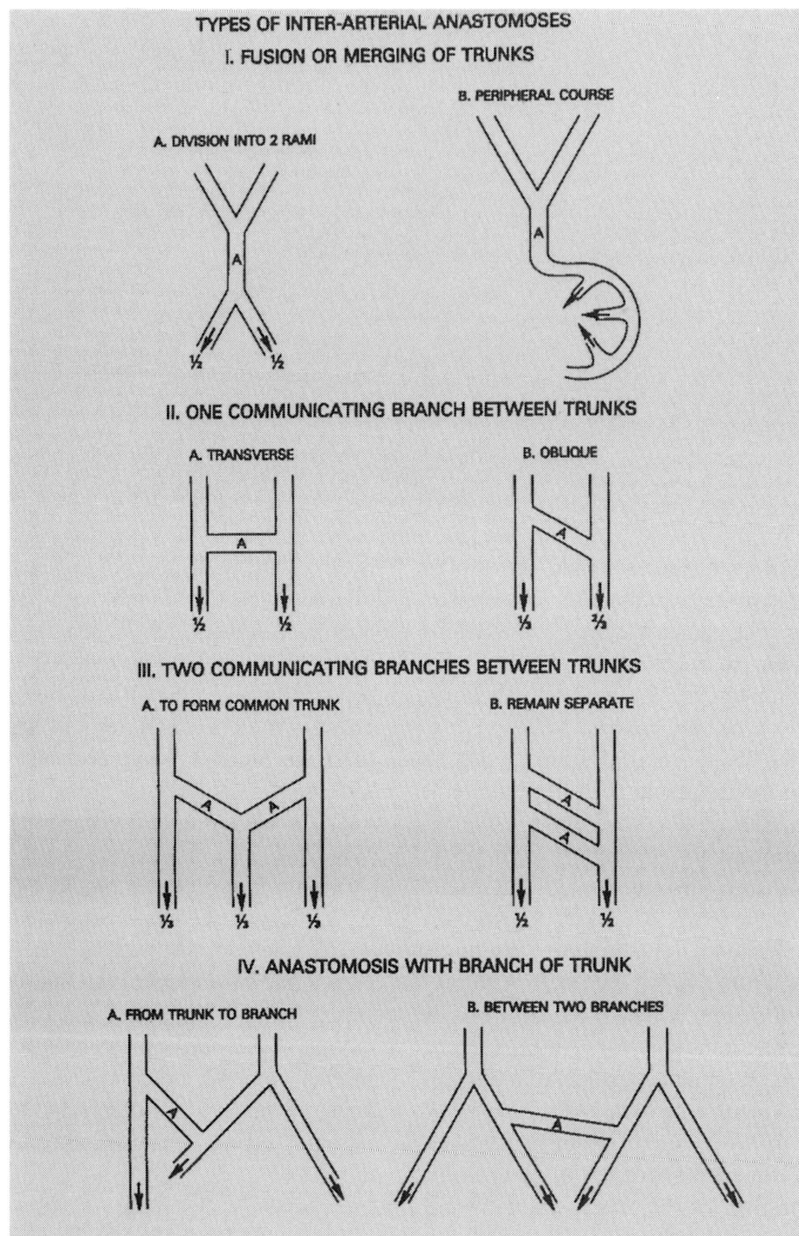

Figure 5–4. Patterns of interarterial anastomoses that are present between the two umbilical arteries near the placental insertion site in 95% of umbilical cords.

found by color Doppler ultrasound, or merely a remnant of a second artery may be seen by microscopic examination (Fig. 5–5); such cases have the same adverse prognostic implications as SUA.[7] The diagnosis should not be based on examination of the distal (placental) end of the cord because in this region the two umbilical arteries may fuse into a single trunk that subsequently redivides on the placental surface into two rami. Similarly, when SUA is noted, its presence should be confirmed at several points along the cord because rare variants of umbilical artery fusion may occur more proximally. Gross examination alone, especially of fresh unfixed cords, may underestimate the frequency of SUA. No evidence of a familial tendency for SUA has been found, suggesting that a genetic cause is unlikely for the majority of cases. SUA occurs slightly more frequently in females than in males, but males are more likely to be malformed. The incidence of SUA in autopsy series is twice that in series of prospective deliveries, indicating the detrimental effect on SUA on fetal survival and well-being.

The incidence of twins among SUA infants is at least three times greater than the overall incidence of twins, and SUA occurs three to four times more frequently among twins than among singletons, regardless of zygosity.[21] Although among twin infants overall the expected incidence of malformations is twice that of singletons, twin SUA infants have no greater incidence of associated malformations than SUA singletons. The adverse prognosis of SUA with respect to associated malformations in all infants (both twins and singletons) overcomes the inherent difference between non-SUA twins and singletons, resulting in the high, but equal, incidence of associated malformation in both groups. Most SUA twins, including those who are monozygotic, are discordant for SUA, with the anomaly usually occurring in the smaller twin. The lack of concordance, especially among monozygotic twins, suggests that environmental rather than genetic factors influence the genesis of SUA. Although concordance for SUA in monozygotic twins is less than 100%, it is substantially greater than among dizygotic twins, indicating that a genetic influence may be combined with an environmental trigger or that the twinning process itself may render each twin more susceptible than singletons to environmental agents, which may have more effect on one twin than the other.

In prospective series of SUA infants the mean perinatal mortality is 20%.[21] Approximately two thirds of the perinatal deaths are stillborn and one third are liveborn; of the stillborn SUA infants approximately 75% die antepartum and 25% die intrapartum. Mortality of SUA infants is related to associated fetal and placental malformations, prematurity and low birth weight, and intrauterine growth retardation. Although associated malformations are the primary cause of the high perinatal mortality, even normally formed SUA infants have an increased mortality rate, suggesting that they are in a more precarious state than non-SUA infants and are less able to withstand the rigors of normal labor.[22]

Approximately 20% of SUA infants (or seven times the number of non-SUA infants) examined prospectively have additional malformations that are often multiple, major, and lethal.[21] These malformations may or may not be sonographically identifiable in the fetus.[23–24] In a large prospective series more than 70% of SUA infants were missing the left artery and only this group had cytogenetic abnormalities and complex congenital anomalies.[23] Because the incidence of malformation in perinatal SUA deaths is twice the already exceedingly high incidence of malformations among the SUA population, associated malformations are largely responsible for the high fetal and neonatal loss in SUA infants.[21] While death is nearly universal in sirenomelia and in acardiac fetuses,[25]

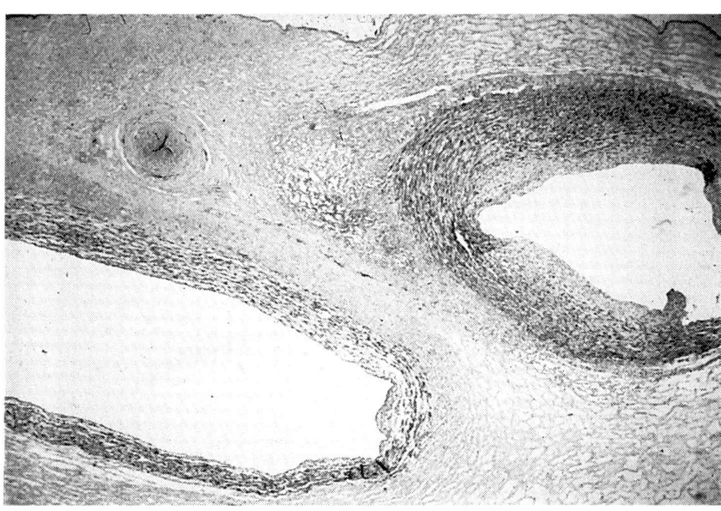

Figure 5–5. Umbilical cord with one markedly hypoplastic artery. Such cases have the same prognostic implications as those with a single umbilical artery.

there is usually no consistent pattern of affected organ systems, although genitourinary anomalies have been described repeatedly and may be detected by routine renal ultrasound in SUA infants without external malformations.[26,27] A teratogenic role for SUA in the production of associated malformations lacks substantiating evidence, although a pathogenetic role has been suggested. The absence of one umbilical artery may impede fetal blood flow to the placenta, causing increased fetal cardiac load and chronic fetal tissue hypoxia. As the functional continuation of the abdominal aorta, the one existing artery may cause a vascular steal from the caudal half of the embryo (caudal defects are more common than cephalic defects in infants with SUA).[28] Rather than being itself teratogenic, SUA is likely to be part of a malformation complex derived from a common teratogen:

1. Since 15% to 20% of malformed infants have multiple malformations,[29] a corresponding percentage of SUA infants would be expected to have an additional malformation.
2. All malformations associated with SUA, including sirenomelia and an acardiac twin, also occur when there are two arteries, and malformations are more likely to occur with two than with one artery.
3. The umbilical arteries arise and attain functional maturity during the critical period of development of many viscera. A teratogenic stimulus of abnormal umbilical artery development during this period may affect these other viscera as well.
4. SUA has been described in one member of conjoined twin sets. SUA could not have caused these malformations, since the formation of conjoined twins is determined several weeks before the umbilical arteries develop.
5. Most SUA infants have no associated malformations and develop normally in extrauterine life.
6. Ligation of one umbilical artery in fetal lambs leads to profound fetal malnutrition, but not to visceral malformations.[30]

No relationship has been found between SUA, or the presence of associated malformations in SUA infants, and maternal age, gravidity, or their interplay (e.g., young or old primigravidas or young or old multigravidas).[21] SUA is associated with maternal hydramnios because of the high incidence of malformations in these infants, as well as with maternal diabetes mellitus and smoking,[31] but the relationship between SUA and toxemia or hypertension remains controversial. SUA is not related to the incidence of previous fetal loss among the mothers, but SUA is associated with a high incidence of abnormal fetal presentation at delivery, largely because of the high incidence of associated malformations, low birth weight, intrauterine growth retardation, and abnormalities of placentation.

In prospective series approximately 25% of SUA infants are premature by dates.[21] Although prematurity among SUA infants is associated with fetal malformations, a premature SUA infant has no poorer prognosis than a premature non-SUA infant. In prospective series approximately 25% of SUA infants weigh less than 2500 g at birth. Low birth weight is far more important than prematurity as a factor in perinatal morality, since even nonmalformed SUA infants are growth retarded in utero and have a significantly lower mean birth weight at all gestational ages than age-matched control infants,[21] possibly because the remaining artery fails to undergo compensatory dilatation.[32] The placentas of SUA infants are also growth retarded, to a degree equivalent to the birth weight retardation. Nonmalformed SUA infants who are growth retarded at birth, however, are likely to attain growth rates indistinguishable from those of non-SUA infants.

SUA infants have a higher incidence of gross placental abnormalities, including placenta extrachorialis, bipartita, and succenturiata, placenta previa, a significant degree of placental infarction, alterations in the usual fetal vascular pattern, and chorangiomas.[21] Marginal and velamentous cord insertion is the placental abnormality most strongly associated with SUA. SUA infants with peripheral cord insertion have a higher incidence of malformations, and in my experience malformed SUA infants show a tendency toward abnormally short umbilical cords and cords with few helicoidal twists.

Although a dominant role for environmental factors in the etiology of SUA is likely, the association of SUA with numerous chromosomal anomalies suggests a multifactorial influence, including genetic factors.[21] Such cases, however, are uncommon, and the presence of SUA may be fortuitous.[33–34] SUA may also result from arteriovascular thrombosis (see below).

In light of the significant risks associated with SUA, as well as the knowledge that SUA occurs frequently with healthy infants who attain normal growth and development, prudent obstetric management after prenatal diagnosis of SUA should include detailed ultrasonographic examination, echocardiography for major fetal malformations and subtle stigmata of aneuploidy, the offer of fetal karyotyping if anatomic defects are detected, periodic enhanced fetal surveillance, and detailed physical examination of the neonate, including renal ultrasonography.[24,33–35]

Supernumerary cord vessels are less common than SUA.[35] Since cord vessels often fork, divide and rejoin, or double back on themselves, causing irregular nodularities (false knots), multiple sections are required to confirm a suspected case of supernumerary vessel. Pseudosupernumerary multiple vascular profiles are relatively common on cross section and have been associated with heavy maternal cigarette smoking and intrauterine distress. They may represent a response to intrauterine hypoxia.[36] When truly supernumerary, additional vessels may be artery, vein (persistent right umbilical vein?), or capillary (persistent vitelline vessels?). Although infants with supernumerary umbilical vessels and additional malformations have been reported, no large series of such cases exist, nor has a consistent pattern of malformations been demonstrated. When both umbilical veins persist, the left provides the fetal circulation with placental blood through the portal system, whereas the right empties directly into the right atrium.[37] On the other hand, persistence of the right umbilical vein with atrophy of the left is associated with SUA and a high incidence of significant fetal visceral anomalies.[38–41]

Vestigial Remnants, Cysts, and Pseudocysts

Remnants of the allantoic and omphalomesenteric (OM) ducts, which generally are completely obliterated by 15 to 16 weeks' of gestation, are present in microscopic sections of approximately 20% of cords at term, primarily near the proximal (fetal) end.[42,43] These vestigial remnants do not usually have clinical importance. Allantoic duct remnants tend to be located between the two umbilical arteries and consist of solid cords of epithelial cells without lumina (urothelium but occasionally mucin-producing epithelium). A smooth muscle investment is rare, but concentric condensation of Wharton's jelly may occur. If the median umbilical ligament (urachus) remains patent, urine-containing cysts may be present.[7,44] An abscess of an allantoic duct remnant in a cord with funisitis has been described,[45] as have allantoic cysts in association with fetal omphalocele.[46]

Cord remnants of the OM duct often have muscular coats, are usually present at the cord's periphery, and may occur in duplicate.[42,43] They may contain a variety of endodermal epithelia, including hepatic, pancreatic, and gastric, in addition to the usual intestinal. Males outnumber females 4 to 1 when OM duct remnants are cystic, and true intestinal walls, complete with ganglion cells, may be found. OM duct cysts and remnants frequently

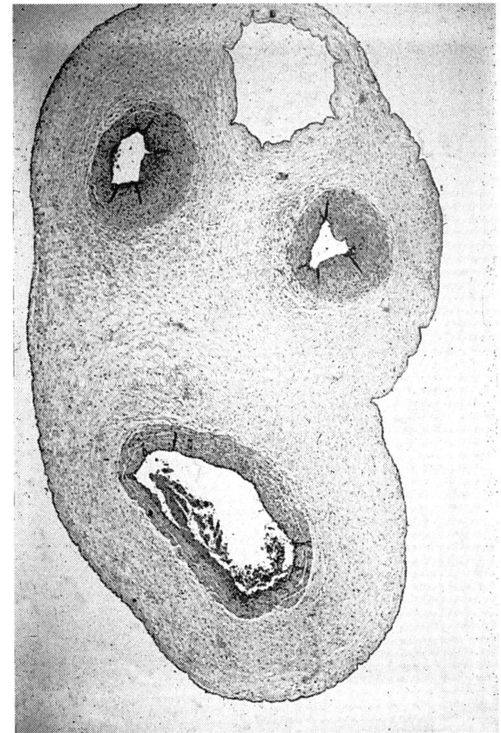

Figure 5–6. Amniotic inclusion "cyst." Serial sections revealed an open communication between the "cyst" and the surface of the cord, indicating that the cystlike appearance was due to a tangential cut of a surface infolding caused by the cord's helicoidal spiraling.

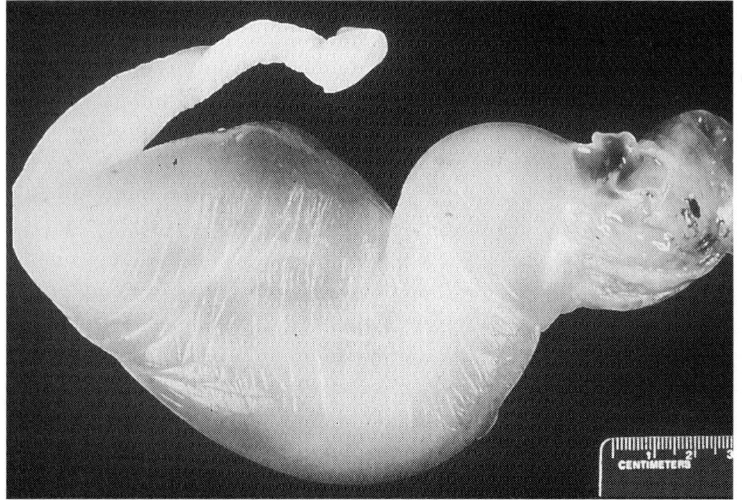

Figure 5–7. Localized edema of the umbilical cord (mucoid degeneration of Wharton's jelly). Cross sections commonly demonstrate a pseudocyst without an epithelial lining. If edema is located at the umbilicus, the cord should be transilluminated before ligation at delivery to search for a possible patent urachus, herniated portion of fetal intestinal tract, or hemangiomatous nodule.

are accompanied by tiny amuscular blood vessels (vitelline capillaries) that may appear angiomatous and contain fetal erythrocytes (Fig. 5–5). Fetal morbidity or mortality from OM duct cysts is rare, except when gastric mucosa is found,[47] but small omphaloceles and potentially serious intraabdominal anomalies of the OM duct (Meckel's diverticulum) may also be present.[48] An association with atresia of the small intestine has been noted.[49]

Amniotic inclusion cysts are lined by cord surface epithelium and are without clinical importance. Most are artifactual tangential cuts of surface infoldings caused by the cord's helicoidal spiraling; however, true cystic entrapment may occur (Fig. 5–6). Localized cord edema (mucoid degeneration of Wharton's jelly) produces a cavitation (pseudocyst) rather than a true cyst, since an epithelial lining is lacking. Local edema is associated with patent urachus, omphalocele, fetal aneuploidy (especially trisomy 18), and cord hemangioma[49–58] and may be responsible for some cases of cord rupture (Fig. 5–7).[59]

Generalized Abnormalities of Cord Diameter

Generalized cord edema is found in 10% of deliveries and is related to prematurity, elective cesarean section, abruption, preeclampsia and eclampsia, rhesus incompatibility, maternal diabetes mellitus, acute chorioamnionitis, and fetal death.[60] Cord edema may be due to low fetal oncotic pressure, raised hydrostatic pressure, low uteroplacental blood flow, or increased fetal total water content. Although most affected infants do not have excessive fetal distress or neonatal asphyxia,[61] they may have increased episodes of transient tachypnea or idiopathic respiratory distress syndrome.[60] When cord distention by edema is severe, it may be accompanied by hydramnios and an excessive number of mast cells.[62]

Although the quantity of Wharton's jelly tends to decrease with gestational age, occasionally a cord is encountered that is remarkably narrow along its entire length, the "thin cord syndrome."[63] Associated findings and risk factors are those associated with fetal-placental growth retardation, including preeclampsia, maternal cigarette smoking, discordance between gestational age and villous appearance, and major fetal malformations. However, the question of cause or effect remains unanswered. An increased frequency of cord prolapse has been reported with a thin cord. In monozygotic twin pregnancies complicated by the twin-twin transfusion syndrome the narrower cord is generally that of the donor.

Stricture of the Umbilical Cord

Cord stricture (coarctation) is a focal deficiency of Wharton's jelly with or without vascular occlusion, usually at the fetal end of the cord and often with superimposed torsion.[64,65] Most strictures are noted with macerated 6- to 8-month fetuses. Because no fetal infarction or congestion is present, most strictures represent postmortem artifacts secondary to autolysis that begins at the fetal end of the cord. Some authors have pointed to the presence of capillaries in Wharton's jelly at the site of stricture as evidence of "collateral" circulation resulting from antemortem gradual stricture formation, but such channels are normally present in the paraumbilical cord segment.[66] Furthermore, the amount of Wharton's jelly usually diminishes gradually as the cord approaches the abdominal surface. This localized "relative" deficiency is compounded after fetal demise (from whatever cause) by maceration, autolysis, and excessive torsion imparted by passive in utero rotation of the dead fetus. Such passively acquired twists congregate in the portion of the cord with the smallest diameter. If stricture and torsion were related to excessive movements of a living fetus, such cases would be expected to have cords of excessive length. Although Benirschke[5] has found this to be true in the majority of his cases of stricture and torsion, my experience has been the opposite.[67] In addition, if most strictures were the cause rather than the result of fetal demise, partial or incomplete strictures would occasionally be noted with either asphyxiated or healthy liveborn infants.[68] I have never seen this phenomenon, and the presence of torsion or stricture in fresh stillbirths is an extremely rare occurrence.[69] Nevertheless, localized thinning of the cord with reduced or absent Wharton's jelly does occur in the absence of torsion and, when present, may predispose to torsion.

I accept as a bona fide cause of fetal demise only those rare cases of stricture and torsion that meet the following criteria: venous congestion and edema distal to the torsion and presence of intravascular antemortem thrombi.[65,70,71] Such criteria are much more likely to be met when the stricture is not at the fetal end and is due to a localized deficiency of Wharton's jelly or the vascular walls,[72] occult prolapse with long-standing compression, or strangulation of the umbilical cord by amniotic bands (Fig. 5–8).[73,74]

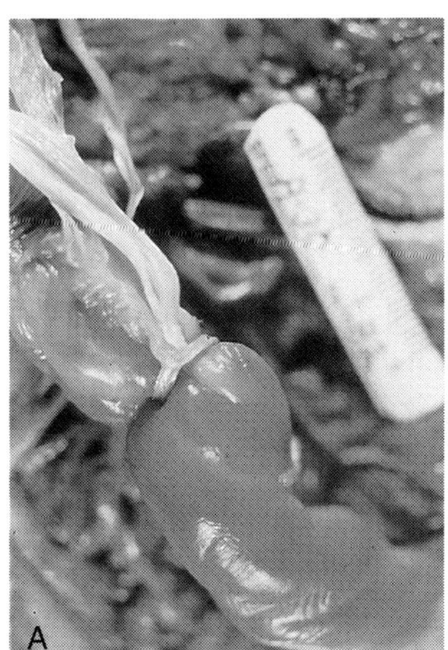

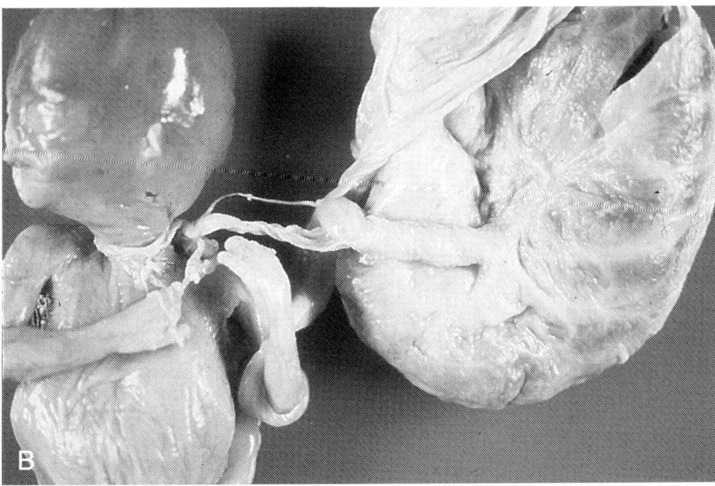

Figure 5–8. A, Strangulation of the umbilical cord by an amniotic band, resulting in true stricture of the cord and in utero fetal demise. **B,** Amniotic band syndrome that led to cord stricture because of fetal entanglement by the cord rather than an amniotic band. An amniotic band encircles the fetal neck, causing jugular venous compression with plethora of the head. Both hands have become entangled with and attached to this band as though the fetus had attempted to relieve the strangulation. However, the cord became entangled about the crook of the right elbow and was compressed by elbow flexion, which could not be relieved because the hand was firmly attached to the fetal neck. The cord stricture that resulted at the elbow was markedly thinner than the cord at either the fetal or placental ends.

Insertion Abnormalities of the Umbilical Cord

The umbilical cord may have a central, eccentric, marginal (battledore), or velamentous (membranous) insertion. Central (one third of cases) and eccentric (two thirds of cases) insertions account for more than 90% of cords and have no clinical importance. Marginal insertions (5% to 7%) may be more susceptible to vessel rupture or compression[75] and have been associated with fetal growth retardation, stillbirth, and neonatal death, but only when placental maturation is unevenly accelerated because of low uteroplacental blood flow.[76] In velamentous insertion (1% to 2%), vessels are divested of and unprotected by Wharton's jelly for a variable distance within the free membranes before reaching the fetal surface (Fig. 5–9*A*). The incidence increases among multiple births, low-lying placentas, SUA and malformed infants, and in vitro fertilization pregnancies and with maternal cigarette smoking, advanced age, or diabetes mellitus.[21,77,78] Velamentous insertion is significantly more common in monochorionic pregnancies complicated by twin transfusion syndrome than in those without the syndrome and usually occurs in the donor twin; the easily compressed membranously inserted vein may cause diversion of blood flow to the co-twin through placental anastomoses and give rise to the syndrome.[79] Rare cord insertions are interposito velamentosa, in which a membranously inserted cord retains its sheath of Wharton's jelly until reaching the fetal surface (Fig. 5–9*B*),[80] and insertio funiculi furcata, in which the insertion site is normal but jelly is lost and vessels branch before reaching the disk surface, thereby exposing them to hazards similar to those of velamentous vessels.[81,82] A forked umbilical cord, common among conjoined twins, occurs when a fused cord divides near the fetal and placental surfaces (Fig. 5–10*A*). The fused cord may contain three, four, five, or six vessels. Cord vessels may also lose their jelly for variable segments at points distant from their insertion site (Fig. 5–10*B*).[59] In rare instances the placental cord insertion is encased by a fold of amnion, a chorda or web, which may be loose or tight, binding the cord to the fetal surface, limiting cord mobility, and

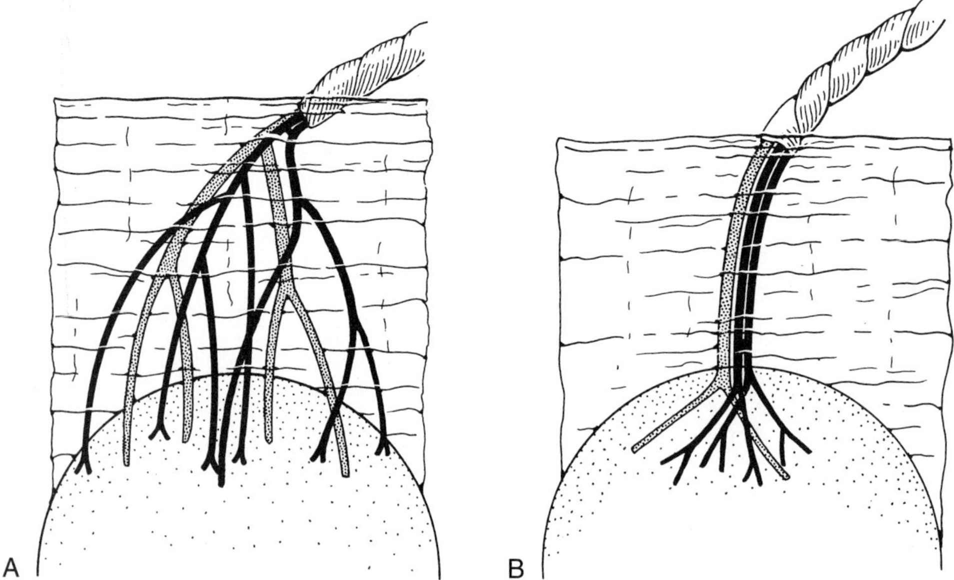

Figure 5–9. Schematic representation of velamentous insertion and interposito velamentosa. **A,** Velamentous insertion. The cord inserts into the membranes at some distance from the placental disk margin. Thereafter the three vessels branch while divested of and unprotected by Wharton's jelly as they course to the disk surface. When vessels branch and lose their jelly before their insertion, but insert directly on the disk surface rather than into the membranes, the condition is termed a furcate cord insertion. **B,** Interposito velamentosa. The membranously inserted cord retains its protective sheath of Wharton's jelly until reaching the placental disk surface.

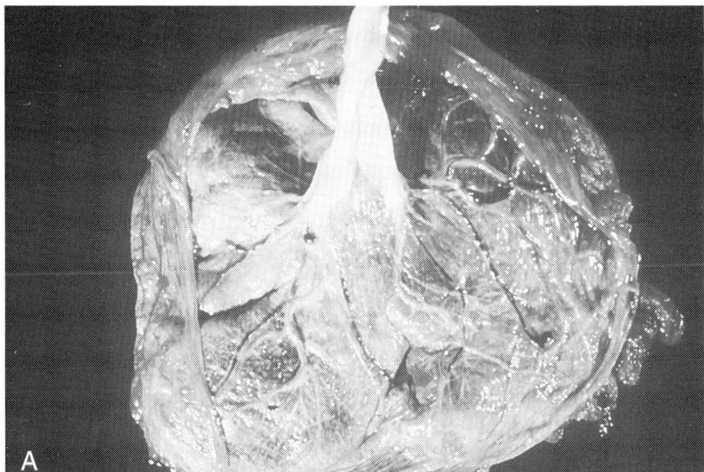

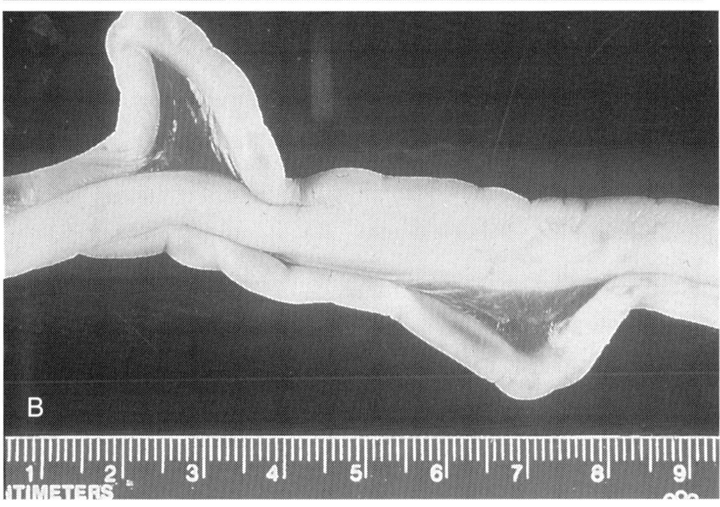

Figure 5–10. A, Forked umbilical cord in thoracopagus twins. The fused common trunk bore five vessels. **B,** Random cord segment with a localized deficiency of Wharton's jelly and separation of the umbilical vessels. Such vessels may be more subject to compression. The cord was entirely normal on either side of this segment, and the infant was alive and well.

possible predisposing to subamniotic vessel hemorrhage.

Velamentous vessels are subject to compression, thrombosis, and tears with fetal (Benkiser) hemorrhage, especially those that pass before the cervical os (vasa previa).[83] Vasa previa in a monochorionic twin with large anastomosing placental vessels may lead to fetal exsanguination of the cotwin by proxy. With blood loss fetal mortality approaches 100%, but vasa previa occurs in only about 2% of cases and, although usually diagnosed retrospectively, is increasingly being diagnosed before catastrophe by color flow Doppler ultrasound, especially with a vaginal transducer.[84-86] Detection of fetal blood in vaginal bleeding is also readily accomplished,[87] but such testing is currently not a "standard of care" in the United States.[88] In addition to fetal exsanguination, velamentous insertion is associated with fetal cerebral white matter necrosis, placental abruption, and unexplained elevation of maternal serum human chorionic gonadotropin (hCG) concentration and may cause neonatal purpura associated with vessel thrombi; affected infants may be mildly growth retarded because peripheral insertions have a relative paucity of fetal surface vessel ramifications[6,35,89-92] and may have an increased incidence of deformations because of in utero restraint of fetal mobility.[93] Since the forces responsible for deformation also may be responsible for velamentous insertion, both may recur in subsequent pregnancies. Intramembranous vessels and vasa previa are not confined to cases of velamentous insertion. Aberrant intramembranous branches may be seen with marginal insertions[75] and occur, by definition, with succenturiate lobes and bipartite placenta.

There has been considerable debate regarding the pathogenesis of peripheral cord insertions, with numerous investigators supporting each of two contradictory theories: abnormal primary implantation (polarity theory),[94] and trophotropism (placental wandering).[95] My view is that more than one mechanism may be responsible and that each of the two proposals may account for a proportion of cases.

The abnormal implantation theory postulates that during nidation of the blastocyst, the embryo, rather than face the endometrium, is obliquely oriented toward the chorion laeve. Thus, when the vascular stalk develops, it must seek its connection with the future placentation site by extending its vessels from the embryo to the chorion frondosum; the vessels must thereby become membranous. If all peripheral insertions were caused by this mechanism, however, their frequency would be as high in the first trimester as in the third. This is not the case among therapeutic abortuses, although peripheral insertions have a higher frequency among spontaneous first-trimester losses than at term, presumably because peripheral insertions correlate with fetal anomalies and low-lying placentas.

The trophotropism theory, in contrast, postulates that marginal atrophy on one side and expansion on the other result in placental "movement" toward better perfused decidua (Fig. 5–11).

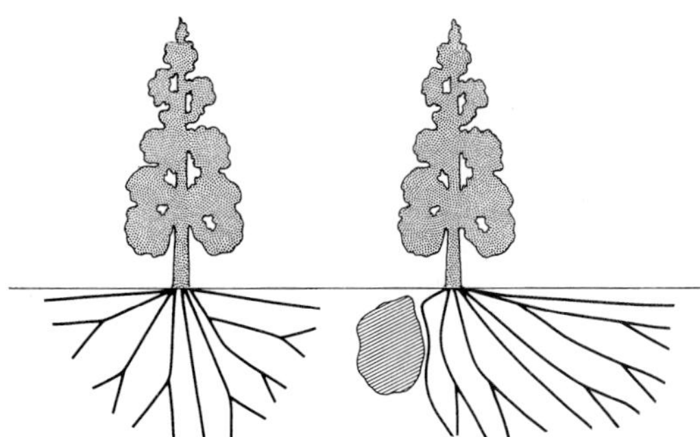

Figure 5–11. Placental trophotropism may be likened to the roots of a tree. Just as roots avoid an obstruction and seek the most fertile soil, the placenta may show marginal atrophy on one side and expansion on the other as it seeks better perfused decidua.

This theory is supported by the higher frequency of peripheral cord insertions in all twin placentas except dichorionic diamniotic twin placentas, as well as their almost invariable presence among higher multiple births. In addition, they are more common when intrauterine contraceptive devices are found in the placental membranes. Eccentric expansion of the placenta during the course of pregnancy has been observed sonographically.[96] Such dynamic placentation accounts for the subsequent disappearance of many instances of first-trimester placenta previa.

Abnormal Length of the Umbilical Cord

The umbilical cord approaches its ultimate length by 28 weeks' gestation, but limited growth continues until delivery, even beyond term.[97] A wide range of cord lengths exists at every gestational age, but the mean at term is 55 to 60 cm, a length that approximates the fetus' crown-heel length, and (anthropologically) one that is sufficient to permit the infant to be put to breast should the placenta remain in utero, with the reflex stimulation of suckling promoting a bloodless third stage of labor. I consider a cord length at term of 70 cm or more to be excessive and of 40 cm or less to be unduly brief. In my experience only about 5% of cords fall into these two extremes.[67] Gardiner calculated that a minimal cord length of 32 cm is necessary to permit a normal vertex delivery.[98]

The range of cord length differences between monochorionic twins is much less than that between same-sex dichorionic twins, indicating that cord length is partly determined by genetic factors.[99] Cord length may be modified by forceful stretching by the developing fetus; the greater the tension, the longer the cord and vice versa.[100,101] The uterine volume and amniotic fluid volume at any given gestational age that would promote or hamper fetal movement and intrinsic fetal factors that would promote or hamper fetal mobility or motility appear to be important factors in the determination of ultimate cord length. Thus slow cord growth rate during the last trimester is explained by reduced intrauterine space available for fetal movement with rapid fetal growth; unduly short cords are explained by maternal or fetal causes of decreased fetal movement, including uterine anomalies or neoplasms, ectopic pregnancy, midtrimester oligohydramnios, amniotic bands, structural limb defects, functional limb defects (Werdnig-Hoffmann syndrome, Down syndrome, maternal β-blocker ingestion), multifetal pregnancy, and multiple malformation syndromes; and cords of excessive length may be explained either as a consequence or as a cause of associated fetal entanglements.[102–105] Short cords have been shown to predict subsequent low intelligence quotient values and psychomotor abnormality,[97] possibly because tension on a short cord may lead to spasm of the umbilical vessels, luminal obliteration, and fetal cerebral hypoxia.[106,107] Neonates with long cords are relatively hyperkinetic when compared with those who have shorter cords. The "stretch hypothesis" does not always apply, however, since I have observed rare instances of long cord with long-standing oligohydramnios and others have been reported.[108]

Both short and long cords are significantly associated with other cord complications, especially entanglements, torsion, and thrombosis.[67] True knots and cord prolapse are associated with long cords, while rupture, hematoma, a high incidence of peripheral insertions, and stricture are associated with short cords. Rupture and hematoma may also occur with greater frequency in long cords that have been converted to relative shortness by fetal entanglements. Other obstetric complications associated with a short cord are delayed completion of the second stage of labor, abruption, uterine inversion, and breech as well as other fetal malpresentations.[97]

Because excessively long or unduly short cords are due to long-standing in utero factors rather than to peripartum or intrapartum events, and because a statistically significant association between short or long cords and fetal cerebral white matter necrosis has been demonstrated,[6] cord length may have profound medicolegal ramifications. Cord length, however, cannot be reliably assessed by routine prenatal ultrasonography[109] or in the pathology laboratory; cord length declines as much as 7 cm during the first few hours after delivery.[110] Obstetricians would be well advised therefore to measure and record the length of all cords at delivery, including any segments removed for blood gas analysis or remaining attached to the neonate. All delivery sets should include an easily sterilized paper tape measure.

Rare instances of absence of the umbilical cord (achordia or body stalk anomaly) have been reported in association with severely malformed abortuses.[111,112] The fetus appears to adhere to the placental surface, and there may be an associated omphalocele.

MECHANICAL LESIONS

Umbilical Cord Coiling and Torsion

The cord vessels are arranged in a spiral or helicoidal fashion along the cord, imparting increased compression-resistant properties to the cord.[113] The average number of cord helices is 11, but as many as 380 have been described. These barber pole–like twists are present as early as 6 weeks' and are well established by 9 weeks' conceptual age.[114] As with cord length, most of the ultimate number of coils are present before the third trimester. At least 75% of cord helices are left-handed (wind counter-clockwise regardless of which direction the cord is viewed),[115] perhaps related to the differing sizes and pressures of the two iliac arteries, but the direction of spirals is not related to the handedness of the fetus or mother.[116] It is plausible to infer that cord spirals are induced by fetal rotation because species with elongated embryos in elongated uterine horns, those with fetal lengthwise fixation in the uterus, and human fetuses with fixation of their bodies to the placental surface (e.g. by amniotic bands) have few or no umbilical helices. A lack of spiraling, present in about 5% of consecutively examined cords,[116,117] may reflect fetal inactivity and possibly central nervous system disturbances. The absence of twists has[116–118] and has not[119] been associated with stillbirth, preterm delivery, fetal distress, karyotypic abnormalities, single umbilical artery, and conditions in which fetal movement is restricted. In general, the more a cord spirals, the greater the likelihood of good pregnancy outcome. However, occasional cases of fetal mortality have been related to excessive twists with constriction of cord vessels, and excessive coiling has been associated with fetal distress,[120] premature delivery, and maternal cocaine use.[119] The "umbilical coiling in-

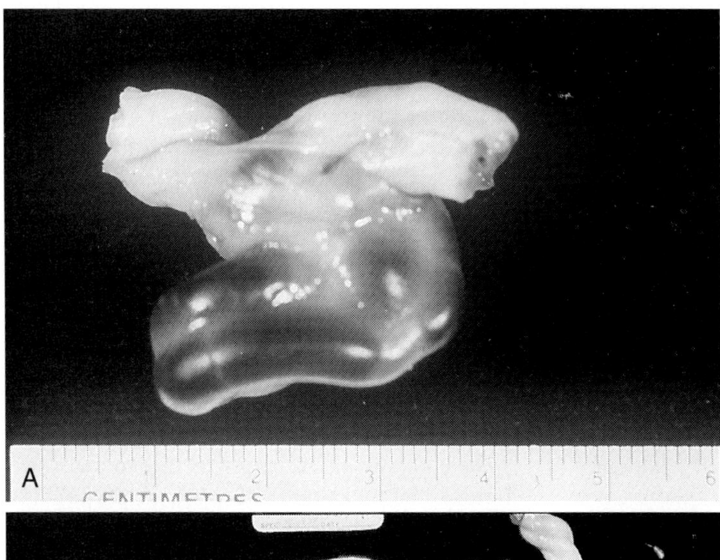

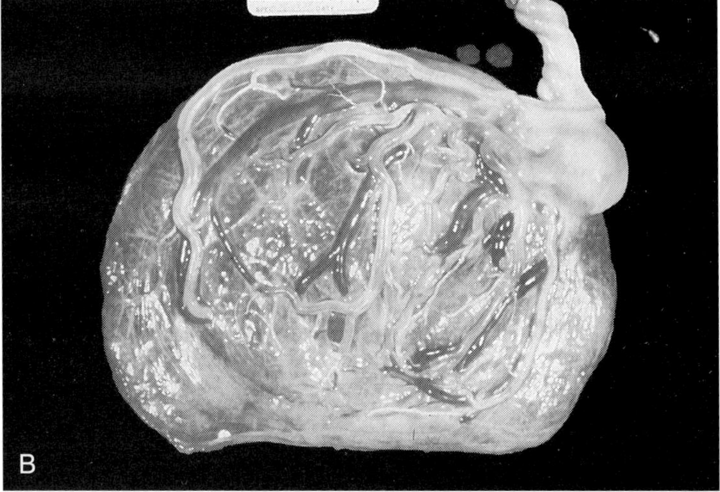

Figure 5–12. A, Thrombosis of redundant umbilical vein varix (false knot). **B,** Umbilical artery aneurysm in its usual location at the placental end of the cord.

dex" has been proposed as an indicator of fetus' at increased risk and perhaps requiring increased antepartum fetal surveillance.[117–120]

Cord torsion is a pathologic accentuation of the normal helicoidal twisting of the cord, most often localized at the fetal end and associated with multigravida and male fetuses. Antemortem examples show congestion, edema, and thrombi.[70,71,121] Torsion may be one cause of nonimmune fetal hydrops because of intermittent cord compression, cardiac arrhythmia, and cardiac failure.[122]

True and False Knots of the Cord

False knots are focal nodular congeries of branched, tortuous (redundant), or ectatic vessels (varicosities) or focal accumulations of Wharton's jelly. They are usually of no clinical importance despite their frequent identification and are not associated with cords of excessive length. Rare instances of thrombotic occlusion may result in fetal death (Fig. 5–12*A*).[58,69,70,123] Arterial aneurysms, usually at the placental end of the cord, are rare but more likely than venous ectasias to adversely affect fetal well-being by their tendency to form thrombi or rupture spontaneously (Fig. 5–12*B*).[124,125]

True knots are found in about 0.5% of cords,[126] but are more common with male fetuses, monoamniotic twins (intertwining), multiparous women, and gestations complicated by fetal growth retardation, hydramnios, or long umbilical cords. Because true knots are formed as a result of the fetus' moving through a loop or loops of cord during its activities in the uterus, the vast majority must form early in gestation, especially those that are highly complex,[127] although some may originate during fetal descent at delivery.[128] Support for the view that most true knots form early in gestation is the observation that the frequency of knots in aborted fetuses is similar to that observed at term.[129]

Except with monoamniotic twins,[130] knots rarely tighten before labor but may do so during fetal descent at delivery. It is also plausible that tightening to a degree insufficient to occlude a vessel might lead to transient umbilical vein stenosis[131] or to vessel spasm and fetal cerebral hypoxia. Despite reports of 8% to 11% perinatal mortality or significant in utero hypoxia with lasting damage,[132] knots are infrequently responsible in my experience and that of others.[133]

Older knots have permanent cord grooving, focal loss of Wharton's jelly, and persistent curling at the site after reduction, whereas those that are clinically significant demonstrate venous distention distal (placental side) to the knot, mural thrombi, especially in the vein, and persistent compression after reduction. Knots suspected of having caused fetal morbidity should be sampled for microscopy through their centers as well as on either side. The significance of a true knot is especially difficult to interpret when present in a macerated stillbirth. Under this circumstance a knot that had no significance while the fetus was alive might tighten after fetal demise from some other cause because of autolysis of Wharton's jelly and loss of the protective turgidity of the umbilical vessels.

Nuchal Coils and Other Fetal Entanglements

Fetal cord entanglements, including nuchal coils, occur in about 20% to 25% of deliveries. They are associated with male fetuses and cords of excessive length. The greater the number of loops or coils, the longer the average cord length. Nuchal cords are significantly more frequent when the placenta is posterior than when it is anterior or fundal.[134]

Whether looping causes or results from the excessive cord length is unclear. Fetal movement and excessive tension on a previously entangled cord may lead to excessive cord length, or a long cord may predispose to looping that may be protective by preventing cord prolapse. Looping has been identified both in early gestation and at term. Of spontaneous abortions, 13.4% have looping and cords of excessive length.[129] Nuchal cords that form early may resolve or persist until term, and coils may form shortly before delivery.[135]

Entanglements can lead to fetal demise by neck compression with obstruction of jugular venous return, congestion of cerebral and meningeal vessels, and intracranial hemorrhage or by obstruction of umbilical venous return, umbilical vascular spasm, or cord rupture when a long cord is converted by entanglement into one of relative brevity (Fig. 5–13). A child coming into the world with a

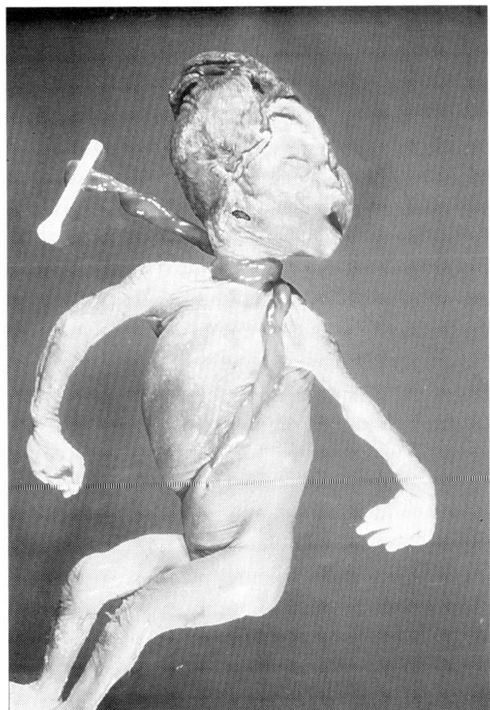

Figure 5–13. Severely macerated 27-week fetus with two nuchal coils that were deemed responsible for the fetal demise because of marked congestion of the cord distal to the entanglement and venous thrombi noted on microscopy. The cord "stricture" at the umbilicus showed no thrombi. The gradually diminishing quantity of Wharton's jelly as the cord approaches the abdomen was due to autolysis, which proceeds from the fetus toward the placenta.

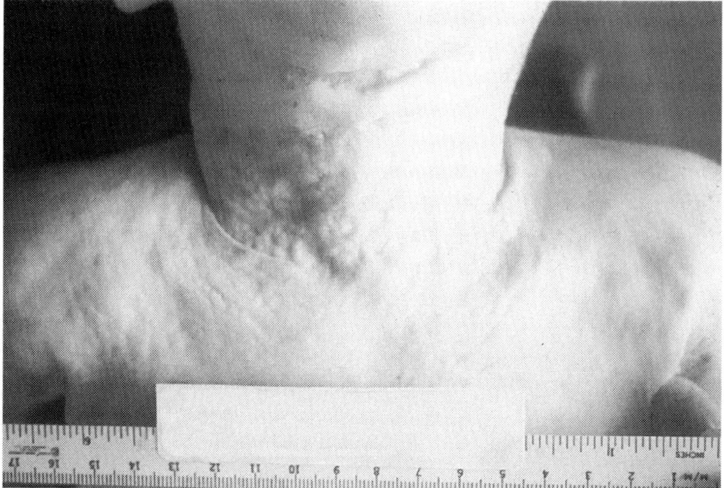

Figure 5–14. Telltale grooves on the fetal neck attest to the double nuchal coil that caused this fresh stillbirth at term.

relatively short cord about his or her neck has been rather colorfully described as "like a roped calf at milking time," or, to use Shakespeare's simile, "like a greyhound straining in the leash."[136] A cord tightly entangled about the neck or other body part may leave a recognizable groove on the skin (Fig. 5–14). As with true knots or cord strictures, a clinically significant entanglement often demonstrates venous distention or cord edema at its placental end, hematoma formation, or vascular thrombi.[137] An increased incidence of neonatal anemia[138] and instances of hypovolemic shock, chronic fetal growth retardation, and fetal distress with nuchal coils may be due to fetoplacental transfusion by chronic relative compression of the umbilical vein.[139–141]

Rupture and Hematoma of the Cord

Complete cord rupture is an instantaneous catastrophic intrapartum event that almost invariably leads to fetal exsanguination, whereas partial rupture refers to vessel tears (usually the vein) with intrafunicular hematoma formation.[142–144] Causes of cord rupture include the following:

1. Absolute or relative shortness of the cord with traction
2. Precipitous unattended delivery, especially when upright or squatting
3. Tight torsion or stricture of the cord
4. Abnormal cord insertion: velamentous, insertio funiculi furcata
5. Inflammation of the cord
6. Trauma: version, forceps, reduction of nuchal coil, assisted breech delivery, amniocentesis, percutaneous umbilical blood sampling, fetal transfusion, prolapse
7. Varix or aneurysm or hematoma of cord
8. Tumultuous fetal movements
9. Paucity of vascular elastic tissue or smooth muscle
10. Vascular thrombi
11. Deficiency of Wharton's jelly
12. Sudden decompression of hydramnios
13. Hemorrhagic disease of the newborn
14. Foreign body: intrauterine contraceptive device
15. Hemangioma of the umbilical cord
16. Omphalomesenteric duct cyst with acid-secreting gastric mucosa

Cord hematomas are purple fusiform swellings that must be distinguished from postdelivery iatrogenic lesions, such as cord clamping or sampling of cord blood. Recently hematomas were found in 1.5% of 341 diagnostic ultrasound–guided percutaneous umbilical blood sampling procedures and were more likely when punctures were attempted in a free loop of cord or when multiple procedures were attempted in any one session.[144]

In my experience hematomas may be found in 1% to 2% of carefully examined consecutively delivered cords but are rarely of clinical importance. Most are of insufficient size to cause umbilical vessel compression or occlusion or fetal cardiovascular embarrassment resulting from loss, but bradycardia secondary to arterial spasm has been observed[145]; large tumefactions that represent substantial fetal blood loss or are capable of causing compression or spasm of adjacent cord vessels are rare. The latter are largely confined to cases of short cord with presumed traction, or long cord with occult or overt prolapse. The sizable perinatal mortality (up to 50%) that is repeatedly cited in the cord hematoma literature[146,147] is related to ascertainment and selection bias.

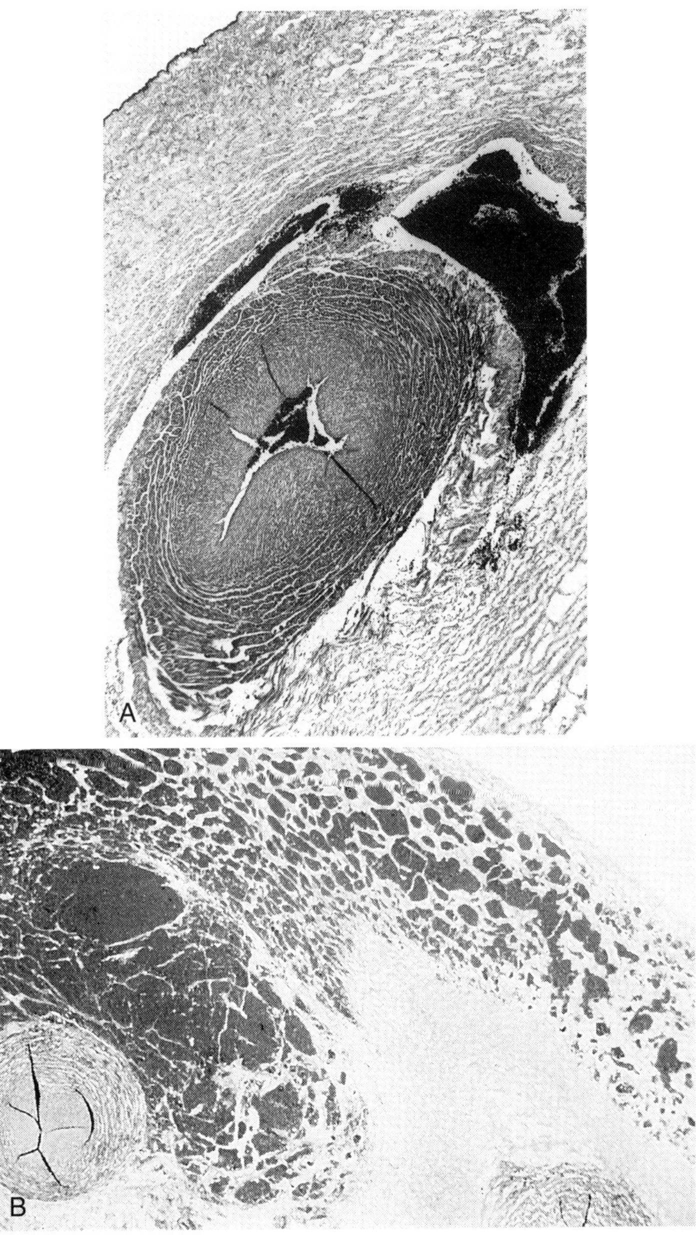

Figure 5–15. A, Periarterial intrafunicular hematoma forming a perivascular lake of extravasated blood. **B,** Periarterial intrafunicular hematoma has dissected through Wharton's jelly, creating an angiomatoid appearance. The spaces lack an endothelial lining, thereby permitting differentiation from true cord hemangioma.

On microscopic study most hematomas are perivascular lakes of extravasated blood, but at times they dissect through Wharton's jelly creating angiomatoid, but non-endothelium-lined, spaces that permit differentiation from true cord hemangiomas (Fig. 5–15).[50]

Prolapse of the Umbilical Cord

Prolapse is a clinical rather than a pathologic entity. In spite of their association with perinatal mortality, prolapsed cords only rarely show morphologic effects of compression. Antecedent risk factors include long cord, thin cord, breech presentation, premature labor, hydramnios, multiparity, major fetal malformations, second-born twin, premature rupture of the fetal membranes, and incompetent cervix.[148,149] Many of these risk factors are related to breech presentation. Prolapse occurs with both very large and very small babies, presumably because of improper engagement of the presenting part.

As with knots, entanglements, and hematomas, the hazard of cord prolapse is related to embarrassment of the umbilical blood flow. Both overt prolapse and occult prolapse are obstetric emergencies associated with a high perinatal death rate. Death results from occlusive compression of the cord against the pelvic wall by the fetus and from the antecedent risk factors such as prematurity and major fetal malformations.[150] No increased frequency of long-term neurologic abnormalities in survivors is found, however, suggesting that when cord prolapse with compression occurs, acute antenatal hypoxia is sufficiently severe to be almost always fatal, and also suggesting that acute hypoxia for up to 60 minutes is unlikely per se to result in long-term neurologic damage.[150]

Thrombosis of Cord Vessels

The incidence of cord thrombosis is 1 in 1300 deliveries with a slight male predominance.[70] Thrombi in veins are more common than in one or both arteries, but poor fetal outcome is more likely with arterial thrombosis. Because of the normally present interarterial anastomosis at the placental end of the cord, a thrombus within one artery may not be detrimental to the fetus unless the placenta is showered by emboli. The strong association in the literature between cord thrombosis and perinatal morbidity and mortality reflects case selection bias and is not noted among prospective cases. When present, however, thrombosis is related to the presence of additional cord abnormalities (long or short cord, entanglements, knots, peripheral insertion, stricture, torsion, funisitis, amniotic bands [Fig. 5–16], and hematoma), obstetric complications (prolapse, breech presentation, and multiple gestations), systemic fetal conditions (fetomaternal hemorrhage, anemia, infants of diabetic mothers, sepsis, and Beckwith-

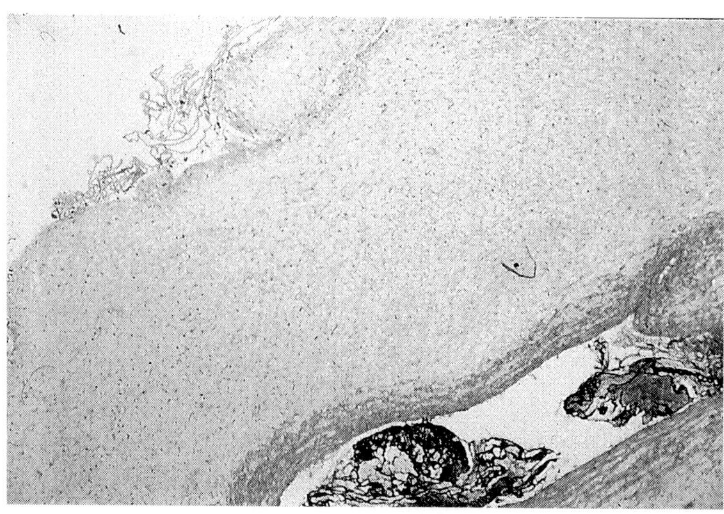

Figure 5–16. Umbilical vein thrombus at the site of cord strangulation by an amniotic band that is seen as the stringy material on the cord surface.

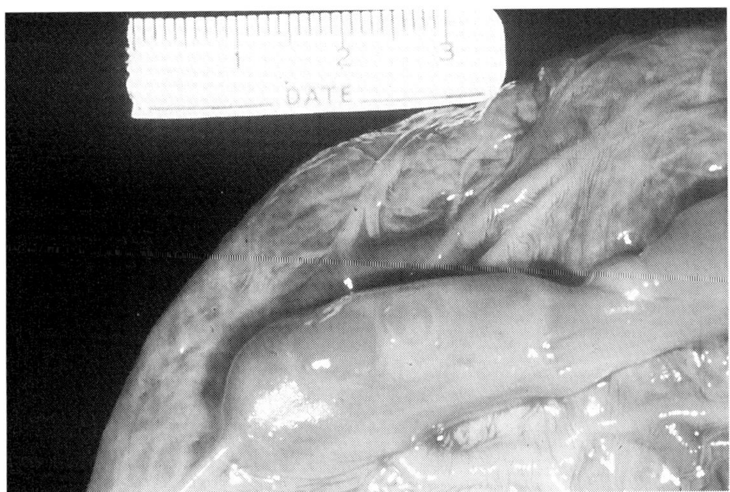

Figure 5–17. Ulceration of the umbilical cord in a child with multiple small intestinal atresias.

Wiedemann syndrome), or iatrogenic factors (amniocentesis, percutaneous umbilical blood sampling, and exchange transfusion) that are the likely cause of both the thrombosis and the poor fetal outcome. In such cases thrombosis may be a marker of the severity of these associated conditions and thrombi may presage fetal distress or demise. Cord thrombi may lead to or result from fetoplacental embolism and be responsible for in utero fetal amputations or a generalized bleeding tendency in the fetus or neonate caused by disseminated intravascular coagulation or protein C or S deficiency.[70,151–154] Thrombi may occur in early pregnancy and lead to single umbilical artery. Because umbilical vessels lack vasa vasorum and receive their nourishment solely from blood flowing within their lumina, occlusive thrombi invariably lead to mural necrosis, at times with superimposed calcification.

ULCERATION

Apart from five case reports of fetal death by exsanguination resulting from cord ulceration and umbilical vein erosion by an adjacent omphalomesenteric duct cyst bearing acid-secreting gastric epithelium,[47] ulceration of the umbilical cord occurs with fetal intestinal atresia or with prolonged exposure to meconium. Five cases of congenital intestinal atresia with cord ulceration and fetal hemorrhage,[155–157] one with cord hemangioma[155] and one with deletion 13q (which has been linked with intestinal atresia),[157] have been reported. Linear cord ulcers, at times with adherent thrombotic material but little if any inflammatory response, follow the spiral groove of the cords between the two arteries (Fig. 5–17). Three pathogenetic mechanisms are possible: (1) abnormal vascular reactivity leading to simultaneous vasospasm of both the umbilical and enteric vasculature with ischemic damage; (2) chemical ulceration of the cord resulting from gastroduodenal reflux into the amniotic fluid because of upper gut atresia (numerous pigment-laden macrophages within the placental membranes of such cases usually contain meconium or bile); and (3) a developmental abnormality of the amniotic epithelium of the cord and the epithelial lining of the gut analogous to the well-known association between epidermolysis bullosa and pyloric atresia.[158]

Meconium-induced vasoconstriction and necrosis of cord and superficial placental vessels, at times with overlying cord epithelial ulceration, occur when meconium has been present in the amniotic cavity for at least 16 hours and are associated with fetal distress, neonatal asphyxia, and severe neurologic damage (Fig. 5–18).[159] Both arterial and venous walls may be affected, from outside inward, and most often only in the portion of the wall oriented toward the cord's surface. Possibly meconium induces vasocontraction, fetal hypoperfusion, and severe neurologic damage even when exposure has been limited to less than the 16 hours required from myocyte necrosis, and therefore the vasoactive effects of meconium may

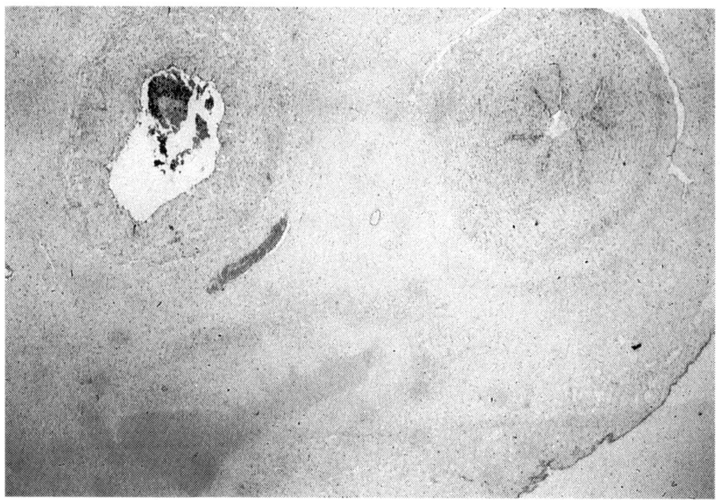

Figure 5–18. Meconium-induced necrosis of one umbilical artery. The portion of the arterial wall oriented toward the surface is most severely affected.

be causally related to neonatal morbidity, including persistent fetal circulation, necrotizing enterocolitis, and renal failure. Meconium passage, therefore, may be the cause of fetal damage under special circumstances.

INFLAMMATION

Acute inflammation of Wharton's jelly, acute funisitis, occurs as a late sequela of the amniotic infection syndrome and is more fully discussed in Chapter 13. Funisitis is almost invariably accompanied by chorioamnionitis and umbilical phlebitis and often includes umbilical arteritis and superficial placental chorionic vasculitis. Funisitis is caused by intraamniotic bacteria–produced leukoattractants that have diffused into the umbilical cord. The intensity of inflammation correlates more with duration of infection and the immunologic status of the fetus than with risk of fetal sepsis. The likelihood of sepsis depends more on the virulence of the infective organism, although there is a direct relationship between the incidence of intrauterine infection, preterm birth, or perinatal death and increasing severity of funisitis.[160] Mounting evidence suggests that funisitis may lead to vasoconstriction, fetal hypoperfusion, and cerebral hypoxia, potentially resulting in neonatal encephalopathy, intraventricular hemorrhage, periventricular leukomalacia, pulmonary vasoconstriction with persistent fetal circulation, necrotizing enterocolitis, and damage to fetal kidneys and liver.[6,161,162] Rarely, funisitis is limited to the cord segment nearest the cervical os or, in the absence of chorioamnionitis, is due to vessel damage by occult prolapse or compression.

Two variants of acute funisitis can be diagnosed by gross examination in the delivery room. *Candida* funisitis appears as discrete 2 to 5 mm yellow plaques on the cord surface that represent microabscesses just beneath the amniotic covering of the cord. The plaques bear candidal yeast and pseudohyphae readily identified with periodic acid–Schiff or silver stain (Fig. 5–19).[163,164] On microscopic examination, inflammatory cells are seen migrating through the walls of the umbilical vessels, indicating their fetal origin. A similar gross and microscopic appearance has been reported with *Torulopsis glabrata,*[165] *Corynebacterium kutscheri,*[166] *Listeria monocytogenes,* and *Haemophilus influenzae.*[167] *Candida* funisitis is related to maternal intrauterine contraceptive devices, cervical instrumentation, or prenatal antibiotic administration and is strongly associated with prematurity. The earlier in gestation that *Candida* funisitis occurs, the greater the likelihood of fetal colonization, especially of the skin, lungs, and gastrointestinal tract (in utero breathing and swallowing of contaminated amniotic fluid).

The grossly visible yellow plaques of *Candida* funisitis must be distinguished from similar grayish plaques of squamous hyperplasia or metaplasia of the cord surface amnion (cord caruncles), which

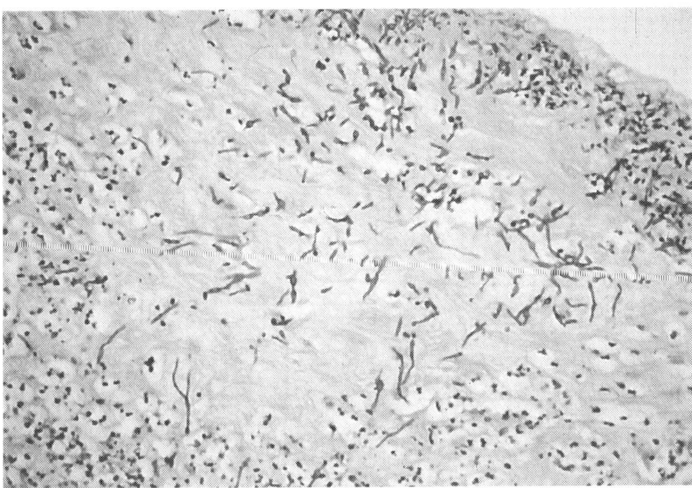

Figure 5–19. Periodic acid–Schiff reaction reveals *Candida* pseudohyphae in superficial (subamniotic) microabscess.

cluster around the placental insertion site and are composed of increased numbers of epithelial layers of keratinizing squamous cells (Fig. 5–20), and from amnion nodosum, which occasionally also affects the cord surface amnion near the placental insertion.

The second macroscopically and microscopically distinctive variant of funisitis is necrotizing (sclerosing) funisitis.[168] On gross examination the cord shows yellowish white chalky stripes that parallel the spiral course of the vessels and on cross section form perivascular rings or crescents or a diffuse brownish discoloration of Wharton's jelly (Fig. 5–21). On microscopic study the intense, usually trivascular, inflammatory cell infiltrate, rather than being continuous and exclusively neutrophilic as in the more prosaic acute funisitis, is commonly discontinuous. The successive waves of inflammatory cells alternate with areas of abundant karyorrhectic and necrotic debris that is susceptible to mineralization, and the neutrophils are frequently accompanied by eosinophils, lymphocytes, and plasma cells. The alternating zones of cellular infiltrate and necrotic debris create the grossly apparent concentric perivascular rings in a manner reminiscent of an Ouchterlony immunodiffusion plate.

Frequently associated pathologic features include necrotizing chorioamnionitis, necrosis of the cord surface amniotic epithelium, mural thrombi,

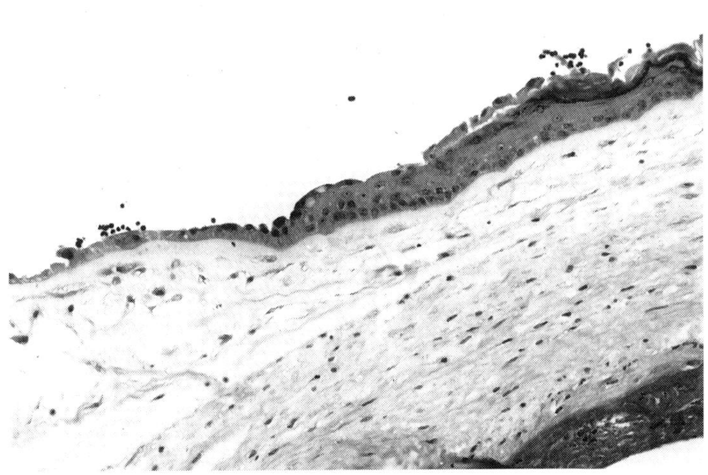

Figure 5–20. Cord caruncle (squamous hyperplasia and metaplasia). Multiple layers of keratinizing squamous epithelial cells arise from the basal layer of the amniotic epithelium and appear to lift the usual cuboidal amniotic epithelium of the cord surface from the underlying Wharton's jelly.

proliferative endovasculitis, and capillary neovascularity. Strong clinical correlations include perinatal infection, prolonged rupture of membranes, prematurity, intrauterine growth retardation, stillbirth, and neonatal necrotizing enterocolitis.[169,170]

Necrotizing funisitis is caused by protracted inflammation of a structure whose normal anatomy (lack of lymphatics, capillaries, and fixed macrophages) precludes removal of inflammatory debris. Both morphologic and clinical features indicate long-standing inflammation, including the high incidence of umbilical arteritis, the lymphoplasmacytic infiltrate, proliferative endovasculitis, capillary neovascularity, and its nearly universal association with fetal or neonatal infection. Although sometimes present in congenital syphilis,[171] necrotizing funisitis is more often absent and is not an "indicator of congenital syphilis"[172] nor does its presence "permit a presumptive diagnosis of congenital syphilis at birth."[173] No single pathogen causes necrotizing funisitis.[174] A strong association exists with latent endometrial herpes simplex virus type 2 (HSV-2) infection, suggesting that whereas the usual ascending (bacterial) infection leads to labor and delivery before necrotizing funisitis has had sufficient time to develop, latent endometrial HSV-2 infection may alter local paracrine factors and delay parturition long enough for necrotizing funisitis, a morphologic hallmark of chronicity, to become apparent.[170]

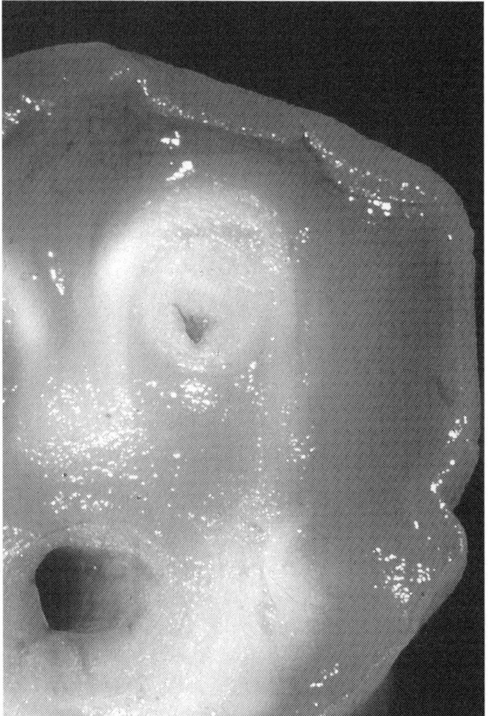

Figure 5–21. Necrotizing funisitis with perivascular rings and crescents composed of calcified necrotic debris.

TRUE TUMORS

Only two true tumors occur in the umbilical cord: angiomas and teratomas.[50] Cord hemangiomas consist of an angiomatous nodule containing and encompassed by edema or cystic myxomatous degeneration of Wharton's jelly that may be up to 15 cm in diameter and exaggerate considerably their apparent dimensions (Fig. 5–22*A*). Hemangiomas tend to occur at the placental end of the cord and arise from one or more of the umbilical vessels (Fig. 5–22*B*). They are composed of anastomosing endothelium-lined vascular channels with variable amounts of mural smooth muscle. They resemble placental chorangiomas and are invariably benign, although death may occur because of obstruction of blood flow or severe in utero hemorrhage. Stromal calcification or osseous metaplasia may be present. Unlike chorangiomas, however, cord hemangiomas are only rarely associated with hydramnios,[175,176] presumably because the transudated fluid remains trapped within Wharton's jelly by the cord surface amnion, which is less permeable than placental or membranous amnion.[50] Elevated levels of α-fetoprotein[177–179] and nonimmune hydrops[180,181] may occur, and our suggestion[50] that they may be associated with fetal hemangiomas at other sites has been confirmed.[180,182]

Teratoma, the only other primary cord tumor, is extremely rare. Only 12 cases have been reported since 1878.[183,184] The teratomas are identical with teratomas of the placenta and invariably benign. There is a marked female preponderance, and several affected infants have had various malformations, especially omphalocele. Germ cells migrate from the yolk sac through the embryonic enteric mesentery within the connecting stalk to the gonadal ridge, and aberrant or arrested migration probably account for the occurrence of teratomas within the placenta and cord. Neuroblastoma

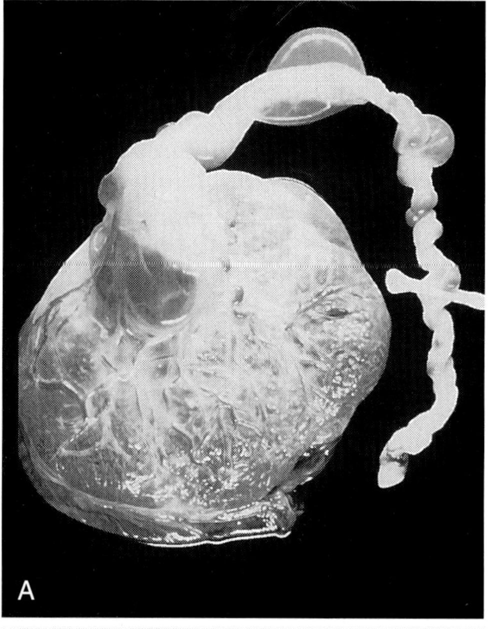

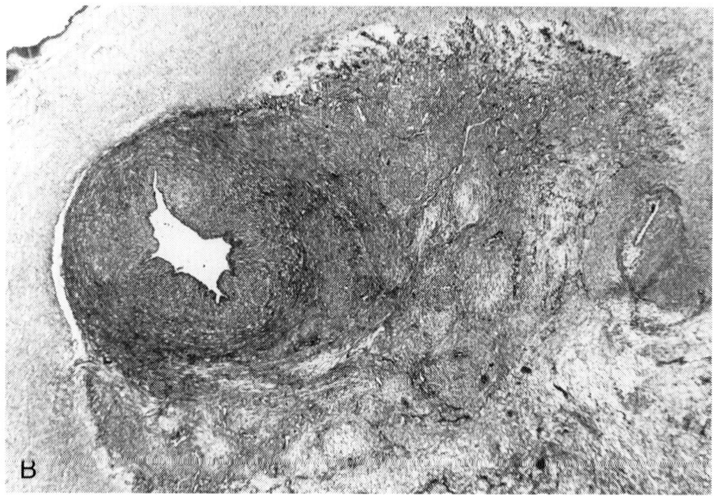

Figure 5–22. A, Hemangioma of the cord. A solid angiomatous nodule near the placental insertion site was associated with massive cystic degeneration of Wharton's jelly. Additional fluid-filled blebs also represent entrapped transudate from the angiomatous nodule. **B,** Cord hemangioma arising from one umbilical artery. Note "pushing" border and marked stromal edema.

metastasizing to the cord from a fetal primary tumor and direct extension to the cord of a giant pigmented nevus have also been described.[185]

REFERENCES

1. Ward CJ: Analysis of 500 obstetric and gynecologic malpractice claims: causes and prevention. Am J Obstet Gynecol 165:298, 1991.
2. Naeye RL: Functionally important disorders of the placenta, umbilical cord and fetal membranes. Hum Pathol 18:680, 1987.
3. Ward CJ: The case for placental examination. The Digest: A Medical Liability and Risk Management Newsletter Fall:1, 1989.
4. Altshuler G: Some placental considerations related to neuro-developmental and other disorders. J Child Neurol 8:78, 1993.
5. Benirschke K: Obstetrically important lesions of the umbilical cord. J Reprod Med 39:262, 1994.

6. Grafe MR: The correlation of prenatal brain damage with placental pathology. J Neuropathol Exp Neurol 53:407, 1994.
7. Dudiak CM, Salomon CG, Posniak HV, et al: Sonography of the umbilical cord. RadioGraphics 15:1035, 1995.
8. Moore KL, Persaud TVN: The developing human. Philadelphia, 1993, WB Saunders.
9. Blackburn W, Cooley W: Umbilical cord. In Stevenson RE, Hall JG, Goodman RM (eds): Human malformations and related anomalies. New York, 1993, Oxford University Press, p. 1275.
10. Reynolds SRM: The proportion of Wharton's jelly in the umbilical cord in relation to distension of the umbilical arteries and veins, with observations on the folds of Hoboken. Anat Rec 113:365, 1952.
11. Takechi K, Kuwabara Y, Mizuno M: Ultrastructural and immunohistochemical studies of Wharton's jelly umbilical cord cells. Placenta 14:235, 1993.
12. Eyden BP, Ponting J, Davies H, et al: Defining the myofibroblast: normal tissues, with special reference to the stromal cells of Wharton's jelly in human umbilical cord. J Submicrosc Cytol Pathol 26:347, 1994.
13. Fox SB, Khong TY: Lack of innervation of human umbilical cord: an immunohistological and histochemical study. Placenta 11:59, 1990.
14. Gebrane-Younes J, Minh HN, Orcel L: Ultrastructure of human umbilical vessels: a possible role in amniotic fluid formation. Placenta 7:173, 1986.
15. Harold JG, Siegel RJ, Fitzgerald GA, et al: Differential prostaglandin production by human umbilical vasculature. Arch Pathol Lab Med 112:43, 1988.
16. McCoshen JA, Tulloch HV, Johnson KA: Umbilical cord is the major source of prostaglandin E2 in the gestational sac during term labor. Am J Obstet Gynecol 160:873, 1989.
17. Boura ALA, Walters WAW: Autoacids and the control of vascular tone in the human umbilical-placental circulation. Placenta 12:453, 1990.
18. Karbowski B, Bauch HJ, Schneider HPG: Functional differentiation of umbilical vein endothelial cells following pregnancy complicated by smoking or diabetes mellitus. Placenta 12:405, 1991.
19. Ulm MR, Plöckinger B, Pirich C, et al: Umbilical arteries of babies born to cigarette smokers generate less prostacyclin and contain less arginine and citrulline compared with those of babies born to control subjects. Am J Obstet Gynecol 172: 1485, 1995.
20. Bankowski E, Sobolewski K, Romanowicz L, et al: Collagen and glycosaminoglycans of Wharton's jelly and their alterations in EPH-gestosis. Eur J Obstet Gynecol Reprod Biol 66:109, 1996.
21. Heifetz SA: Single umbilical artery: a statistical analysis of 237 autopsy cases and review of the literature. Perspect Pediatr Pathol 8:345, 1984.
22. Bryan EM, Kohler HG: The missing umbilical artery. I. Prospective study based on a maternity unit. Arch Dis Child 49:844, 1974.
23. Abuhamad AZ, Shaffer W, Mari G, et al: Single umbilical artery: does it matter which artery is missing? Am J Obstet Gynecol 173:728, 1995.
24. Persutte WH, Hobbins J: Single umbilical artery: a clinical enigma in modern prenatal diagnosis. Ultrasound Obstet Gynecol 6:216, 1995.
25. Stocker JT, Heifetz SA: Sirenemelia: a morphological study of 33 cases and review of the literature. Perspect Pediatr Pathol 10:7, 1987.
26. Feingold M, Fine RN, Ingall D: Intravenous pyelography in infants with single umbilical artery. N Engl J Med 270:1178, 1964.
27. Bourke WG, Clarke TA, Mathews TG, et al: Isolated single umbilical artery—the case for routine renal screening. Arc Dis Child 68:600, 1993.
28. Stevenson RE, Jones KL, Phelan MC, et al: Vascular steal: the pathogenetic mechanism producing sirenomelia and associated defects of the viscera and soft tissues. Pediatrics 78:451, 1986.
29. Neel JV: A study of major congenital defects in Japanese infants. Am J Hum Genet 10:398, 1958.
30. Emmanoulides GC, Townsend DE, Bauer RA: Effects of single umbilical artery ligation in the lamb fetus. Pediatrics 42:919, 1968.
31. Monica G, Lilja C: Single umbilical artery and maternal smoking. Br Med J 302:569, 1991.
32. Bronshtein M, Zimmer EZ: Are measurements of the umbilical vessels a reliable method in diagnosing a single umbilical artery? Ultrasound Obstet Gynecol 8:5, 1996.
33. Khong TY, George K: Chromosomal abnormalities associated with a single umbilical artery. Prenatal Diagn 12:965, 1992.
34. Saller DN Jr, Neiger R: Cytogenetic abnormalities among perinatal deaths demonstrating a single umbilical artery. Prenatal Diagn 14:13, 1994.
35. Bjoro K Jr: Vascular anomalies of the umbilical cord. I. Obstetric implications. II. Perinatal and pediatric implications. Early Hum Dev 8:119, 279, 1983.
36. Gupta I, Hillier VF, Edwards JM: Multiple vascular profiles in the umbilical cord; an indication of maternal smoking habits and intrauterine distress. Placenta 14:117, 1993.
37. Bell AD, Gerlis LM, Variend S: Persistent right

umbilical vein—case report and review of the literature. Int J Cardiol 10:167, 1986.
38. Jeanty P: Persistent right umbilical vein: an ominous prenatal finding? Radiology 177:735, 1990.
39. Hill LM, Mills A, Peterson C, Boyles D: Persistent right umbilical vein: sonographic detection and subsequent neonatal outcome. Obstet Gynecol 84:923, 1994.
40. Kinare AS, Ambardekar ST, Bhattacharya D, Pande SA: Prenatal diagnosis with ultrasound of anomalous course of the umbilical vein and its relationship to fetal outcome. Clin Ultrasound 24:333, 1996.
41. Moore L, Toi A, Chitayat D: Abnormalities of the intra-abdominal fetal umbilical vein: reports of four cases and a review of the literature. Ultrasound Obstet Gynecol 7:21, 1996.
42. Heifetz SA, Rueda-Pedraza ME: Omphalomesenteric duct cysts of the umbilical cord. Pediatr Pathol 1:325, 1983.
43. Jauniaux E, DeMunter C, Vanesse M, et al: Embryonic remnants of the umbilical cord: morphological and clinical aspects. Hum Pathol 20:458, 1989.
44. Sepulveda W, Bower S, Dhillon HK, Fisk NM: Prenatal diagnosis of congenital patent urachus and allantoic cyst: the value of color flow imaging. J Ultrasound Med 14:47, 1995.
45. Baill IC, Moore GW, Hedrick LA: Abscess of allantoic duct remnant. Am J Obstet Gynecol 161:334, 1989.
46. Fink IJ, Filly RA: Omphalocele associated with umbilical cord allantoic cyst: sonographic evaluation in utero. Radiology 149:473, 1983.
47. Blanc WA, Allan GW: Intrafunicular ulceration of persistent omphalomesenteric duct with intra-amniotic hemorrhage and fetal death. Am J Obstet Gynecol 82:1392, 1961.
48. Jona JZ: Congenital hernia of the cord and associated patent omphalomesenteric duct: a frequent neonatal problem? Am J Perinatol 13:223, 1996.
49. Petrikovsky BM, Nochimson DJ, Campbell WA, Vintzileos AM: Fetal jejunoileal atresia with persistent omphalomesenteric duct. Am J Obstet Gynecol 158:173, 1988.
50. Heifetz SA, Rueda-Pedraza ME: Hemangiomas of the umbilical cord. Pediatric Pathol 1:385, 1983.
51. Quartero HWP, v.d. Berg W, Kolkman PH: A prenatal diagnosis of umbilical cord oedema made by ultrasound: a case report. Eur J Obstet Gynecol Reprod Biol 17:409, 1984.
52. Iaccarino M, Baldi F, Persico D, Pulagiano A: Ultrasonographic and pathologic study of mucoid degeneration of umbilical cord. J Clin Ultrasound 14:127, 1986.
53. Jauniaux E, Jurkovic D, Campbell S: Sonographic features of an umbilical cord abnormality combining a cord pseudocyst and a small omphalocele; a case report. Eur J Obstet Gynecol Reprod Biol 40:245, 1991.
54. Kalter CS, Williams MC, Vaughn V, Spellacy WN: Sonographic diagnosis of a large umbilical cord pseudocyst. J Ultrasound Med 13:487, 1994.
55. Sepulveda W, Pryde PG, Greb AE, et al: Prenatal diagnosis of umbilical cord pseudocyst. Ultrasound Obstet Gynecol 4:147, 1994.
56. Chen C-P, Jan S-W, Liu F-F, et al: Prenatal diagnosis of omphalocele associated with umbilical cord cyst. Acta Obstet Gynecol Scand 74:832, 1995.
57. Ramirez P, Haberman S, Baxi L: Significance of prenatal diagnosis of umbilical cord cyst in a fetus with trisomy 18. Am J Obstet Gynecol 173:955, 1995.
58. Shipp TD, Bromley B, Benacerraf BR: Sonographically detected abnormalities of the umbilical cord. Int J Gynecol Obstet 48:179, 1995.
59. Labarrere C, Sebastiani M, Siminovich M, et al: Absence of Wharton's jelly around the umbilical arteries: an unusual cause of perinatal mortality. Placenta 6:555, 1985.
60. Coulter JBS, Scott JM, Jordan MM: Oedema of the cord and respiratory distress in the newborn. Br J Obstet Gynaecol 82:453, 1975.
61. Rolschau J: The relationship between some disorders of the umbilical cord and intrauterine growth retardation. Acta Obstet Gynecol Scand Suppl 72:15, 1978.
62. Howorka E, Kapczynski W: Unusual thickness of the fetal end of the umbilical cord. J Obstet Gynaecol Br Commonw 78:283, 1971.
63. Hall SP: The thin cord syndrome: a review with a report of two cases. Obstet Gynecol 18:507, 1961.
64. Kiley KC, Perknis CS, Penney LL: Umbilical cord stricture associated with intrauterine fetal demise: a report of two cases. J Reprod Med 31:154, 1986.
65. Sun Y, Arbuckle S, Hocking G, Billson V: Umbilical cord stricture and intrauterine fetal death. Pediatr Pathol Lab Med 15:723, 1995.
66. Krawczuk-Rybakowa M, Lotocki W: Accessory blood vessels of the umbilical cord in the third trimester of physiological pregnancy, abstracted. Rocz Akad Med Bialymstoku 25:163, 1980.
67. Heifetz SA: The placenta. In Stocker JT, Dehner LD (eds): Pediatric pathology. Philadelphia, 1992, Lippincott, p 387.
68. Weber J: Constriction of the umbilical cord as a cause of foetal death. Acta Obstet Gynecol Scand 42:259, 1963.

69. Ghosh A, Woo JS, MacHenry C, et al: Fetal loss from umbilical cord abnormalities—a difficult case for prevention. Eur J Obstet Gynecol Reprod Biol 18:183, 1984.
70. Heifetz SA: Thrombosis of the umbilical cord: analysis of 52 cases and literature review. Pediatr Pathol 8:37, 1988.
71. Glanfield PA, Watson R: Intrauterine death due to umbilical cord torsion. Arch Pathol Lab Med 110:357, 1986.
72. Qureshi F, Jacques SM: Marked segmental thinning of the umbilical cord vessels. Arch Pathol Lab Med 118:826, 1994.
73. Heifetz SA: Strangulation of the umbilical cord by amniotic bands: report of six cases and literature review. Pediatr Pathol 2:284, 1984.
74. Kanayama MD, Gaffey TA, Ogburn PL Jr: Constriction of the umbilical cord by an amniotic band, with fetal compromise illustrated by reverse diastolic flow in the umbilical artery: a case report. J Reprod Med 40:71, 1995.
75. Cordero DR, Helfgott AW, Landy HJ, et al: A nonhemorrhagic manifestation of vasa previa: a clinicopathologic case report. Obstet Gynecol 82:698, 1993.
76. Salafia CM, Vintzileos AM: Why all placentas should be examined by a pathologist in 1990. Am J Obstet Gynecol 163:1282, 1990.
77. Englert Y, Imbert MC, van Rosendall E, et al: Morphological anomalies in the placentae of IVF pregnancies: preliminary report of a multicentric study. Hum Reprod 2:155, 1987.
78. Jauniaux E, Englert Y, Vanesse M, et al: Pathologic features of placentas from singleton pregnancies obtained by in vitro fertilization and embryo transfer. Obstet Gynecol 76:61, 1990.
79. Fries MH, Goldstein RB, Kilpatrick SJ, et al: The role of velamentous cord insertion in the etiology of twin-twin transfusion syndrome. Obstet Gynecol 81:569, 1993.
80. Ottow B: Interposito velamentosa funiculi umbilicalis, eine bisher übersehene Nabelstranganomalie, ihre entstehung und klinische Bedeutung. Arch Gynäkol 116:176, 1922.
81. Herberz O: Uber die insertio furcata funiculi umbilicalis. Acta Obstet Gynecol Scand 18:336, 1938.
82. Swanberg H, Wiqvist N: Rupture of the umbilical cord during pregnancy: a report of a case. Acta Obstet Gynecol Scand 30:323, 1951.
83. Paavonen J, Jouttunpää K, Kangasluoma P, et al: Velamentous insertion of the umbilical cord and vasa previa. Int J Gynaecol Obstet 22:207, 1984.
84. Raga F, Ballester MJ, Osborne NG, Bonilla-Musoles F: Role of color flow Doppler ultrasonography in diagnosing velamentous insertion of the umbilical cord and vasa previa: a report of two cases. J Reprod Med 40:804, 1995.
85. Clerici G, Burnelli L, Lauro V, et al: Prenatal diagnosis of vasa previa presenting as amniotic band: "a not so innocent amniotic band." Ultrasound Obstet Gynecol 7:61, 1996.
86. Daly-Jones E, Hollingsworth J, Sepulveda W: Vasa previa: second trimester diagnosis using colour flow imaging. Br J Obstet Gynaecol 103:284, 1996.
87. Apt L, Darney W: Melena neonatorum: the swallowed blood syndrome; a simple test for differentiation of adult and fetal hemoglobin in blood stool. J Pediatr 47:6, 1955.
88. Messer RH, Gomez AR, Yambao TJ: Antepartum testing for vasa previa: current standard of care. Am J Obstet Gynecol 156:1459, 1987.
89. Davies BR, Casanueva E, Arroyo P: Placentas of small for dates infants: a small controlled series from Mexico City. Mex Obstet Gynecol 149:731, 1984.
90. Nordenvall M, Sandstedt B, Ulmsten U: Relationship between placental shape, cord insertion, lobes and gestational outcome. Acta Obstet Gynecol Scand 67:611, 1988.
91. Heinonen S, Ryynänen M, Kirkinen P, Saarikoski S: Perinatal diagnostic evaluation of velamentous umbilical cord insertion: clinical, Doppler, and ultrasonic findings. Obstet Gynecol 87:112, 1996.
92. Heinonen S, Ryynänen M, Kirkinen P, Saarikoski S: Velamentous umbilical cord insertion may be suspected from maternal serum alpha-fetoprotein and hCG. Br J Obstet Gynaecol 103:209, 1996.
93. Robinson LK, Jones KL, Benirschke K: The nature of structural defects associated with velamentous and marginal insertion of the umbilical cord. Am J Obstet Gynecol 146:191, 1983.
94. Franque O von: Zur Pathologie der Nachgeburtsheile. Ztschr Geburtsh Gynäkol 43:463, 1900.
95. Strassmann P: Placenta praevia. Arch Gynäkol 67:112, 1902.
96. King DL: Placental migration demonstrated by ultrasonography: a hypothesis of dynamic placentation. Radiology 109:167, 1973.
97. Naeye RL: Umbilical cord length: clinical significance. J Pediatr 107:278, 1985.
98. Gardiner JP: The umbilical cord: normal length; length in cord complications; etiology and frequency of coiling. Surg Gynecol Obstet 34:252, 1922.
99. De Silva N: Zygosity and umbilical cord length. J Reprod Med 37:850, 1992.

100. Moessinger AC: Fetal akinesis deformation sequence: an animal model. Pediatrics 72:857, 1983.
101. Moessinger AC, Mills JL, Harley EE, et al: Umbilical cord length in Down's syndrome. Am J Dis Child 140:1276, 1986.
102. Grange DK, Ayra S, Opitz JM, et al: The short umbilical cord. Birth Defects 23:191, 1987.
103. Katz V, Blanchard G, Dingman C, et al: Atenolol and short umbilical cords. Am J Obstet Gynecol 156:1271, 1987.
104. Soernes T, Bakke T: The length of the human umbilical cord in twin pregnancies. Am J Obstet Gynecol 154:1086, 1986.
105. Katsumata T, Miyake A, Tadaatsu A, et al: Length of the human umbilical cord in multiple pregnancy. Eur J Obstet Gynecol Reprod Biol 40:25, 1991.
106. Dunn PM: The placental venous pressure during and after the third stage of labour following early cord ligation. J Obstet Gynecol Br Commow 73:747, 1966.
107. Bain C, Eliot BW: Fetal distress in the first stage of labour associated with early fetal heart rate decelerations and a short umbilical cord. Aust NZ J Obstet Gynaecol 16:51, 1976.
108. Fujinaga M, Chinn A, Shepard TH: Umbilical cord growth in human and rat fetuses: evidence against the "stretch hypothesis." Teratology 41:333, 1990.
109. Collins J: First report: prenatal diagnosis of long cord (letter). Am J Obstet Gynecol 165:1901, 1991.
110. Manci EA, Ulmer DR, Nye DM, et al: Variations in normal umbilical cord length following birth, abstracted. Mod Pathol 6:p6p, 1993.
111. Lockwood CJ, Scioscia AL, Hobbins JC: Congenital absence of the umbilical cord resulting from maldevelopment of embryonic body folding. Am J Obstet Gynecol 155:1049, 1986.
112. Giacoia GP: Body stalk anomaly: congenital absence of the umbilical cord. Obstet Gynecol 80:527, 1992.
113. Malpas P, Symonds EM: Observations on the structure of the human umbilical cord. Surg Gynecol Obstet 123:746, 1966.
114. Chaurasia BD, Agarwal BM: Helical structure of the human umbilical cord. Acta Anat 103:226, 1979.
115. Fletcher S: Chirality in the umbilical cord. Br J Obstet Gynaecol 100:234, 1993.
116. Lacro RV, Jones KL, Benirschke K: The umbilical cord twist: origin, direction and relevance. Am J Obstet Gynecol 157:833, 1987.
117. Strong TH Jr, Elliott JP, Radin TG: Non-coiled umbilical blood vessels: a new marker for the fetus at risk. Obstet Gynecol 81:409, 1993.
118. Ercal T, Lacin S, Altunyurt S, et al: Umbilical coiling index: is it a marker for the foetus at risk? Br J Clin Pract 50:254, 1996.
119. Rana J, Ebert GA, Kappy KA: Adverse perinatal outcome in patients with an abnormal umbilical coiling index. Obstet Gynecol 85:573, 1995.
120. Strong TH Jr, Jarles DL, Vega JS, Feldman DB: The umbilical coiling index. Am J Obstet Gynecol 170:29, 1994.
121. Ben-Arie A, Weissman A, Steinberg Y, et al: Oligohydramnios, intrauterine growth retardation and fetal death due to umbilical cord torsion. Arch Gynecol Obstet 256:159, 1995.
122. Collins JH: Prenatal observation of umbilical cord torsion with subsequent premature labor and delivery of a 31-week infant with mild nonimmune hydrops. Am J Obstet Gynecol 172:1048, 1995.
123. Schröcksnadel H, Holböck E, Mitterschiffthaler G, et al: Thrombotic occlusion of an umbilical vein varix causing fetal death. Arch Gynecol Obstet 248:213, 1991.
124. Siddiqi TA, Bendon R, Schultz DM, Miodovnik M: Umbilical artery aneurysm: prenatal diagnosis and management. Obstet Gynecol 80:530, 1992.
125. Fortune DW, Ostor AG: Umbilical artery aneurysm. Am J Obstet Gynecol 131:339, 1978.
126. McLennan H, Price E, Urbanska M, et al: Umbilical cord knots and encirclements. Aust NZ J Obstet Gynaecol 28:116, 1988.
127. Robins JB: A complex true knot of the umbilical cord. Br J Clin Pathol 49:164, 1995.
128. Blickstein I, Shoham-Schwartz Z, Lancet M: Predisposing factors in the formation of true knots of the umbilical cord: analysis of morphometric and perinatal data. Int J Gynaecol Obstet 25:395, 1987.
129. Javert CT, Barton B: Congenital and acquired lesions of the umbilical cord and spontaneous abortion. Am J Obstet Gynecol 63:1065, 1952.
130. Change D-Y, Change R-Y, Chen R-J, et al: Triplet pregnancy complicated by intrauterine fetal death of conjoined twins from an umbilical cord accident of an acardius. J Reprod Med 41:459, 1996.
131. Gembruch U, Baschat AA: True knot of the umbilical cord: transient constrictive effect to umbilical venous blood flow demonstrated by Doppler sonography. Ultrasound Obstet Gynecol 8:53, 1996.
132. Matorra R, Diez J, Pereira JG, et al: True knots in the umbilical cord: clinical findings and fetal consequences. J Obstet Gynaecol 10:383, 1990.
133. Sepulveda W, Shennan AH, Bower S, et al: True

knot of the umbilical cord: a difficult prenatal ultrasonographic diagnosis. Ultrasound Obstet Gynecol 5:106, 1995.
134. Collins JH: An association between placental location and nuchal cord occurrence (letter). Am J Obstet Gynecol 167:570, 1992.
135. Collins JH, Collins CL, Weckwerth SR, DeAngelis L: Nuchal cords: timing of prenatal diagnosis and duration. Am J Obstet Gynecol 173:768, 1995.
136. Elmore JP: Shortening of the umbilical cord from coiling around the fetal neck. New Orleans Med Surg J 62:911, 1909-1910.
137. Collins JR: Two cases of multiple umbilical cord abnormalities resulting in stillbirth: prenatal observation with ultrasonography and fetal heart rates. Am J Obstet Gynecol 168:125, 1993.
138. Shepherd AJ, Richardson CJ, Brown JP: Nuchal cord as a cause of neonatal anemia. Am J Dis Child 139:71, 1985.
139. Vanhaesebrouck P, Vanneste K, dePraeter C, van Trappen Y: Tight nuchal cord and neonatal hypovolemic shock. Arch Dis Child 62:1276, 1987.
140. Hakura A, Kurauchi O, Mizutani S, Tomoda Y: Intrauterine growth retardation and fetal distress associated with the excessively long (160 cm) umbilical cord. Arch Gynecol Obstet 255:99, 1994.
141. Larson JD, Rayburn WF, Crosby S, Thurnau GR: Multiple nuchal cord entanglements and intrapartum complications. Am J Obstet Gynecol 173:1228, 1995.
142. Summerville JW, Powar JS, Ueland K: Umbilical cord hematoma resulting in intrauterine fetal demise: a case report. J Reprod Med 32:213, 1987.
143. Chénard E, Bastide A, Fraser WD: Umbilical cord hematoma following diagnostic funipuncture. Obstet Gynecol 76:994, 1990.
144. Duchatel F, Oury JF, Mennesson B, Muray JM: Complications of diagnostic ultrasound-guided percutaneous umbilical blood sampling: analysis of a series of 341 cases and review of the literature. Eur J Obstet Gynecol Reprod Biol 53:95, 1993.
145. Moise KJ, Carpenter RJ, Huhta JC, Deter RL: Umbilical cord hematoma secondary to in utero intravascular transfusion for Rh isoimmunization. Fetal Ther 2:65, 1987.
146. Gregora MG, Lai J: Umbilical cord hematoma: a serious pregnancy complication. Aust NZ J Obstet Gynaecol 35:212, 1995.
147. Sizun J, Soupre D, Broussine L, et al: L'hématome spontané du cordon: une cause rare de souffrance foetale aiguë. Arch Pédiatr (Paris) 2:1182, 1995.
148. Koonings PP, Paul RH, Campbell K: Umbilical cord prolapse—a contemporary look. J Reprod Med 35:690, 1990.
149. Critchlow CW, Leet TL, Benedetti TJ, Daling JR: Risk factors and infant outcomes associated with umbilical cord prolapse: a population-based case-control study among births in Washington State. Am J Obstet Gynecol 170:613, 1994.
150. Murphy DJ, MacKenzie IZ: The mortality and morbidity associated with umbilical cord prolapse. Br J Obstet Gynaecol 102:826, 1995.
151. Wolf, PL, Jones KL, Longway SR, et al: Prenatal death from acute myocardial infarction and cardiac tamponade due to embolus from the placenta. Am Heart J 109:603, 1985.
152. Hoyme HE, Jones KL, VanAllen MI, et al: Vascular pathogenesis of transverse limb reduction defects. J Pediatr 101:839, 1982.
153. Marco-Johnson MJ, Marlar RA, Jacobson LJ, et al: Severe protein C deficiency in newborn infants. J Pediatr 113:359, 1988.
154. Cook V, Weeks J, Brown J, Bendon R: Umbilical artery occlusion and fetoplacental thromboembolism. Obstet Gynecol 83:870, 1995.
155. Dombrowski MP, Budev H, Wolfe HM, et al: Fetal hemorrhage from umbilical cord hemangioma. Obstet Gynecol 70:439, 1987.
156. Bendon RW, Tyson RW, Baldwin VJ, et al: Umbilical cord ulceration and intestinal atresia: a new association? Am J Obstet Gynecol 164:582, 1991.
157. Khong TY, Ford WDA, Haan EA: Umbilical cord ulceration in association with intestinal atresia in a child with deletion 13q and Hirschsprung's disease. Arch Dis Child 71:F212, 1994.
158. Chang C-H, Perrin EV, Bove KE: Pyloric atresia associated with epidermolysis bullosa: special reference to pathogenesis. Pediatr Pathol 1:449, 1983.
159. Altschuler G, Arizawa M, Molnar-Nadasdy G: Meconium-induced umbilical cord vascular necrosis and ulceration: a potential link between the placenta and poor pregnancy outcome. Obstet Gynecol 79:760, 1992.
160. vanHoeven KH, Anyaegbunam A, Hochster H, et al: Clinical significance of increasing histologic severity of acute inflammation in the fetal membranes and umbilical cord. Pediatr Pathol Lab Med 16:731, 1996.
161. Hyde S, Smotherman J, Moore JI, Altschuler G: A model of bacterially induced umbilical vein spasm, relevant to fetal hypoperfusion. Obstet Gynecol 73:966, 1989.
162. Romero R, Avila C, Edwin SS, Mitchell MD: Endothelin-1,2 levels are increased in the amniotic fluid of women with preterm labor and mi-

crobial invasion of the amniotic cavity. Am J Obstet Gynecol 166:95, 1992.
163. Schwartz DA, Reef S: *Candida albicans* placentitis and funisitis: early diagnosis of congenital candidemia by histopathologic examination of umbilical cord vessels. Pediatr Infect Dis J 9:661, 1990.
164. Qureshi F, Jacques SM, Bendon RW, et al. *Candida* funisitis: a clinicopathologic study of 30 cases. Pediatr Pathol Lab Med, In Press.
165. Sander CH, Martin JN, Rogers AL, et al: Perinatal infection with *Torulopsis glabrata:* a case associated with maternal sickle cell anemia. Obstet Gynecol 61S:21S, 1983.
166. Fitter WF, deSa DJ, Richardson H: Chorioamnionitis and funisitis due to *Corynebacterium kutscheri.* Arch Dis Child 54:710, 1979.
167. deSa DJ: Diseases of the umbilical cord. In Perrin (ed): Pathology of the placenta. New York, 1984, Churchill Livingstone, p 121.
168. Navarro C, Blanc WA: Subacute necrotizing funisitis: a variant of cord inflammation with a high rate of perinatal infection. J Pediatr 85:689, 1974.
169. Jacques SM, Qureshi F: Necrotizing funisitis: a study of 45 cases. Hum Pathol 23:1278, 1992.
170. Heifetz SA, Bauman M: Necrotizing funisitis and herpes simplex infection of placental and decidual tissues: study of four cases. Hum Pathol 25:715, 1994.
171. Schwartz DA, Larsen SA, Beck-Sague C, et al: Pathology of the umbilical cord in congenital syphilis: analysis of 25 specimens using histochemistry and immunofluorescent antibody to *Treponema pallidum.* Hum Pathol 26:784, 1995.
172. Knowles S, Frost T: Umbilical cord sclerosis as an indicator of congenital syphilis. J Clin Pathol 42:1157, 1989.
173. Fojaco RM, Hensley GT, Moskowitz L: Congenital syphilis and necrotizing funisitis. JAMA 261:1788, 1989.
174. Wright JR Jr, Stinson D, Wade A, et al: Necrotizing funisitis associated with *Actinomyces meyeri* infection: a case report. Pediatr Pathol 14:927, 1994.
175. Mishriki YY, Vanyshelbaum Y, Epstein H, Blanc W: Hemangioma of the umbilical cord. Pediatr Pathol 7:43, 1987.
176. Armes JE, Billson VR: Umbilical cord hemangioma associated with polyhydramnios, congenital abnormalities and perinatal death in a twin pregnancy. Pathology 26:218, 1994.
177. Yavner DL, Redline RW: Angiomyxoma of the umbilical cord with massive cystic degeneration of Wharton's jelly. Arch Pathol Lab Med 113:935, 1989.
178. Jauniaux E, Moscoso G, Campbell S, et al: Correlation of ultrasound and pathologic findings of placental anomalies in pregnancies with elevated maternal serum alpha-fetoprotein. Eur J Obstet Gynecol Reprod Biol 37:219, 1990.
179. Brühwiler H, Rabner M, Lüscher KP: Pränatale Diagnose eines Nabelschnur: Hämangioms bei erhöhtem Alpha fötoprotein. Ultraschall Med 15:140, 1994.
180. Seifer DB, Ferguson JE II, Behrens CM, et al: Nonimmune hydrops fetalis in association with hemangioma of the umbilical cord. Obstet Gynecol 66:283, 1985.
181. Corles D, Maugey-Laulom B, Roux D, et al: Anasarque foetoplacentaire létale secondaire à un hémangiome du cordon ombilical. Ann Pathol 14:244, 1994.
182. Weyerts LK, Jones MC, Grafe M, Scioscia AL: Umbilical cord haemangioma associated with an eruptive cutaneous haemangioma in a female infant. Prenatal Diagn 13:61, 1993.
183. Wagner H, Baretton G, Wisser J, et al: Teratom der Nabelschnur; Kasuistik Mit Literatureübersicht. Pathologe 14:395, 1993.
184. Kreczy A, Alge A, Menardi G, et al: Teratoma of the umbilical cord; case report with review of the literature. Arch Pathol Lab Med 118:934, 1994.
185. Andersen HJ, Hariri J: Congenital neuroblastoma in a fetus with multiple malformations: metastasis in the umbilical cord as a cause of intrauterine death. Virchows Arch (A) 400:219, 1983.

6

Placental Membranes

Steven H. Lewis and Enid Gilbert-Barness

The diverse structural and functional complexity of the placental membranes as reflected in their pathologic alterations is simpler to understand with knowledge of their embryologic origins, normal anatomy, and histologic features.

The placental membranes are composed of the amnion and chorion. In the developing gestation they form the membranous compartment housing the fetus, cord, and amniotic fluid. The amnion is the inner layer. Peripheral to this, the chorion contains the chorionic vasculature and villi, which interface with the uterine decidua.

EMBRYOLOGY AND ANATOMY

At implantation, at the endometrial aspect of the blastocyst's inner cell mass, the basal chorion as cell cords and villi forms the chorion frondosus. This eventually becomes the placental parenchyma. Opposite to the implantation pole, the extraembryonic trophoblastic cells form the capsular chorion and make up the chorionic sac. Villous degeneration begins here as early as the third week after conception. With this degeneration the intervillous spaces on the capsular chorion are obliterated. Capsular decidua covers its surface and with expansion abuts the parietal decidua of the endometrium opposite and adjacent to the implantation pole. Fusion occurs here at about 15 to 20 weeks after conception. Therefore the chorion forms a sac with the chorionic plate above the chorion frondosum at the implantation site and the chorion laeve, which makes up the bulk and remainder of the chorionic sac (Fig. 6–1).[1]

The chorionic villi are invested with embryonic mesoderm, which forms soon after implantation during the lacunar stage of development.[2,3] These mesodermal derivatives are the scaffolding for villi and the connective tissue of the inner surface of the chorion, where they house vessels in the chorionic plate (forming the connection between umbilical cord and chorionic villous vasculature) and a connective tissue layer of the chorion laeve adjacent to the amnion.

The third component of the membranes (in addition to the chorion and its mesodermal investments) is the amnion, which forms the innermost aspect of the placental membranes. During implantation a cavity forms between the early embryo (embryoblast) and basal trophoblast (developing chorion frondosum). This cavity is enclosed by amniogenic cells. As it expands, it parallels the development of the yolk sac, allantois, and umbilical vessels. These constituents eventually form a tubular structure (the yolk stalk), which becomes the umbilical cord. The early amniotic cavity surrounds them as the embryo prolapses into the cavity beneath it. From 6 to 12 weeks after conception this amniotic epithelium begins fusion first with the umbilical cord, then with the chorionic plate, and eventually with the remainder of the chorionic sac.[1]

Thus placental membranes form the amnion and chorion. As viewed on gross examination, the amnion is translucent with a bluish sheen. The chorion is relatively more opaque. The layers may be separated in specimens along either natural or artifactual cleavage planes in the region of their fusion. On histologic examination their layers are distinct and should be understood as they relate to the chorion frondosum (at the chorionic plate) and the chorion laeve (of the so-called free membranes).

Within the amniotic sac are the fetus and amniotic fluid. Fluid volume increases until about 34

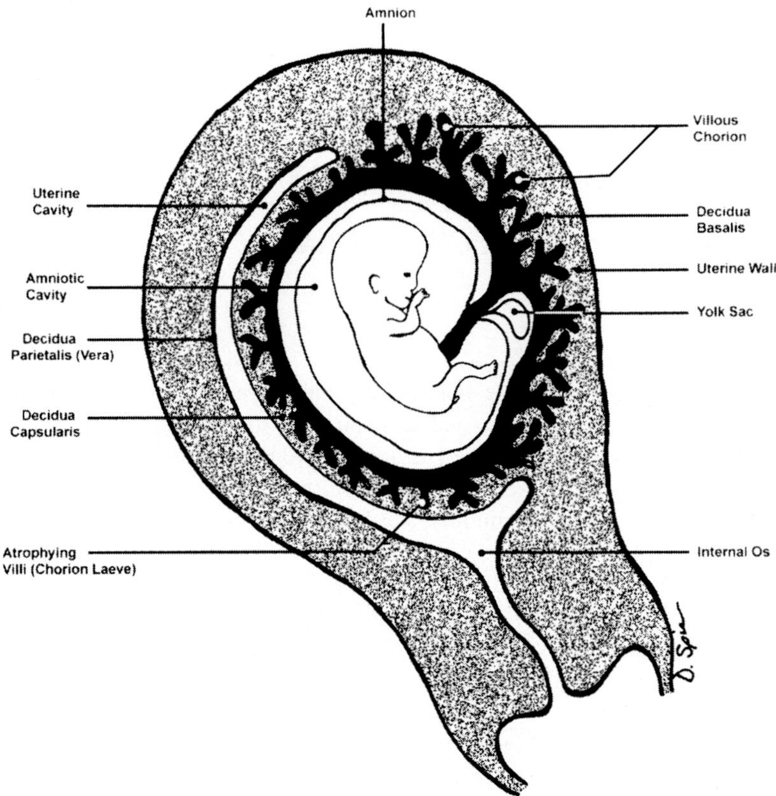

Figure 6–1. Relationships of the fetus, placenta, membranes, and decidua in early development (embryonic period).

weeks' gestation, when it measures nearly 1 L. Thereafter volume declines until birth. A large variation is noted from pregnancy to pregnancy, but calculations of fluid volume based on ultrasonography allow a reasonably accurate identification of marked deviations from norm, indicating either oligohydramnios or polyhydramnios. The fluid is derived from decidual vascular filtration (through the chorion laeve), filtration from the vessels of the chorionic plate and umbilical cord, and fetal urine. The amnionic fluid is composed of water, glucose, proteins, globulins, lipids, urea, creatinine, bilirubin, and uric acid, all in characteristic quantities. Amniotic fluid contains cytologic elements including squames and fetal urothelial cells.[4]

BIOCHEMISTRY

A discussion of the biochemistry of the fetal membranes is beyond the scope of this chapter. In the recent literature are scores of articles pertaining to biochemical mechanisms potentially involved in infectious and immune activities of the fetal membranes, as well as mechanisms potentially related to parturition. Their significance is probably debatable. Of key interest here is that unlike the sheep model, in humans the onset of labor is not related to cortisol production. Prostaglandins probably play an important role, since it has long been known that a variety of physical membrane insults (e.g., "stripping" of the membranes, rupture of membranes, infection, infusion of saline) result in the initiation of uterine contractions. Glycerophospholipids (phosphatidylinositol and phosphatidylethanolamine) and arachidonic acid (a prostaglandin precursor) are present in the fetal membranes. Arachidonic acid is released from storage by phospholipases A and C, which are activated by calcium and a not yet fully characterized molecule derived from fetal urine. In its released form, arachidonic acid is readily converted to prostaglandins. Oxytocin also stimulates decidual prostaglandins $F_{2\alpha}$ and E_2. Corticosteroids and catecholamines interact to modulate uterine activity. The stage is thus set for the initiation of labor through maternal, fetal, and membrane interaction. Despite the vast array of biochemical data, the final word on human parturition remains elusive.[5]

HISTOLOGY

Amnion

The amnion is the innermost membrane component lining the amnionic cavity. Its surface at this inner aspect is covered by a usually single layer of amnionic epithelial cells that are situated on a basement membrane. This basement membrane adheres to a layer of connective tissue. Beneath the connective tissue layer is the chorion, which is further described below (Fig. 6–2).[6]

The amnion possesses no vasculature and measures only 35 to 60 μm in greatest thickness. It is nourished by the magma reticulare (a thixotropic gel containing mesenchymal-epithelial cells that is present between the chorion and amnion until their fusion at 12 weeks' gestation), the amniotic

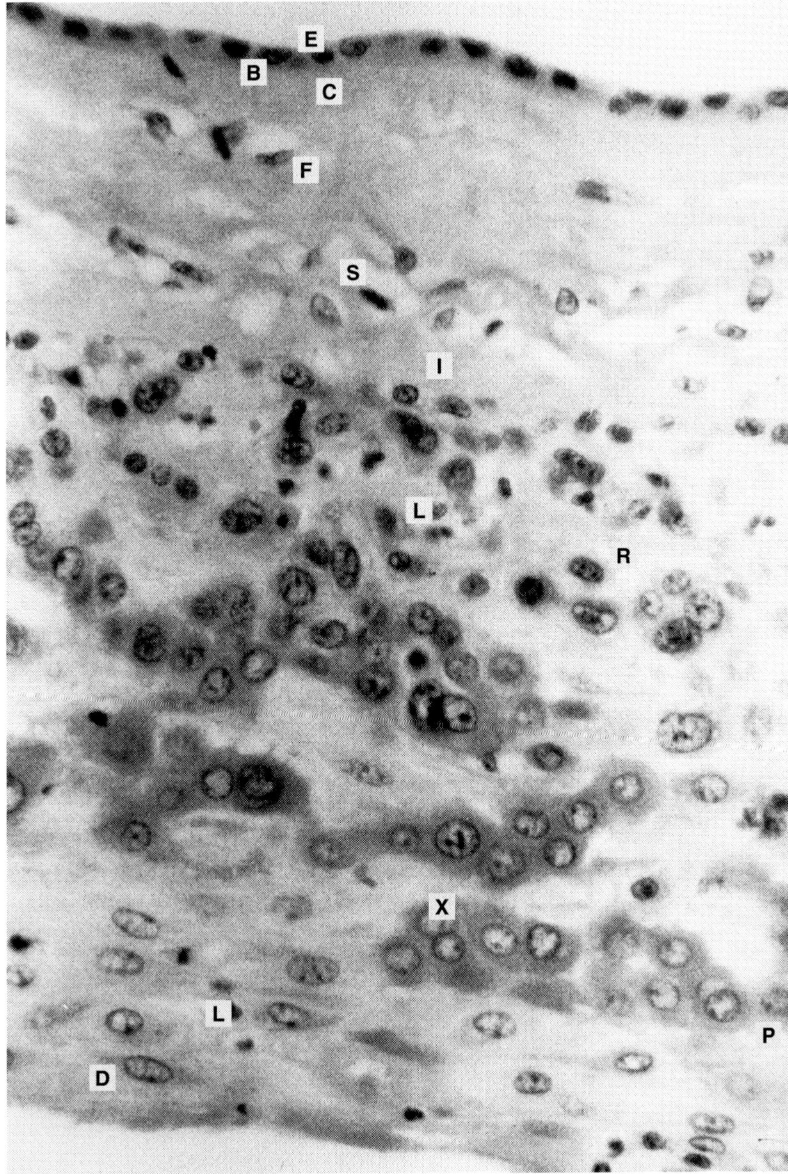

Figure 6–2. Microscopic layers of the amnion and chorion (reflected membranes). **Amnion** (from above): amnionic epithelium (*E*), basement membrane (*B*), compact layer (*C*), fibroblastic layer (*F*), spongy layer (*S*). **Chorion:** incomplete cellular zone (*I*), reticular layer (*R*), pseudo–basement membrane (*P*), trophoblast X cells (*X*), decidua (*D*). Note acute leukocytic (*L*) infiltrate in the decidua and chorion indicating chorionitis.

fluid, and surface fetal vasculature. Although the amnion is epithelial in origin, it stains not only for cytokeratin and CA125 but also for vimentin. These dual staining characteristics are also found in the stellate cells of the magma reticulare.[7,8]

The several cell types that may be observed in the amnion are the subject of speculation. It is currently believed that only a single cytologic element is present. This cell type may take on varying appearances because of its localization, degrees of degeneration, and other artifactual aberrancies. Amnionic epithelial cells are usually squamoid to cuboidal. More columnar cells can be identified at the margin of the chorionic plate, and more squamoid cells are observed at greater distances radially from the center of the placenta. Varying histologic stages of squamous metaplasia with cell proliferation to several layers, including parakeratosis and hyperkeratosis, can be found. Metaplasia is most commonly seen near the cord insertion.[4,9–12]

Amniotic cells divide by mitosis, which accounts for their sometimes polyploid appearance. Dividing cells may contaminate amniotic fluid and confound cytogenetic studies.[13–15] Spaces between amnionic cells represent cell loss or "dropout" and probably are not indicative of channels for fluid equilibration. Microvilli, rough endoplasmic reticulum, glycogen, pinocytotic vesicles, and lipid are found with electron microscopy of amnionic cells. The origins of intraamnionic lipid, as well as the diversity of other biochemical and immunologic mediators and their roles in physiology and initiation of parturition, are complex and not fully understood. Amnionic cytologic relationships with leukotrienes, interleukins, prostaglandin synthesis enzymes, endothelien, and growth factors are vital, and their roles in intrauterine gestational homeostasis continue to be studied.[4,16–19] Amniotic fluid pH, CO_2 resorption, and amniotic fluid transfer are also influenced by the amnion. That the amnion is avascular and requires nutritional support through diffusion to accomplish all of these activities further complicates the understanding of this complex epithelium.[4,20,21]

Amnionic cells are attached to one another by desmosomes. Beneath amnionic epithelial cells lies a basement membrane. Deep to this is a connective tissue layer with an upper compact zone (the strongest layer of the amnion) and a lower fibroblastic zone (which contains macrophages). Beneath this and directly overlying the chorion is a spongy layer with relative absence of fibroblastic cells.[6]

Chorion

As described, the amnion fuses with the chorion during expansion of the amniotic cavity. The chorion is made up of connective tissue and trophoblast. The chorionic mesenchyme carries the fetal vasculature (the chorionic vessels). The inner aspect of the chorion is bordered by the outer layer of the amnion, and the outer layer of the chorion is in conjunction with trophoblastic villi that sprout from its surface and are in contact with decidua of varying names depending on the site of the chorion and the degree of development. The decidua basalis is beneath the chorion frondosum, and the decidua capsularis is beneath the chorion laeve. The capsular decidua fuses with the parietal decidua of the uterine wall when the chorionic sac grows to occupy the entire endometrial cavity. Therefore there are two contiguous aspects of the chorion that relate to the placenta: one associated with the chorion laeve or the reflected membranes (sandwiched between amnion and decidua) and one associated with the surface of the placental disk or the chorionic plate (here also covered by amnion but bordered beneath by trophoblast associated with the parenchyma or chorion frondosum of the placenta) (Fig. 6–1).[6]

The exact embryologic derivation of the chorionic mesenchyme is unknown, but it is believed to develop from primitive streak and not trophoblast. As with the amnion, several distinct layers have been described. From inner to deep, these are an inner cellular layer, a reticular layer, a pseudo-basement membrane, and an outer trophoblastic layer (Fig. 6–2).[6,22]

Macrophages, degenerated endothelia, mesenchymal cells rich in endoplasmic reticulum, acid mucopolysaccharides, and type IV collagen are all found in the chorion. Inherent in its structure is its function, which is to serve as a scaffold for the chorionic vessels, support for the amnion, interdigitation and apposition with the decidua, and a way station for degradation and pathologic depositions, as discussed below.[23,24]

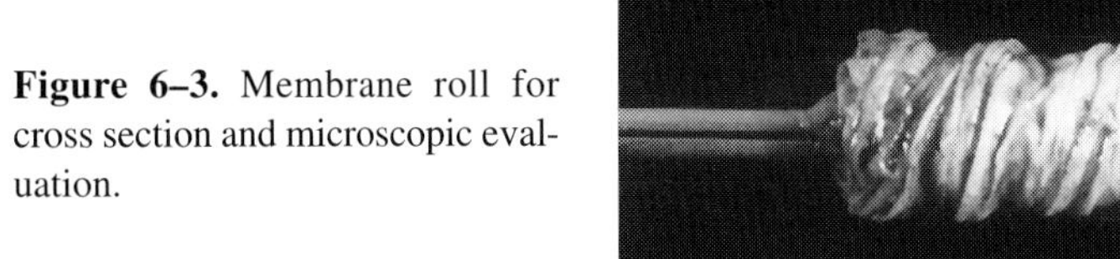

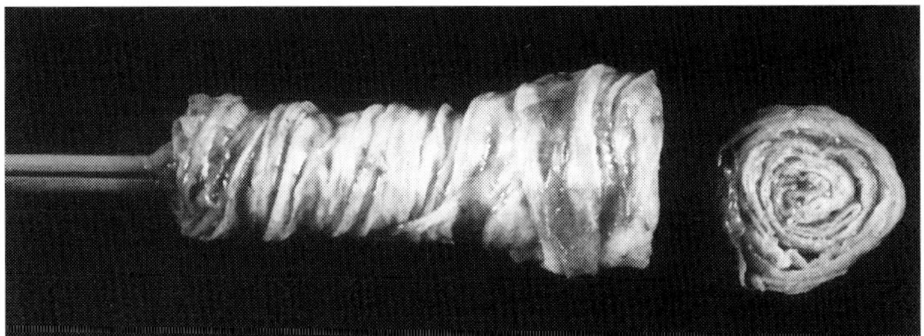

Figure 6–3. Membrane roll for cross section and microscopic evaluation.

GROSS INSPECTION

In the delivery room or the pathology laboratory the placental membranes should be examined in a systematic fashion. Most commonly, during the delivery of the placenta (in the third stage of labor), the membrane sac everts over the placental disk so that the fetal surface (the inner aspect of the membranes) is demonstrated. Obstetricians call the glistening surface of the amnion "shiny Schultze." Whether this or its less common counterpart, "dirty Duncan" (seen when the membranes of the placenta retain their normal anatomic relations), occurs is of no known clinical significance. The membranes should be manually reflected to their normal anatomic location and assessed for completeness. The absence of a complete sac does not necessarily indicate that portions of membranes have been retained in utero. Often small amounts of membranes detach during removal of the placenta at delivery, and these are usually teased from the introitus or cervical os with a ring forceps and unfortunately discarded. Next, the narrowest width is identified. This distance measures the shortest span from the opening in the membranes (the point of rupture through which the fetus is delivered) to the placental disk margin. In cases in which this numerical value approaches zero, a low-lying or marginal placental previa is implied. This does not apply in cesarean births, since often amniotomy is performed cephalad to the cervix in the lower uterine segment before extraction of the fetus.

The membranes are subsequently examined for their transparency, color, sheen, membranous vessels, additional lobes, and important surface irregularities. In the pathology laboratory the membranes are next trimmed from the disk and a membrane roll is constructed by grasping the membranes at the point of rupture with a "toothed pickups" and rolling them concentrically. The resultant roll can be immersed in fixative for 8 to 24 hours (Bouin's is best for this) so that it becomes sufficiently hard to be sectioned easily for microscopy. Having the point of rupture at the center permits identification of early chorioamnionitis with neutrophils confined to this region. The roll creates a relatively large transsectional surface area for evaluation. Interestingly, it is the membrane roll that provides the best evaluation of the maternal decidua. Much more decidua is adherent to this aspect of the chorion than to chorion attached to the villous parenchymal disk.[6]

Microscopic disorders of the decidua are usually identified in sections of membrane roll unless specimens from the seldom performed uterine bed biopsy are available (Fig. 6–3).

PATHOLOGY

The pathologic conditions of the membranes can be broken down into entities that affect the amnion, the chorion, and the chorionic vessels. The peculiarities of membrane relations in multiple gestations are also of pathologic interest. Some conditions affect one, two, or all aspects, depending on nature or severity (Table 6–1) and are discussed further below.

Severe Metaplasia of the Amnion

Squamous metaplasia of the amnion is truly a part of its normal histology. When the amnion becomes excessively metaplastic, pathologic conditions should be suspect. Chronic abrasion or trauma to the amnion, not resulting in its rupture, produces an ichthiotic picture. Metaplasia may be easily seen on gross examination as plaques or

Table 6–1. Pathology of the Membranes

Severe metaplasia
Amnion nodosum
Amnionitis (chorionitis and chorioamnionitis)
Meconium change
Membrane edema
Amnionic bands
Extrachorial placentation
Extramembranous gestation
Gastroschisis-associated change
Chorionic vascular thrombi
Placenta membranacea
Chorionic cysts
Membranous vessels
Retromembranous hemorrhage
Multiple gestations
Amniotic fluid embolus

patches of white on the amnion. These areas cannot be easily removed by scraping and when immersed in water do not hydrate well. On histologic examination the metaplasia ranges from immature to frank hyperkeratosis. In the example provided, a large encephalocele with surface abrasion was seen in conjunction with the dramatic metaplasia (Fig. 6–4).[6]

Amnion Nodosum

Amnion nodosum is the placental corollary of oligohydramnios. The causes or sequelae of no or low amniotic fluid are renal agenesis (Potter se-

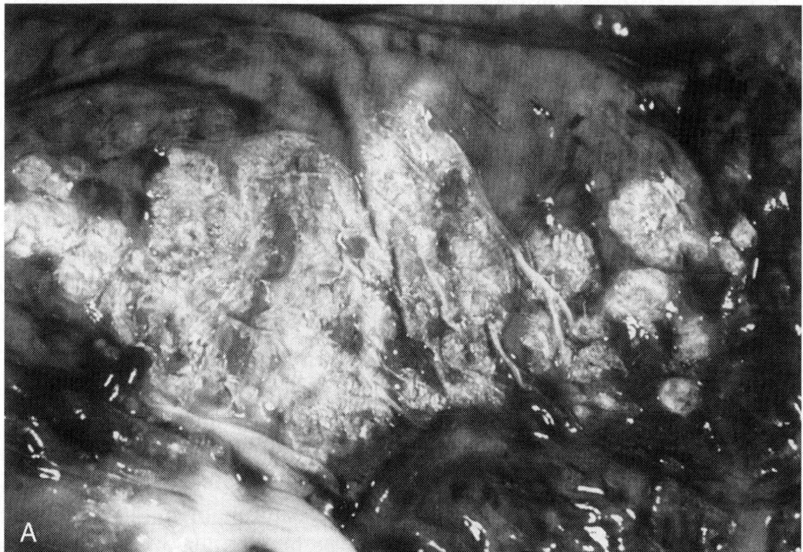

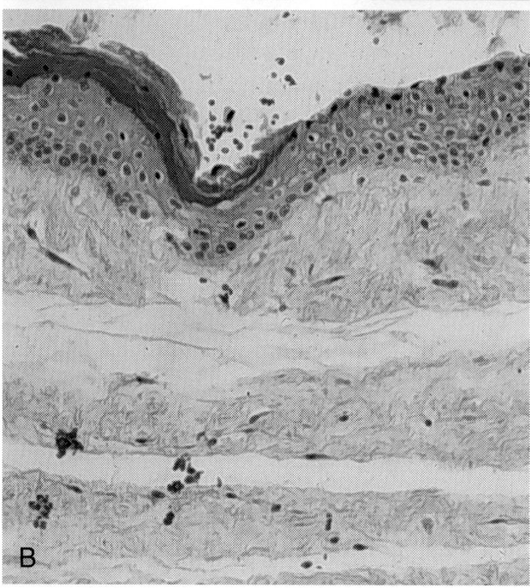

Figure 6–4. Squamous metaplasia of the amnion. **A,** Extensive metaplasia caused by chronic trauma from an encephalocele. **B,** Microscopic squamous metaplasia. (**A** from Lewis SH, Benirschke K: The placenta. In Sternberg S [ed]: Histology for pathologists. New York, 1997, Raven Press.)

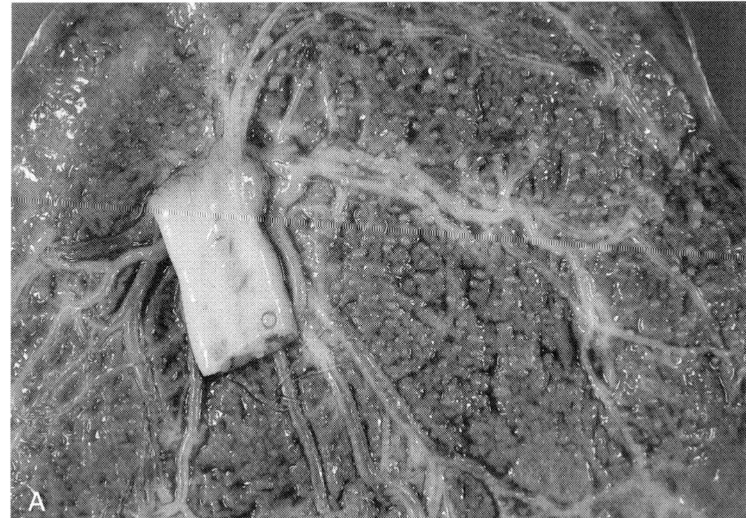

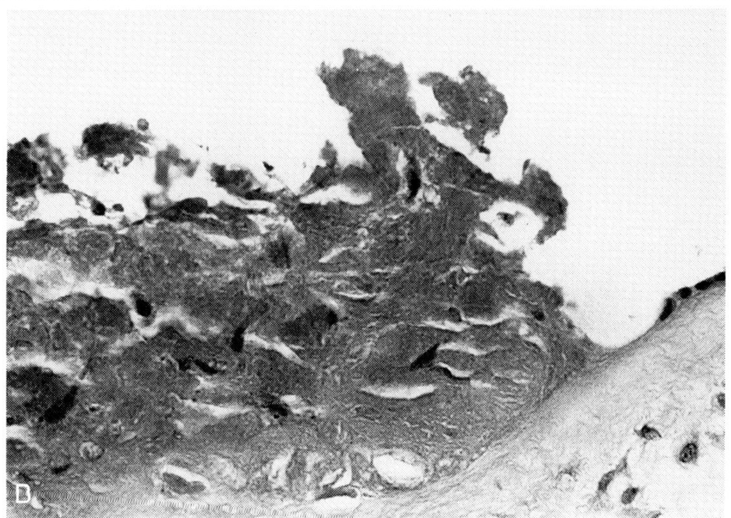

Figure 6–5. A, Innumerable papules of amnion nodosum. **B,** Microscopic amnion nodosum. Note the fetal squames and debris, which characterize the lesion. (**A** courtesy K. Benirschke, San Diego, California.)

quence) with resultant pulmonary hypoplasia, amniotic infection syndrome, and intrauterine growth retardation. These clinical events are the consequence and manifestation of either low production or chronic leakage of amniotic fluid. Absence or dramatic diminishment of amniotic fluid causes desquamated fetal epithelium and associated debris (vernix) to accumulate as whitish papules on the surface of the amnion. These lesions are easily abraded, and in fact rough handling and sponging may remove some or most of the evidence. Unlike metaplastic lesions, lesions of amnion nodosum can be hydrated when immersed in water (Fig. 6–5).[4,25–27]

Yolk Sac Remnant

The remnant of the yolk sac can be seen in many placentas. The reason for this is unknown. Identification of the yolk sac remnant is of no clinical significance other than to highlight the importance of embryologic concerns related to placental development (as described above) and to ensure that the remnant is distinguished from other entities such as squamous metaplasia and amnion nodosum. The residua of the yolk sac appears as a single white to yellow nodule or plaque about 3 to 4 mm in diameter. It will be peripheral to the cord and histologically it is composed of amorphous

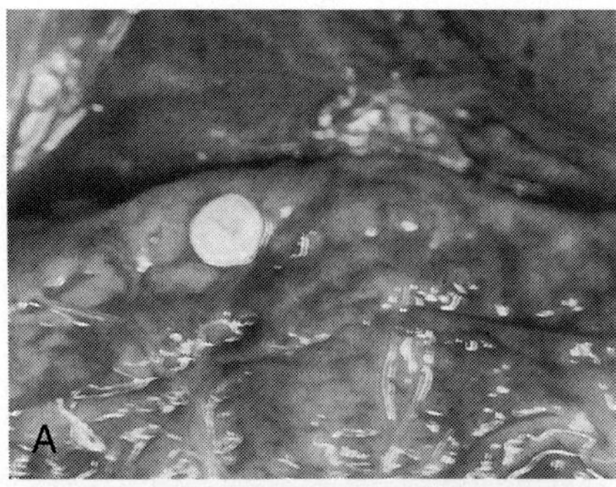

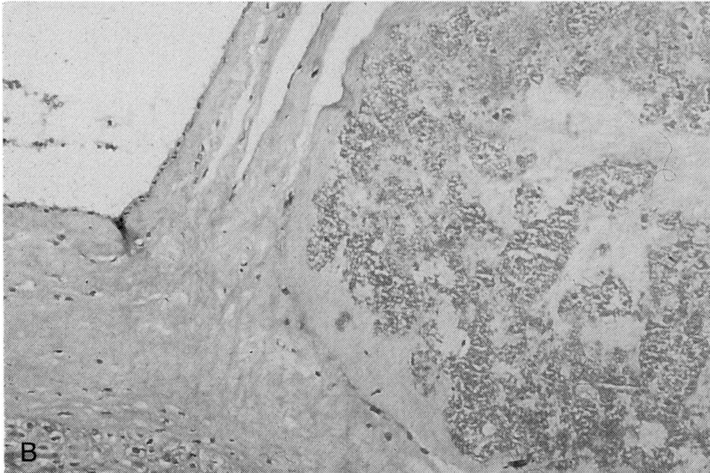

Figure 6–6. A, Yolk sac. **B,** Microscopic yolk sac with characteristic amorphous material. **A** from Lewis SH, Benirschke K: The placenta. In Sternberg S [ed]: Histology for pathologists. New York, 1997, Raven Press.)

degenerated material from former hematopoietic elements and early endoderm (Fig. 6–6).

AMNIONITIS, CHORIONITIS, AND DECIDUITIS

Amnionitis is inflammation of the amnion. It represents the advanced stage of polymorphonuclear leukocyte (PMN) migration in response to bacterial antigens. Ascending infection or hematogenously spread bacteria result in immunologic response by both the fetus and the mother. In the former case PMNs marginate in chorionic vessels in the chorionic plate (acute chorionic vasculitis) and invade the chorion (chorionitis) and eventually the amnion (chorioamnionitis) chemotactically toward the presence of bacterial antigens in the amniotic cavity (Fig. 6–7*A*).[4] Maternal PMNs migrate from decidual vessels to effect a similar response in the reflected membranes (Fig. 6–7*B*). Decidually derived PMNs additionally percolate up around villi and collect in aggregates beneath the chorionic plate. With chronic infection these collections migrate into the chorion and amnion and eventually the amniotic cavity.

Intense inflammation of the amnion may give the membranes a whitish appearance (Fig. 6–7*C*). In severe infection the amnion may become necrotic and amniotic epithelial cells may be difficult to identify histologically (Fig. 6–7*D*). Frank membrane necrosis may occur in the setting of chorioamnionitis. However, necrosis does not necessarily indicate infection; other associations in the absence of inflammation include meconium, postmaturity, increased fetal movement, and fetal anomalies. The histologic identification of PMNs in the amnion confirms the diagnosis of chorioamnionitis (since neutrophils must migrate through the chorion to reach the amnion). The grading of chorioamnionitis is of some clinical significance because there is correlation with the duration of infection.[31] Parenthetically, it is paradoxical that inflammation associated with group B β-streptococci is usually slight, whereas the clinical outcome when fetal sepsis results from it is usually severe.[28,29]

The development of ascending infection and the potential for involvement of a wide diversity of commensal bacteria are well documented. Recent associations with bacterial vaginosis, as well as the development of detection and prevention strategies, underscore this principle.[30] In the collaborative Perinatal Study, chorioamnionitis was twice as common when membranes ruptured within 4 hours before the onset of labor as when membrane rupture occurred after the onset of labor. It is evident that premature rupture of membranes is often associated with chorioamnionitis.[31]

In addition to bacteria, other infectious disease organisms, such as *Candida,* may affect the placental membranes (Fig. 6–8). Prematurity and morbidity associated with infection and premature rupture of membranes are discussed further in Drs. Hyde and Altshuler's chapter on infection (Chapter 13).

Meconium Amniotic Epithelial Degeneration, Membrane Macrophage Ingestion, and Chorionic Vascular Medial Degeneration

Meconium is toxic to the amnion. On gross examination membranes exposed to meconium have a greenish hue. After several hours meconium causes amniotic epithelial degeneration characterized by elongation to columnar forms in association with coarse cytoplasmic vacuolization (Fig. 6–9*A*).[4,6,32] In addition, meconium may become ingested within the macrophages in the amniotic (Fig. 6–9*B*) (within 1 hour of exposure) and chorionic (after 3 hours) connective tissue, indicating longer exposure. (Heme pigments may also be found in macrophages. If a pigment's origin is uncertain, an iron stain such as Prussian blue is helpful in identifying nonmeconium pigment.) Granules of meconium are identified at later stages in the decidua capsularis. With prolonged exposure the amnion may become frankly necrotic and the umbilical cord is deeply stained. The temporal re-

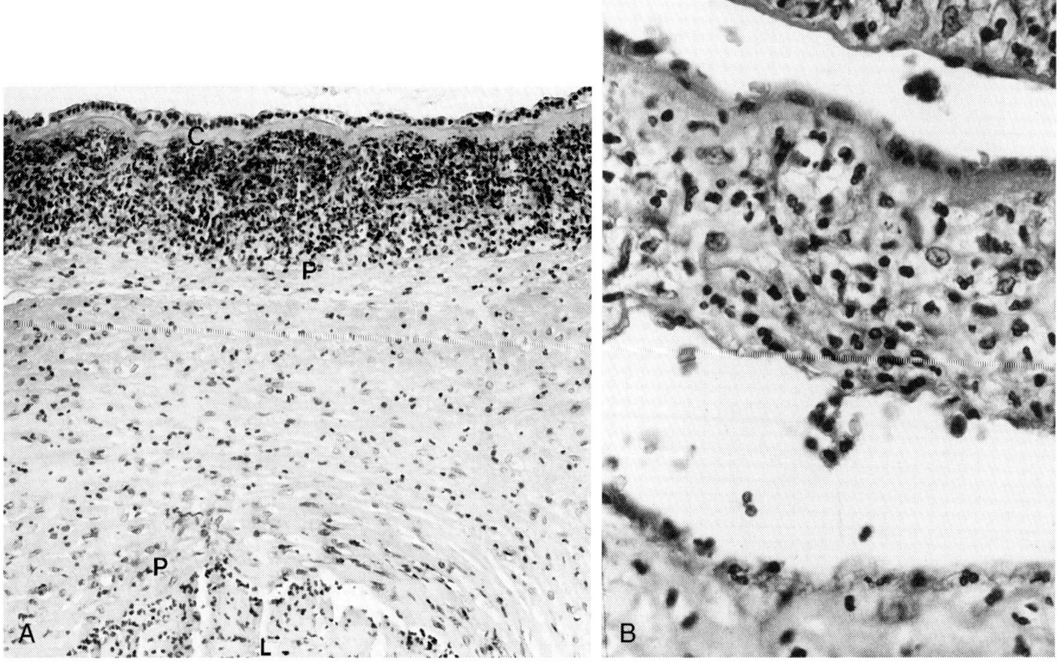

Figure 6–7. A, Intense chorioamnionitis with vasculitis of the chorionic plate. Polymorphonuclear cells (*P*) are marginating along chorionic vasculature lumina (*L*) and migrating toward the amnion. In this case they appear trapped beneath the compact layer (*C*) of the amnion, its strongest and most impervious layer. **B,** Acute chorioamnionitis involving the reflected membranes. (*A* from Benirschke K, Kauffmann R: Pathology of the human placenta. New York, 1995, Springer-Verlag. *B* from Lewis SH, Benirschke K: The placenta. In Sternberg S [ed]: Histology for pathologists. New York, 1997, Raven Press.)

Illustration continued on following page

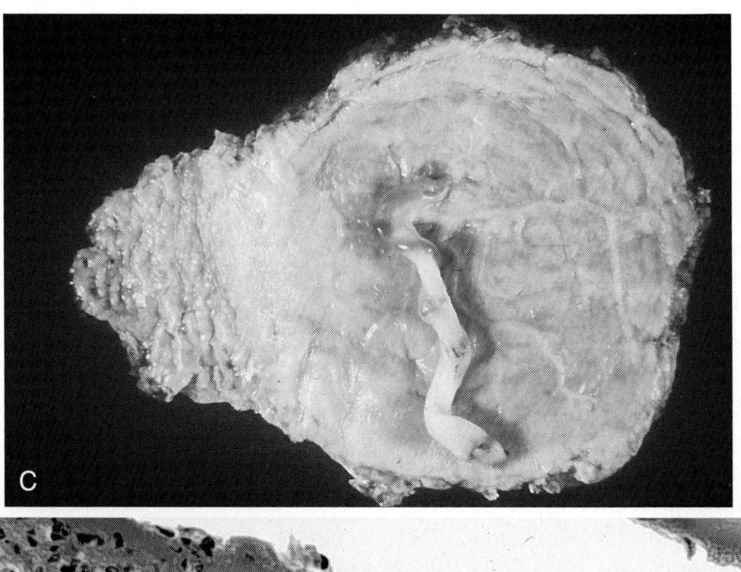

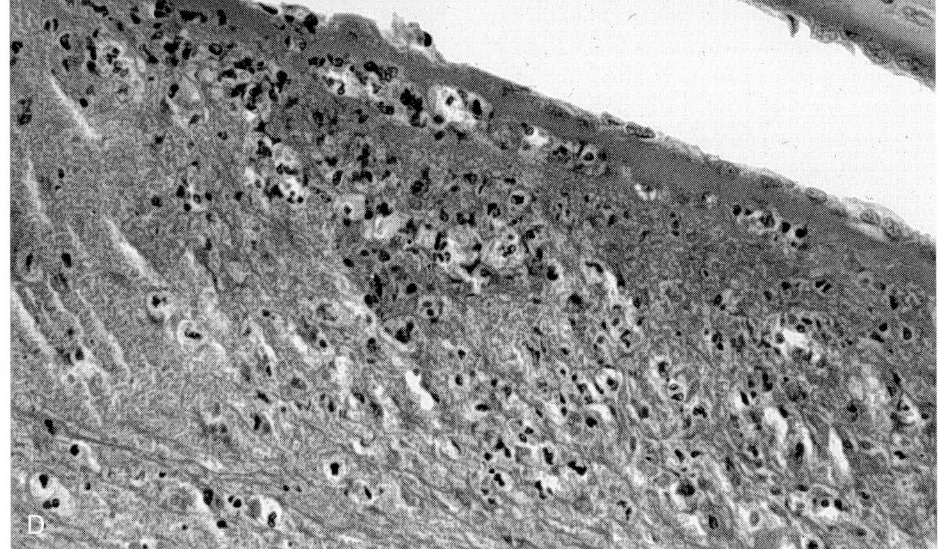

Figure 6–7 *Continued* **C,** Infected "white" membranes. **D,** Chorioamnionitis with amnion necrosis.

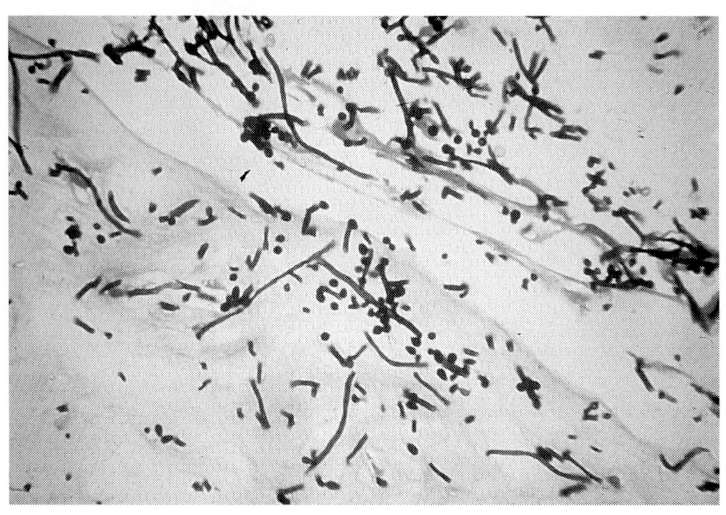

Figure 6–8. *Candida* membranitis (GMS).

lations of meconium effects on the placenta are not fully understood and are complicated by the fact that the fetus discharges meconium at varying intervals.[4]

Meconium passage, once thought to be solely due to fetal stress, is now known to be also a result of normal gut maturation and motilin secretion. Umbilical and chorionic vascular musculature undergo necrosis with prolonged exposure, causing vasospasm and insufficiency that in some cases lead to fetal stress. These findings have been confirmed in vitro (Fig. 6–9*C*).[33] Meconium may also cause significant morbidity and mortality through aspiration in utero or at delivery, resulting in meconium aspiration syndrome.[4]

Membrane Edema

Both gross and microscopic edema of the membranes is seen in about 5% to 6% of births. Preeclampsia, eclampsia, and infection are common associates. Edema is also common in the placentas of stillbirths (Fig. 6–10).[31]

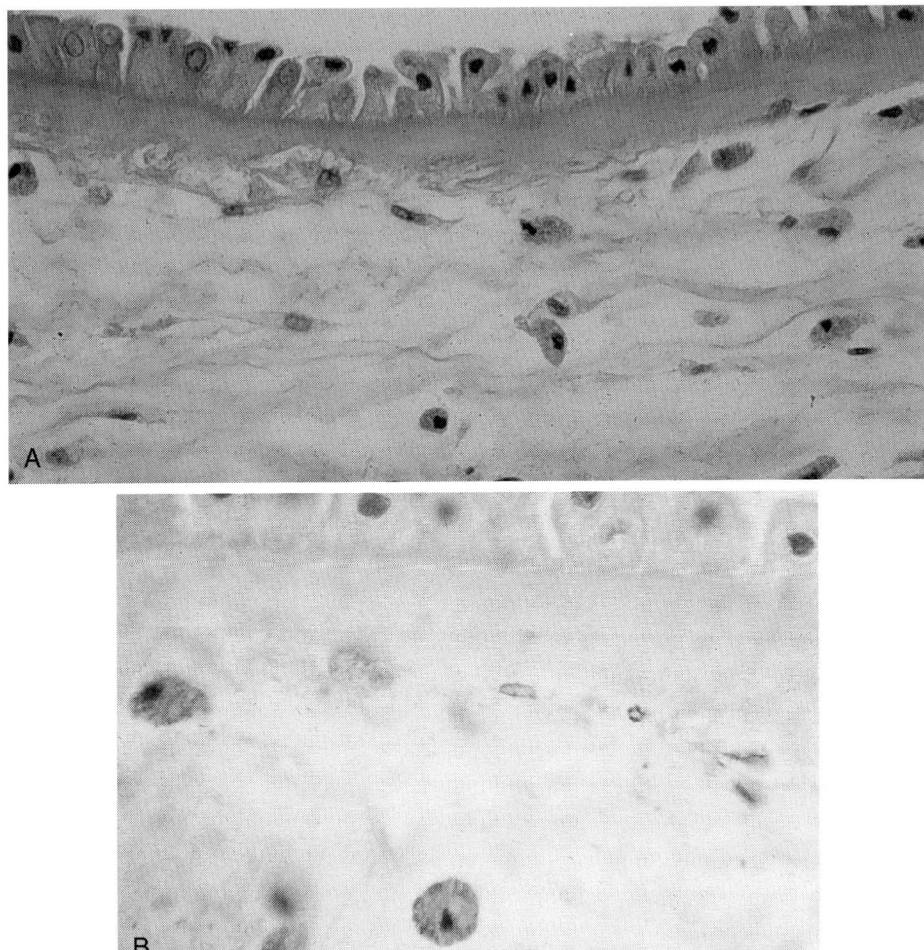

Figure 6–9. A, Amnionic epithelial degeneration caused by meconium. Note the elongation (to columnar forms) and early degeneration of epithelial cells. **B,** Meconium in macrophages. (*B* from Lewis SH, Benirschke K: The placenta. In Sternberg S [ed]: Histology for pathologists. New York, 1997, Raven Press.)

Illustration continued on following page

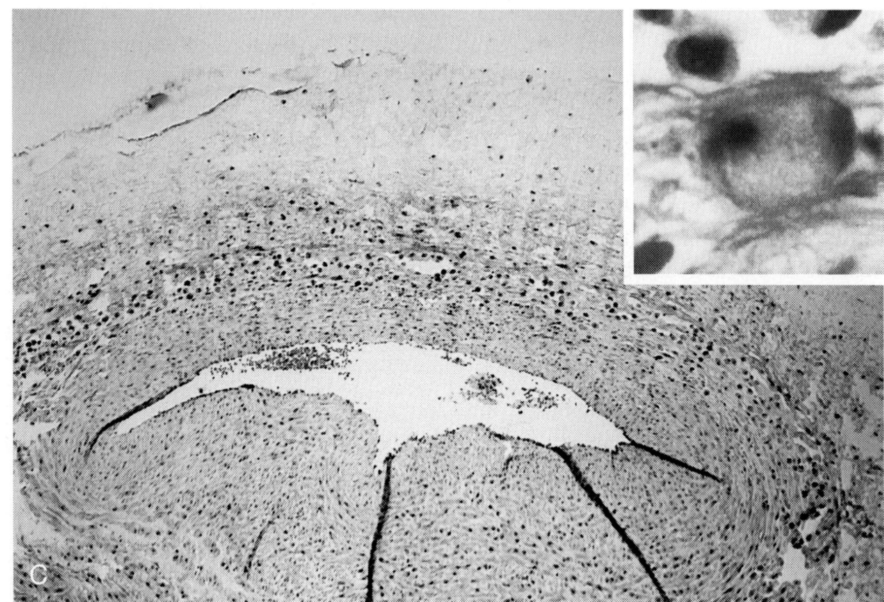

Figure 6–9 *Continued* **C,** Meconium vascular medial necrosis. Note degenerated "globular" myometrial cells magnified (inset). (From Altshuler G, Hyde S: J Child Neurol 4:137, 1989.)

Amniotic Bands

The presence of amniotic bands may lead to fetal anomalies, amputations, and death. Bands may amputate limbs or digits and obstruct the umbilical cord (Fig. 6–11*A* and *B*).[4,34] More complex anomalies usually result from sheets often broadly attached to the facies or head (Fig. 6–11*C*).[4,35] Early rupture of the amnion occurs from unknown causes and usually without an antecedent history of trauma. Defective amniotic tissue or excessive fetal activity may be causal. With rupture of the amnion, bands and sheets of amniotic tissue remain adherent to the base of the cord, to which the amnion always firmly adheres, rendering even manual removal during examination difficult (Fig. 6–11*D*). Tethered against this base these formations cause mechanical constriction and adhesion. On gross examination the fetal surface of the placenta appears opaque, since there is no covering

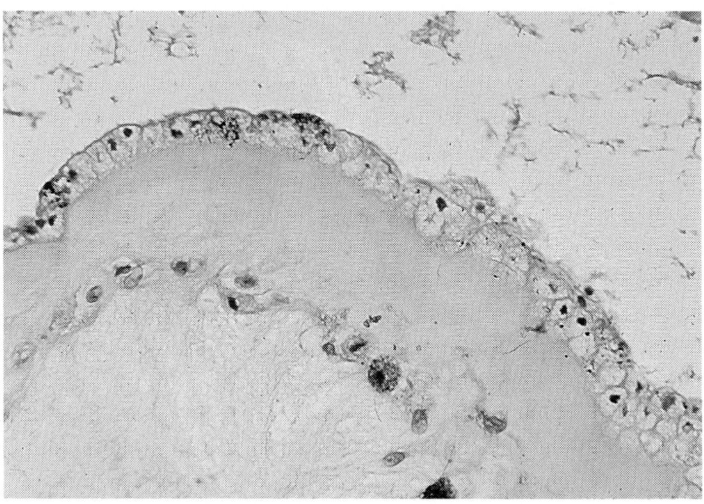

Figure 6–10. Membrane edema caused by meconium. Note vacuolated amnionic epithelial degeneration and marked edema of the compact and fibroblastic layers. Meconium is seen in macrophages.

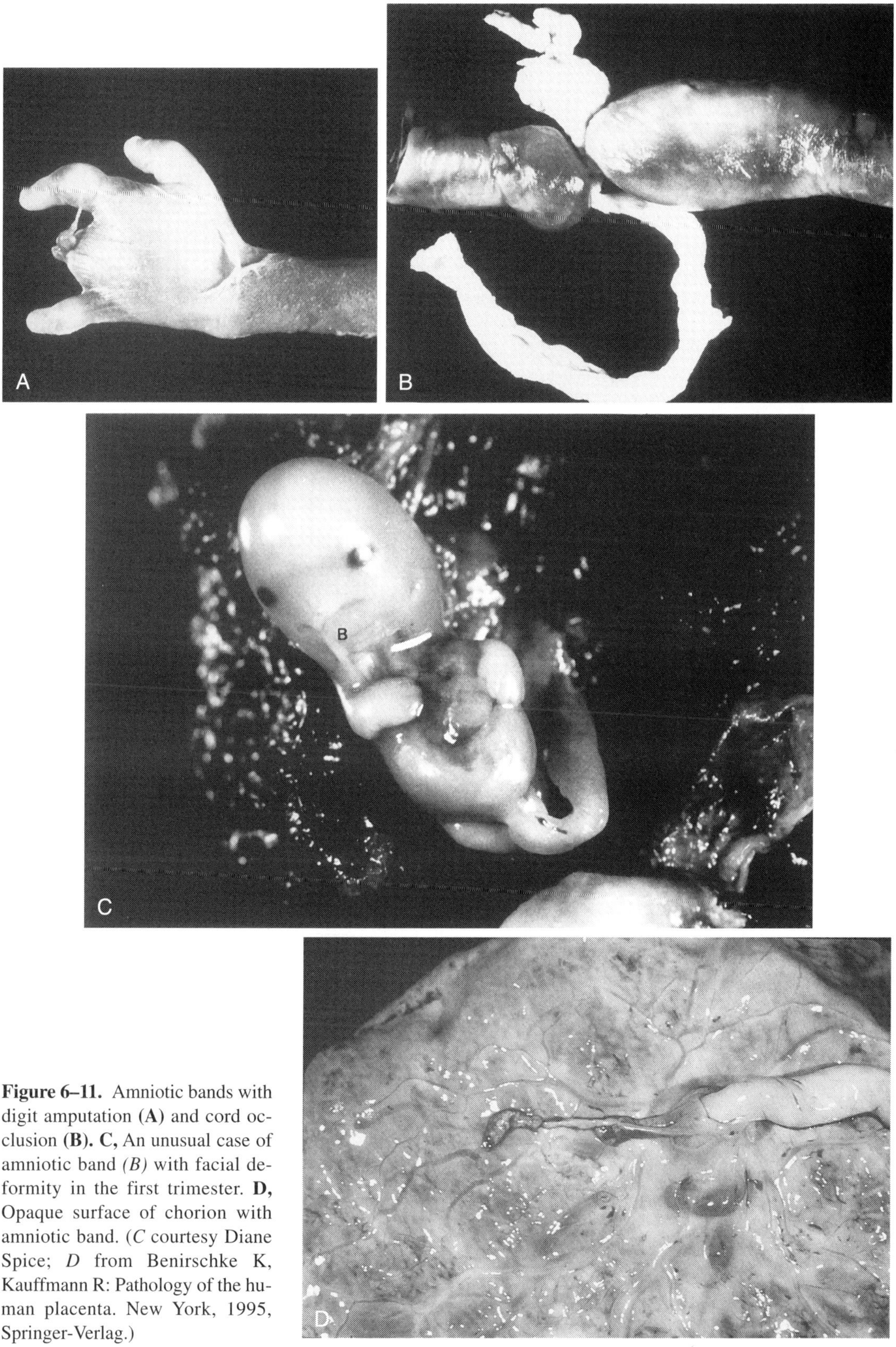

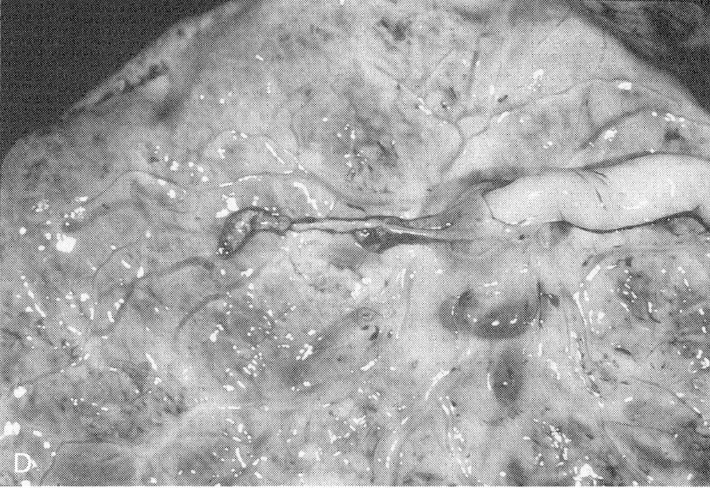

Figure 6–11. Amniotic bands with digit amputation **(A)** and cord occlusion **(B). C,** An unusual case of amniotic band *(B)* with facial deformity in the first trimester. **D,** Opaque surface of chorion with amniotic band. (*C* courtesy Diane Spice; *D* from Benirschke K, Kauffmann R: Pathology of the human placenta. New York, 1995, Springer-Verlag.)

amnion (Fig. 6–11*D*). The gestation has taken place partially or completely in the chorionic cavity. Histologic examination confirms that the bands and sheets are amniotic tissue.

Extramembranous Gestation

With rupture of both the amnion and chorion, the fetus may develop within the endometrial cavity. This is a rare condition usually associated with chronic leakage of amniotic fluid. Fetal demise and premature delivery usually result. The placentas in these cases are circumvallate with slight amnion nodosum. Fetuses have anomalies that are positional in origin and often have pulmonary hypoplasia.[4,36,37]

Extrachorial Membranes

Extrachorial membranes are characterized by *circumvallate* and *circummarginate* placentas. Rather than inserting at the disk margin, the chorion laeve (or reflected membranes) inserts at varying degrees inside that margin. The edge of the placenta then is only loosely covered by membrane. A ring of fibrin underlies the point of membrane attachment and indicates prior bleeding. The ring does not always form a complete circle inside the disk margin, indicating varying degrees of extrachoriality. When the membranes fold back on themselves before departing the chorionic plate, the term "circumvallate placenta" applies. When the reflected membranes leave the surface without folding back, a circummarginate placenta is present. The genesis of this condition is speculative. Superficial implantation is often touted as causal, but other factors (such as decreased amniotic fluid pressure and antecedent hemorrhage) may also play a role (Fig. 6–12*A*).

Circumvallation occurs in about 6% (reported incidence 2% to 18%) of pregnancies. Multiparity, early fluid loss, antenatal bleeding, smoking, preeclampsia, decidual necrosis, and fetal growth retardation are seen in association with this abnormality (Fig. 6–12*B*).[4] Circumvallation may be diagnosed with prenatal ultrasound.[38]

Circummarginate placentas are seen in about 4% (reported incidence 3% to 25%) of pregnancies and have similar associations as do circumvallate placentas, except that growth retardation is not a statistically significant concomitant (Fig. 6–12*C*).[4]

Gastroschisis

Infants affected by gastroschisis have a membrane change that is peculiar to this condition. The amnion is characterized by innumerable uniform, fine vacuoles containing lipid. The origin of their composition remains obscure, since the intestines of affected infants are covered by fibrinous material and not lipid (Fig. 6–13).[4]

Chorionic Vascular Thrombi

Thrombosis of the chorionic vasculature is caused by infection, coagulation disorders, and pressure phenomenon. Inflammatory mediators often cause localized vascular pathologic alterations resulting in thrombosis. Hypercoagulability as seen in maternal anticardiolipin, lupus anticoagulant, protein S and C deficiency, and the factor V Leiden mutation is probably also causal. When membranous vessels are present (as with velamentous cord insertion and accessory lobes), poorly cushioned or protected vessels are prone to thrombosis because of pressure from adjacent fetal parts. The resultant thrombosis causes major deficits in perfusion of the underlying villous structures, effectively removing these zones from participation in nutrient, waste, and oxygen exchange. Such major effects are the reason for a high degree of association with neurologic morbidity in cases where chorionic thrombi are identified.[4,39,40]

On gross examination thrombosis is noted as vascular occlusion that varies in color according to chronicity. Fresh thrombi are dark red, and older thrombi are yellow-white. Occlusion may be complete or partial (endothelial cushion). With complete occlusion the vessel may be distended. With partial occlusion a streak of thrombotic material may be seen running parallel to the periphery of the vascular lumen (Fig. 6–14). These thrombi are fragile and should be handled gently during examination to avoid artifactual dissolution. Findings are confirmed microscopically.

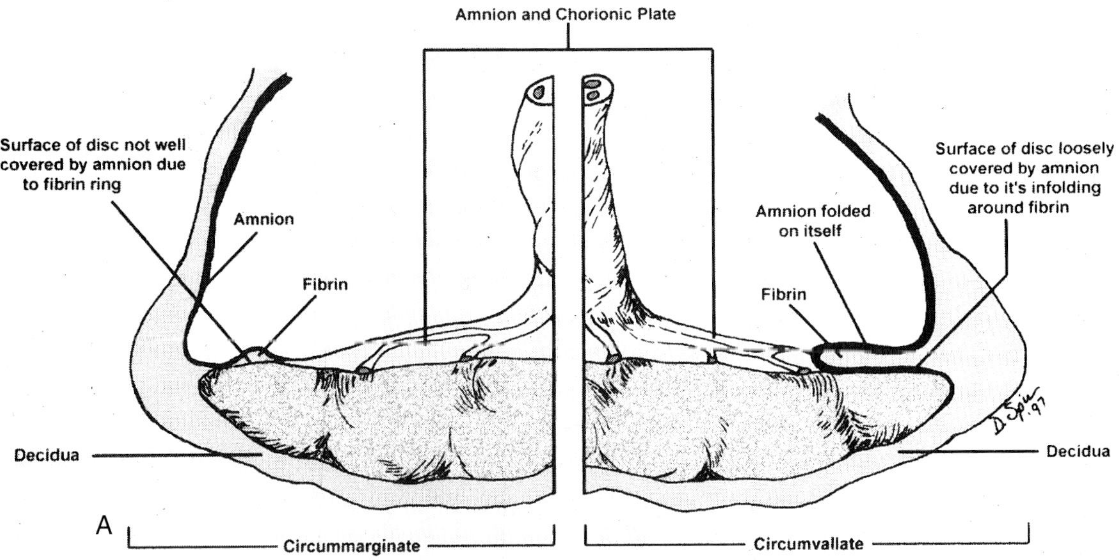

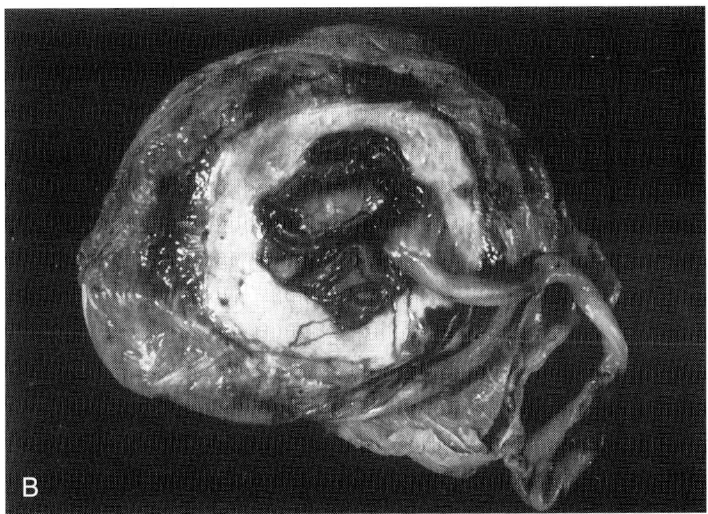

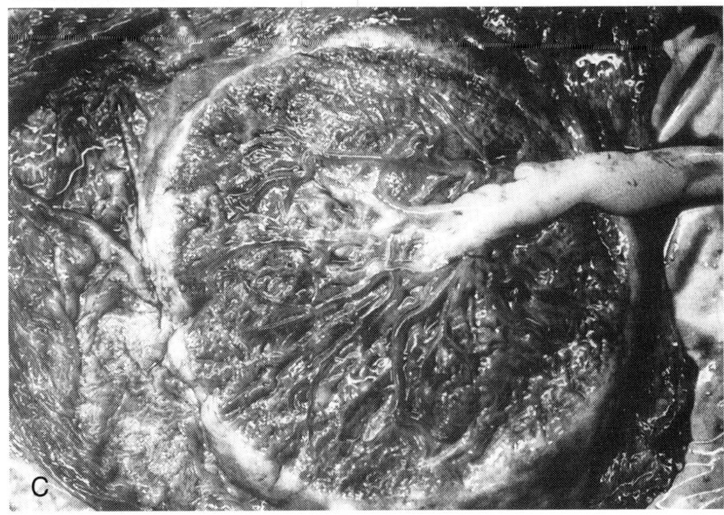

Figure 6–12. A, Cross-sectional diagram of circummargination and circumvallation. **B,** Circumvallation. **C,** Circummargination. (*C* from Lewis SH, Benirschke K: The placenta. In Sternberg S [ed]: Histology for pathologists. New York, 1997, Raven Press.)

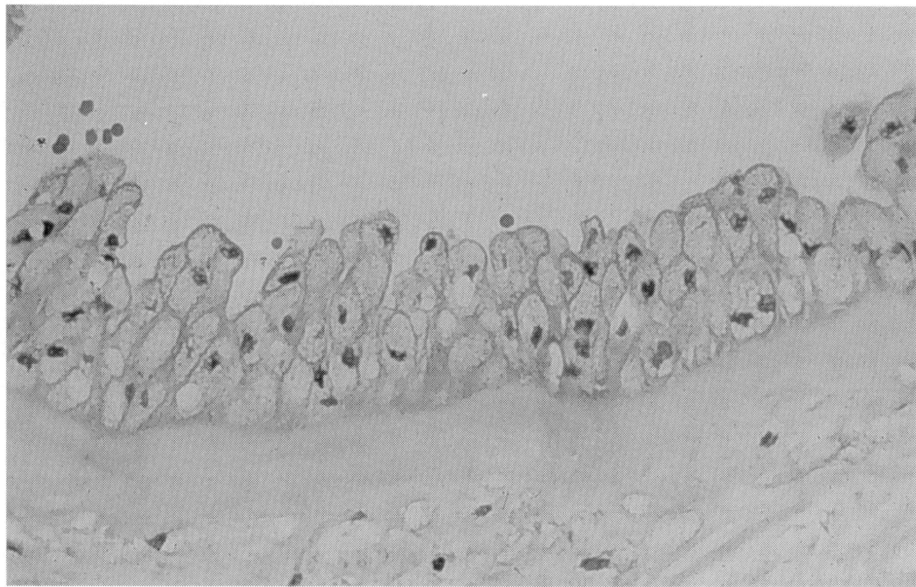

Figure 6–13. Gastroschisis amnionic vacuolization. Vacuolated epithelial cells are in turn filled with innumerable smaller vacuoles. (From Benirschke K, Kauffmann R: Pathology of the human placenta. New York, 1995, Springer-Verlag.)

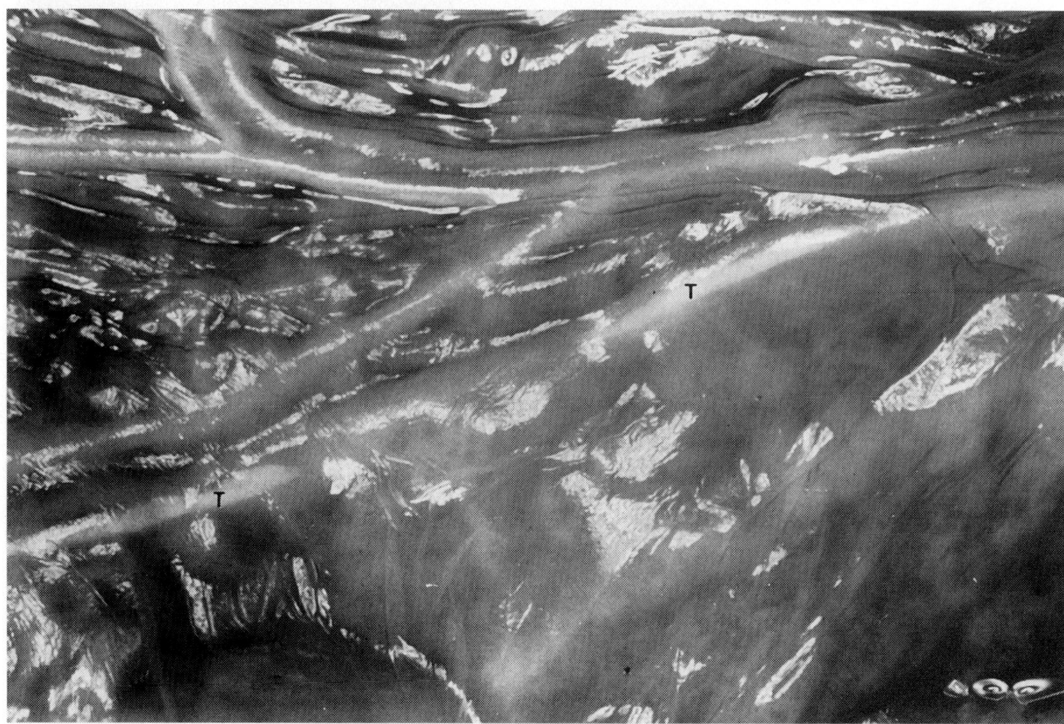

Figure 6–14. Chorionic vascular thrombi (*T*). (From Benirschke K, Kauffmann R: Pathology of the human placenta. New York, 1995, Springer-Verlag.)

Placenta Membranacea

Placenta membranacea is a rare anomaly of the placenta that has an occurrence of about 1 in 3000 to 4000 gestations. It is caused by failure of resorption of the chorionic villi beneath the chorion laeve. The resultant placenta has little or no free reflected membranes, since nearly the entire surface is covered with villi. The villous parenchyma is diffusely thin throughout, only about 1 to 2 cm deep. The condition is often manifested in the second trimester with bleeding placenta previa, and premature delivery. Many cases of placenta membranacea result in placenta accreta. The pathologist often receives a placenta with the uterus, since uncontrollable bleeding in placenta accreta often necessitates hysterectomy (Fig. 6–15).[4,41,42]

Subchorionic Cysts

Cystic structures found within placental septa and within the chorion have been termed subchorionic cysts. In the delivered placenta these structures often have a striking appearance. They may be single or multiple, often measuring up to 3 or 4 cm in diameter and rarely as large as 10 cm. Seen from the fetal surface, these cysts distend the chorion and amnion from the subchorionic zone where aggregates of chorionic cell islands composed of extravillous trophoblast (X cells) cavitate and form these characteristic structures. The cysts become filled with a thick fluid rich in major basic protein (a cytotoxic substance, derived from X cells and characterized as a nonglycosylated protein, that is elevated in the serum during pregnancy and rises in concentration before labor). With one exception they have no known clinical significance. There is speculation that these structures are associated with the genesis of maternal floor infarction, since placentas so affected often have abundant extravillous trophoblast and cyst formation (Fig. 6–16).[4,6,43]

Membranous Vessels

The term "membranous vessels" refers to the finding of chorionic vasculature that aberrantly lies outside the chorionic plate. There is no associated villous parenchyma beneath this vasculature. This condition is due to accessory (or succenturiate) lobes and velamentous cord insertions. In the former, chorionic vasculature courses between placental lobes in the chorion. In the latter, chorionic vessels insert from the umbilical cord away from the chorionic plate and also course through the chorion until they reach the parenchymal disk.

Occasionally, small-caliber vessels are seen that leave the chorionic plate, travel for several centimeters, and are not associated with velamentous cords or accessory lobes. They are probably remnants of vasculature associated with the involuted chorionic villi of the chorion laeve.

As described above, membranous vessels are prone to thrombosis, probably from pressure phenomena. In addition, these vessels are subject to

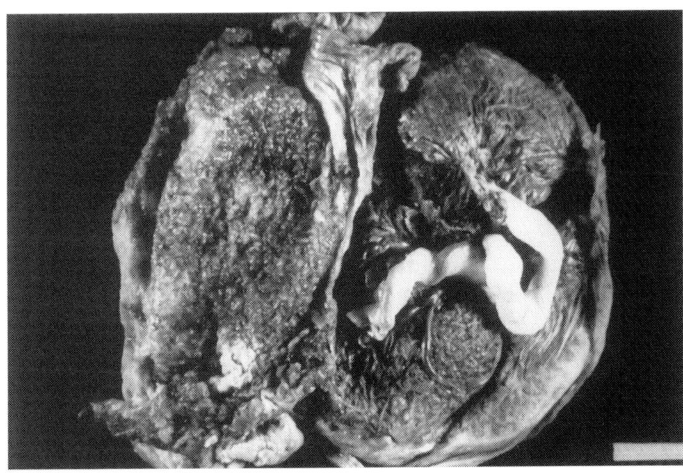

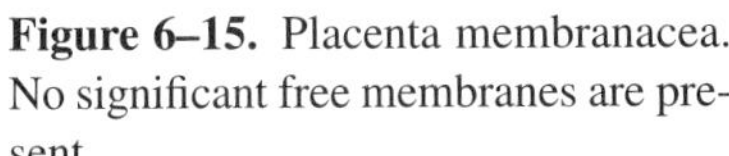

Figure 6–15. Placenta membranacea. No significant free membranes are present.

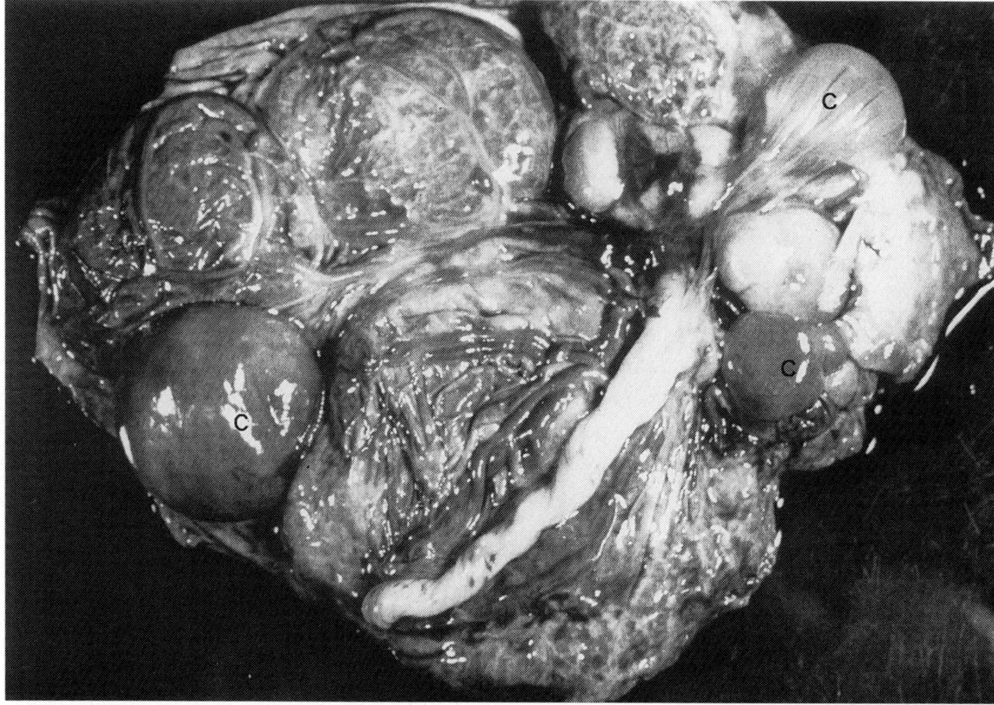

Figure 6–16. Subchorionic cysts (*C*). The two lower cysts are associated with increased fibrin deposition. (From Lewis SH, Benirschke K: The placenta. In Sternberg S [ed]: Histology for pathologists. New York, 1997, Raven Press.)

hemorrhage from trauma. Trauma occurs from iatrogenic causes, including amniocentesis and amniotomy. Disruption of vasculature and resultant hemorrhage possibly occur from fetal activity and laceration by fetal parts such as fingernails (Fig. 6–17).[4]

Retromembranous Hemorrhage

In inspection of the membranes, not all that appears green is necessarily meconium. Old hemorrhage sometimes collects beneath the chorion and leaves a greenish brown plaque usually several centimeters in diameter. The color of the hemorrhage and its amount of contained fibrin depend on its duration. Heme-derived pigments account for the green-brown hue. Bleeding may have any number of causes. Conditions include clinically evident or subclinical manifestations of placenta previa and abruptio placentae. Other causes are membranous vessels, intrauterine devices in situ, amniocentesis, decidual necrosis, so-called trophotropism (or placental wandering), and disrupted venous lakes (Fig. 6–18).[4,44]

Multiple Gestations

The relations of the placental membranes in multiple gestations are important for understanding zygosity and potential complications. In multiple gestations, evaluation of the intervening membrane is of great assistance in assigning zygosity.

If no intervening membrane is present, the gestations are monozygous. These pregnancies are termed monoamnionic monochorionic (MoMo). They are associated with a 50% incidence of fetal demise caused by cord entanglements. Vascular anastomoses between the two fused placentas may occur but less frequently than in diamnionic monochorionic (DiMo) placentas (see below).[6]

If the intervening membrane has no chorion between two amnions, the gestation is monozygous and termed DiMo (Fig. 6–19*A*). The chief mor-

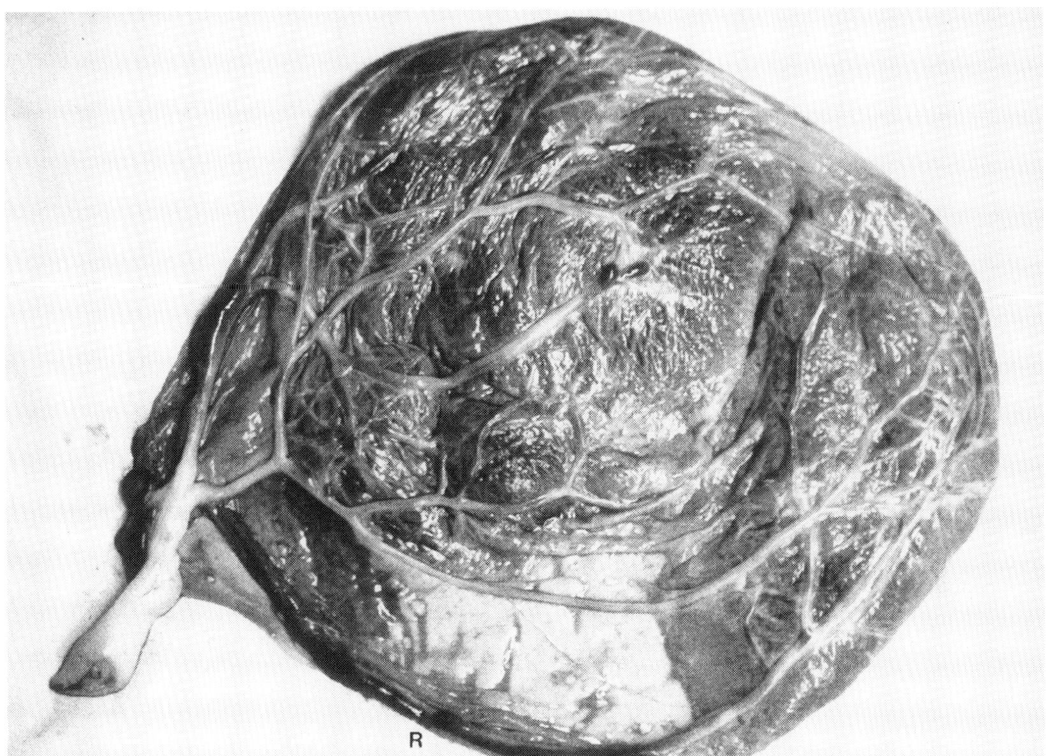

Figure 6–17. Ruptured vasa previa (*R*) (velamentous vessels) from amniotomy resulting in catastrophic fetal hemorrhage. (From Lewis SH, Benirschke K: The placenta. In Sternberg S [ed]: Histology for pathologists. New York, 1997, Raven Press.)

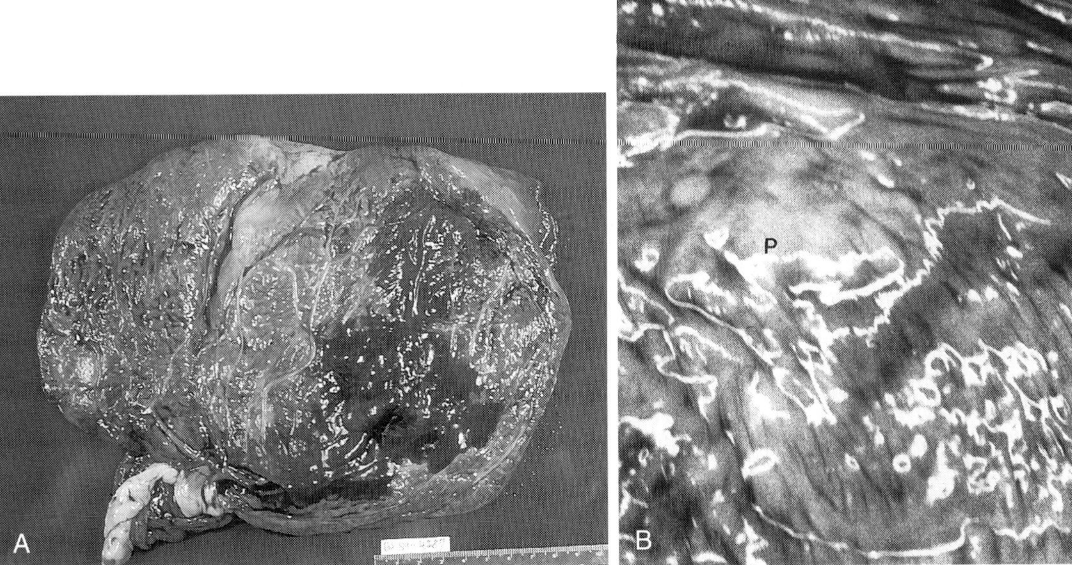

Figure 6–18. A, Acute retromembranous hemorrhage from amniocentesis. **B,** Older plaque *(P)* of retromembranous hemorrhage seen from the fetal surface in conjunction with a circummarginate placenta.

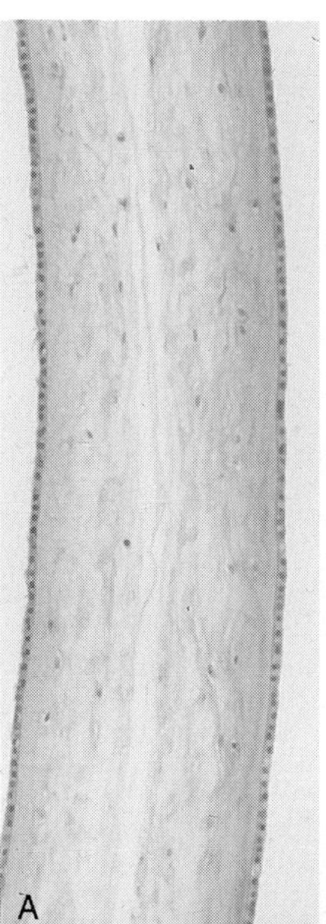

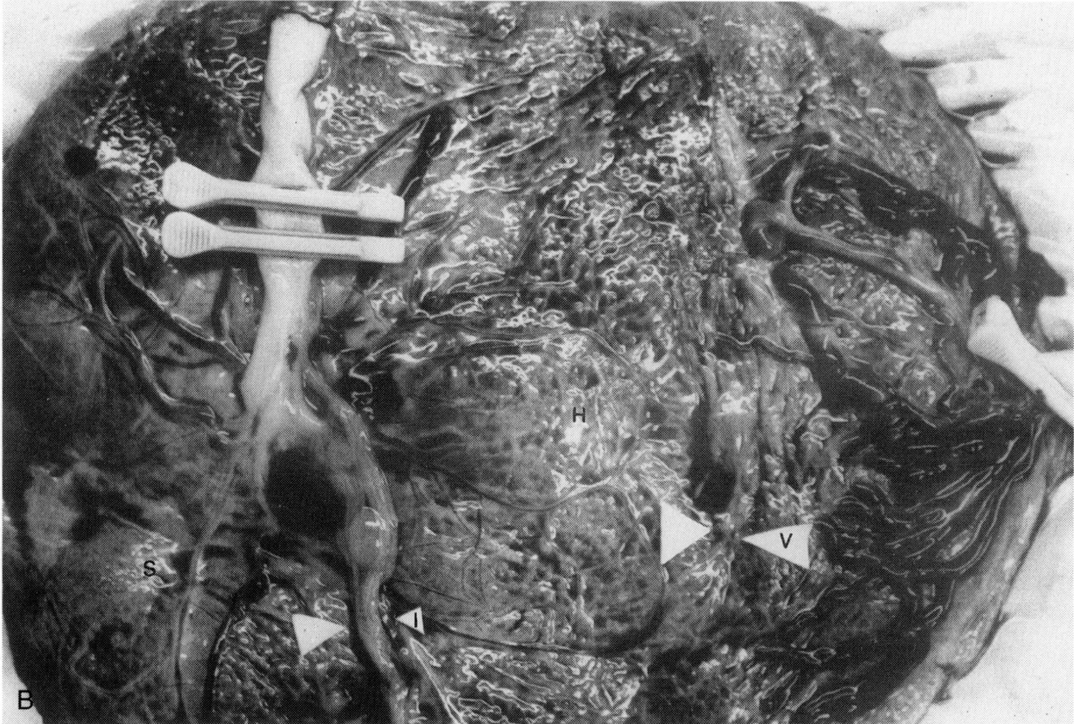

Figure 6–19. A, DiMo intervening membrane. Note the absence of intervening chorion. This is diagnostic of a monozygotic pregnancy. **B,** DiMo twin-twin transfusion twins and placenta. The equator of the intervening membrane *(I)* is different from the vascular equator *(V)* of the fused placenta. This is due to amniotic fluid discrepancies characteristic of transfusion syndrome and resulting in hydramniotic *(H)* and "stuck" *(S)* twin amniotic sacs. (*A* from Lewis SH, Benirschke K: The placenta. In Sternberg S [ed]: Histology for pathologists. New York, 1997, Raven Press.)

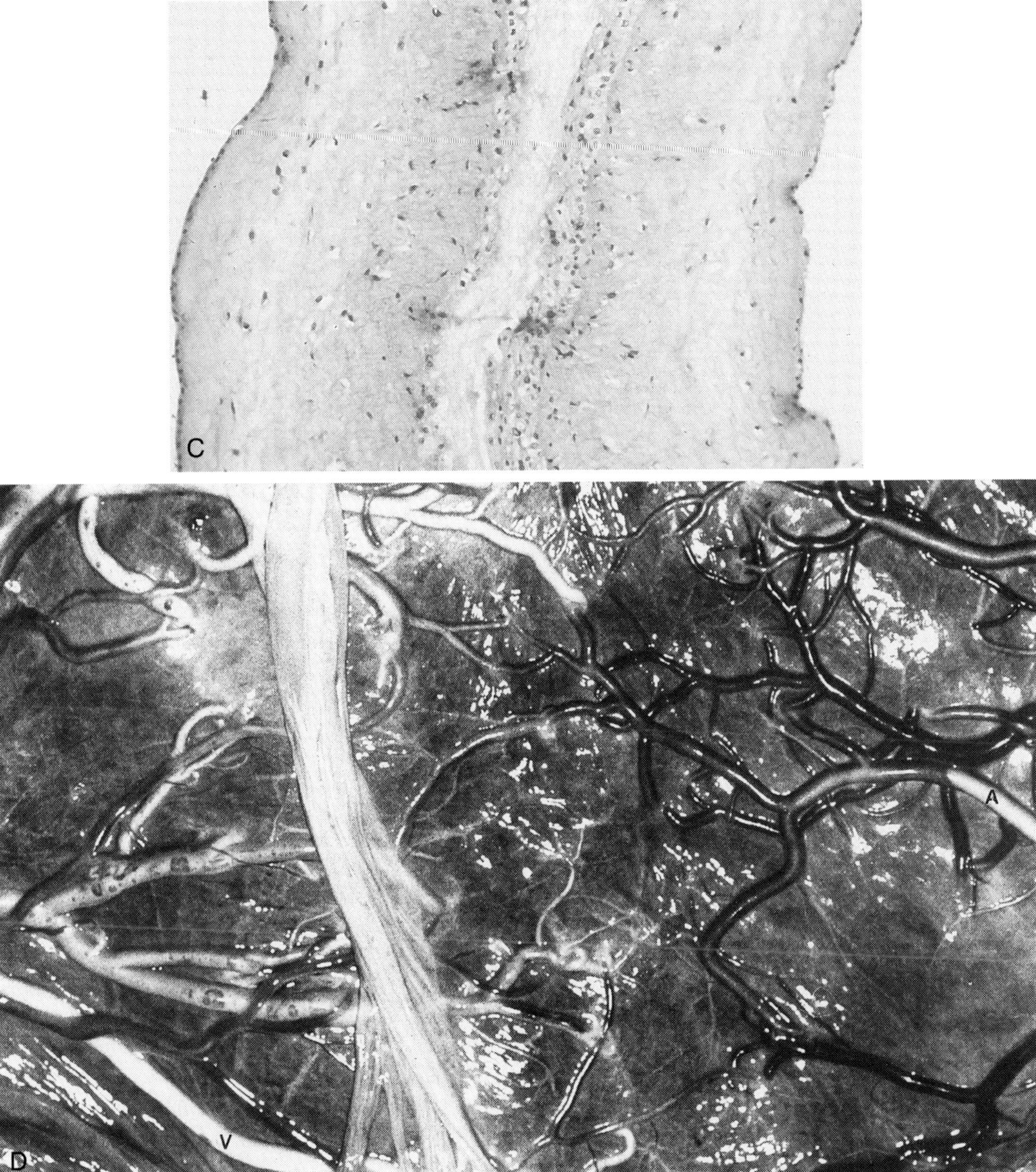

Figure 6–19 *Continued* **C,** DiDi intervening membrane (amnion-chorion/chorion-amnion). **D,** Injection studies with artery *(A)* to vein *(V)* anastomoses. Arteries course over veins, enabling distinction and characterization of the anastomoses. (*C* from Lewis SH, Benirschke K: The placenta. In Sternberg S [ed]: Histology for pathologists. New York, 1997, Raven Press.)

Illustration continued on following page

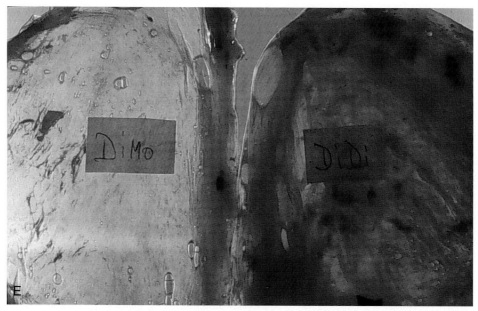

Figure 6–19 *Continued* **E,** Transillumination of DiDi and DiMo intervening membranes. (*E* courtesy K. Benirschke, San Diego, California.)

bidity is due to vascular anastomoses. In decreasing order of occurrence, vein-to-vein, artery-to-artery and artery-to-vein anastomoses are found. The first two probably rarely account for morbidity during gestation, since there are no associated pressure gradients to direct aberrant flow. At delivery, with manipulation of the fetuses and cords, blood volume distributions may shift from these channels. When artery-to-vein anastomoses occur, the classic transfusion syndrome may be found.[6] In this condition the artery of the anemic donor transfers blood to the vein of the plethoric recipient. The donor placenta is often pale with hydropic villi, nucleated red blood cells in villous vasculature, and increased villous macrophages. The recipient placenta is often deep red with villous congestion. The "stuck" (from oligohydramnios) donor twin weighs less, as do its organs when compared with its recipient sib, which often has hydramnios (Fig. 6–19*B*). The classic findings in twin-twin transfusion syndrome are not always seen. Alterations caused by highly complex anastomoses or shifts in flow at delivery may obscure the diagnosis and render apparently contradictory data when these factors are analyzed in affected twins.[4]

If the intervening membrane has a chorion between two amnions, the gestation is dizygous in about two thirds of cases and monozygous in the remaining third. These gestations are termed diamnionic dichorionic (DiDi) (Fig. 6–19*C*). Vascular anastomoses do not occur. They are reportable if identified. Zygosity may be determined by sex determination, blood typing, and human leukocyte antigen and DNA fingerprint analysis.

Vascular anastomoses are identified in utero by Doppler ultrasound or by injection studies performed in the delivered placenta. Cannulating a vessel on the chorionic plate with a needle and syringe filled with milk or dye allows the injection and identification of filling in the chorionic vessels or villous district of the associated twin placenta. It is important to recall that chorionic arteries always overlie veins when evaluating these relations (Fig. 6–19*D*).

Although histologic evaluation of the intervening membrane establishes chorionicity, gross inspection is often also useful. By transilluminating the intervening membrane, the observer may look for filamentous vessels (white streaks) representing the remnants of chorionic vessels. This is diagnostic of a DiDi placenta with the chorion between two amnions. These vessels are not seen in DiMo placentas, since the amnion is avascular and the intervening membrane is composed only of two amnions and no chorion (Fig. 6–19*E*).

Additional morbidity associated with the membranes of multiple gestations is due to the increased incidence of velamentous cord insertions and the problems associated with membranous vessels.

The membrane associations described above also pertain to multiple gestations greater than twins. In analysis of such cases, each intervening membrane and vascular relation between adjacent sibs should be described and preferably illustrated to ascertain their associated dynamics.

Amniotic Fluid Embolism

The amniotic fluid contents may find their way to the maternal circulation and result in embolism, a life-threatening condition. Fetal vernix enters the maternal circulation through disruption of placental membranes and open venous channels. Tempestuous deliveries and placenta accreta or previa are causal. Dissection of vernix beneath the amnion, which is seen in many cases, is probably not the cause. Maternal findings include hypotension, respiratory failure, disseminated intravascular coagulation, and death. Finding vernix in peripheral blood smears is diagnostic. The identification of vernix in maternal lungs is hampered by contaminants (dandruff), resulting in false-positive findings.[4,45]

CONCLUSION

The complexity of the fetal membranes is seen in their diverse functional roles and in the wide range of pathologic conditions that affect them. This chapter describes these relationships and displays the findings associated with their pathologic alterations. Not merely a bag of waters, the fetal membranes are an integral component of placental-fetal homeostasis.

ACKNOWLEDGMENT

It is with great appreciation that we acknowledge Dr. Kurt Benirschke's gracious review of this manuscript.

REFERENCES

1. Wynn RM: Morphology of the placenta. In Biology of gestation. Orlando, Fla., 1968, Academic Press.
2. Kaufmann P, Scheffen I: Placental development. In Neonatal and fetal medicine. Orlando, Fla., 1992, WB Saunders.
3. Hertig AT: Human trophoblast. Springfield, Ill., 1968, Charles C. Thomas.
4. Benirschke K, Kauffmann R: Pathology of the human placenta. New York, 1995, Springer-Verlag.
5. American College of Obstetrics and Gynecology: Update in obstetrics and gynecology V, 1994, The College.
6. Lewis SH, Benirschke K: The placenta. In Sternberg S (ed): Histology for pathologists. New York, 1997, Raven Press.
7. Michael H, Ulbright TM, Brodhecker C: Magma reticulare–like differentiation in yolk sac tumor and its pluripotential nature. Mod Pathol 1:63A, 1988.
8. Nanbu Y, Fujii S, Konishi I, et al: Cal25 in epithelium closely related to the embryonic ectoderm: the periderm and the amnion. Obstet Gynecol 161:462, 1989.
9. Schmidt W: The amniotic fluid compartment: the fetal habitat. Adv Embryol Cell Biol 127:1, 1992.
10. King BF: Developmental changes in the fine structure of rhesus monkey amnion. Am J Anat 157:285, 1980.
11. Hoyes AD: Fine structure of the amnionic epithelium following short term preservation in vitro. J Anat 111:43, 1972.
12. King BF: Cell surface specializations and intercellular junctions in human amnionic epithelium: an electron microscopic and freeze-fracture study. Anat Rec 203:73, 1982.
13. Kalousek DK, Dill FJ: Chromosomal mosaicism confined to the placenta in human conceptions. Science 221:665, 1983.
14. Verjaal M, Leschot NJ, Wolf NJ, et al: Karyotypic differences between cells from placenta and other fetal tissues. Prenat Diagn 7:343, 1987.
15. Butler WJ, Schwartz CE, Sauer SM, et al: Discordance in DNA analysis of the fetus and trophoblast. Am J Obstet Gynecol 158:642, 1988.

16. Rote NS, Menon R, Swan KF, et al: Expression of IL-1β and IL-6 protein and mRNA in amniochorionic membrane. Placenta 14A:63, 1993.
17. Fuchs AR, Periysamy S, Alexanddrova M, et al: Correlation between oxytocin in pregnant myometrium: effects of ovarian steroids. Endocrinology 113:742, 1983.
18. Benedetto MT, de Cicco, Rosielli F, et al: Oxytocin receptor in human fetal membranes. J Steroid Biochem 35:205, 1990.
19. Rees MCP, diMarzo V, Lopez Bernal A, et al: Leukotriene release by human fetal membranes, placenta and decidua in relation to parturition. J Endocrinol 118:497, 1988.
20. Crescimanno C, Muhlhauser J, Castellucci M, et al: Immunocytochemical expression patterns of carbonic anhydrase isoenzyme in human placenta cord and membranes. Placenta 14:All, 1993.
21. Muhlhauser J, Crescimanno C, Rajaniemi H: Immunohistochemistry of carbonic anhydrase in human placenta, cord and membranes. Histochemistry 101:91, 1994.
22. Bourne GL: The microscopic anatomy of the human amnion and chorion. Am J Obstet Gynecol 79:1070, 1960.
23. Malak TM, Okleford CD, Bell SC, et al: Confocal immunofluorescence localization of collagen type-I, type-III, type-IV, type-V and type VI and their ultrastructural organization in term human fetal membranes. Placenta 14:385, 1993.
24. Hessle H, Engvall E: Type IV collagen. J Biol Chem 259:3955, 1984.
25. Blanc WA: Vernix granulomatosis of amnion in oligohydramnios: lesion associated with urinary anomalies, retention of dead fetuses, and prolonged leakage of amniotic fluid. NY State J Med 61:1492, 1961.
26. Landing BH: Amnion nodosum: a lesion of the placenta apparently associated with deficient secretion of fetal urine. Am J Obstet Gynecol 60:1339, 1950.
27. Barss VA, Benacerraf BR, Frigoletto FD: Second trimester oligohydramnios, a predictor of poor fetal outcome. Obstet Gynecol 64:608, 1984.
28. Altshuler G: Placenta infection and inflammation. In Perrin EVDK (ed): Pathology of the placenta. New York, 1984, Churchill Livingstone.
29. Novak RW, Platt MS: Significance of placental findings in early-onset group B streptococcal neonatal sepsis. Clin Pediatr 24:256, 1985.
30. Hauth JC, Goldberg RL, Andrews WW, et al: Reduced incidence of preterm delivery with metronidazole and erythromycin in women with bacterial vaginosis. N Engl J Med 28:333, 1995.
31. Naeye RL: Disorders of the placenta, fetus, and neonate. St. Louis, 1992, Mosby.
32. Rubovits WH, Taft E, Neuwelt F: The pathologic properties of meconium. Am J Obstet Gynecol 36:501, 1938.
33. Altshuler G, Hyde S: Meconium induced vasoconstriction: a potential cause for cerebral and other hypoperfusion and of poor pregnancy outcome. J Child Neurol 4:137, 1989.
34. Torpin R: Fetal malformations caused by amnion rupture during gestation. Springfield, Ill., 1968, Charles C Thomas.
35. Moerman P, Fryns J, Vandenberg K, et al: Constrictive amniotic bands, amniotic adhesions, and limb-body wall complex: discrete disruption sequences with pathogenic overlap. Am J Med Genet 42:470, 1992.
36. Hofbauer J: Extrachoriale Fruchtentwicklung, in situ beobachtet. Arch Gynecol 135:332, 1929.
37. Benirschke K: Effects of placental pathology on the embryo and the fetus. In Handbook of teratology. New York, 1977, Plenum Press.
38. McCarthy J, Thurmond AS, Jones MK, et al: Circumvallate placenta: sonographic diagnosis. J Ultrasound Med 14:21, 1995.
39. DeSa DJ: Intimal cushions in foetal placental veins. J Pathol 110:347, 1973.
40. Altshuler G: Some placental considerations related to neurodevelopmental and other disorders. J Child Neurol 8:78, 1993.
41. Fox H, Sen DK: Placenta extrachorialis: a clinicopathologic study. J Obstet Gynaecol Br Commonw 79:32, 1972.
42. Hurley VA, Beischer NA: Placenta membranacea: case reports. Br J Obstet Gynaecol 94:798, 1987.
43. Maddox DE, Kephart GM, Coulam CB, et al: Localization of a molecule immunochemically similar to eosinophil major basic protein in human placenta. J Exp Med 158:1211, 1983.
44. Pozniak MA, Cullenward MJ, Zickuhr D, et al: Venous lake bleeding: a complication of chorionic villous sampling. J Ultrasound Med 7:297, 1988.
45. Haddad FS: Amniotic fluid embolism: a review of the literature and a case report with recovery. J Indian Med Assoc 17:76, 1985.

7

Disorders of the Placental Parenchyma

Raymond W. Redline

The placental parenchyma can be defined in several ways. For the purposes of this chapter the parenchyma has been separated into three compartments: the fetal vasculature distal to the umbilical cord, the supporting stroma of the chorionic villous tree, and the interhemal membrane separating maternal blood in the intervillous space from vascularized fetal connective tissue in the villi. The fetal vasculature can in turn be separated into four physiologically distinct segments: large and small arteries of the chorionic plate and primary and secondary stem villi, which transport deoxygenated fetal blood to the terminal villous unit without themselves participating in gas exchange; arterioles of the tertiary stem villi, which regulate access to the terminal villous unit; the capillary bed of the terminal villous unit, where substrate exchange occurs; and the draining venous system, which transmits oxygenated fetal blood back to the fetus. The second compartment, chorionic villous stroma, is a fibroblastic connective tissue that surrounds the fetal vasculature, separating it from the trophoblastic epithelium of the interhemal membrane. Adjacent to large vessels in the chorionic plate and stem villi this stroma is dense, sparsely cellular, and rich in collagen, while in tertiary stem villi and terminal villous units it is a loose connective tissue devoid of collagen, rich in extracellular fluid, and populated by abundant tissue macrophages known as Hofbauer cells. One characteristic feature of advancing placental development is a decreased percentage of villous stroma in terminal villi relative to other components of the parenchyma (i.e., fetal vessels and trophoblastic epithelium). This developmental change decreases the diffusion distance for substrate and is one of the criteria for assessing placental dysmaturity (see below). The interhemal membrane consists of trophoblastic epithelium, the perivillous space immediately adjacent to its apical surface, and the basement membrane underlying its basal surface. Villous trophoblast is composed of discrete trophoblast proliferative units, which together cover the chorionic villous tree.[1] Each trophoblast proliferative unit consists of 10 to 13 syncytiotrophoblast nuclei dispersed in a single cytoplasmic envelope overlying a single stem cell, the villous cytotrophoblast. Syncytiotrophoblast possesses numerous specialized transport systems for different types of substrate. Its apical surface has the additional protective function of inhibiting activation of the maternal immune and coagulation systems and thereby preventing tissue damage and ensuring free circulation in the intervillous space.

In respiratory organs the primary function of parenchyma is to serve as a scaffolding separating two circulations. This has two implications. First, any process that alters parenchymal architecture will have profound effects on placental function by changing the diffusion distance. Second, since the parenchyma is primarily supportive and has limited independent functions, pathologic lesions are more likely to reflect disease processes occurring in the fetus or the mother than primary abnormalities of the parenchyma itself. Nevertheless, patterns of injury in the placental parenchyma when taken in context with the clinical history are extremely useful in understanding many of the complications of pregnancy.

FETAL VASCULAR LESIONS

Lesions of Large and Medium-sized Vessels

Fetal thrombotic arteriopathy[2] (obstructive fetal vasculopathy,[3] fetal vascular obliteration,[4] endarteritis obliterans,[5] thrombosclerosing placentitis[6]) refers to lesions resulting from localized or diffuse thrombosis of chorionic or stem villous arteries. Because of the difficulty in identifying discrete thrombi on gross examination and the three-dimensional architecture of the villous tree, arterial thrombi are most readily identified by their downstream effects on the villous tree. Thrombi in fetal arteries result in well-circumscribed zones of downstream avascular villi conforming to the dependent portion of the affected villous tree (Fig. 7–1). These avascular villi show a densely collagenized (hyalinized) stroma, generally without the mineralization, karyorrhexis, fibroblasts, or inflammatory cells seen in fibrotic villi associated with villitis of unknown etiology (VUE), venous obstructive lesions, or uteroplacental underperfusion (see below). Attesting to the strong association between avascular villi and arterial thrombosis is the fact that despite the sampling problems described above, almost two thirds of placentas in a recently published series of cases with avascular villi had thrombi identified in one or more fetal arteries.[2] Other fetal vascular lesions sometimes observed in cases of fetal thrombotic arteriopathy include platelet fibrin thrombi and venous throm-

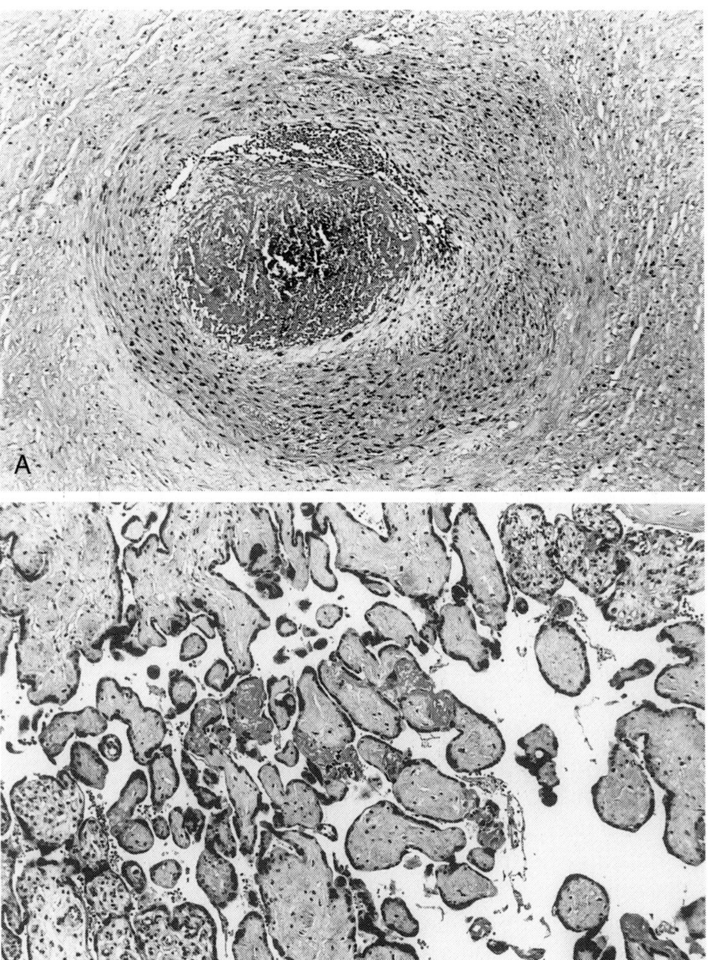

Figure 7–1. A, Occlusive chorionic artery thrombus of the type often associated with focally avascular villi. **B,** Focally avascular villi related to upstream arterial occlusion show bland homogeneous collagenized stroma and interdigitate with normally vascularized villi.

boocclusive changes (see below). Thrombotic arteriopathy is significantly increased in placentas with coexistent membrane hemosiderin deposition and VUE, suggesting that chronic marginal separation and activation of maternal lymphoid cells in the fetal stroma may place arteries at risk for thrombosis.[2]

The three best-established risk factors for arterial thrombosis are platelet activation, hypercoagulability, and critical stenosis of the arterial lumen. Consonant with the first two risk factors several authors have described fetal thrombotic arteriopathy in association with antiplatelet antibodies (autoimmune or alloimmune), anticoagulant factor deficiencies (protein C, protein S, antithrombin III), and various hypercoagulability syndromes (antiphospholipid antibody, acute promyelocytic leukemia, activated factor V resistance).[2,6–8] The cause of arterial thrombosis in patients without hemostatic abnormalities is less clear. One mechanism worthy of consideration relates to the third risk factor, critical stenosis. Fetal arteries are known to close rapidly after delivery by the constriction of specialized spiral folds in the arterial wall (so-called folds of Hoboken).[9] Transient flow decreases or hypoxia during gestation might prematurely trigger this reflex pathway, leading to localized areas of critical stenosis.

Thrombotic arteriopathy has been associated with intrauterine growth retardation (IUGR), intrauterine fetal demise (IUFD), nonimmune hydrops, acute and chronic fetal monitoring abnormalities, neonatal asphyxia, and thromboembolic disease in various studies.[2,7] However, many placentas with thrombotic arteriopathy are not associated with adverse outcomes. Features correlated with worse outcome in my experience include many numerous small foci of avascular villi rather than single large lesions, the presence of platelet fibrin thrombi, and the coexistence of other placental lesions such as VUE, maternal vascular lesions, or increased nucleated red blood cells.[2] The risk for thrombotic arteriopathy in subsequent pregnancies is increased with genetic coagulation factor abnormalities and antibody-mediated coagulopathies in the mother. A search for such abnormalities is most fruitful in severe cases of fetal arteriopathy associated with bad fetal outcome.

Venous thromboocclusive lesions (hemorrhagic endovasculitis,[10,11] fibrinous vasculosis,[12] intimal fibrin cushions,[13] obstructive fetal vasculopathy[4]) involving the umbilical, chorionic, and stem villous veins are among the most controversial lesions in placental pathology. In part this controversy relates to the gradual transition between stasis and thrombosis, which leads to a continuum of upstream effects on draining villi. One noncontroversial venous thromboocclusive lesion is *occlusive thrombosis* of a major chorionic vein, which can often be identified on gross examination as a darkly discolored and focally dilated vessel showing an abrupt transition at the point of occlusion (reviewed in Benirschke and Kaufmann[14]). A second easily recognized lesion is the *intimal fibrin cushion,* which occurs in chorionic plate and stem villous veins and is characterized by insudation of fibrin beneath the endothelium (Fig. 7–2*A*).[13] Intimal cushions may be a cause of later thrombosis, and some intimal fibrin cushions may represent thrombi that have been incorporated into the vessel wall. With time intimal fibrin cushions can undergo mineralization, leading to mural calcification of chorionic plate or stem vessels (Fig. 7–2*B*).[15] The more controversial lesions are those representing secondary effects of upstream stasis on villous morphology. These changes, as might be anticipated, are recapitulated in placentas from intrauterine fetal deaths and in suboptimally handled placentas (inadequately fixed or nonrefrigerated), which can undergo artifactual postdelivery changes. The stereotypical sequence of villous changes related to venous stasis has been well documented in stillborns and by in vitro placental organ culture.[16,17] Reflex arterial vasospasm leads to incorporation of red blood cells into the arterial wall (so-called hemorrhagic endovasculitis).[10,11] Fibrotic strands bridge the lumen of small to medium-sized veins (so-called recanalization lesion), eventually leading to occlusion. Villous capillary endothelial cells and circulating nucleated fetal cells undergo karyorrhexis with spillage into the villous stroma. The resulting combination of villous edema, necrotic debris, and siderocalcific deposits forms a dirty background that stands out from normally perfused villi in other parts of the placenta (Fig. 7–3). Villous heterogeneity and focal involvement in appropriately processed placentas are the best indicators that these changes represent predelivery events and not post delivery artifacts.

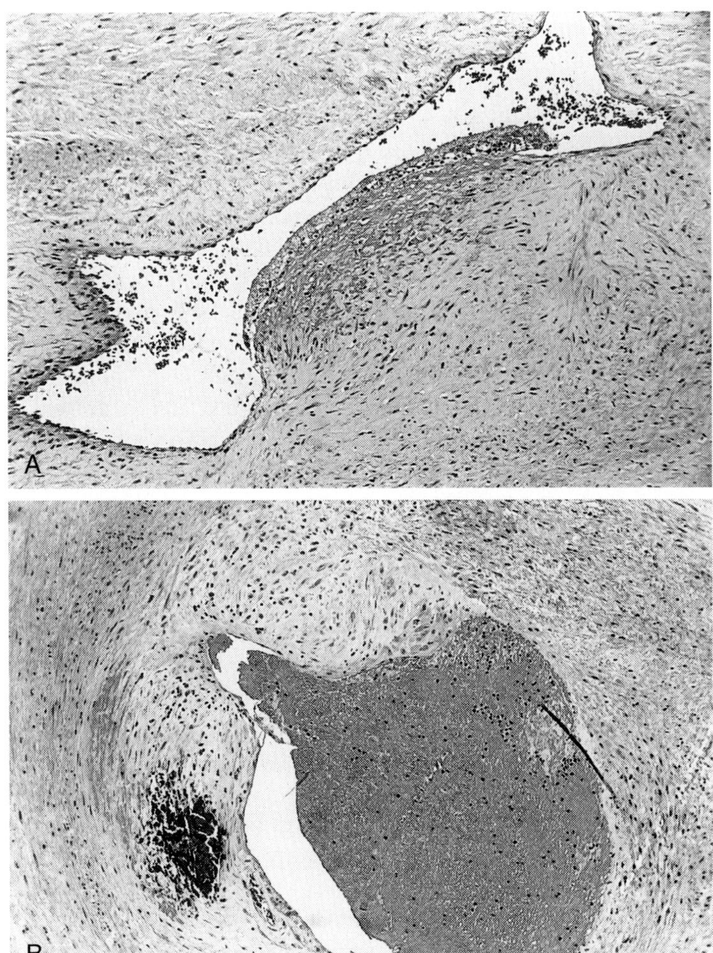

Figure 7–2. **A**, Recent intimal fibrin cushion in a chorionic vein. This type of mural abnormality is thought to represent pressure-related insudation of plasma through damaged endothelium. **B**, Mural calcification in the muscularis of a large chorionic vein reflecting the chronic organizing stage of intimal fibrin cushion.

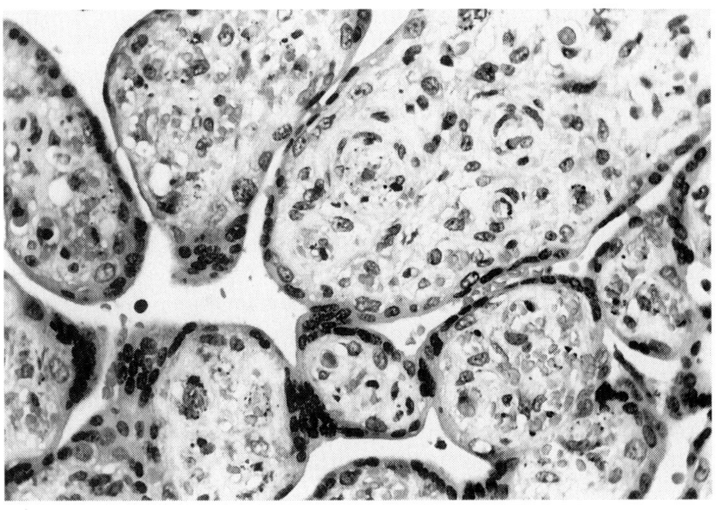

Figure 7–3. Venous thromboocclusive changes ("hemorrhagic endovasculitis"). Obstruction of the draining venous vasculature leads to villous vascular-stromal hemorrhage, degeneration, macrophage accumulation, and karyorrhexis.

Established risk factors for venous thrombosis include stasis, endothelial damage, and an imbalance between coagulation factors and anticoagulant mechanisms. Many venous lesions in the placenta probably result from acute and chronic umbilical cord occlusion related to either direct pressure or torsion.[10,11,18] Cord compression preferentially affects the thinner-walled umbilical vein, leading to increased transmural pressure and stasis in upstream veins. Increased transmural pressure may be particularly important in the generation of intimal fibrin cushions, whereas stasis is more often related to luminal fibrosis and changes in villous morphology.[13] Infants with in utero heart failure (hydrops fetalis) are at increased risk for venous thrombosis because of their baseline low flow state.[19] Acquired procoagulant antiphospholipid antibodies are associated with both arterial and venous thrombi in other organ systems, and recent work suggests that the long-known susceptibility of diabetic fetuses to umbilical vein thrombi may be the consequence of antiphospholipid antibodies in their mothers.[20,21]

Patients with venous thromboocclusive disease are at risk for IUFD and neonatal asphyxia.[10,11,18] Some studies suggest that they are also more likely to have cerebral palsy.[22] IUGR and prematurity are not strongly related to venous thromboocclusive disease. Recurrence risk is generally limited to patients with underlying coagulopathies, which, as for arterial thrombotic disease, should be pursued in the context of severe placental involvement, bad outcome, or poor obstetric history.

Acute degenerative vessel wall lesions include intense chorionic vasculitis[23] and meconium-related peripheral vascular necrosis.[24] *Intense chorionic vasculitis* is an acute degenerative change affecting the vessel wall in cases of long-standing chorioamnionitis. Amniotic fluid infections stimulate the chemotaxis of fetal inflammatory cells, resulting in migration through the vessel wall. This so-called vasculitis occurs most commonly with long duration of infection and in mature fetuses. Intense chorionic vasculitis in preterm gestations often has a prominent component of eosinophils. Although occasional inflammatory cells in the vessel wall may be relatively innocuous, intense infiltration and possibly local activation can lead to mural edema and vascular smooth muscle degeneration, which may cause vasospasm. Intense chorionic vasculitis is not infrequently associated with nonocclusive recent thrombi (Fig. 7–4*A*).[2] Meconium alone can be associated with chorionic vasculitis,[25] but the intensity of vasculitis is particularly intense in cases of both chorioamnionitis and meconium exposure. Another degenerative vessel wall lesion associated with prolonged exposure of the umbilical cord or chorionic vessels to large amounts of meconium is *meconium-related peripheral vascular necrosis* (Fig. 7–4*B*).[21] This distinctive lesion is characterized by myonecrosis of periadventitial vascular smooth muscle cells, resulting in degenerating circular cells with intensely eosinophilic cytoplasm and a shrunken hyperchromatic central nucleus.

A number of in vitro experiments support the concept that acute degenerative lesions associated with infection or meconium may cause fetal vasospasm.[26,27] In these experiments fetal vessels exposed to bacterial extracts and meconium suspensions develop a contractile response. Activation of leukocytes associated with cytokines and chemokines in other systems is also well known to cause endothelial damage and vessel wall injury.[28]

Lesions of Small Arteries and Arterioles

Small artery lesions associated with abnormal pulsed-flow Doppler studies include fetal arteriolar hypertrophy,[29] degenerative changes in small arteries,[30] small artery obliteration,[31] and peripheralization of arterial smooth muscle.[32] There is no a priori reason that placentas grouped on the basis of increased vascular resistance as defined by abnormal pulsed-flow Doppler testing should show any one characteristic lesion. Attempts to define such a Doppler-associated lesion have relied on morphometry, leading to considerable variation from study to study depending on the methods used. Changes described in these studies reflect group averages and may have little predictive value in any given placenta. Despite these caveats a few common themes have emerged. Affected placentas are generally small for gestational age and show a relative undergrowth of excessively small terminal villi.[33,34] Three types of small arterial lesions have been described. First is a deficiency of small arteries, which has variably been considered a primary developmental abnormality

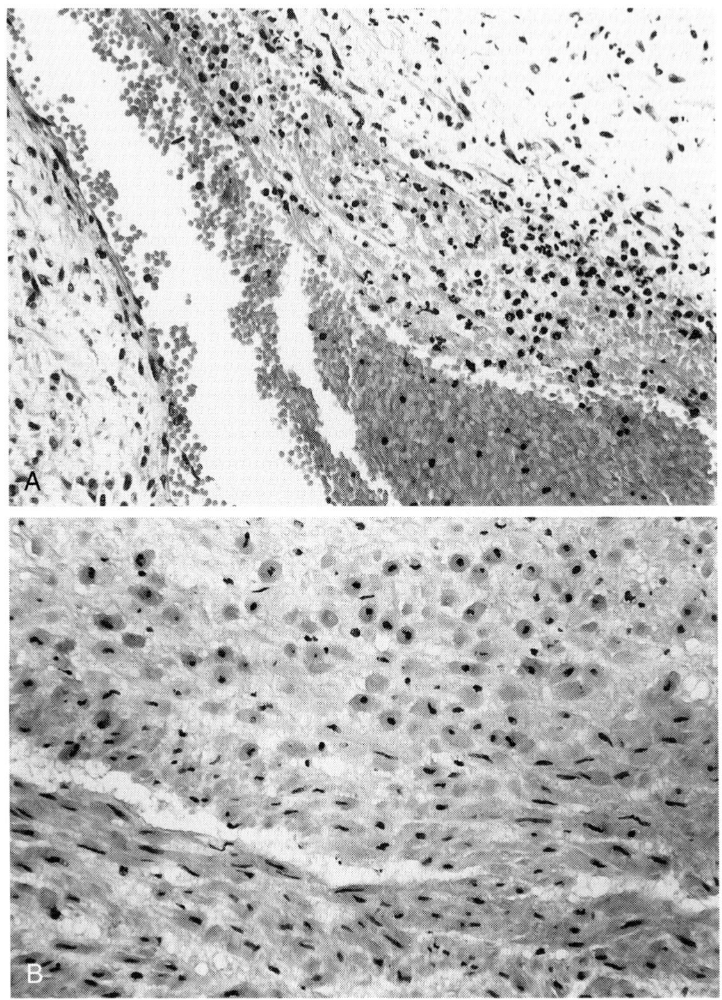

Figure 7–4. **A**, Intense chorionic vasculitis related to amniotic fluid infection with associated recent nonocclusive thrombosis. **B**, Meconium-related peripheral vascular smooth muscle necrosis involving a chorionic vein. Note the rounded apoptotic myocytes showing intense cytoplasmic eosinophilia and nuclear pyknosis.

or a secondary obliterative phenomena related to fetal platelet activation.[35,36] This type of abnormality requires morphometry for definition, which is difficult to apply in practice. The second lesion is distalization of arterial smooth muscle into the terminal villous vasculature, which resembles changes seen with pulmonary hypertension.[32,37] This distalization of smooth muscle depends on immunostaining with antibodies to muscle-specific actin. The third and most diagnostically useful pattern is a diffuse abnormality of small arteries and arterioles characterized by mural thickening and degeneration of the vessel wall, sometimes associated with hypovascular and fibrotic distal villi (Fig. 7–5).[30] This diagnosis of small artery fetal vasculopathy should be made with caution, preferably based on severe involvement and a strong supporting clinical history, because of overlap with lesions caused by postdelivery arterial vasospasm.

Maternal vascular insufficiency seems to be the underlying lesion in most cases of IUGR with abnormalities on pulsed-flow Doppler.[34] The most plausible underlying abnormality is chronic placental underperfusion leading to both underdevelopment of tertiary stem-terminal villous units and arteriolar vasoconstriction followed by vascular remodeling.[38] Arterial adaptations are similar to those seen with pulmonary hypertension: vasospasm, mural hypertrophy, peripheralization of smooth muscle, and eventually arterial dropout.

The clinical scenarios associated with pulsed-flow Doppler abnormalities are IUGR, severe early-onset preeclampsia, and chromosomal abnormali-

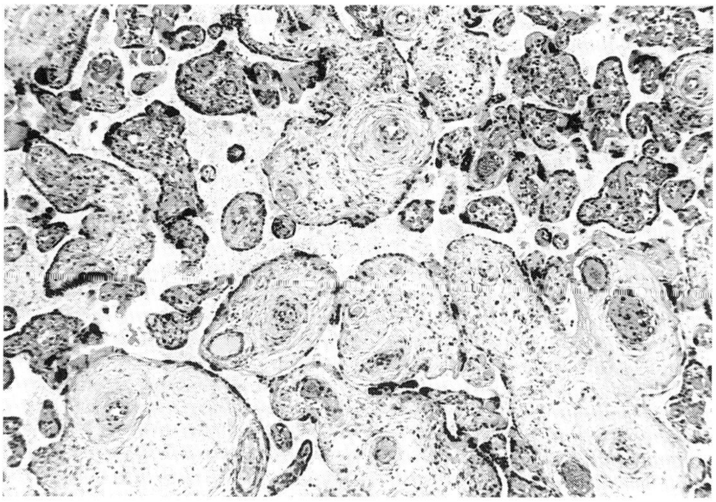

Figure 7–5. Small artery lesions associated with abnormal pulsed-flow Doppler studies. Secondary and tertiary stem villi show prominent small arteries and arterioles with marked concentric hypertrophy and stenosis.

ties.[35,39,40] Whether some cases are due to confined placental chromosomal mosaicism (see Chapter 14) is an interesting question. Recurrence risks depend on the underlying cause; many of the above syndromes have a high incidence of recurrence.

Lesions of Terminal Villous Capillaries

Villous chorangiosis (hypercapillarization) has been defined by the rule of 10s.[41] More than 10 terminal villi having more than 10 capillaries in cross section should be seen in 10 or more medium-power fields in at least three areas of the placenta. In reality the low-power appearance of hypercapillarized villi is sufficiently distinct that actual counting is seldom necessary (Fig. 7–6). Chorangiosis has been subjectively graded, but the criteria used for grading have not been specified. Placentas with chorangiosis are often large for gestational age and characterized by delayed villous maturation (see below). These characteristics are commonly seen in diabetic placentas, which have been shown to have increased capillaries.[42] Prominence of capillaries caused by venous congestion should be carefully excluded. This can be more difficult than it might seem, since only about 50% of any capillary bed is normally filled, with the remainder filling only with increased pressure.[43] A helpful diagnostic point is that many villi

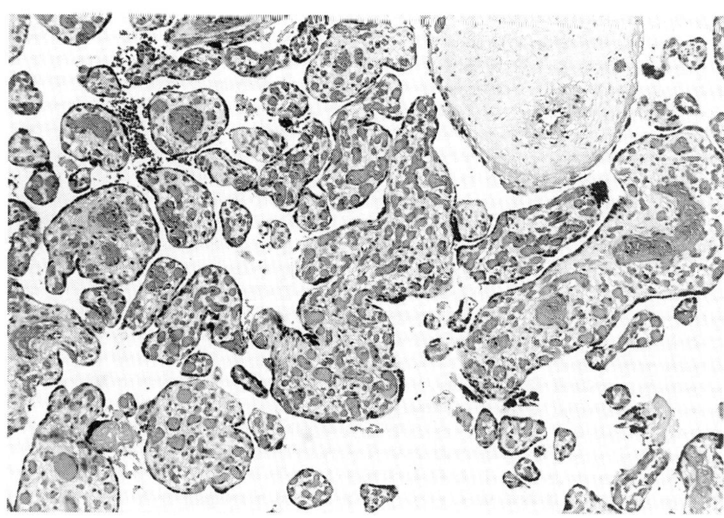

Figure 7–6. Villous chorangiosis defined as hypercapillarization of terminal and tertiary stem villi with greater than 10 capillaries per villous cross section.

in placentas with true chorangiosis have up to 20 capillaries, a number difficult to account for by capillary reserve alone.

Chorangiosis is distinguished from the benign vascular tumor known as chorangioma by virtue of the tumorous nature and prominent perithelial and stromal proliferation in the latter (see Chapter 12). Rarely, an intermediate lesion known as *chorangiomatosis* or *infiltrating chorangioma* is seen.[44] Chorangiomatosis is characterized by diffuse endothelial and perithelial proliferation in multiple stem and terminal villi. The few cases of chorangiomatosis I have encountered have been associated with preeclampsia or cocaine abuse.

The central question never addressed in chorangiosis is whether the lesion represents direct stimulation of capillary growth or the elongation, coiling, and distention of existing capillaries. Persistent terminal villogenesis in continuously growing third-trimester placentas occurs by herniation of coiled capillary loops through the perimeters of existing villi.[45,46] Cross sections of these coiled capillaries might simulate capillary proliferation in existing villi. Clearly congestion and hypoxia may be difficult to differentiate in situations such as umbilical vein occlusion. An analogous situation may be seen in the lung where hypercapillarization of alveolar septa is sometimes seen in cases of chronic congestive heart failure. Nevertheless, several arguments support the hypothesis that chorangiosis is an adaptive proliferative response to hypoxia or chronic inflammation. Chorangiosis is increased in placentas delivered from pregnancies occurring at high altitude and in placentas showing chronic villous inflammation.[41,47–49] Furthermore, villi have been shown to express angiogenic growth factors and receptors that are upregulated in response to low oxygen tension (vascular endothelial growth factor, platelet-derived growth factor–β) and activation of inflammatory cells (tumor necrosis factor–α, tumor growth factor–β, interleukin–6).[50–55]

The true prevalence of chorangiosis is unknown. Since it is largely confined to placentas older than 37 weeks, available figures fail to account for the 80% to 90% of term placentas that are not submitted for pathologic examination. Overall prevalence in Altshuler's study was 74/1350 (5.5%),[41] which is in agreement with my data from Boston (36/606, 5.9%) and Cleveland (69/1349, 5.1%). Associations with acute and chronic placental ischemia, congenital anomalies, chronic villitis, placentomegaly, and cord lesions have been described.[41] I believe that chorangiosis represents a reaction pattern rather than a primary disease process. Although not a direct cause of a bad outcome, severe chorangiosis is commonly seen in abnormal pregnancies.

CHORIONIC-VILLOUS STROMAL LESIONS

Inflammatory Lesions

Acute infectious placentitis includes acute villitis and abscesses.[3,4] Acute placentitis can be either an unusual manifestation of a relatively common infection (e.g., *Escherichia coli* or *Haemophilus influenzae* chorioamnionitis) or a predictable pattern associated with unusual organisms such as *Listeria monocytogenes, Campylobacter* spp., nonsyphilitic spirochetes, *Coccidioides immitis, Francisella tularensis,* or *Brucella abortus.*[56,57] This pattern is characterized by acute and chronic suppurative villitis and perivillitis with prominent villous necrosis, sometimes progressing to frank villous abscess formation (Fig. 7–7). Organisms and neutrophils are frequently seen in fetal villous capillaries. Chorioamnionitis is almost always present. Careful examination of the inflammatory infiltrate reveals a polymorphous character, including eosinophils, plasma cells, and macrophages, Silver impregnation stains (Dieterle, Steiner, Warthin-Starry) occasionally reveal the offending organism in areas of perivillitis.

Chronic infectious placentitis (chronic villitis, specific) describes a group of placental lesions associated with documented chronic fetal infections. Unlike VUE (see below), these placentas generally show a panplacentitis with inflammatory changes and organisms in membranes, decidua, umbilical cord, and villous stroma. In the United States chronic infectious placentitis is most commonly associated with organisms of the TORCH group (toxoplasmosis, rubella, cytomegalovirus, and herpes simplex). Two distinct patterns are seen: excessively large placentas with villous edema (most common with syphilis, toxoplasmosis, and occasionally cytomegalovirus [CMV])

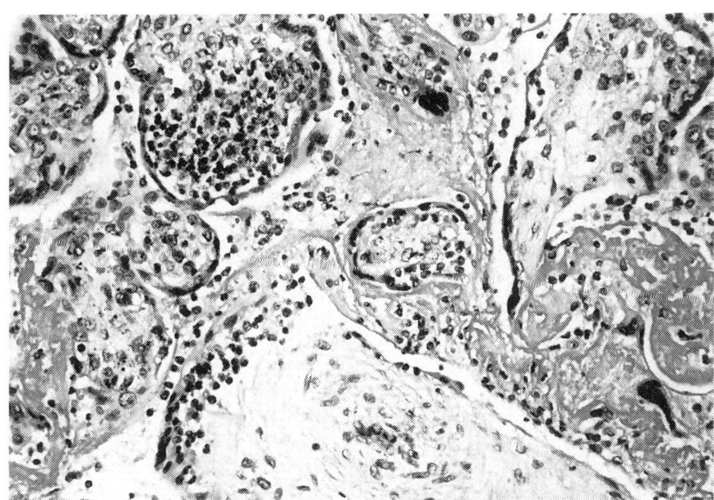

Figure 7–7. Acute infectious placentitis with acute villitis and abscesses. A polymorphous acute and chronic inflammatory infiltrate including neutrophils is centered below the villous trophoblastic basement membrane. Inflammatory cells fill fetal capillaries and spill over into the intervillous space where they are embedded in inflammatory-type perivillous fibrin.

and excessively small placentas with villous sclerosis (herpes simplex virus, varicella zoster virus, rubella, and most cases of CMV). Among the TORCH group, CMV and syphilis are by far the most common. Pathologic changes in chronic infections are described in greater detail in Chapter 13. Parenchymal lesions in *syphilitic placentitis* include chronic chorionitis, a proliferative stem arteritis with occasional lymphoblasts and plasma cells, and edematous villi with increased macrophages.[58,59] Stainable spirochetes are usually confined to the umbilical cord.[60] The parenchyma in *CMV placentitis* typically shows diffuse villitis with prominent sclerosis, calcification, and hemosiderin deposition.[61] Villous plasma cells, which are rare in VUE and other infections, are often prominent with CMV.[62] Typical CMV inclusions are seen in about 50% of cases. The suggestive histologic picture can usually be confirmed in the remainder of cases by immunostaining or paraffin-based polymerase chain reaction.

Villitis of unknown etiology (chronic villitis, nonspecific[3]; idiopathic villitis) is defined as a destructive inflammatory process affecting predominantly terminal and stem villi in the absence of a histologic pattern, clinical history, or laboratory findings suggestive of a specific infection.[63] The overall prevalence of VUE is 3% to 5%, with most cases occurring in placentas at or near term.[64,65] VUE is easily identified with low-power microscopy by the characteristic pallor, agglutination, and inflammatory fibrosis of groups of affected villi. On higher power a nonuniform chronic mononuclear cell infiltrate can be appreciated (Fig. 7–8). Either small lymphocytes or macrophages may predominate. Immunostaining shows the lymphocytes to be exclusively T cells. Other cell types such as eosinophils or plasma cells are rare. On occasion a granulomatous picture predominates. Despite multiple attempts, mycobacteria or fungi are virtually never identified by special stains in granulomatous VUE and the cost-effectiveness of performing these stains must be questioned. Although scattered plasma cells are often seen in the decidua basalis, severe chronic inflammation of the decidua, chorion, or umbilical cord is rare in VUE. Various grading schemes have been proposed.[64,65] The one we use separates VUE into focal, multifocal, patchy, and diffuse subgroups. Focal VUE (fewer than five villi per focus; foci on one slide only) and multifocal VUE (fewer than five villi per focus; multiple slides involved) are relatively innocuous, while patchy (more than five villi per focus) and diffuse VUE (greater than 5% of all terminal villi involved) are commonly associated with IUGR. Other placental lesions associated with VUE include a moderate reduction in placental weight, increased perivillous fibrin deposition without X cell proliferation (inflammatory fibrin [see below], villous chorangiosis, decidual plasma cells, and chronic intervillositis).

The etiology and pathogenesis of VUE have stirred up needless controversy. Several facts are clear: VUE is common, has a stereotypical histologic appearance, and is associated with diffuse in-

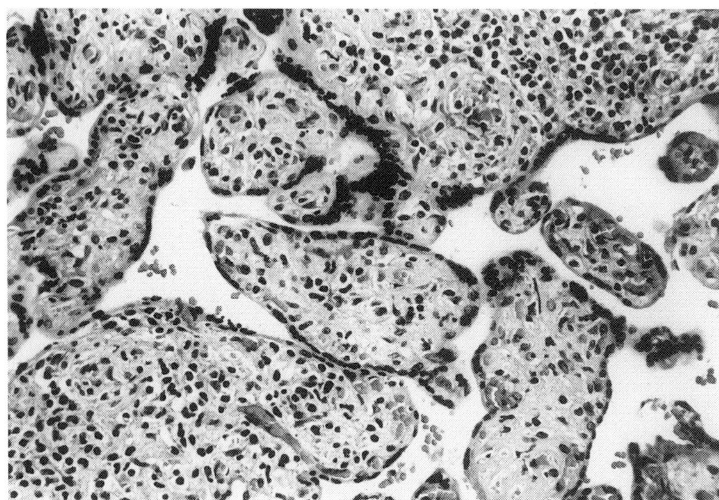

Figure 7–8. Chronic villitis of unknown etiology. The villous stroma is distorted by a nonuniform infiltrate of small lymphocytes.

filtration of fetally derived villous stroma by maternally derived T lymphocytes.[66,67] Also clear is that despite intensive investigation no infectious symptoms (fetal or maternal), seasonal variation, specific exposure history, serologic abnormality, or electron microscopic evidence of an associated pathogen has been found in VUE. Although an unrecognized pathogen can never be absolutely excluded, the important feature of VUE is not the stimulus leading to maternal lymphocytic infiltration of villi, but rather the inflammatory reaction accompanying it. Whether the etiology is infectious or noninfectious, it is likely that host-versus-graft reactivity plays a significant role in the inflammatory reaction, which interferes with gas exchange across the interhemal membrane. The initial breach of the interhemal membrane by maternal T cells is probably a chance occurrence. The ultimate magnitude of the resulting inflammatory reaction depends on the number of transferred cells, the strength of the accompanying inflammatory reaction, and the activation of adhesion molecules on adjacent villi.

VUE is the most frequent pathologic finding in cases of IUGR in nonhypertensive term pregnancies.[68] The risk of IUGR is directly proportional to the extent of villitis and is somewhat dependent on the magnitude of associated findings such as intervillositis and perivillous fibrin deposition.[63,64] VUE is one of the common lesions in the placentas of patients having serum α-fetoprotein levels at midtrimester.[69] VUE is occasionally seen in association with IUFD or prematurity, but in these contexts it is usually accompanied by other changes such as thrombotic arteriopathy, maternal vascular lesions, massive perivillous fibrin, or prominent stem villitis or vasculitis.[70] Patients with recurrent VUE have worse outcomes than those with isolated VUE of the same severity, at least in part because of earlier onset during pregnancy.[71] In our somewhat selected series we found an overall recurrence risk of 17% for VUE, with 7% of patients having three or more affected pregnancies. Patients with recurrent VUE also had an increased incidence of autoimmune disease, infertility, and recurrent spontaneous abortion.

Basal villitis (anchoring villitis) is a distinct form of VUE affecting primarily anchoring villi in the basal plate.[63,71] Basal VUE is generally associated with diffuse basal lymphoplasmacytic deciduitis (lymphocytes and plasma cells in the decidua basalis) (Fig. 7–9). Cases of VUE involving both terminal and basal villi should not be placed in this category. Isolated basal VUE is less common than VUE (18/1349 placentas [1.4%] submitted for pathologic examination in our unpublished series). Further attesting to the distinct nature of the two patterns, patients with recurrent villitis generally have the same pattern, diffuse or basal, in all affected pregnancies.[71] Recurrent basal villitis is more strongly associated with recurrent pelvic infections and low socioeconomic status than with autoimmunity or infertility. The association with pelvic infection and the intensity of the associated endometritis suggest that anchoring villi may be damaged and infiltrated by inflammatory cells responding to persistent microbial antigen in the uterus. Basal villitis is more common than VUE in premature infants and may contribute to premature labor in some instances.

Villous Dysmaturity

Villous dysmaturity has been used to describe a discrepancy between the maturity of the villous tree as assessed by histologic criteria and the true gestational age as determined by clinical history and fetoplacental weights.[3,4] In general, gestational age can be determined within ±2 weeks by assessing the relationships among the size, number, and morphology of stem and terminal villi. The underlying abnormality in dysmature placentas relates primarily to the nature and extent of terminal villogenesis.[72]

Placentas with *delayed maturation* (abnormal maturation, retarded for dates) show continuing growth and branching of incompletely differentiated terminal villi, which retain features typical of immature intermediate villi, including increased size, abundant loose cellular stroma, central capillaries, persistent villous cytotrophoblast, and densely cellular syncytiotrophoblast with decreased syncytial knots (Fig. 7–10*A*). The terminal/stem villous ratio is increased, and placentas are often large for gestational age. Delayed maturation is seen with hydrops, diabetes, and fetal macrosomia. The common denominator seems to be excessive villous stromal volume that results from edema, increased insulin, or overnutrition and leading to compensatory trophoblast proliferation.

Placentas with *accelerated maturation* (abnormal maturation, accelerated for dates) show premature and truncated formation of mature terminal villi with features including increased syncytial knots, scant fibrotic stroma, patchy trophoblastic necrosis with agglutination, and fibrinoid aggregates (so-called fibrinoid necrosis of villi) (Fig. 7–10*B*). Accelerated maturation is seen with maternal vascular diseases such as preeclampsia, essential hypertension, insulin-dependent diabetes, collagen vascular disease, and antiphospholipid antibody syndrome and is believed to represent an adaptive mechanism to maximize gas exchange (reviewed in Redline[73]).

In rare cases features of both delayed and accelerated maturation *(irregular maturation)* are seen in the same placenta, suggesting a milieu favoring continuing villous growth in the face of maternal vascular lesions causing uteroplacental insufficiency. One scenario in which this pattern is seen is insulin-dependent diabetes with maternal vascular disease.

Miscellaneous Lesions of the Chorionic Villous Stroma

Villous infarcts are caused by separation of the intervillous space from its underlying maternal

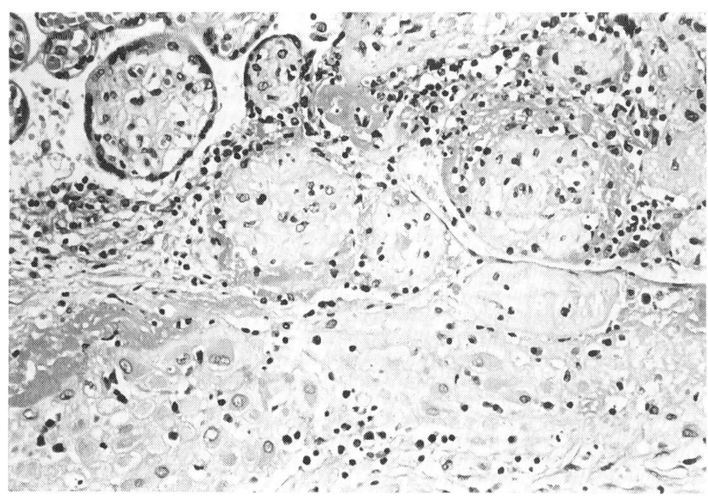

Figure 7–9. Basal villitis with basal lymphoplasmacytic deciduitis. A plasma cell–rich decidual infiltrate spills over into anchoring villi but fails to extend into so-called floating villi.

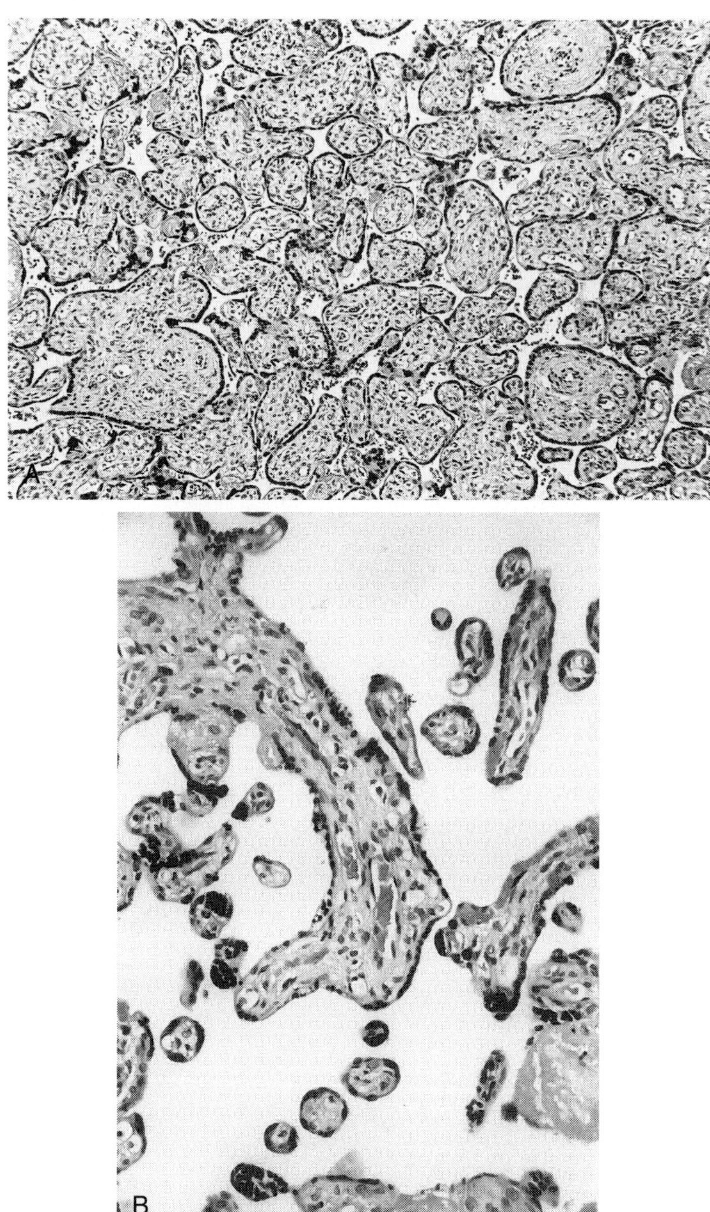

Figure 7–10. Villous dysmaturity. **A**, Delayed maturation. Terminal villi in a term placenta show characteristics of immature intermediate villi with loose edematous stroma, central capillaries, and cellular villous trophoblast. **B**, Accelerated maturation. Long, thin stem villi with stromal fibrosis give rise to tiny, sparse, terminal villous projections, many of which lack capillaries and others of which show increased syncytial knots.

blood supply either by occlusion of one or more spiral arteries or by premature separation of the placenta from the uterus.[74] Villous infarcts often occur in the context of underlying maternal vascular lesions, which can either be pregnancy specific and associated with inadequate arterial remodeling as in preeclampsia or be due to chronic maternal vascular diseases such as essential hypertension or connective tissue disease. Infarcts are recognized on gross examination as firm, wedge-shaped, granular lesions with one margin clearly aligned with and adjacent to the basal plate

(Fig. 7–11*A*). Recent infarcts are dark red. With time infarcts become white and more clearly delineated from the adjacent parenchyma. The keys to histologic identification are collapse of the intervillous space with juxtaposition of villi plus eosinophilic degeneration and karyorrhexis of villous trophoblast (Fig. 7–11*B*). Lesions that can mimic true infarcts include placental atrophy, plaques of perivillous fibrin, intervillous thrombi, and chorangiomas. Although the percentage of total parenchyma showing infarction has been emphasized, a more relevant issue is often the volume and quality of the remaining noninfarcted placental tissue. Most observers consider any villous infarct in a preterm placenta to be abnormal. In term placentas marginal infarcts or infarcts less than 3 cm in diameter are sometimes underemphasized, but as always these lesions should be considered in context with findings in the remainder of the placenta.

Villous edema has been used to described two unrelated lesions. The first is *villous hydrops,* which is associated with hydrops fetalis, either immune or nonimmune. This pattern is characterized by enlarged edematous terminal and stem villi showing features of delayed maturation.[75] The villous stroma shows symmetric displacement of fibroblasts by edema fluid, increased villous macrophages (Hofbauer cells), and an unusually prominent villous trophoblastic layer (Fig. 7–12*A*). This prominence is due to several factors, including persistence of cytotrophoblast, increased density of syncytial cell nuclei, thickening of the basement membrane, and an artifactual separation

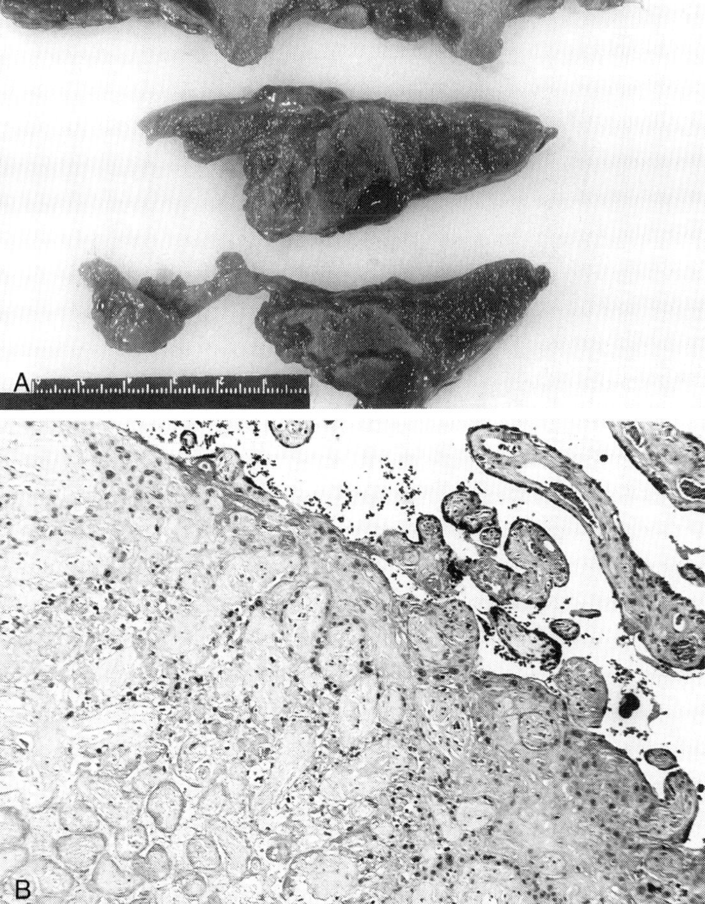

Figure 7–11. Maternal villous infarct. **A**, Gross pathology. Pale, firm, granular, wedge-shaped lesions with their broad base paralleling the basal plate reflect total occlusion of one or more decidual arterioles. **B**, Microscopic pathology. Ghostlike eosinophic villi are collapsed on one another, show trophoblast karyorrhexis, and are sharply demarcated from adjacent normal parenchyma.

of the epithelium from the underlying stroma. The second pattern, *villous edema (nonhydropic),* was initially described by Naeye[76] and occurs only in preterm placentas. Nonhydropic villous edema represents an exaggeration of the normal lacunar interstitial spaces seen in immature intermediate villi and results in a distinctive bubbly, popcorn-like appearance (Fig. 7–12*B*). This lesion has been hypothesized to increase the diffusion distance for oxygen and other substrates across the interhemal membrane. The initial report of villous edema suggested an association with decreased Apgar scores and a higher incidence of respiratory distress syndrome. This lesion is seen only in preterm placentas without accelerated maturation. Since the majority of placentas in this subgroup have histologic chorioamnionitis, the two lesions are commonly seen together.

Villous stromal hemorrhage (intravillous hemorrhage[3]), most commonly of recent onset, is seen predominantly in preterm placentas with clinically suspected abruption. It is the finding most commonly associated with early mortality in preterm infants.[77] Acute stromal hemorrhage is most likely due to sudden ischemia and hemodynamic shifts within the villous circulation, leading to the rupture of capillary walls, and may be considered the placental equivalent of germinal matrix and intraalveolar hemorrhages, both of which are commonly associated with vascular instability in very

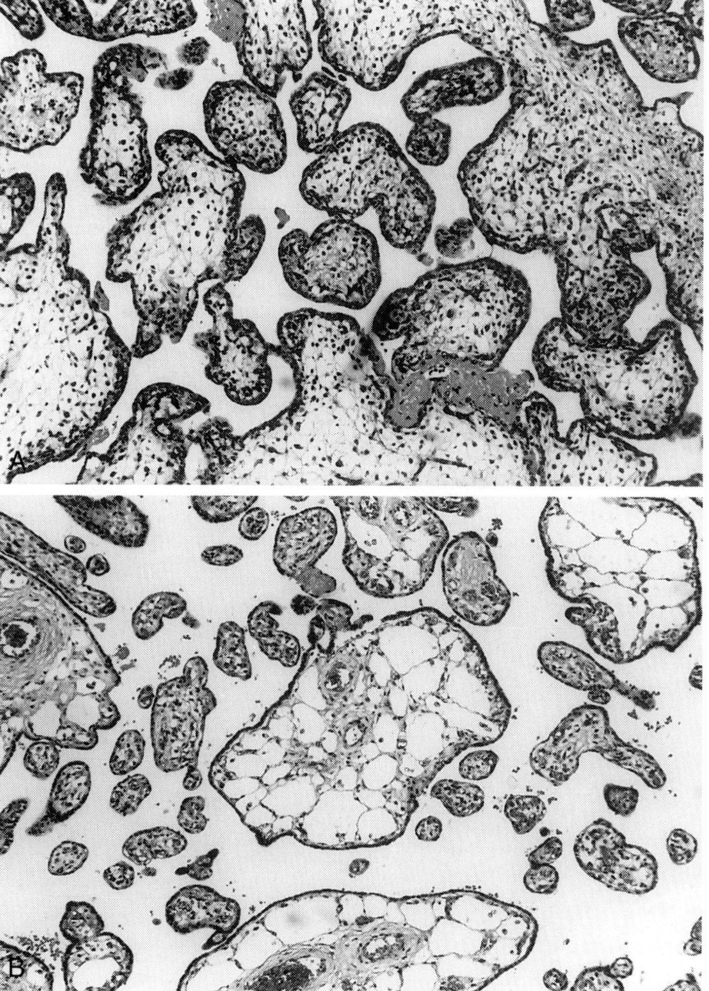

Figure 7–12. A, Villous hydrops showing diffuse interstitial edema of stem and terminal villi with peripheralization of capillaries and a thickened, irregular villous trophoblast layer. **B**, Villous edema (nonhydropic) is characterized by an exaggeration of the normal lacunae seen in immature intermediate tertiary stem villi of late second- and early third-trimester placentas.

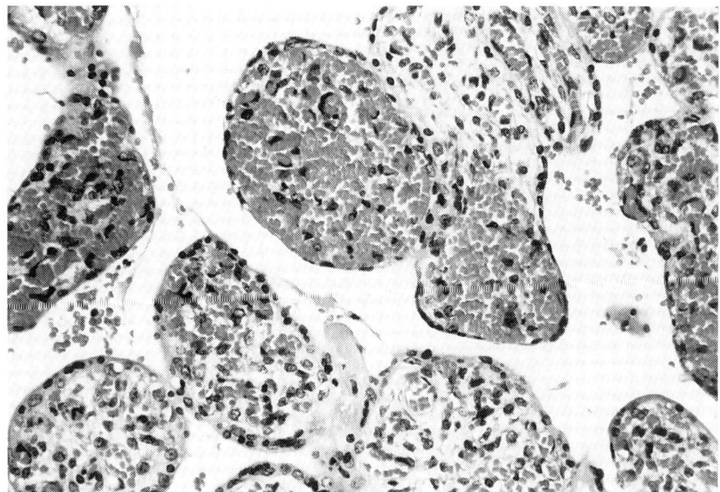

Figure 7–13. Villous stromal hemorrhage. Recent capillary rupture with intravillous spread often accompanying sudden anoxia as seen with placental abruption ("shock villi").

low birth weight infants (Fig. 7–13). Whether stromal hemorrhage is seen in situations other than abruption is not clear.

Increased nucleated red blood cells (NRBCs) (villous normoblastemia) in third-trimester placentas is an important feature that often goes unrecognized. While not a primary or causal factor in adverse outcomes, increased nucleated red blood cells can be helpful in understanding the chronicity and timing of antenatal events.[78] Although more objectively assessed by neonatal blood counts, an increase in NRBCs will not be detected by any other method in stillborns, term infants for whom blood counts are not performed, and premature or asphyxiated infants whose first blood counts are performed long after birth. Only rare NRBCs are normal after the first trimester. The presence of NRBCs in more than two capillaries in a random 10× field represents a mild elevation, whereas the finding of NRBCs in a majority of capillaries is a marked elevation (Fig. 7–14). Although circulating fetal lymphocytes occasionally confuse the picture, elevation of lymphocyte counts is also a feature of fetal hypoxia and so may have similar connotations.[78] Increased NRBCs are the consequence of either anemia or hypoxia, generally of at least 6 to 12 hours' duration. This timing may depend somewhat on the magnitude of the insult, with more severe hypoxia leading to a more rapid elevation. Differentiation between hypoxia and anemia as the causative factor depends on additional data such as fetal hema-

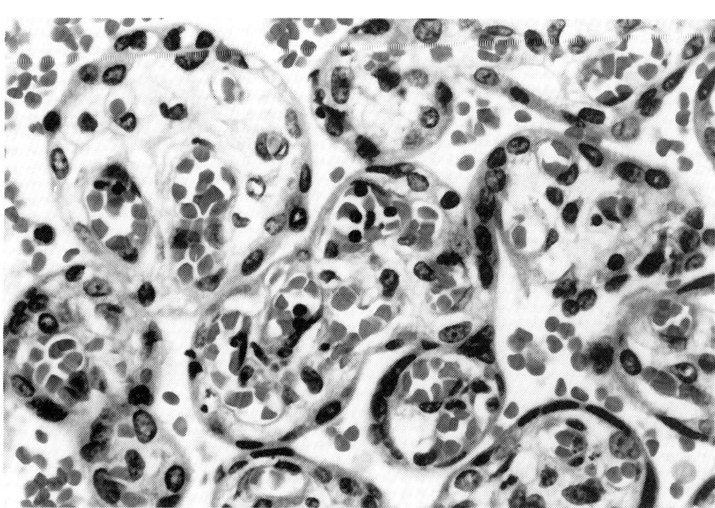

Figure 7–14. Increased nucleated red blood cells. Multiple villous capillaries in one low-power field showing normoblasts with perfectly round nuclei, featureless hyperchromatic chromatin, and glassy eosinophilic cytoplasm.

tocrit, maternal Kleihauer-Betke test, and presence or absence of fetal hydrops. The mechanism of increased NRBCs is an acute increase in erythropoietin in response to hypoxia followed by increased erythropoiesis and premature release of immature nucleated red blood cells from the bone marrow. Persistent low-grade hypoxia can lead to tonically elevated erythropoietin levels and NRBC counts and is common with severe IUGR.[79,80]

PROCESSES INVOLVING THE INTERHEMAL MEMBRANE

INTERVILLOUS FIBRIN

Maternal floor infarction[81–83] (maternal floor fibrin deposition,[3] excessive basal perivillous fibrin with X cell proliferation,[84] increased intervillous fibrin—severe) is a rare, distinctive clinicopathologic entity with a wholly inappropriate name that is unfortunately deeply ingrained in the literature. Maternal floor infarction is not a true infarct but rather an accumulation of excessive fibrin(oid) material that resembles the material in Nitabuch's layer of the basal plate and that expands the basal plate, envelopes the anchoring villi, and surrounds large numbers of basal and periseptal terminal villi. Placentas with maternal floor infarction are small for gestational age and have a distinct 0.5 to 2 cm rind on the maternal surface. On cut section the basal and periseptal parenchyma is often marbled by firm, smooth, lacy bands of fibrinoid (Fig. 7–15*A*). On microscopic examination terminal villi are enveloped in fibrin(oid), which is infiltrated by large numbers

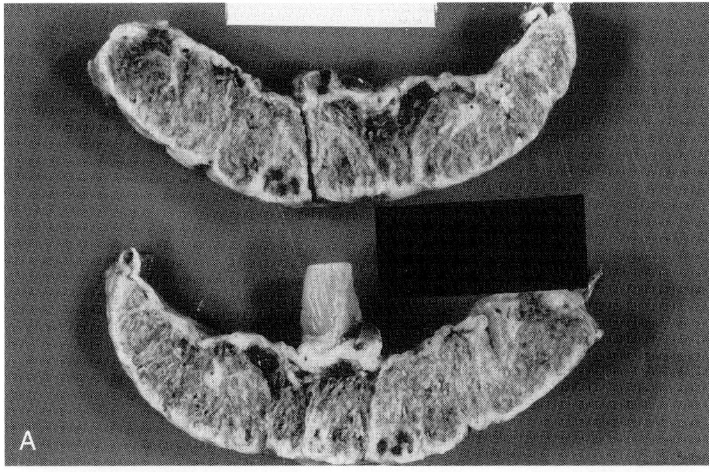

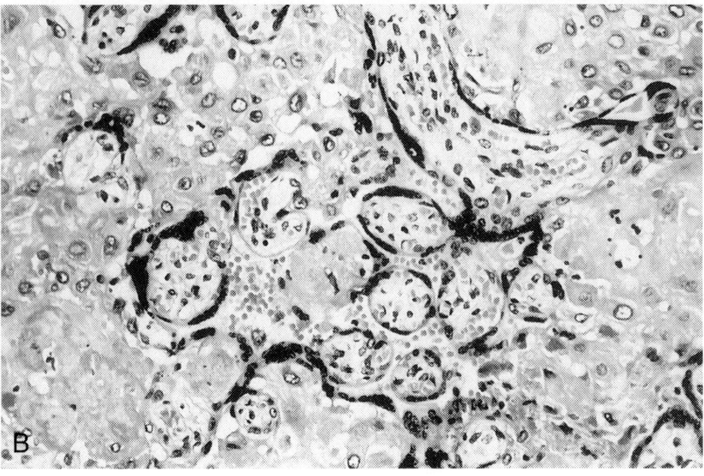

Figure 7–15. **A**, Maternal floor infarction (gross). Thickening of the basal plate, septal infoldings, and paraseptal villi secondary to diffuse deposition of extracellular matrix and fibrin. **B**, Increased perivillous fibrin deposition with X cells. Terminal villi are embedded in a smooth blue-red sea of extracellular matrix or fibrin or both. The matrix is colonized by infiltrating intermediate trophoblast (X cells) differentiating along the invasive trophoblastic pathway normally seen in the basal plate.

of intermediate trophoblastic cells (X cells) growing out from the entrapped villi (Fig. 7–15*B*). Placental fibrin(oid) can be separated into two groups[85]: true fibrin deposits composed of coagulation cascade products that support villous trophoblast repair [86] but not intermediate trophoblast (X cell) growth and fibrinoid deposits that contain little or no fibrin but rather are rich in extracellular matrix products such as fibronectin, basement membrane collagen, and laminin, all of which support intermediate trophoblast (X cell) growth.[87] Although the composition of the fibrin(oid) in maternal floor infarction has not been studied, its frequent association with X cells differentiates it from the perivillous fibrin that commonly accompanies inflammatory lesions such as VUE.

Accumulation of fibrin(oid) on the interhemal membrane of terminal villi could be either passive and related to stasis or active with a local stimulus for coagulation or extracellular matrix deposition. Evidence thus far argues more strongly for stasis caused by decreased maternal perfusion pressure. Perivillous fibrin deposition is commonly associated with maternal vascular disease and a failure to expand the maternal circulating blood volume in the early stages of pregnancy.[82,83] Occasional cases associated with autoimmunity and antiphospholipid antibodies argue for the alternative explanation of a coagulation disturbance.[88] Since many pregnancy-associated maternal vascular diseases, particularly when recurrent, may be associated with coagulation abnormalities, both of the proposed mechanisms could be operative.[89,90]

The classic maternal floor infarction syndrome occurs in 1 to 5 of 1000 pregnancies and is highly associated with severe early IUGR, IUFD, and preterm delivery.[82,83] Recent reports have described typical ultrasound findings that may be useful in diagnosing maternal floor infarction antenatally.[91] These studies are particularly important because of the high recurrence rate for maternal floor infarction (12% to 78%) in various series.[82,83,91] It should be stressed that typical findings of maternal floor infarction can also be seen in first- and second-trimester spontaneous abortion specimens from these patients. Other abnormalities in antenatal testing include elevated midtrimester α-fetoprotein levels and high-resistance pulsed-flow Doppler studies. Preliminary results with aspirin and antiplatelet drugs have been promising.[92]

Gitterinfarkt (increased perivillous fibrin—severe without basal predominance) is a term used by some for cases of massive perivillous fibrin deposition that lack the basal component seen with maternal floor infarction.[93] In our series in Boston and Cleveland this gitterinfarkt pattern was as common as maternal floor infarction (3 of 1000 delivered placentas, 0.6 of 1000 deliveries for each) and had a similar clinicopathologic profile. Of note, however, were two placentas that had the gitterinfarkt pattern (normal basal plate) and were associated with severe fetal growth retardation but were extremely large for gestational age (two to three times expected weight). This striking increase in placental weight contrasts sharply with the small placentas usually seen in maternal floor infarction and may favor active fibrin(oid) deposition as opposed to stasis in these unusual cases.

In our experience maternal floor infarction and gitterinfarkt represent the most severe end of a continuum. Cases of *increased perivillous fibrin—mild to moderate*—are somewhat more frequently encountered (14.5 per 1000 placentas examined, 2.9 per 1000 deliveries in our series). These milder cases with lesser but still significant amounts of perivillous fibrin (placentas with greater than 5% but less than 20% of terminal villi enveloped by fibrin[oid] and lacking other major placental lesions such as maternal vasculopathy or VUE) may not be recognized at gross examination and may or may not show the basal predominance seen with maternal floor infarction. Similar but lesser degrees of association with preterm delivery, IUGR, prior obstetric losses, and decreased uteroplacental perfusion have been noted in these cases.[68,84]

Until we learn more about the underlying etiology of these lesions our preference has been to diagnose all of the above lesions as *increased perivillous fibrin,* adding the qualifiers "mild-moderate or severe," "diffuse" or "basal predominant," and "with" or "without X cell proliferation" after the diagnosis, and to append the terms "maternal floor infarction" or "gitterinfarkt" in parentheses when appropriate. Pointing out in a note the high recurrence rate in severe cases is particularly important since many obstetricians are not familiar with these unusual lesions.

INTERVILLOSITIS

Infectious intervillositis is often seen with villitis as a component of acute or chronic placental infection.[56,57] Infectious intervillositis limited to the intervillous space is much less common and is associated predominantly with placental malaria.[94,95] In malarial placentas parasitized RBCs accumulate and adhere to trophoblast by specific trophoblastic cell membrane receptors.[96] This accumulation of parasitized RBCs is accompanied by large numbers of intervillous monocyte-macrophages and associated perivillous fibrin. The combined effects of parasitized intervillous RBCs and macrophages can lead to IUGR or perinatal death.[97]

Massive chronic intervillositis, idiopathic (MCIV), is a rare placental lesion characterized by the accumulation of large numbers of mononuclear inflammatory cells in the intervillous space without VUE or evidence of infection (Fig. 7–16).[98–100] Lesional cells are virtually all of the monocyte-macrophage lineage staining positively for CD68, a pan-macrophage marker, and Mac387, which is more selective for immature monocyte-macrophages. Occasional CD3-positive T lymphocytes may be present.[57,100] Perivillous fibrin and villous trophoblast necrosis can be extensive. Changes consistent with decreased uteroplacental perfusion (increased syncytial knots, acute atherosis, small placental size) accompany MCIV in many cases. Villi may show nonspecific alterations such as stromal fibrosis, hypovascularity, or increased Hofbauer cells but lack clear-cut chronic inflammation.

MCIV is associated with infertility, recurrent spontaneous abortion, and autoimmune maternal vascular disease.[99,100] The recurrence rate is high, and specimens from early spontaneous abortion often show the same pattern seen in later placentas. Detailed workup in one typical patient revealed increased production of an embryotoxic factor by cultured maternal peripheral blood mononuclear cells.[101] Production of this factor, believed to be γ-interferon, can be downregulated in some patients by progesterone treatments.[102] γ-Interferon, also known as macrophage-activating factor, is a T cell–derived cytokine known to upregulate the expression of adhesion molecules on macrophages.[103] Of note is that syncytiotrophoblast expresses large numbers of γ-interferon receptors.[104] The preliminary evidence favors a hypothesis that patients with MCIV have a population of sensitized T cells reactive with either autoantigens or fetal alloantigens expressed in the uteroplacental environment. On activation these cells might produce high levels of γ-interferon, promoting macrophage-trophoblast interactions in the intervillous space.

FETOMATERNAL HEMORRHAGE

Intervillous thrombi (fetomaternal hemorrhage—small vessel type) are spherical accumu-

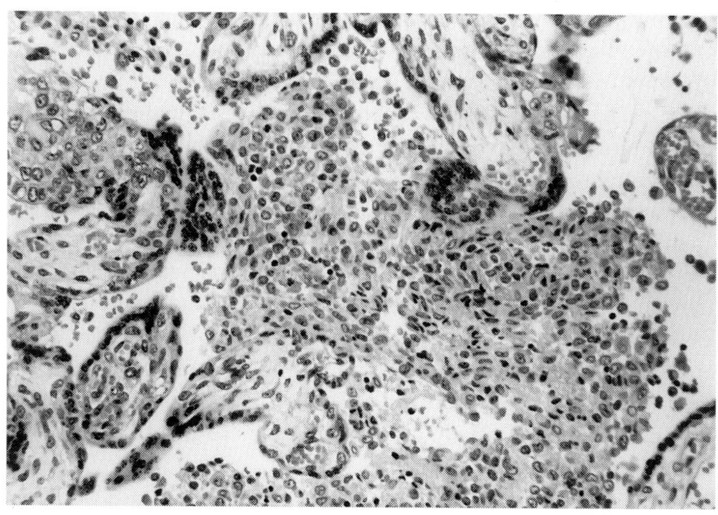

Figure 7–16. Massive chronic intervillositis. Normal terminal villi are separated by sheets of monocytoid cells that adhere to the villous trophoblastic apical membrane.

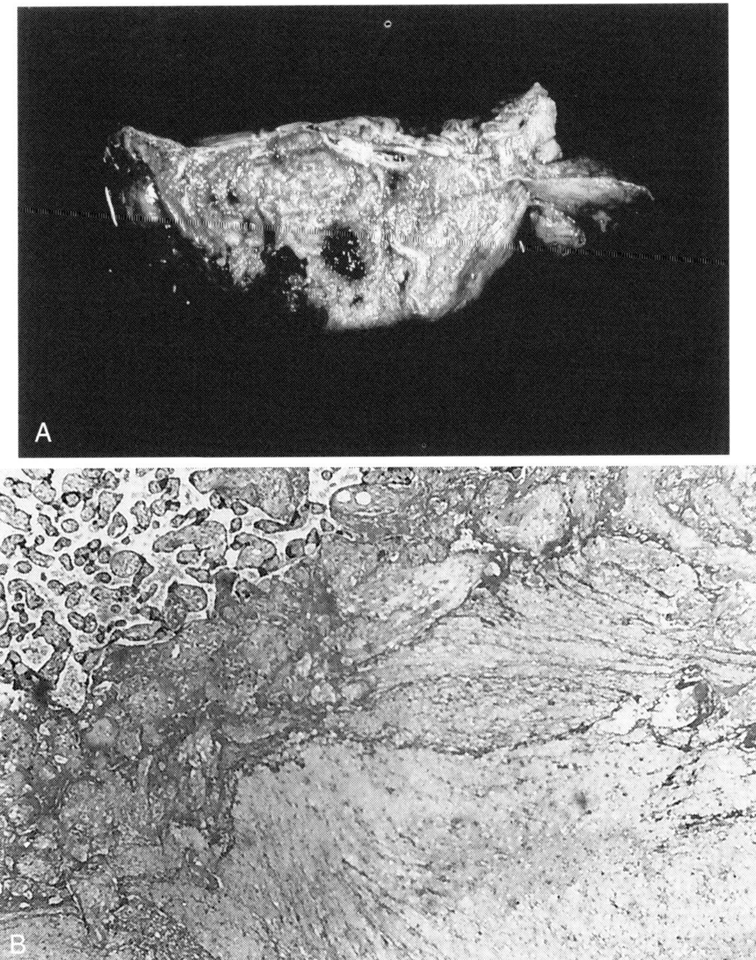

Figure 7–17. Intervillous thrombus. **A**, Space-occupying spherical accumulation of blood symmetrically displacing the villous parenchyma. **B**, The blood products have become laminated (H&E, ×40).

lations of clotted blood in the intervillous space that displace and are completely surrounded by terminal villi (Fig. 7–17). Typical intervillous thrombi represent foci of fetomaternal hemorrhage (see below).[105] Small amounts of fetomaternal hemorrhage are common during gestation, and with a diligent gross examination typical intervillous thrombi can be seen in many placentas.[106,107] The thrombi become laminated as they age. The risk of clinically significant fetomaternal hemorrhage is increased with the finding of multiple or large intervillous thrombi.[108] Associated placental findings in clinically significant cases include increased NRBCs and villous hydrops.[109] Supportive clinical data include a positive Kleihauer-Betke test, neonatal anemia, or frank hydrops fetalis. Atypical intervillous thrombi that are irregularly shaped or border on the basal plate, placental septa, or chorionic plate may be foci of fetomaternal hemorrhage but can also represent intervillous extension of retroplacental hematomas associated with abruptio placentae. Other lesions to be differentiated from intervillous thrombi include nodular subchorionic fibrin, hemorrhage into placental septal cysts, and infarcts with central hemorrhagic necrosis.

Typical intervillous thrombi have been shown to represent sites of fetomaternal hemorrhage by immunoperoxidase staining that demonstrated fetal hemoglobin containing RBCs in the maternal

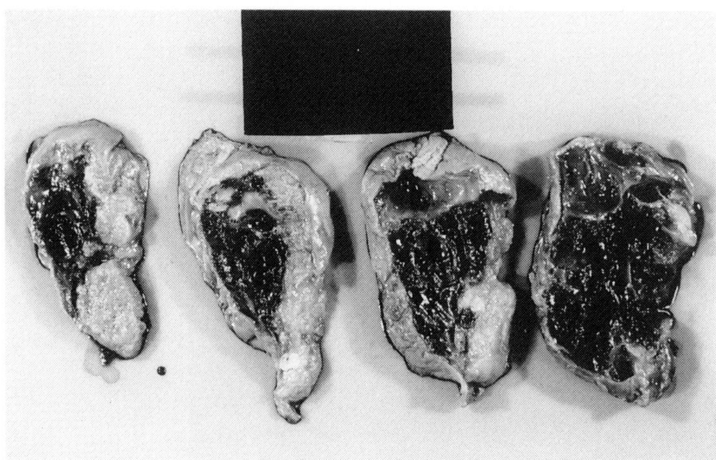

Figure 7–18. Subchorial thrombus. Laminated enlarging hematoma separating the villous parenchyma from the chorionic plate with substantial elevation of the latter structure.

intervillous space.[105] Such hemorrhages usually are random events, but conditions leading to friability of terminal villi such as increased syncytial knotting in preterm infants and delayed villous maturation in term infants may increase the risk of villous rupture (Unpublished Data). Significant fetomaternal hemorrhage is a major cause of IUFD near term and may be a significant factor in some cases of unexplained adverse neurologic outcome.[110,111] Intervillous thrombi are not generally associated with IUGR, preterm delivery, or recurrent reproductive failure.

Massive subchorial thrombosis (fetomaternal hemorrhage—large vessel type) is an extremely large, atypical intervillous thrombus that underlies and elevates the chorionic plate while displacing the underlying villous parenchyma downward (Fig. 7–18).[112] Massive subchorial thrombi are often laminated with both old and recent blood clot, suggesting repeated episodes of bleeding. Massive subchorial thrombi have generally been assumed to represent rupture of large fetal vessels in the chorionic plate or larger stem villi. Massive subchorial thrombosis is associated with late abortion and preterm IUFD. These associations are so strong that for many years the lesion was considered an artifact developing after fetal death. Several examples of severely impaired liveborn infants with this placental lesion have led to the conclusion that massive subchorial thrombosis is a catastrophic and most likely random event that is unlikely to recur in subsequent pregnancies.

REFERENCES

1. Simpson RA, Mayhew TM, Barnes PR: From 13 weeks to term, the trophoblast of human placenta grows by the continuous recruitment of new proliferative units: a study of nuclear number using the disector. Placenta 13:501, 1992.
2. Redline RW, Pappin A: Fetal thrombotic vasculopathy: the clinical significance of extensive avascular villi. Hum Pathol 26:80, 1995.
3. Kaplan C, Lowell DM, Salafia C: College of American Pathologists Conference XIX on the Examination of the Placenta: Report of the working group on the definition of structural changes associated with abnormal function in the maternal/fetal/placental unit in the second and third trimesters. Arch Pathol 115:709, 1991.
4. Langston C, Kaplan C, Macpherson T, et al: Practice guideline for examination of the placenta. Placental Pathology Practice Guideline Development Task Force of the College of American Pathologists. (In Press.)
5. Fox H: Pathology of the placenta. London, WB Saunders, 1978, p 181.
6. Benirschke K, Driscoll SG: Pathology of the human placenta. New York, Springer-Verlag, 1967, p. 236.
7. Rayne SC, Kraus FT: Placental thrombi and other vascular lesions: classification, morphology, and clinical correlations, Pathol Res Pract 189:2, 1993.
8. Alles AJ, Longtine J, Roberts DJ: The incidence of factor V Leiden in fetal thrombotic events. Mod Pathol 10:1P, 1997.

9. Rocklein G, Kobras G, Becker V: Physiological and pathological morphology of the umbilical and placental circulation. Pathol Res Pract 186:187, 1990.
10. Sander CH: Hemorrhagic endovasculitis and hemorrhagic villitis of the placenta. Arch Pathol Lab Med 104:371, 1980.
11. Sander CH, Stevens NG: Hemorrhagic endovasculitis of the placenta: an indepth morphologic appraisal with initial clinical and epidemiologic observations. Pathol Annu 37, 1984.
12. Scott JM: Fibrinous vasculosis of the human placenta. Placenta 4:87, 1983.
13. DeSa DJ: Intimal cushions in foetal placental veins. J Pathol 110:347, 1973.
14. Benirschke K, Kaufmann P: Pathology of the human placenta, 3rd ed. New York, 1994, Springer-Verlag, p 360.
15. Redline RW: Placenta and adnexa in late pregnancy. In Reed GB, Claireaux AE, Cockburn F (eds): Disease of the fetus and newborn, 2nd ed. London, 1995, Chapman & Hall, p 330.
16. Genest DR: Estimating the time of death in stillborn fetuses. 2. Histologic evaluation of the placenta—a study of 71 stillborns. Obstet Gynecol 80:585, 1992.
17. Silver MM, Yeger H, Lines LD: Hemorrhagic endovasculitis–like lesion induced in placental organ culture. Hum Pathol 19:251, 1988.
18. Shen-Schwarz S, MacPherson TA, Mueller-Heubach E: The clinical significance of hemorrhagic endovasculitis of the placenta. Am J Obstet Gynecol 159:48, 1988.
19. Novak PM, Sander CM, Yang SS, et al: Report of 14 cases of nonimmune hydrops-fetalis in association with hemorrhagic endovasculitis of the placenta. Am J Obstet Gynecol 165:945, 1991.
20. Triplett DA: Antiphospholipid-protein antibodies: clinical use of laboratory test results (identification, predictive value, treatment). Haemostasis 26:358, 1996.
21. Boddi M, Prisco D, Fedi S, et al: Antiphospholipid antibodies and pregnancy disorders in women with insulin dependent diabetes. Thromb Res 82:207, 1996.
22. Sander CH, Kinnane L, Stevens NG: Hemorrhagic endovasculitis of the placenta: a clinicopathologic entity associated with adverse pregnancy outcome. Comp Ther 11:66, 1985.
23. Blanc WA: Pathology of the placenta and cord in ascending and in haematogenous infection. In Perinatal infections (CIBA Foundation Symposium 77). London, 1977, Excerpta Medica.
24. Altshuler G, Arizawa M. Molnar-Nadasdy G: Meconium-induced umbilical cord vascular necrosis and ulceration: a potential link between the placenta and poor pregnancy outcome. Obstet Gynecol 79:760, 1992.
25. Burgess AM, Hutchins GM: Inflammation of the lungs, umbilical cord, and placenta associated with meconium passage in utero—review of 123 autopsied cases. Pathol Res Pract 192:1121, 1996.
26. Hyde S, Smotherman J, Moore JI, Altshuler G: A model of bacterially induced umbilical vein spasm, relevant to fetal hypoperfusion. Obstet Gynecol 73:966, 1989.
27. Altshuler G, Hyde S: Meconium-induced vasocontraction: a potential cause of cerebral and other fetal hypoperfusion and of poor pregnancy outcome. J Child Neurol 4:137, 1989.
28. Cotran RS: New roles for the endothelium in inflammation and immunity. Am J Pathol 129:407, 1987.
29. Redline RW: Placenta and adnexa in late pregnancy. In Reed GB, Claireaux AE, Cockburn F (eds): Disease of the fetus and newborn, 2nd ed. London, 1995, Chapman & Hall, p 319.
30. Fok RY, et al: The correlation of arterial lesions with umbilical artery Doppler velocimetry in the placentas of small-for-dates pregnancies. Obstet Gynecol 75:578, 1990.
31. Giles WB, Trudinger BJ, Baird PJ: Fetal umbilical artery flow velocity waveforms and placental resistance: pathological correlation. Br J Obstet Gynaecol 92:31, 1985.
32. Macara L, Kingdom JCP, Kohrn G, et al: Elaboration of stem villous vessels in growth restricted pregnancies with abnormal umbilical artery Doppler waveforms. Br J Obstet Gynaecol 102:807, 1995.
33. Karsdorp VHM, Dirks BK, van der Linden JC, et al: Placenta morphology and absent or reversed end diastolic flow velocities in the umbilical artery: a clinical and morphometrical study. Placenta 17:393, 1996.
34. Trudinger BJ, Giles WB, Cook CM: Uteroplacental blood flow velocity-time waveforms in normal and complicated pregnancy. Br J Obstet Gynaecol 92:30, 1985.
35. Rochelson B, et al: A quantitative analysis of placental vasculature in the third-trimester fetus with autosomal trisomy. Obstet Gynecol 75:59, 1990.
36. Wilcox GR, Trudinger BJ: Fetal platelet consumption: a feature of placental insufficiency. Obstet Gynecol 77:616, 1991.
37. Rabinovitch M, Haworth SG, Vance Z, et al: Early

pulmonary vascular changes in congenital heart disease studied in biopsy tissue. Hum Pathol 11:499, 1980.

38. Jackson MR, Walsh AJ, Morrow RJ, et al: Reduced placental villous tree elaboration in small-for-gestational-age pregnancies: relationship with umbilical artery Doppler waveforms. Am J Obstet Gynecol 172:518, 1995.
39. Trudinger BJ, Giles WB, Cook CM, et al: Fetal umbilical artery flow velocity waveforms and placental resistance: clinical significance. Br J Obstet Gynaecol 92:23, 1985.
40. Doppler ultrasound in obstetrics. Lancet 339:1083, 1992.
41. Altshuler G: Chorangiosis: an important placental sign of neonatal morbidity and mortality. Arch Pathol Lab Med 108:71, 1984.
42. Mayhew TM, Sorensen FB, Klebe JG, et al: Growth and maturation of villi in placentae from well-controlled diabetic women. Placenta 15:57, 1994.
43. Guyton AC: Textbook of medical physiology, 5th ed. Philadelphia, 1976, WB Saunders, p. 237.
44. Jaffe R, Siegal A, Rat L, et al: Placental chorioangiomatosis—high risk pregnancy. Postgrad Med J 61:453, 1985.
45. Benirschke K, Kaufmann P: Pathology of the human placenta, 3rd ed. New York, 1994, Springer-Verlag, p 138.
46. Demir R, Kaufmann P, Castellucci M, et al: Fetal vasculogenesis and angiogenesis in human placental villi. Acta Anat 136:190, 1989.
47. Lee R, Mayhew TM: Star volumes of villi and intervillous pores in placentae from low and high altitude pregnancies. J Anat 186:349, 1995.
48. Soma H, Watanabe Y, Hata T: Chorangiosis and chorangioma in three cohorts of placentas from Nepal, Tibet and Japan. Reprod Fertil Dev 7:1533, 1996.
49. Reshetnikova OS, Burton GJ, Milovanov AP, et al: Increased incidence of placental chorioangioma in high-altitude pregnancies: hypobaric hypoxia as a possible etiologic factor. Am J Obstet Gynecol 174:557, 1996.
50. Clark DE, Smith SK, Sharkey AM, et al: Localization of VEGF and expression of its receptors flt and KDR in human placenta throughout pregnancy. Hum Reprod 11:1090, 1996.
51. Holmgren L. Glaser A, Pfeifer-Ohlsson S, et al: Angiogenesis during human extraembryonic development involves the spatiotemporal control of PDGF ligand and receptor gene expression. Development 113:749, 1991.
52. Chen H-L, Yang Y, Hu X-L, et al: Tumor necrosis factor alpha, mRNA, and protein are present in human placental and uterine cells at early and late stages of gestation. Am J Pathol 139:327, 1991.
53. Yelavarthi KK, Hunt JS: Analysis of p60 and p80 tumor necrosis factor-α receptor messenger RNA and protein in human placentas. Am J Pathol 143:1131, 1993.
54. Lysiak JJ, Hunt J, Pringle GA, et al: Localization of transforming growth factor β and its natural inhibitor decorin in the human placenta and decidua throughout gestation. Placenta 16:221, 1995.
55. Nishino E, Matsuzaki N, Masuhiro K, et al: Trophoblast-derived interleukin-6 (IL-6) regulates human chorionic gonadotropin release through IL-6 receptor on human trophoblasts. J Clin Endocr Metab 71:436, 1990.
56. Gersell DJ, Kraus RF, Reffle M: Diseases of the placenta. In Kurman RJ (ed): Blaustein's pathology of the female genital tract, 3rd ed. New York, 1987, Springer-Verlag, p 769.
57. Redline RW: Recurrent villitis of bacterial etiology. Pediatr Pathol 6:995, 1996.
58. Russell P, Altshuler G: Placental abnormalities of congenital syphilis. Am J Dis Child 128:160, 1974.
59. Qureshi F, Jacques SM, Reyes MP: Placental histopathology in syphilis. Hum Pathol 24:779, 1993.
60. Knowles S, Frost T: Umbilical cord sclerosis as an indicator of congenital syphilis. J Clin Pathol 42:1157, 1989.
61. Moustofi-Zadeh M, et al: Placental evidence of cytomegalovirus infection of the fetus and neonate. Arch Pathol Lab Med 108:403, 1984.
62. LePage F, Schramm P: Aspects histologiques du placenta et des membranes dans la maladies des inclusions cytomegaliques. Gynecol Obstet 57:273, 1958.
63. Altshuler G, Russell P: The human placental villitides: a review of chronic intrauterine infection. In Grundmann, Kirstein (eds): Current topics in pathology. Berlin, 1975, Springer-Verlag.
64. Russell P: Inflammatory lesions of the human placenta. Placenta 1:227, 1980.
65. Knox WF, Fox H: Villitis of unknown aetiology: its incidence and significance in placentae from a British population. Placenta 5:395, 1984.
66. Redline RW, Patterson P: Villitis of unknown etiology is associated with major infiltration of fetal tissue by maternal inflammatory cells. Am J Pathol 143:473, 1993.
67. Labarrere CA, Faulk WP: Maternal cells in chorionic villi from placentae of normal and abnormal human pregnancies. Am J Reprod Immunol 33:54, 1995.

68. Redline RW, Patterson P: Patterns of placental injury: correlations with gestational age, placental weight, and clinical diagnosis. Arch Pathol Lab Med 118:698, 1994.
69. Salafia CM, Silberman L, Herrera NE, et al: Placental pathology at term associated with elevated midtrimester maternal serum alpha-fetoprotein concentration. Am J Obstet Gynecol 158:1064, 1988.
70. Driscoll SG: Autopsy following stillbirth: a challenge neglected. In Ryder OA, Byrd ML (eds): One medicine. Berlin, 1984, Springer-Verlag, p 20.
71. Redline RW, Abramowsky CR: Clinical and pathological aspects of recurrent placental villitis. Hum Pathol 16:727, 1985.
72. Benirschke K, Kaufmann P: Pathology of the human placenta, 3rd ed. New York, 1994, Springer-Verlag, p 170.
73. Redline RW: Placental pathology: the neglected link between basic disease mechanisms and untoward pregnancy outcome. Curr Opin Obstet Gynecol vol 7, 1995.
74. Wallenburg HCS, Stolte LAM, Jannsens J: The pathogenesis of placental infarction. I. A morphologic study in the human placenta. Am J Obstet Gynecol 116:835, 1973.
75. Fox H: Pathology of the placenta. London, 1978, WB Saunders, p 172.
76. Naeye RL, et al: The clinical significance of placental villous edema. Pediatrics 71:588, 1983.
77. Genest D, Ringer S: Placental findings correlate with neonatal death in extremely premature infants (24-32 weeks): a study of 150 cases. Lab Invest 68:126A, 1993.
78. Naeye RL, Localio AR: Determining the time before birth when ischemia and hypoxemia initiated cerebral palsy. Obstet Gynecol 86:713, 1995.
79. Maier RF, Gunther A, Vogel M, et al: Umbilical venous erythropoietin and umbilical arterial pH in relation to morphologic placental abnormalities. Obstet Gynecol 84:81, 1994.
80. Soothill PW, Nicolaides KH, Campbell S: Prenatal asphyxia, hyperlacticaemia, hypoglycaemia, and erythroblastosis in growth retarded fetuses. Br Med J 294:1051, 1987.
81. Clewell WH, Manchester DK: Recurrent maternal floor infarction: a preventable cause of fetal death. Am J Obstet Gynecol 147:346, 1983.
82. Naeye RL: Maternal floor infarction. Hum Pathol 16:823, 1985.
83. Andres RL, Kuyper W, Resnik R, et al: The association of maternal floor infarction of the placenta with adverse perinatal outcome. Am J Obstet Gynecol 163:935, 1990.
84. Salafia CM, Minior VK, Pezzullo JC, et al: Intrauterine growth restriction in infants of less than thirty-two weeks gestation: associated placental pathologic features. Am J Obstet Gynecol 175: 1049, 1995.
85. Frank HG, Malekzadeh F, Kertschanska S, et al: Immunohistochemistry of two different types of placental fibrinoid. Acta Anat 150:55, 1994.
86. Nelson DM, et al: Trophoblast interaction with fibrin matrix: epithelialization of perivillous fibrin deposits as a mechanism for villous repair in the human placenta. Am J Pathol 136:855, 1990.
87. Damsky CH, Fitzgerald ML, Fisher SJ: Distribution patterns of extracellular matrix components and adhesion receptors are intricately modulated during first trimester cytotrophoblast differentiation along the invasive pathway, in vivo. J Clin Invest 89:210, 1992.
88. Bendon RW, Hommel AB: Maternal floor infarction in autoimmune disease: two cases. Pediatr Pathol Lab Med 16:293, 1996.
89. Dekker GA, de Vries JIP, Doelizsch PM, et al: Underlying disorders associated with severe early onset preeclampsia. Am J Obstet Gynecol 173:1042, 1995.
90. Preston FE, Rosendaal FR, Walker ID, et al: Increased fetal loss in women with heritable thrombophilia. Lancet 348:913, 1996.
91. Mandsager NT, et al: Maternal floor infarction of placenta: prenatal diagnosis and clinical significance. Obstet Gynecol 83:750, 1994.
92. Fuke Y, Aono T, Imai S, et al: Clinical significance and treatment of massive intervillous fibrin deposition associated with recurrent fetal growth retardation. Gynecol Obstet Invest 38:5, 1994.
93. Benirschke K, Kaufmann P: Pathology of the human placenta, 3rd ed. New York, 1994, Springer-Verlag, p 409.
94. Walter PR, Garin Y, Blot P: Placental pathologic changes in malaria: a histologic and ultrastructural study. Am J Pathol 109:330, 1982.
95. Leopardi O, Naughten W, Salvia L, et al: Malaric placentas—a quantitative study and clinico-pathological correlations. Pathol Res Pract 192:892, 1996.
96. Fried M, Duffy PE: Adherence of *Plasmodium falciparum* to chondroitin sulfate A in the human placenta. Science 272:1502, 1996.
97. McGregor IA: Epidemiology, malaria and pregnancy. Am J Trop Med Hyg 33:517, 1984.
98. Valderrama E: Massive chronic intervillositis: report of three cases. Lab Invest 66:10, 1992.
99. Jacques SM, Qureshi F: Chronic intervillositis of the placenta. Arch Pathol Lab Med 117:1032, 1993.

100. Doss BJ, Greene MF, Hill J, et al: Massive chronic intervillositis associated with recurrent abortions. Hum Pathol 26:1245, 1995.
101. Ecker JL, Laufer MR, Hill JA: Measurement of embryotoxic factors is predictive of pregnancy outcome in women with a history of recurrent abortion. Obstet Gynecol 81:84, 1993.
102. Hill JA, Polgar K, Harlow BL, et al: Evidence of embryo-toxic and trophoblast-toxic cellular immune response(s) in women with recurrent spontaneous abortion. Am J Obstet Gynecol 166:1044, 1992.
103. Adams DO, Hamilton TA: The cell biology of macrophage activation. Annu Rev Immunol 2:283, 1984.
104. Peyman JA, Hammond GL: Localization of IFN-τ receptor in first trimester placenta to trophoblasts but lack of stimulation of HLA-DRA, –DRB, or invariant chain mRNA expression by 1-N-τ. J Immunol 149:2675, 1992.
105. Kaplan C, Blanc WA, Elias J: Identification of erythrocytes in intervillous thrombi: a study using immunoperoxidase identification of hemoglobins. Hum Pathol 13:554, 1982.
106. Medearis AL, Hensleigh PA, Parks DR, et al: Detection of fetal erythrocytes in maternal blood post partum with the fluorescence-activated cell sorter. Am J Obstet Gynecol 148:290, 1984.
107. Batcup G, Tovey LAD, Longster G: Fetomaternal blood group incompatibility studies in placental intervillous thrombosis. Placenta 4:449, 1983.
108. Devi B, Jennison RF, Langley FA: Significance of placental thrombi in transplacental hemorrhage. J Clin Pathol 21:322, 1968.
109. Redline RW, Driscoll SG: The placenta and adnexa. In Reed G, Bain AD, Claireaux A (eds): Diseases of the fetus and newborn. London, 1989, Chapman & Hall, p 41.
110. Laube DW, Schauberger CW: Fetomaternal bleeding as a cause for "unexplained" fetal death. Obstet Gynecol 60:649, 1982.
111. de Almeida V, Bowman JM: Massive fetomaternal hemorrhage: Manitoba experience. Obstet Gynecol 83:323, 1994.
112. Shanklin DR, Scott JS: Massive subchorial thrombohaematoma (Breus' mole). Br J Obstet Gynaecol 82:476, 1975.

8

Disorders of the Decidua and Maternal Vasculature

Carolyn M. Salafia and Robert Pijnenborg

A successful pregnancy requires that the conceptus have a normal developmental program, a normal fetoplacental vasculature that allows nutrient transport via the villous trophoblast to the fetus, and a normal maternal vasculature that enables nutrient transport to the intervillous blood space at a volume adequate for fetal needs and that has flow characteristics permitting normal placental growth and development.

An abnormal developmental program often results in early embryo failure. Placental details of embryonic pathology are considered in Chapter 4. The intraplacental vasculature is considered in more detail in Chapter 7.

VASCULAR ANATOMY OF THE NONPREGNANT UTERUS

The most obvious property of the future uteroplacental arteries is their peculiar shape, hence the term "curling arteries" (coined by their discoverer, William Hunter, 1774) or "spiral arteries" as they are now known. Since they undergo extensive changes during the menstrual cycle, they are considered one of the most labile vascular systems in the body. They arise from the radial arteries at the inner third of the myometrium, while the radial arteries themselves branch from the arcuate system that forms the stratum vasculare at the outer third. In addition to these main arteries, small basal arteries arise from the radial arteries and nourish the basal layer of the endometrium. They are important for tissue regeneration after shedding at menstruation or delivery. Basal arteries are relatively unresponsive to hormonal stimuli, although they cannot be considered completely inert.[1] Along the endometrial segments of the spiral arteries arise minor side branches, which are the same caliber as the basal arteries but seem to supply more superficial tissue layers. Our main focus is on the spiral arteries, which represent the future uteroplacental arteries.

Histologic variation occurs along the length of the vessels. Within the endometrium, segments close to the endometrial-myometrial junction have a more defined muscular coat than that of the higher, superficial parts, and the most solid wall structure is within the myometrial segments. The apparent shift in muscular coat structure from myometrial to endometrial segments is also reflected in the gradual disappearance of elastica staining in the spiral arteries when they enter the endometrium.[2] Therefore the first arterial structures encountered by invading trophoblast in early pregnancy are the least differentiated, which allows easier perforation of the vessels. As discussed later, however, the deeper segments of the spiral arteries play an important role during pregnancy. Split and reduplicated elastic lamellae are commonly present in spiral arteries of multiparous women in which pregnancy-associated changes had not completely been resolved post partum.[2]

GESTATIONAL MODIFICATIONS OF THE UTERINE VASCULAR ANATOMY

A dramatic feature of uteroplacental vasculature during pregnancy is the invasion of spiral arteries by extravillous trophoblast, leading to marked changes in vascular architecture that are essential for successful pregnancy. Trophoblast invasion proceeds by two pathways: interstitial and endovascular. Both are derived from the proliferating tips of the anchoring villi, and it can be assumed that the distal ends of spiral arteries, which possess a relatively undifferentiated wall structure, are easily penetrated by "interstitial" trophoblast, which them becomes "endovascular" and begins retrograde migration along the vascular lumen. The ultimate fate of both populations of invading cells is different: whereas interstitial trophoblastic cells fuse to form multinuclear giant cells at the end of their itinerary, the endovascular trophoblastic cells remain essentially mononuclear and are buried in an amorphous, acidophilic "fibrinoid" material.

An outline of vascular anatomy during the first weeks of gestation is provided by Harris and Ramsey,[3] but detailed histologic descriptions are not available for this early period. At 8 weeks vascular changes are well established in the decidua, resulting in a vessel wall composed of "fibrinoid" with embedded trophoblastic cells.[4] It is therefore assumed that invasion and endovascular migration take place soon after implantation and are interrupted at the deciduomyometrial junction. Only after 14 to 15 weeks does endovascular trophoblast migration proceed into the myometrial segments of the spiral arteries; this is regarded as a second wave of endovascular migration. Histological descriptions of this period are available and note degenerative changes in vessel wall structure, including disruption of the medial smooth muscle layers and fragmentation of elastic tissue before the appearance of endovascular trophoblast. These changes have been related to the presence of interstitial trophoblast invading the myometrium from 8 weeks onward, which is thought to have a disruptive action on the spiral arteries.[5] The end result of these processes is a physiologic change in which the original musculoelastic tunica media of the spiral arteries is replaced by mononuclear trophoblast embedded in fibrinoid (Fig. 8–1).[6] The diameter of the artery is increased, converting it from a high-resistance/low-capacitance circuit to a high-capacitance system that can carry large volumes of blood to the intervillous space.[7] Moreover, the absence of musculoelastic tissue should prevent the spiral arteries from responding to vasoactive stimuli, which protects the fetus from undesired fluctuations in maternal blood supply. A commonly held opinion is that the tunica media is destroyed by the invading endovascular trophoblast: according to our data this vascular layer disintegration occurs before the trophoblast invasion and is probably affected by the interstitial trophoblast.[5] This view is supported by the complete medial disruption in noninvaded areas of partially converted spiral arteries. Hamilton and Boyd[8] describe marked vascular alterations as the spiral arteries approach the trophoblastic shell, including marked endothelial hypertrophy that disrupts the normal smooth contour of the vessel lumen and increasing attenuation of the media to the point that the lining endothelium is surrounded only by a layer of reticular or collagen fibers. The explo-

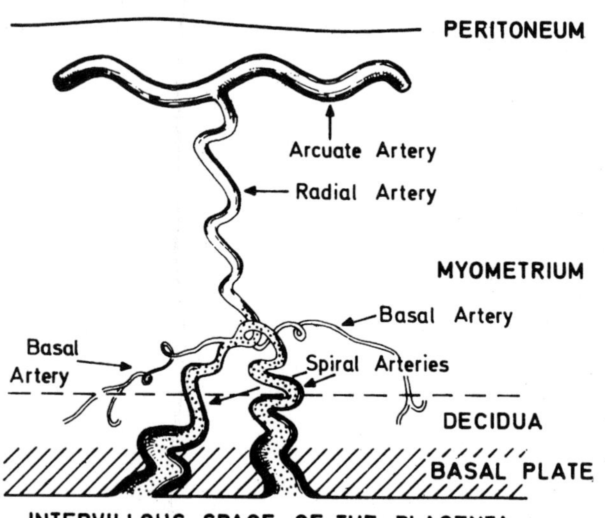

Figure 8–1. Anatomy of interstitial and endovascular trophoblast invasion in pregnancy. (From Brosens I, Robertson WB, Dixon HG: J Pathol Bacteriol 93:569, 1967.)

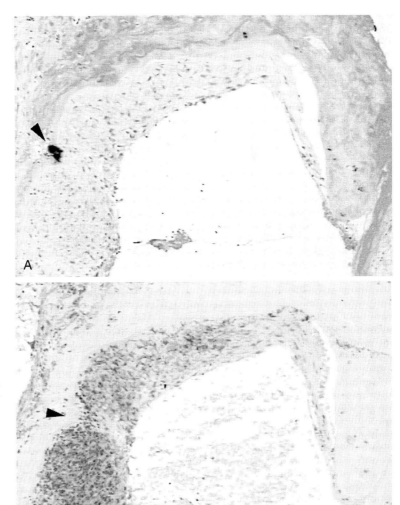

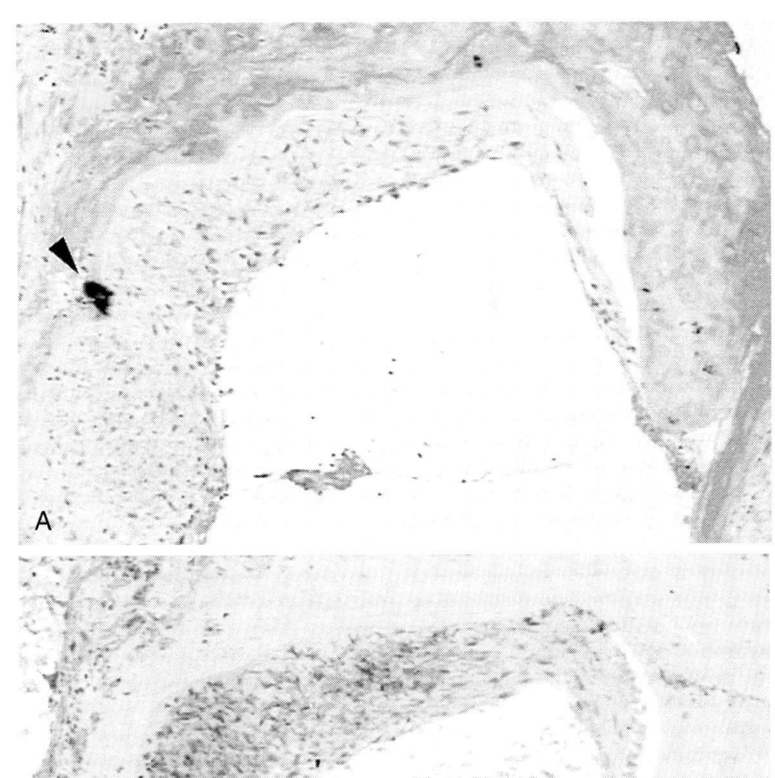

Figure 8–2. **A**, Placental bed biopsy from term normotensive delivery, showing a converted uteroplacental vessel with trophoblasts embedded within the amorphous fibrinoid wall *(arrowhead)* and areas of intimal proliferation *(single arrowheads)* (immunohistochemical stain for cytokeratin, with H & E counterstain [courtesy of Lisbet Vercruysse], ×20). **B**, Same view. Note α-actin positive areas of intimal proliferation (compared with 2A). No actin is found in the vicinity of the single endovascular trophoblast (immunohistochemical stain for α-actin, ×20).

ration of non trophoblast-dependent (and potentially preimplantation) uterine vascular changes may lead to improvements in in vitro fertilization, which may increase the chance of successful pregnancy.

The degenerative changes in the vessel wall are affected by a loss in tissue integrity, with a falling apart of different tissue components, including the smooth muscle cells. Therefore, although individual (actin-positive) smooth muscle cells may still be present, the functional capacity of a well-organized muscular tissue has been lost. In many converted vessels thickened intimal cushions appear, which probably result from local tissue repair. These intimae contain so-called myofibroblasts, which are α-actin positive but do not contribute to any contractile function of the blood vessel at that stage of development (Fig. 8–2). This feature is not pathologic. In a normal pregnancy more than 90% of the vessels have undergone the physiologic conversion at term,[9] while at 16 to 18 weeks only one third of the arteries have been invaded. It can therefore be assumed that between 18 weeks and term the remainder of the vessels are invaded in normal pregnancy; failure to complete late conversion may underlie a wide range of obstetric pathology (see below).

It is remarkable that the elaboration of vascular changes is restricted to the arteries, while the veins do not seem to be involved. In the very superficial layers of the placental bed, facing the intervillous space, the most distal venous segments may show replacement of endothelium by trophoblast,[10] which may be considered an outgrowth from the syncytiotrophoblastic covering of the placental floor and therefore should not be seen as extravillous trophoblast. A similar phenomenon is described in the rhesus monkey.[11] However, evidence suggests that some interstitial trophoblastic cells attach to venules from the outside, leading to occasional insertion of isolated trophoblastic cells in the endothelial layer of the vessel. The significance of this process is not clear (Pijnenborg R et al, unpublished observations, 1996). The different behavior of trophoblast versus arteries and veins is intriguing, and some evidence has been provided for the importance of physical (hemodynamic) flow stress in inducing retrograde trophoblast migration in blood vessels.[12]

UTEROPLACENTAL VASCULAR PATHOLOGY

In complicated pregnancies "normal" uteroplacental vascular adaptation takes place only *partially* within any one vessel; it does not extend to the maximum *depth* or it occurs in a limited total *number* of placental bed arteries. The wide range of pregnancy compromise that has been associated with poor uteroplacental vascular conversion—from first-trimester pregnancy loss[13] to prematurity[14–16] and late fetal growth restriction—most likely reflects different combinations of these potential problems, different strengths of deleterious influences, and different times of onset in gestation. These combinations have been associated with (any may be causally related to) early pregnancy loss, intrauterine growth retardation (IUGR) at term, and every clinical manifestation of obstetric compromise in between.

Placental Bed

Placental bed biopsy specimens are not easy to obtain, and their interpretation may be even more complicated than placental histopathologic examination. However, given the recent increased appreciation of the role of uteroplacental vascular pathology in obstetric compromise, biopsy samples from the placental bed may become a more common specimen, especially in university centers. Also, since the endometrial segments available for review in the basal plate of delivered placentas represent the end-vascular distributions of these myometrial arteries, an understanding of this deeper anatomy and physiology can aid in the understanding of basal plate uteroplacental vascular lesions.

The most outstanding uteroplacental defect is the complete or partial absence of physiologic conversion of spiral arteries (Fig. 8–3). Restriction of trophoblastic invasion and associated physiologic change has been documented most extensively in preeclampsia.[17] The classic view is that the second wave of endovascular trophoblast invasion, which occurs in the myometrial segments of the spiral arteries from about 15 weeks, does not take place in patients in whom preeclampsia will develop.[18] Direct observations within the critical time period, from the late first through the second trimester, are lacking. Only one observation of a hysterectomy specimen at 15 to 18 weeks with complete absence of endovascular trophoblast in the myometrial spiral arteries has been reported,[19] but of course it is impossible to tell whether preeclampsia would have developed later in this woman's pregnancy. There is no evidence of restricted interstitial invasion in preeclampsia as indicated by often high numbers of interstitial trophoblastic cells in the myometrium,[20] and therefore a failure to disrupt spiral artery walls before the arrival of endovascular trophoblast cannot be implied. Lack of physiologic conversion is apparent not only in the myometrial segments of spiral arteries, but also in the decidual parts of some of the vessels, so that a proportion of spiral arteries do not undergo trophoblast invasion and physiologic change.[21] Whether such vessels end up in the intervillous space is not clear. Since unconverted vessels retain high-resistance/low-capacitance properties, the effect on maternal blood supply to the placenta may be dramatic. Noninvaded arteries may continue to have a normal arterial structure but may also show a disorganized muscular coat or, at least in hypertensive cases, medial hyperplasia. Such nonconverted vessels may subsequently be prone to atherotic lesions, characterized by fibrinoid necrosis, infiltrating leukocytes and macrophages, and lipid-containing foam cells.[22] Although the presence of trophoblast has often been regarded as protecting an artery from the development of atherotic lesions, rem-

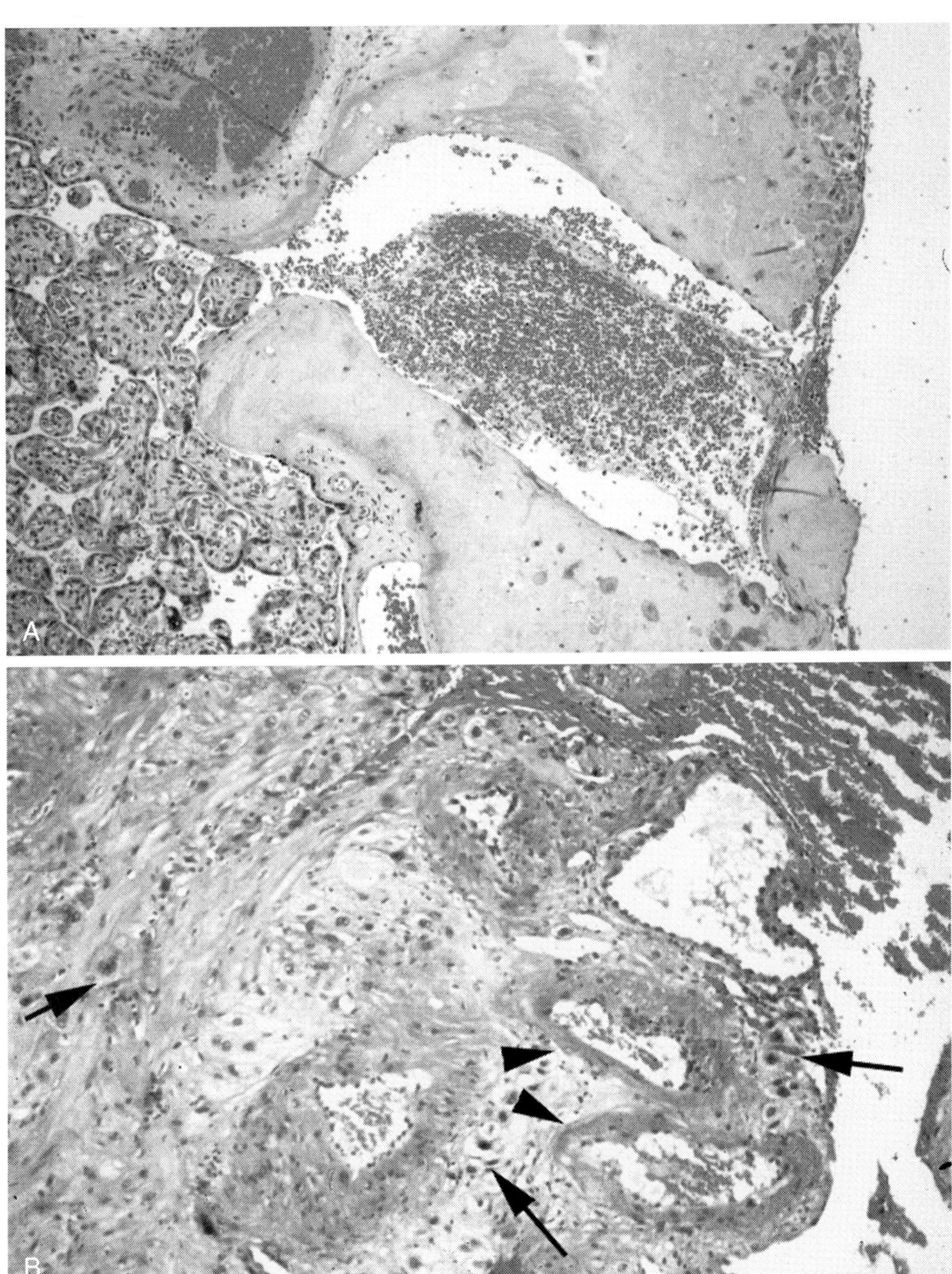

Figure 8–3. **A**, Basal plate from delivered placenta, showing a converted uteroplacental vessel with trophoblasts embedded within the amorphous fibrinoid wall. The vessel empties into the intervillous blood space. (H & E, ×10.) **B**, Basal plate from delivered placenta, showing multiple loops of spiral arteries with circumferential persistence of a muscular media. Focal thinning and disorganization of the media are visible *(arrowheads)*. Note numerous interstitial trophoblasts *(arrows)* (H & E, ×10). (*A* courtesy of E.J. Popek, D.O., Houston, Texas.)

nants of trophoblastic cells are occasionally observed in atherotic vessels.[23,24] Atherotic vessels often end up in areas of decidual necrosis and may be associated with placental infarction.[25] This lesion therefore may also seriously compromise the normal blood supply to the placenta.

Defects in endovascular trophoblast invasion occur not only in preeclampsia, but also in other hypertensive conditions of pregnancy. In various conditions trophoblast invasion and physiologic changes may be partial or isolated, rather than occurring along the whole circumference of the vessel.[23,26] Restricted trophoblast invasion also occurs in miscarriage[13] and IUGR.[27–29] Therefore limitation of trophoblast invasion is associated with defective placentation but cannot be viewed as specific for preeclampsia or pregnancy-induced hypertension. Endovascular trophoblast invasion and associated conversion of spiral arteries is not an all-or-none phenomenon but may show different degrees within normal and abnormal pregnancy, with the balance tipping to a more complete invasion in normal pregnancy.

Abnormalities in the three-dimensional architecture and size of placental bed arteries have been noted in preeclampsia.[1] Computer-assisted morphometry has demonstrated that, at least in certain cases, preeclamptic spiral and basal arteries of the placental bed can be more tortuous and densely distributed than normal placental bed arteries. Intrinsic differences in anatomic distribution and caliber of placental bed arteries may be an anatomic basis for some cases of familial preeclampsia. Alternatively, the three-dimensional distribution of placental bed arteries may be altered by abnormal growth of the preeclamptic placenta. Normal placental expansion in the early trimesters deforms the placental bed arteries.[30] Failure of normal placental implantation and placental growth may prevent the placental bed from stretching sufficiently, leading to a tortuous and hemodynamically vulnerable architecture (Fig. 8–4). We speculate that endothelial damage in preeclampsia may be caused by shear forces in these tortuous, small-caliber arteries. Physiologic vasoconstriction and myointimal hypertrophy would only exacerbate the poor hemodynamic situation within the preeclamptic placental bed. Spiral arterial wall disorganization may occur in different degrees, with or without intimal or medial hyperplastic changes in the absence of intravascular or even local trophoblast.[26] In preeclampsia these early and possibly trophoblast-independent vascular modifications may occur but are not followed by trophoblast invasion and vascular remodeling. Normal tissue repair mechanisms may fail to stabilize the modified spiral arteries or may simply prove inadequate in preeclampsia. Further study is necessary to determine whether preeclampsia in different demographic groups has different features and to delineate the three-dimensional architecture in cases of spontaneous preterm birth with uteroplacental vascular pathology. One mental image of the anatomy of placental bed arteries may not suffice to categorize the vasculature of the placental bed in pathologic conditions.

A complete understanding of the defects in the placental bed in complicated pregnancies requires insight into the factors that regulate trophoblast migration and associated maternal tissue responses. A potentially important factor that may regulate invasion is the composition of the extracellular matrix within the successive uterine tissue layers, which acts as a substrate for attachment and invasion. Decidualization of the endometrium is associated with marked changes in matrix composition, including deposition of laminin and collagen IV around decidual cells and an overall loss of the cross-linking collagen VI within the stroma.[31] These matrix changes have a substantial role in directing trophoblast invasion in early pregnancy. So far no differences in matrix composition have been reported in hypertensive pregnancies. The increased plasma levels of fibronectin in preeclamptic patients are usually related to overall endothelial damage,[32–34] but it is difficult to draw a direct correlation with local processes in the placental bed. However, trophoblast itself contributes significantly to fibronectin production during pregnancy, as indicated by observations in vitro[35] and in vivo.[36] Furthermore, preeclamptic placental beds show marked deposition of fibronectin within atherotic spiral arteries, but a possible relation of this deposition with increased blood levels of fibronectin is not clear.

Interaction of invading cells with extracellular matrix requires the expression of appropriate receptors, notably specific integrins. Invasive trophoblastic cells, arising within the cell columns in early pregnancy, show a loss of the laminin receptor α6/β4, which may facilitate their migration through the decidua and later into the myometrium.[37,38] Zhou and colleagues[39] noticed a defect in this integrin shift in preeclampsia (specifically a failure to downregulate α6/β4 and upregulate α1/β1 receptors), but these observations could not be confirmed by Divers and associates.[40] On the other hand, experiments in vitro show defective attachment of isolated third-trimester trophoblast to matrix proteins.[41] However, isolated (villous) placental trophoblast does not necessarily reflect the properties of extravillous trophoblast. In addition, all studies of preeclamptic trophoblast must rely on third-trimester material, although the key events of abnormal invasion occur during the first and early second trimester of pregnancy.

An essential aspect of trophoblast invasion is the secretion of proteinases, including urokinase-type plasminogen activator and various metalloproteinases, and associated inhibitors (plasminogen activator inhibitor [PAI] 1 and 2, tissue inhibitors of metalloproteinases [TIMPs], which are assumed to confer additional control over the invasion process.[42,43] Expression of various metalloproteinases by invading trophoblast has been shown in immunohistochemical and in situ hybridization studies,[44–46] but no information is available yet on the placental bed in hypertension. In vitro culture of trophoblast from preeclamptic placentas showed an altered secretion of gelatinase β and decreased activity of surface plasminogen activator,[47] but whether the same is true in the extravillous trophoblast of the placental bed remains to be proved.

All the functions inherent in invasion processes, such as the expression of adhesion molecules and secretion of matrix-degrading enzymes, are regulated by cytokines. Invasive trophoblast does express tumor necrosis factor–α (TNF-α),[48] tumor growth factor–α (TGF-α),[49] interleukin-1 (IL-1),[50] and TGF-β.[51,52] Furthermore, the receptors for macrophage colony–stimulating factor (M-CSF)[53] and IL-1[50] have been localized in these cells. Epidermal growth factor receptor is expressed in proliferating trophoblastic cell columns, while the closely related protooncogene product c-*erb* B2 is present in the invading extravillous cells.[54] Trophoblast proliferation and invasion may therefore be regulated via an autocrine stimulatory loop. Some of the cytokines mentioned are equally present within decidual stromal cells (TNF-α, TGF-β, IL-1), which may indicate paracrine interactions. Limited data are available concerning the placental bed macrophages, but they are reported to express IL-1[50] and the receptor for M-CSF.[53] All the immunolocalization studies mentioned so far deal with normal placentation, and little information is available for complicated pregnancies. One of the few studies on pathologic cases showed a significantly stronger expression of IL-2 in decidual cells of preeclamptic patients than in normotensive control subjects.[55] Since increased serum levels of TNF-α indicate a role of this cytokine in preeclampsia,[56–59] we performed immunolocalization studies for TNF-α in placental bed biopsy specimens from both normotensive and preeclamptic pregnancies. Apart from confirming the presence of TNF-α in invasive extravillous trophoblast (endovascular trophoblast in spiral arteries, as well as interstitial cytotrophoblast), the studies showed clear localization in the macrophage-derived foam cells of atherotic arteries.[60] It is tempting to relate the latter observation to the increased serum levels of this cytokine, but clear evidence of such a correlation will not be easy to provide. The association of TNF-α with both invasive trophoblast and foam cells of atherotic vessels may also sustain the idea of a dual action of this cytokine in placentation, stimulatory on the one hand and inhibitory on the other.[61]

Placental Basal Plate

In the everyday clinical setting, principal questions concerning the uteroplacental vasculature include: Is there histologic evidence of uteroplacental vascular pathology? Is the pathology (in the most general terms) "acute" or "chronic"? Is there associated placental damage that might have impaired placental function (and therefore fetal well-being)? These questions can generally be answered by careful and thoughtful examination of the delivered placenta without placental bed biopsy. Although lesions of the end-vascular distribution of the uteroplacental circulation (in the basal plate) may not accurately represent the myometrial pathology, biopsy of the placental bed can provide only a small, focal sample of the placental bed, within which there is a great deal of regional

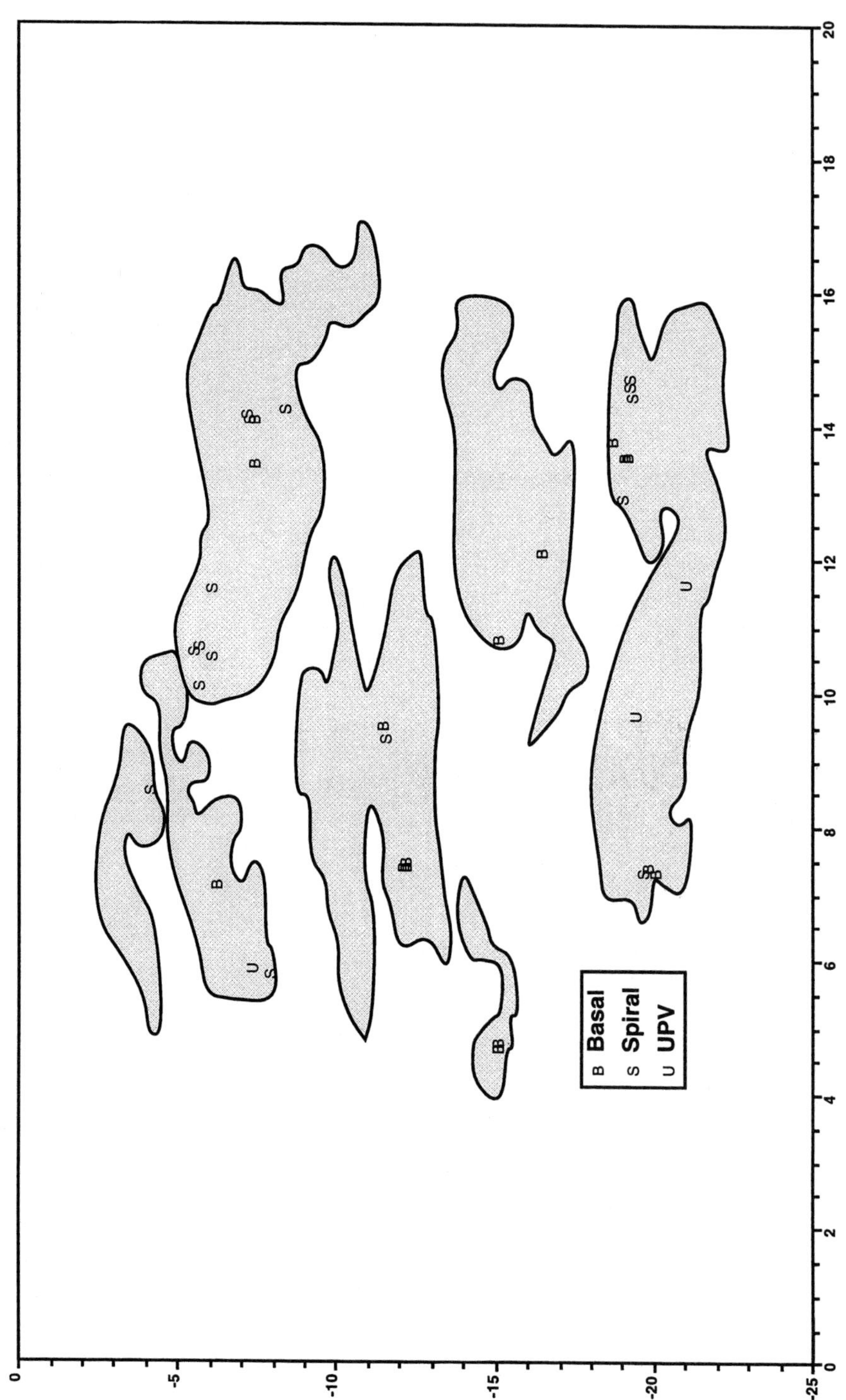

B Basal
S Spiral
U UPV

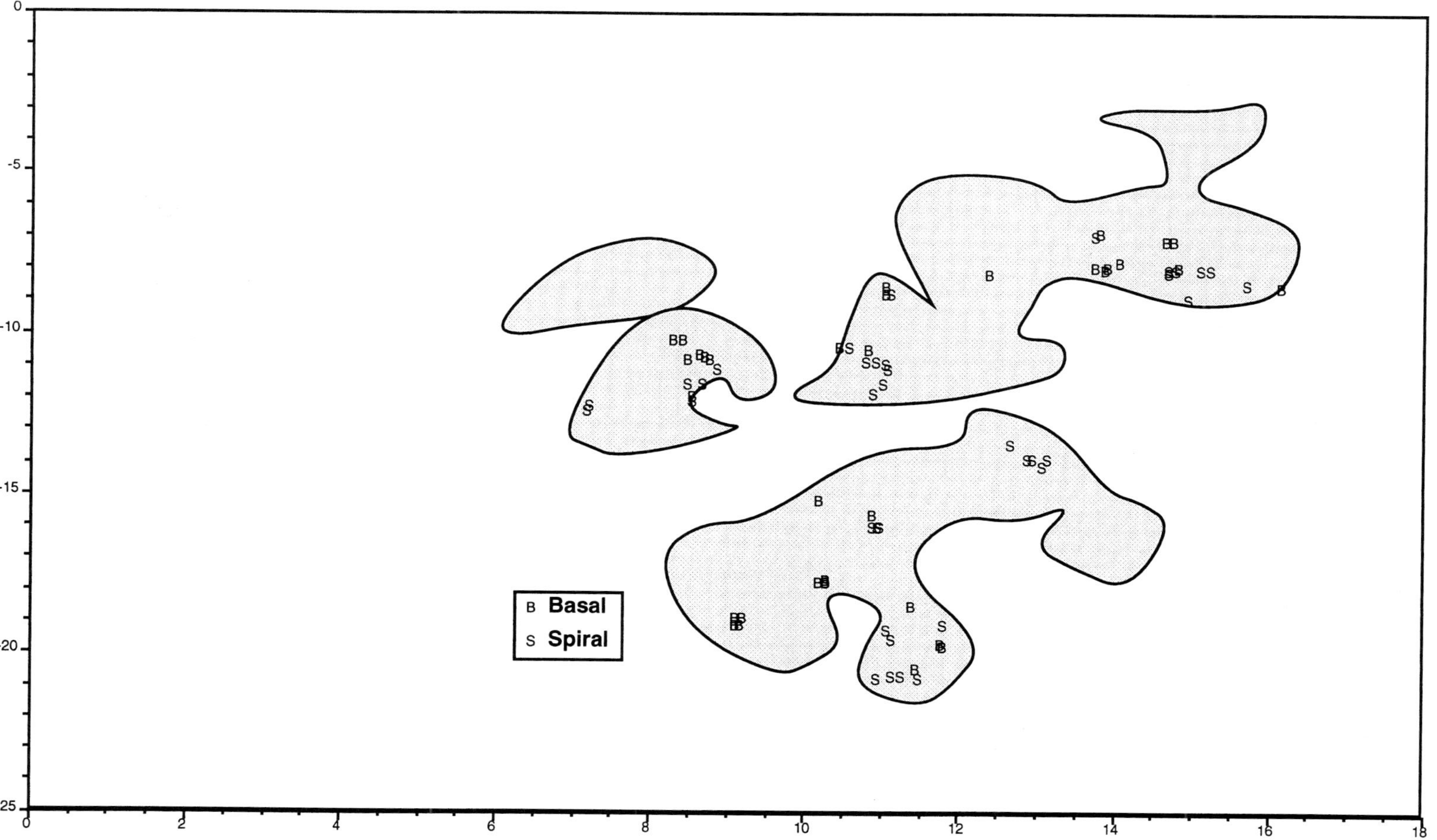

Figure 8–4. **A**, Field map of vessel lumina, drawn from placental bed biopsy obtained from term normotensive delivery. The microscope slide was scanned into the computer to obtain tissue contours. Each vessel lumen was identified using an x-y stage, and coordinates superimposed on the tissue contour map. **B**, Field map of vessel lumina, drawn from placental bed biopsy obtained from preterm preeclamptic delivery, prepared like **A**.

variation.[30] Placental bed biopsy specimens are therefore difficult to interpret except when procured by an experienced operator. Uteroplacental arteries are generally easily seen in the basal plate of the delivered placenta. End-vascular samples should be provided for review whenever the question of uteroplacental vascular insufficiency is clinically relevant. Four or five enface slices of the basal plate (which can all fit into a single cassette) may include the distal (basal plate) segments of several different uteroplacental arteries, located at different sites in the placental bed, which is an improvement over the view of the uteroplacental vasculature provided by a placental bed biopsy.[62] Variation in uteroplacental vascular anatomy and pathology implies also that one section of the placental villi may not be representative of placental function. Identification of failure of uteroplacental vascular adaptation, fibrinoid necrosis or atherosis, persistence of endovascular trophoblasts, thrombosis, and chronic vasculitis in the basal plate may shed light on the nature and mechanisms of uteroplacental vascular pathology. This information has proved useful for selecting appropriate therapy in subsequent pregnancies.[63]

In the basal plate or the placental bed, uteroplacental arteries with absent, incomplete, or failed adaptation have variable persistence of vascular muscle and elastic lamina. This leads to increased uterine vascular resistance, decreased capacitance, and decreased total blood flow to the placenta. Doppler and isotope studies in human beings suggest that uteroplacental flow is decreased to between 50% and 70% of normal, which may explain the often associated fetal IUGR.[64,65] While it now appears likely that trophoblast vascular conversion may continue well into the second and even the early third trimester, endovascular trophoblast in the endometrial (basal plate) uteroplacental arteries after the early midtrimester may reflect a disturbance in the normal process of uteroplacental vascular conversion. Fibrinoid necrosis of the vessel wall with mural foamy cells (atherosis [Fig. 8–5*A*]) is accompanied by dense lipoprotein(a) deposition within the vascular wall (Fig. 8–5*B*), clearly reflecting a vascular pathology akin to that seen in atherosclerosis. Other common uteroplacental arterial lesions are thrombosis and chronic vasculitis (Fig. 8–5*C*). In cases of preeclampsia, in which uteroplacental vascular pathology is common, Redline and Patterson[66] explored the hypothesis that a generalized maturation defect in the extravillous trophoblast increases accumulation of trophoblast in the superficial layers of the implantation site, in contrast to the normal process of progressive invasion through the endometrium to the myometrium. By immunostaining with proliferating cell nuclear antigen, they were able to distinguish increased thickness of basal cytotrophoblast and increased cytotrophoblast proliferation in preeclamptic placentas studied from 24 to 40 weeks compared with cases at term. It is unlikely that trophoblast accumulation at the placental-decidual interface reflects an intrinsic invasive defect, since placental bed biopsies in preeclampsia show normal interstitial trophoblast invasion even at that deep level (and an apparently selective defect in vascular invasion). Cytotrophoblast has been demonstrated to proliferate in conditions of low oxygen tension; the basal plate findings are more likely an additional histologic marker of generally poor uteroplacental perfusion, which can be assessed in the delivered placenta.

Uteroplacental thrombosis is required at the time of placental separation during parturition to protect the mother from exsanguination. On the other hand, uteroplacental thrombosis cannot occur during gestation without risk to placental—and fetal—well-being. In our experience, single thrombotic lesions in the uteroplacental arteries that occlude greater than 50% of the lumen and that are not accompanied by villous evidence of abnormal uteroplacental perfusion are fairly common at term. The association of intimal proliferation and often a chronic inflammatory infiltrate has suggested to us that some involutional change of the uteroplacental vasculature occurs as part of the preparation for parturition.[67] However, the uterine vasculature appears to be particularly susceptible to thrombosis, possibly because its endothelium is *normally* eroded and basement membranes and decidual stromal collagen are *normally* exposed to circulating maternal platelets for up to at least 24 weeks. As a central player in clinically significant allograft rejection,[68,69] coagulation has also been implicated in the pathogenesis of obstetric compromise, including antiphospholipid antibody–related fetal death[70] and preeclampsia.[71] The characteristic cause of pregnancy loss in these condi-

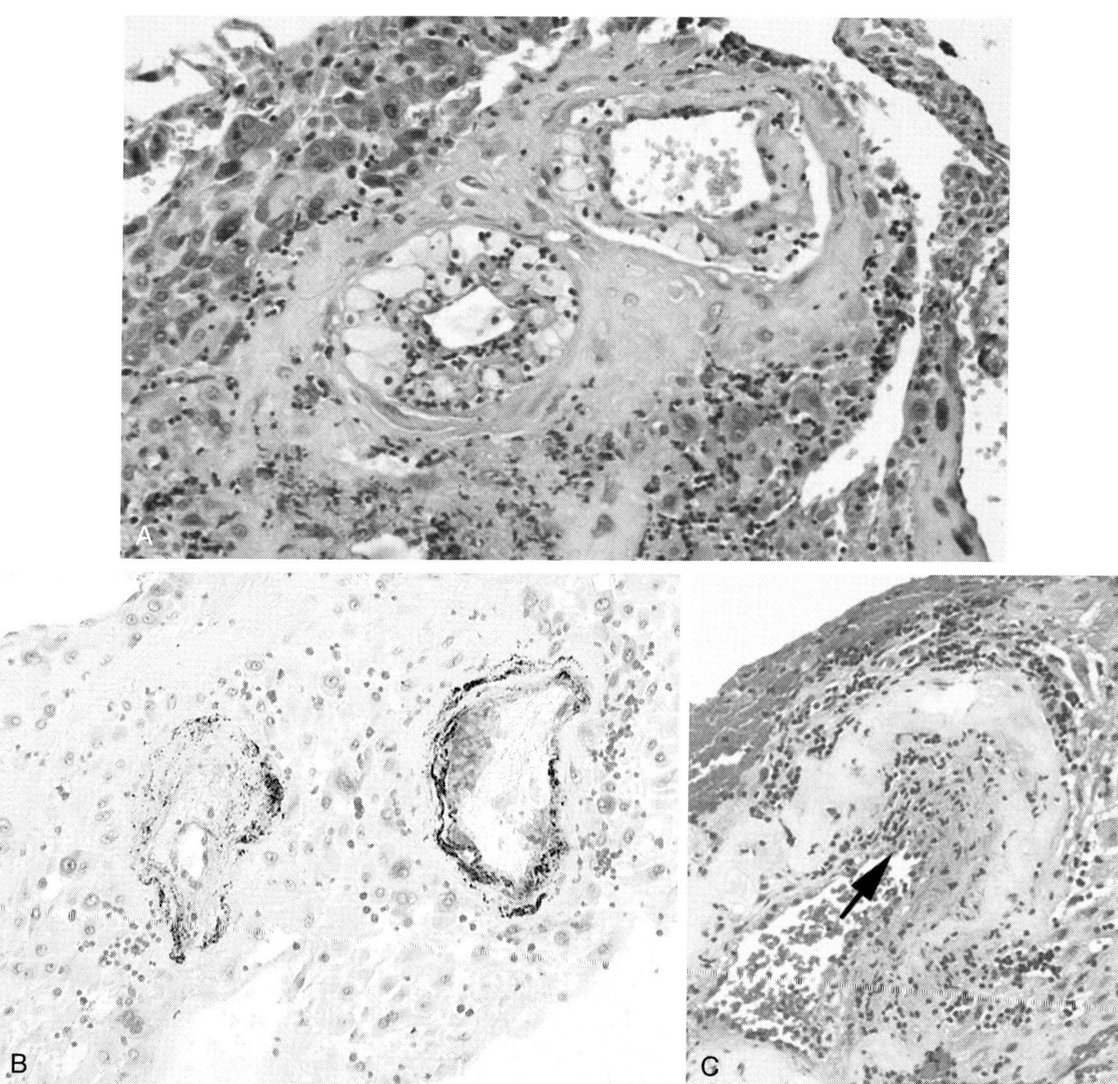

Figure 8–5. **A**, Basal plate of delivered placenta, uteroplacental artery with fibrinoid necrosis and atherosis. Note numerous foamy macrophages ("atherosis," *arrows)* within the homogeneous eosinophilic wall of the vessel. Dense chronic vasculitis is associated with the foamy macrophages. The infant was growth restricted at term, the mother was normotensive, and there were no clinical risk factors (H & E, ×40). **B**, Immunohistochemical stain for lipoprotein(a), with intense mural immunoreactivity in the wall of atherotic spiral artery of the decidua capsularis. Fetal growth restriction associated with preeclampsia, delivery at 35 weeks, no other clinical risk factors (×40). **C**, Basal plate, delivered placenta, chronic uteroplacental vasculitis in spontaneous preterm birth at 34 weeks' gestation. Numerous lymphocytes are within the fibrinoid of the otherwise normally converted vessel and also within a focus of myointimal proliferation *(arrow)* (H & E, ×10.)

tions, uteroplacental thrombosis and placental infarction,[72] is not pathognomonic of a positive test for lupus anticoagulant as opposed to cardiolipin antibody. It is likely that our serologic investigations of gestation-associated coagulopathy do not test for critical (but as yet unidentified) antibodies; on the other hand, coagulation is a nonspecific response to a wide variety of pathologic stimuli and would not likely be uniquely associated with any one clinical or laboratory test abnormality. Failed regrowth of the maternal endothelium over the converted uteroplacental vascular wall of fibrinoid material and embedded trophoblasts, as well as protracted exposure of the maternal vascular wall to the maternal circulation, has been identified in preeclampsia.[73] Potential targets for pathologic coagulation include the (maternal) uteroplacental vasculature, the basal plate (including Nitabuch's fibrin), the intervillous space, the villous (syncytiotrophoblast) surface, and the fetoplacental vasculature. In our clinical (and unfortunately, anecdotal) experience, maternal anticoagulant therapy is most effective when the maternal vasculature is the target of pathologic coagulopathy and is specifically not effective when coagulation is initiated on the villous trophoblast surface or within the fetoplacental vasculature.

There is no uteroplacental arterial lesion that distinguishes among the clinical conditions associated with uteroplacental vascular pathology.[14,74] If uteroplacental vascular damage is part of the pathophysiology of obstetric compromise, molecular markers that have been localized to areas of vascular injury, such as lipoprotein(a), might be found in the uteroplacental vasculature.[75] In support of this speculation, Berg and associates[76] reported a patient with a serum lipoprotein(a) level greater than 99th percentile for her population who delivered three consecutive very low birth weight infants with placentas described as "small and ischemic." Meekins and associates[77] demonstrated that lipoprotein(a) deposition in the placental bed spiral arteries is greater in preeclamptic women than in normotensive control subjects and is directly related to the severity of histologic disruption of nonconverted spiral arteries. These observations were recently expanded to include placental basal plate arteries from consecutive births in March–June 1995 in normal term births, term preeclampsia, preterm preeclampsia, spontaneous preterm birth, and postpartum curettage and peripartum hysterectomy samples.[67] Results of this study are presented in Table 8–1.

Lipoprotein(a) deposition in the uteroplacental vasculature appears to be essentially ubiquitous, at least in cases in which maternal bleeding ceases within a few heartbeats of placental separation and delivery. Some preparation of the placental bed, including development of a more thrombogenic vascular environment, may be critical for normal placental separation to occur without maternal exsanguination. If basal plate lipoprotein(a) deposition is present in most normal term deliveries, involution-related changes must develop either before parturition or as part of normal parturition (perhaps secondary to the mechanical trauma of

Table 8–1. Distribution of Lipoprotein(a) Immunoreactivity in Uteroplacental Vessels of the Placental Bed and Basal Plate

	Number (%) Lipoprotein(a)-Reactive Uteroplacental or Spiral Arteries	*p* Value	OR (95% CI)
Placental bed biopsy			
Normotensive	2/69 (3%)		
Preeclampsia	71/179 (40%)	<.0001*	22 (5-134)
Basal plate			
Normal term	14/35 (40%)		
Term preeclampsia	20/21 (95%)	.0001†	30 (3.5-670)
Preterm preeclampsia	10/10 (100%)	.003†	150 (N/A)
Spontaneous prematurity	49/56 (88%)	<.0001†	10.5 (3-34)
Remote postpartum implantation site	65/70 (93%)	.0001†	19.5 (6-72)
Massive peripartum hemorrhage	0/40 (0%)	<.0001‡	>1000 (N/A)

OR, Odds ratio; CI, confidence interval.
*Significance compared with normotensive placental bed biopsies.
†Significance compared with normal term basal plate.
‡Significance compared with involuting implantation sites.

labor). If lipoprotein(a) deposition occurs within the restricted period from labor to delivery, we should expect primarily early (endothelial) lesions,[78] rather than the smooth muscle cell deposition characteristic of chronic vascular damage. Our cases of uncomplicated term births, all of which delivered after labor, demonstrate both patterns, suggesting a more chronic vasculopathy. Preparation for uteroplacental involution may develop before clinical parturition, just as myometrial activity increases before onset of clinical labor.[79] Precocious or more extensive antepartum development of uteroplacental involution may explain cases of decreased fetal growth in the third trimester. Similarly, in term preeclampsia the more extensive lipoprotein(a) deposition in the basal plate may represent uteroplacental involution to a degree that results in placental ischemia (a potential trigger of preeclampsia).[80] In preterm preeclampsia, placental bed arteries show the effects of failed trophoblast invasion in the early to middle second trimester, and lipoprotein(a)-reactive uteroplacental arteries have been seen in all cases of preterm preeclampsia. Chronic vascular pathology may facilitate early vascular wall uptake of lipoprotein(a). The progressive increase in uteroplacental flow throughout gestation may contribute to a vicious cycle in which abnormally converted uteroplacental arteries produce a high-resistance/low-capacitance circulation and vascular damage enhances thrombus formation, further reducing capacitance and uteroplacental perfusion. We would apply the same arguments to the cases of preterm labor and premature membrane rupture. Since in all these cases the mothers received tocolytic therapy (prolonging the period of clinical myometrial activity), a deleterious effect of mechanical trauma on the uteroplacental vasculature cannot be excluded. Alternatively, we have shown that placentas from preterm labor and premature membrane rupture contain fewer and less severe uteroplacental lesions and less widespread placental ischemic damage than placentas in preterm preeclampsia.[74] We hypothesize that lipoprotein(a) deposition in preterm labor and premature membrane rupture is the result of vascular damage initiated by chronic low-level uteroplacental vascular pathology, which may then be exacerbated by the mechanical trauma of labor.

If we consider the findings of hematoxylin and eosin studies of normal uteroplacental involution, the similarity to atherosclerosis becomes clearer. Normal uteroplacental vascular involution is accompanied by thrombosis, leukocytic infiltration of the vascular wall, and apparent proliferation or migration of endothelia and vascular smooth muscle[81]; similar changes in the vascular microenvironment are induced in atherosclerosis.[78] A significant role of lipoprotein(a) in processes related to uteroplacental vascular wall damage would explain the recent clinical observation of homocysteinuria in patients with preeclampsia.[82] Harpel and Borth[83] have recently shown that sulfhydryl-containing compounds (including homocysteine) increase the affinity between lipoprotein(a) and fibrin. The up to 84-fold increase in affinity seen in the presence of homocysteine may explain the increased prevalence of vascular pathologic conditions, placental ischemia, and preeclampsia in patients with homocysteinuria. Interestingly, homocysteine has been studied as a marker of atherosclerotic vascular processes.

PLACENTAL EFFECTS OF ABNORMAL UTEROPLACENTAL PERFUSION

Endovascular trophoblast invasion has been considered to establish, from the earliest days of gestation, a maternal circulation providing the conceptus with nutrients. This circulation originally was thought to be a sluggish capillary-derived blood pool that evolves with trophoblast remodeling of the spiral arteries into a high-volume/low-resistance circuit. Hustin and Schaaps[84,85] have challenged this theory based on their failure to identify intervillous circulation either on direct visualization of the intervillous space or in perfused hysterectomy specimens, in which they demonstrated occlusion of the uteroplacental circulation by trophoblastic plugs until the twelfth week of pregnancy. They speculated that these trophoblastic plugs protect the young conceptus from the force of maternal arterial blood flow until implantation is well established. Since then, it has been proposed that precocious initiation of maternal arterial perfusion of the intervillous space may be responsible for early pregnancy loss.[86] A cogent rebuttal has been provided by Moll,[87] who suggested that fixation artifact and intervillous flow rates (below the current limits of Doppler resolution) may explain most of the observations. Whether most or all of embryogenesis occurs in the absence of contact with the maternal circulation awaits final resolution.

The potential for mechanical factors to remodel and deform the evolving intraplacental vasculature cannot be overestimated. Intraluminal direction and volume of fetoplacental flow are major determinants of arterial as opposed to venous differentiation of the placental vasculature. Recently Burton and co-workers[88] confirmed the mechanical effect of intraplacental and maternal perfusion pressures on villous capillary growth. Increasing intraplacental perfusion pressure from 40 to 100 mm Hg resulted in more proliferating endothelial nuclei, suggesting that mechanical factors affect villous angiogenesis and the formation of terminal villi. Similarly, if a sufficiently high pressure is generated in the intervillous space, the elastic and deformable placental capillaries may be compressed.

When uteroplacental vascular lesions are present, the resultant disturbance in resistance and capacitance and the increased fragility of the vasculature predispose to uteroplacental vascular accidents such as placental infarcts[28] or abruption.[89] Abruption is essentially a hemorrhagic infarct. However, marginal separation of the placenta may be related to prematurity.[90] When uteroplacental arteries are occluded, intervillous flow ceases, the intervillous space collapses, and villi become compressed and undergo ischemic necrosis (an infarct [Fig. 8–6]). The gross appearance of placental infarcts varies with the age of the infarct; older lesions, in which blood is more extensively degraded, may appear tan to pink-tan. More recent lesions may be the same color as the adjacent noninfarcted placenta but simply have a firm feel, consistent with the collapse of intervillous space. The boundaries of an infarct, with the compressed villi, often can be clearly demarcated by the unassisted eye (Fig. 8–6, *top section*). Older lesions are characterized histologically by complete loss of nuclear detail (Fig. 8–6*B*). Central infarcts are believed to be more significant to the fetus, given the greater dependence of the fetus on the central, most healthy area of villous parenchyma. One of us (C.S.) grossly examined 500 consecutive placentas from uncomplicated term deliveries in a community hospital; 10% of placentas had an infarct. Ninety percent of the lesions were at the placental margin; 90% were less than 1 cm^3 in dimension. Therefore we consider placentas with more than one infarct, infarcts located centrally, and infarcts greater than 1 cm^3 to be outside the range of normal. Such lesions only rarely compromise more than 50% of the placenta, which is the criterion for "placental insufficiency" based on estimated placental reserve. However, they reflect an abnormal uteroplacental vascular environment because the 40 to 60 placental functional units are served by 100 to 150 uteroplacental vessels, providing a redundancy of perfusion (collateral flow) that should prevent placental infarct. The presence of an infarct therefore means that collateral flow in the intervillous space is insufficient to protect the placental parenchyma if a single uteroplacental vessel becomes occluded or otherwise compromised. As a corollary, in placentas with central, large, or multifocal infarcts, viable villi most commonly show evidence of chronic and diffuse uteroplacental malperfusion. Central, large, or multifocal infarcts generally do not occur in the context of noninfarcted placental villi with normal syncytial knotting, no cytotrophoblast proliferation, normal (nonfibrotic) villous stroma, and well-developed terminal villous capillary networks.

In abruption the placenta is forcibly separated from the uterine wall by retroplacental hemorrhage from abnormal uteroplacental vessels.[91] Placental compression by a retroplacental hematoma (Fig. 8–7*A*) increases fetal blood volume and may be associated with villous stromal hemorrhage (Fig. 8–7*B*).[92] In some settings villous stromal hemorrhage may indicate the effects of placental trauma, essentially as a bruise. Villous stromal hemorrhage may also be a precursor of or a lesion underlying fetomaternal transfusion. In our experience, in cases of fetomaternal blood group *compatibility* (in which preformed maternal antibodies to fetal blood do not exist), an acute abruption that is clinically stabilized may be followed by fetal decompensation caused by a chronic fetomaternal transfusion and severe fetal anemia, which may lead to fetal death. Separation from the uterine lining precludes effective blood flow to the involved placental area, acutely reducing fetoplacental oxygen availability.[91] Endothelial damage

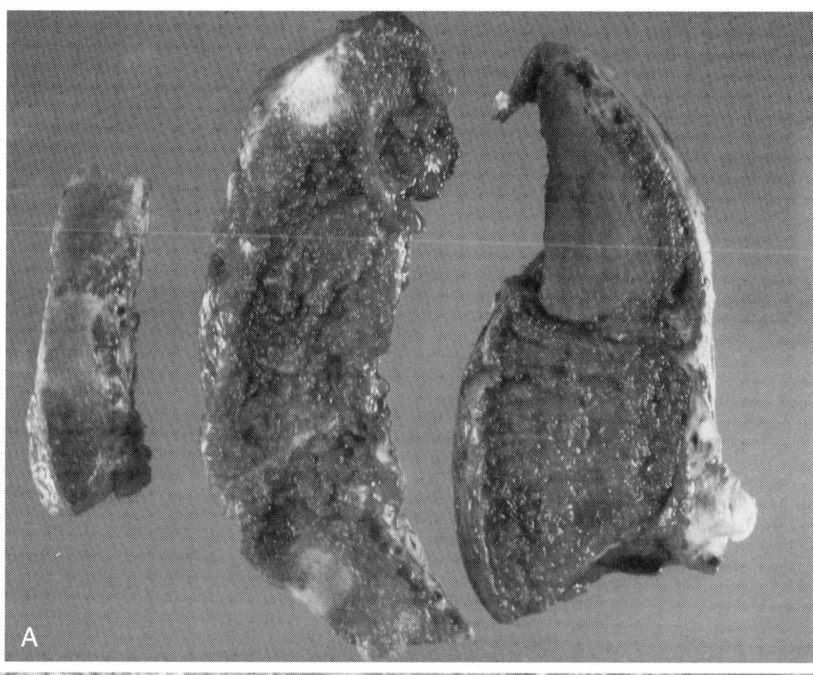

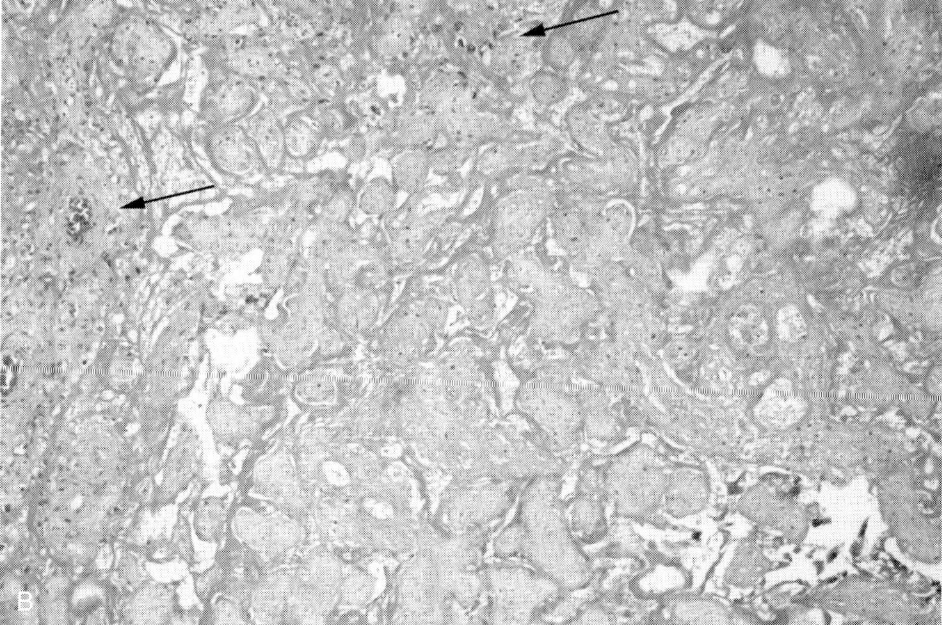

Figure 8–6. **A**, Delivered placenta from 28-week stillborn infant of nonhypertensive mother. Histologic examination of the placenta showed multifocal lesions of fibrinoid necrosis or atherosis, despite the absence of clinical preeclampsia. The varying ages of the lesions are reflected in the range of color from tan (second section, extreme right, most blood hemolyzed and degraded) to pink-tan (top section, and second section, extreme left) to dark purple, essentially a condensation of normally blood-filled villi (third section, extreme right, at placental margin). **B**, Infarct from same patient as in **A**. Nuclear detail is absent centrally but is partly preserved at the periphery of the lesions *(arrows)*. (H & E, ×4.)

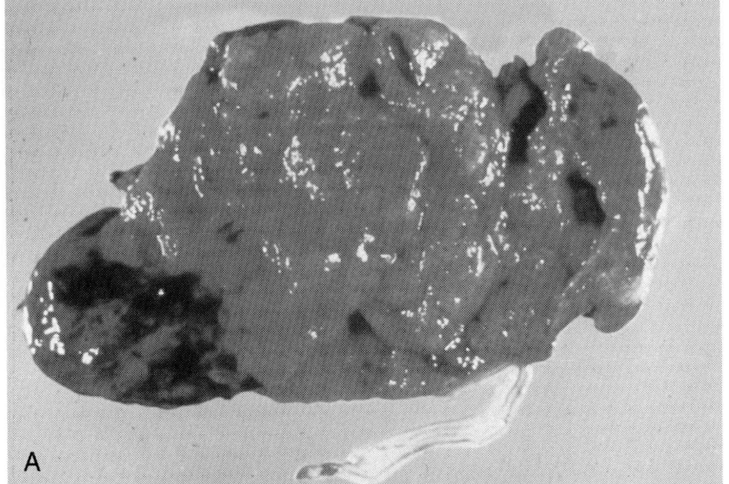

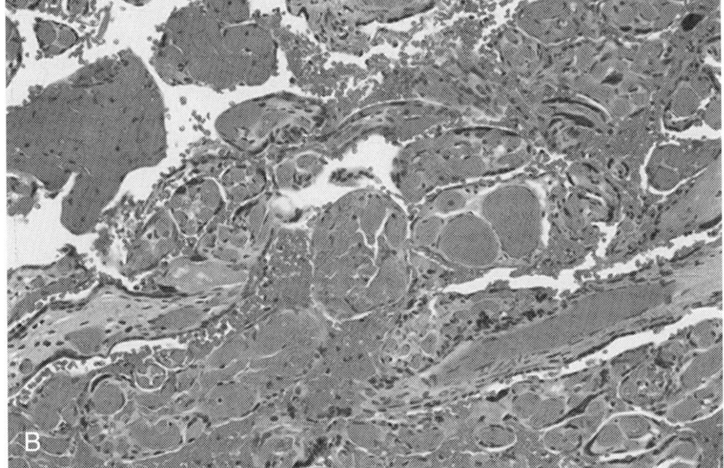

Figure 8–7. A, Abruption with marginal attached retroplacental hematoma. The date of this specimen (1984) reflects the increasing rarity of these types of subacute lesion. Most commonly in our practice we now see "chronic abruptions," with old, laminated, pale tan retroplacental hemorrhage and placental infarct, or acute "clinical abruptions," in which case an abrupt change in fetal status results in crash delivery before the blood may even have the chance to adhere. Often in these cases only basal plate disruption, intervillous congestion, and villous stromal hemorrhage can provide anatomic support for a clinical acute abruption. **B**, Focus of villous stromal hemorrhage at the margin of an acute placental abruption. (H & E, ×10.)

caused by hypoxia, complicated by increased intravascular volume resulting from placental compression, may explain the common correlate of extensive visceral and germinal matrix hemorrhages in abruption.[91] Basal intervillous thrombi are primarily maternal blood[93]; these lesions may be mild forms of abruption-type pathology.

In addition to large-scale placental lesions, chronically abnormal uteroplacental vascular perfusion may impair the growth and development of the placenta or alternatively lead to diffuse villous lesions that cannot be identified on gross examination. Scarred, shrunken, fibrotic, hypovascular villi, with reduced number or caliber of placental capillaries, have been proposed to result from destruction of growing villous capillaries by abnormal uteroplacental flow (Fig. 8–8).[95] Such capillary damage may lead to fetomaternal hemorrhage. Given the uteroplacental vascular pathology common in hypertensive pregnancies, it is not surprising that fetomaternal hemorrhages in the midtrimester are more common in hypertensive pregnancies.[95] Tenney-Parker changes of the terminal villi, an increase in syncytial nuclear clumping and basophilia (Fig. 8–8*C*), are common in cases of chronic uteroplacental malperfusion. However, it is often forgotten that these syncytial histologic features accompany abnormal placental perfusion of either maternal *or* fetal origin. Avascular villi (villi devascularized from intraplacental vascular lesions) commonly have excess syncytial knotting compared with their normally vascularized neighbors. Experimental ligation of a fetal artery in the monkey placenta appeared to increase syncytial knotting in the villi so rendered avascular.[96]

The small size of placentas delivered in the con-

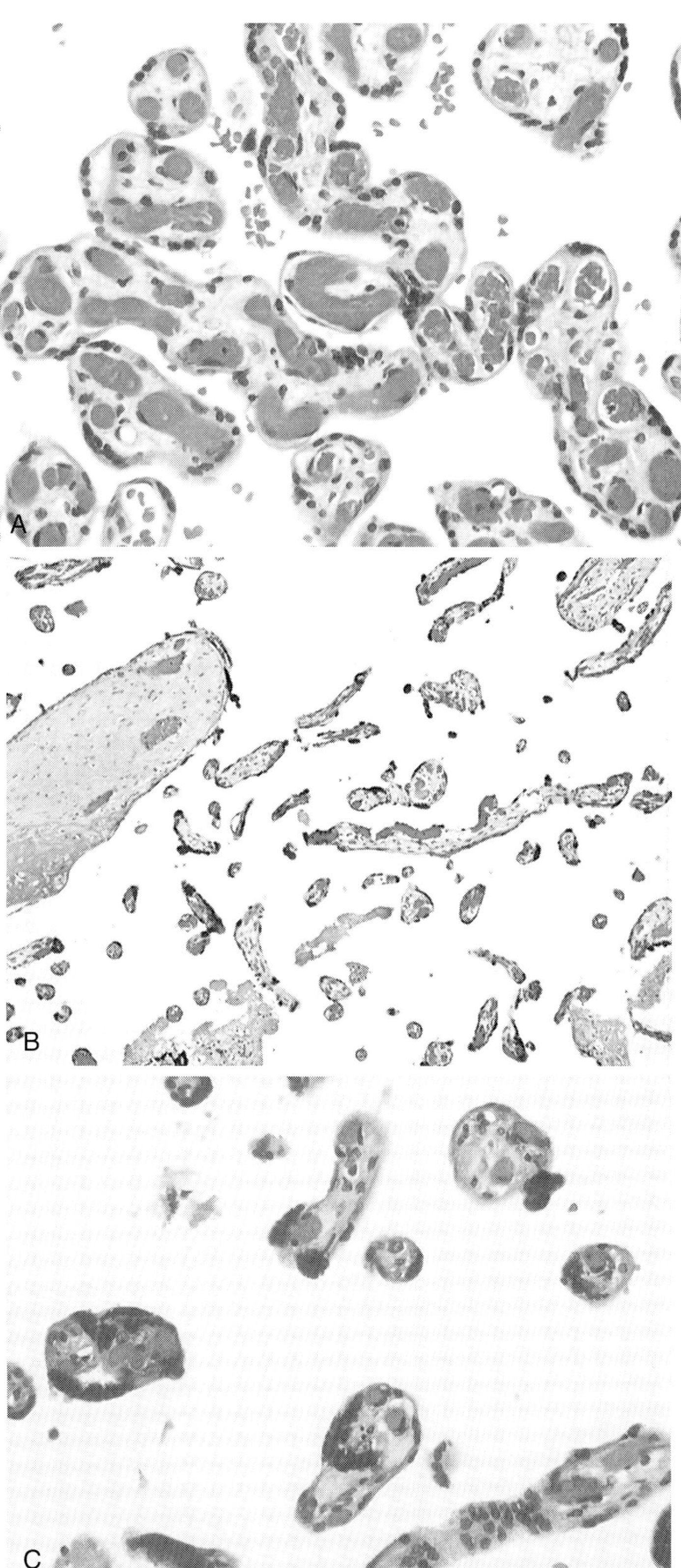

Figure 8–8. **A**, Normal terminal villi from a case of fetal growth restriction following maternal ethanol abuse. (H & E, ×10.) **B**, Decreased terminal villous arborization in fetal growth restriction delivered at 32 weeks with no clinical risk factors. Placenta demonstrated extensive uteroplacental vascular lesions. (H & E, ×4.) **C,** Same case as in **B.** Vascular development is irregular, with poorly vascularized villi and one villus with multiple capillary lumina *(arrow)*. (H&E, ×40.)

text of long-standing poor uteroplacental perfusion suggests that chronic placental nutritional deprivation impairs terminal villous arborization. This is supported by the microscopic impression of increased intervillous volume and decreased villous parenchymal volume. In these cases the placenta may fail to develop adequate mass, rather than be destroyed by abnormal perfusion patterns. Either way, the total villous capillary bed is reduced, producing an anatomy analogous to the emphysematous lung, with parallel compromise of placental respiratory sufficiency. Just as significant to the fetus is the potential for increased placental resistance and increased cardiac work, since 500 ml/min of fetal cardiac output is directed to the placenta. An indirect reflection of umbilical-placental resistance is the umbilical systolic-diastolic (S/D) ratio. The S/D ratio approaches infinity, and end-diastolic flow in the umbilical artery may be negative when the placental capillary bed is reduced by more than 50%.[94] A reduction in the total fetoplacental capillary bed necessitates a like reduction in fetoplacental volume. This may lead to reduced fetal glomerular filtration rate and

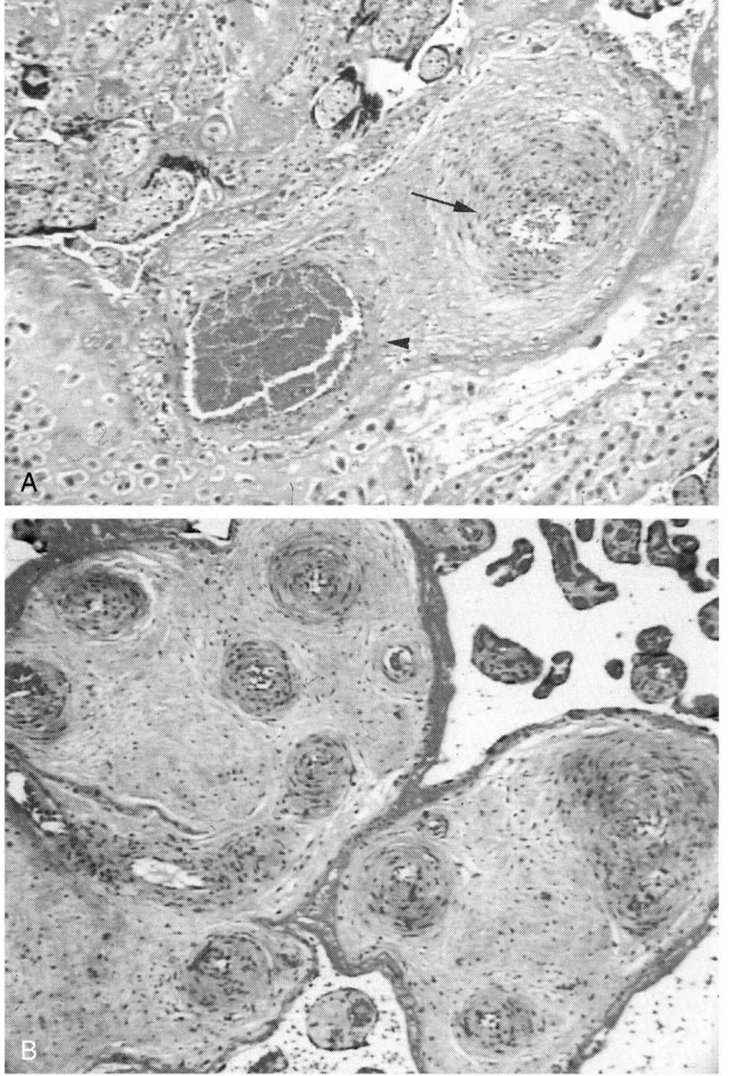

Figure 8–9. **A**, Fetal stem containing a thicker-walled artery *(arrow)* and a thin-walled vein *(arrowhead).* Normal term delivery. (H & E, ×4.) **B**, Fetal stem containing vessels that can no longer be distinguished as artery or vein. A relative decrease in lumen calibers (compared with **A**) accompanies the medial hypertrophy. The placenta was delivered at 34 weeks, fetal growth restriction, abnormally high systolic/diastolic ratio on umbilical artery Doppler ultrasonography (end-diastolic flow present), no maternal risk factors. (H & E, ×4.)

oligohydramnios.[97] Arabin[98] and Laurini[99] and their associates have related histologic evidence of uteroplacental ischemia to abnormal Doppler velocimetry of the umbilical artery. Perfusion of the placenta at abnormally low oxygen tension is associated with increased basal perfusion pressure, consistent with placental vasoconstriction.[100] Chronic vasoconstriction (and increased intraluminal pressure) could lead to vascular obliteration (Fig. 8–9) through progressive mural hyperplasia. Increased intraluminal pressure could predispose to endothelial damage and luminal obliteration by lesions of the hemorrhagic endovasculitis type.

PATHOLOGY OF THE MATERNAL-PLACENTAL INTERFACE

At the eighth week the basal plate is composed of a dense mixture of extravillous trophoblastic and decidual cells intermingled with a few trophoblastic giant cells. By the midtrimester a nearly complete layer of extravillous cytotrophoblast cells is largely separated from the decidual cells by Nitabuch's fibrinoid. This layer is believed to mark the border of placental and decidual tissues but is generally not the exact plane of cleavage of the placenta. Identification of *fas* and c-*myc* gene products in Nitabuch's fibrinoid suggests that apoptosis may be a mechanism by which this acellular zone is formed. Basal plate extravillous cytotrophoblast produces TNF-α,[60] which may be an important promoter of villous trophoblast apoptosis recently demonstrated by Nelson and Swanson.[101] Whether Nitabuch's fibrinoid is formed as part of the process that permits normal placental separation is not clear, but animal models suggest that the prospective separation zone (located slightly below Nitabuch's fibrinoid in human beings) is devoid of intact cells 1 to 2 days before parturition.[102] The cellular zone has been replaced by a loosely arranged fibrin network, which may facilitate wound healing after placental separation. Premature and too extensive cell loss in the basal plate and placental bed may destabilize placental implantation and lead to pathologic placental separation (e.g., abruption). In our studies of the basal plate in preterm abruption, we have had great difficulty identifying uteroplacental vessels because of extensive decidual destruction. At the time we attributed that difficulty to tissue injury from the abruption process.[74] Apoptosis in the basal plate probably contributes to pathologic placental separation. We have reanalyzed that dataset to determine the distribution of noninflammatory cell loss at the interface of the chorionic trophoblast and extraplacental decidua (which we have termed laminar chorionic necrosis). Of 33 cases of clinical abruption before 32 weeks, 17 (48.5%) had laminar chorionic necrosis, as compared with 78 (22%) of 354 cases of premature membrane rupture or preterm labor delivering at less than 32 weeks' gestation ($p < .01$). Assessment of the role of apoptosis, a process with extremely rapid onset and cell clearance, in rupture of the extraplacental membranes is complicated by the interval between clinical presentation and delivery (especially in preterm cases in which prolongation of pregnancy is commonly a clinical aim) and the mechanical trauma and vascular stresses to which the membranes are subject during delivery.

Fibrin and fibrinoid deposition in the basal plate has been proposed to result from maternal-placental immunologic interactions; increased basal plate coagulation has been identified in cases of pregnancy compromise believed to be of immunologic origin.[103] Increased basal coagulation results in a thick band of basal plate fibrin and fibrinoid, replacing the normal zone of extravillous cytotrophoblasts, and may even extend to involve several layers of entrapped and necrotic basal villi. Chronic anchoring villitis can often be seen in the surviving villi, perched atop the pile of necrotic and fibrinoid material. The noninflammatory lesions of encroaching basal fibrinoid may represent milder forms of the uncommon lesion maternal floor infarct (Fig. 8–10*A*). These possibly milder forms have also been observed to recur in successive pregnancies of women with recurrent poor pregnancy outcome. This lesion tends to be unaffected by maternal aspirin and heparin therapy. We have frequently observed a subjective increase in basal cytotrophoblast in such cases, a finding that may be reflected in the observations of Redline and Patterson[66] of increased basal cytotrophoblast in preeclampsia. Especially in recurrent poor pregnancy outcome, it is tempting to speculate that trophoblast invasion is impaired by an abnormal basal matrix or immunologic environment. Bendon and Hommel[104] have reported two cases of se-

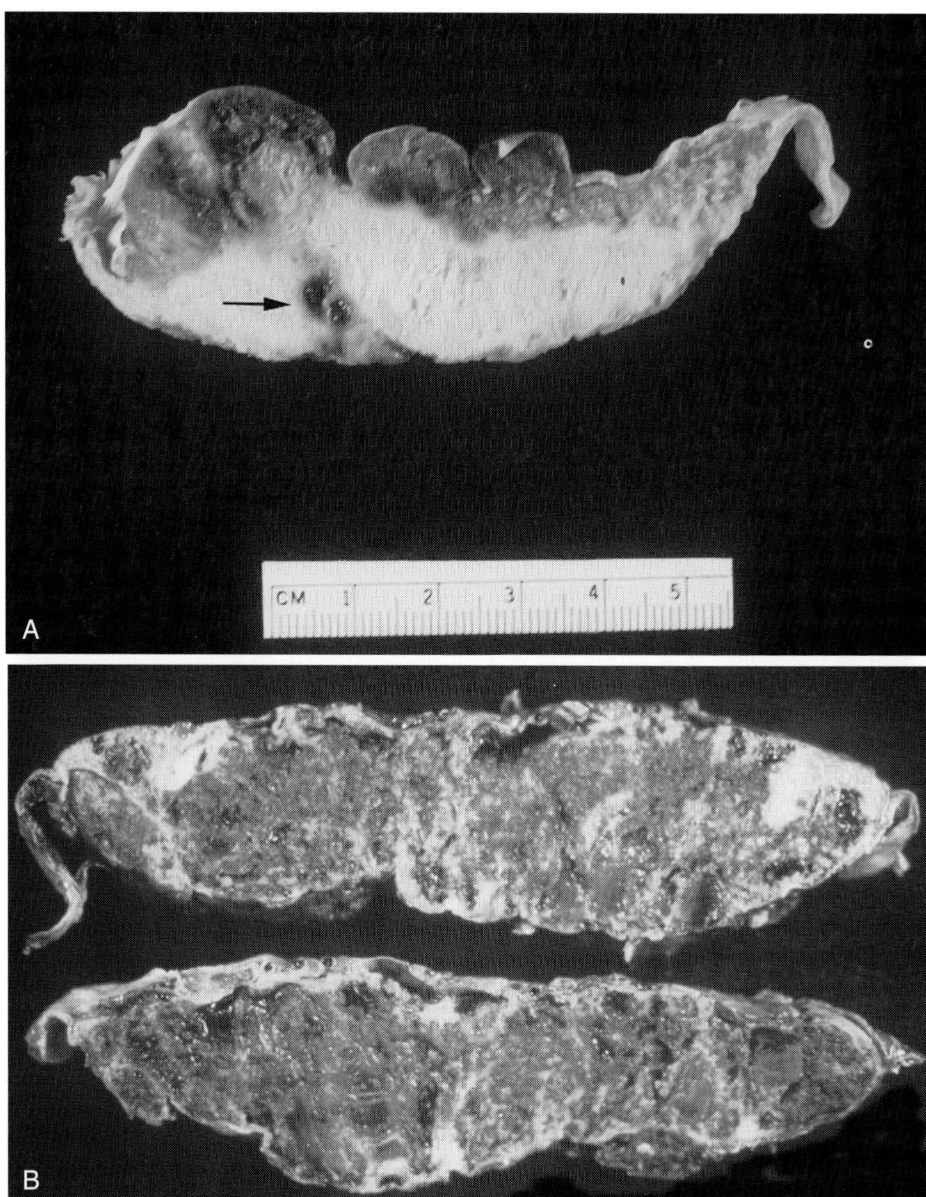

Figure 8–10. **A**, Section of placenta with maternal floor infarct. Note lumen of large (and histologically normal) uteroplacental vessel *(arrow)*. Clinically there was fetal growth restriction and abnormal antepartum testing, necessitating crash cesarean section. The mother had two prior spontaneous first-trimester losses (no pathologic diagnoses available). **B**, Excessive perivillous fibrin deposition, irregularly distributed throughout the villous parenchyma. No clinical data are available.

vere maternal floor infarct without villitis or deciduitis in a patient with multiple autoantibodies. They suggested that this lesion may be a rare complication of maternal autoimmunity caused by antibodies against the placental urokinase-plasmin system. Excessive perivillous fibrin or fibrinoid deposition (Fig. 8–10*B* and *C*) may be considered a generic response to any type of syncytial injury. As such, this lesion may reflect, among other disorders, chronic uteroplacental malperfusion or immune-associated trophoblast injury (as may be seen in phospholipid antibody syndrome). The

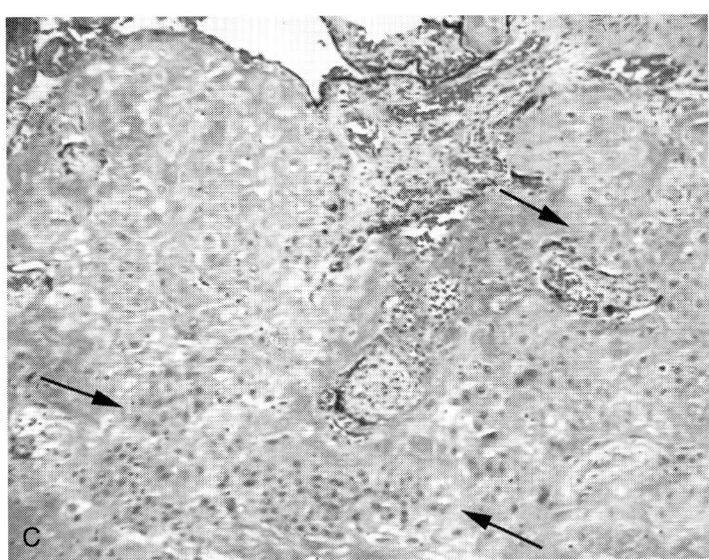

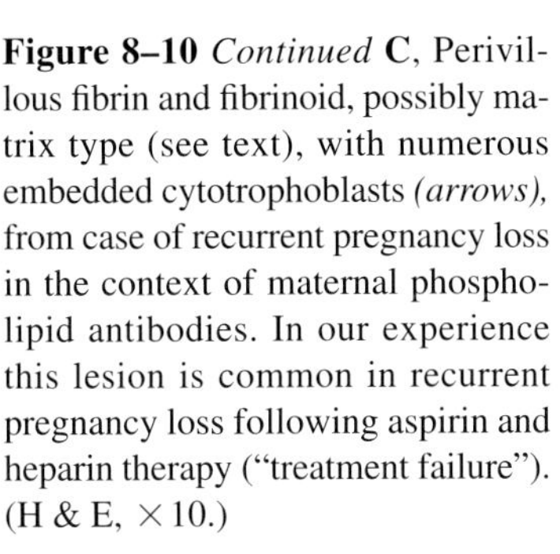
Figure 8–10 *Continued* **C**, Perivillous fibrin and fibrinoid, possibly matrix type (see text), with numerous embedded cytotrophoblasts *(arrows)*, from case of recurrent pregnancy loss in the context of maternal phospholipid antibodies. In our experience this lesion is common in recurrent pregnancy loss following aspirin and heparin therapy ("treatment failure"). (H & E, ×10.)

concurrence of other villous lesions reflecting chronic uteroplacental malperfusion or, conversely, of chronic villitis can help place this lesion in its proper context.

Recently two different types of placental fibrinoid have been distinguished,[105] a fibrin type and a matrix type. Fibrin-type fibrinoid was characterized by immunoreactivity for fibrin and cellular fibronectin, but for no other matrix component, and never contained extravillous cytotrophoblastic cells. In contrast, matrix-type fibrinoid was essentially fibrin negative and immunoreactive for oncofetal fibronectin, collagen IV, laminin, and tenascin. Matrix-type fibrinoid contained nonproliferative cytotrophoblasts, which the authors speculated secreted the matrix in a nonpolarized fashion. Matrix-type fibrinoid was generally covered by fibrin-type fibrinoid toward the intervillous space, with cytotrophoblast providing a line of demarcation between the two types of fibrinoid. The authors proposed that fibrin-type fibrinoid helps to adapt the intervillous space to maternal hemodynamics and temporarily replaces damaged syncytiotrophoblast as a transport and immune barrier, while matrix-type fibrinoid may be related to properties of trophoblast invasiveness. Both maternal floor infarcts and more restricted lesions of perivillous fibrin and fibrinoid we have observed in the 10 years we have consulted for pregnancy loss evaluation services generally have numerous cytotrophoblasts embedded in the perivillous material (Fig. 8–10*C*). A predominantly matrix derivation of the fibrinoid material would be consistent with its apparent resistance to anticoagulant therapy.

Chronic Inflammation of the Decidua

A few decidual lymphocytes are normally present in the decidua of the basal plate and the extraplacental membranes. One component of the normal decidual leukocyte population, the large granular lymphocytes, may play a major role in limiting trophoblastic penetration of maternal tissues.[106] In uncomplicated term pregnancies, clustering of maternal lymphocytes near anchoring villi and even sparse infiltration—with preservation of the anchoring villous structure—are common (Fig. 8–11*A*). In our experience in complicated gestations, chronic destructive anchoring villitis is more common, especially in the context of fetal growth restriction or maternal preeclampsia (Fig. 8–11*B*). Such cases often have other chronic inflammatory lesions (see below). The stimulus to the villitis is unknown, but this response has been suggested to indicate underlying maternal-placental immunopathology and to be more common in patients with poor reproductive outcome.[103]

A diagnosis of chronic choriodeciduitis and amnionitis indicates not only a denser distribution of

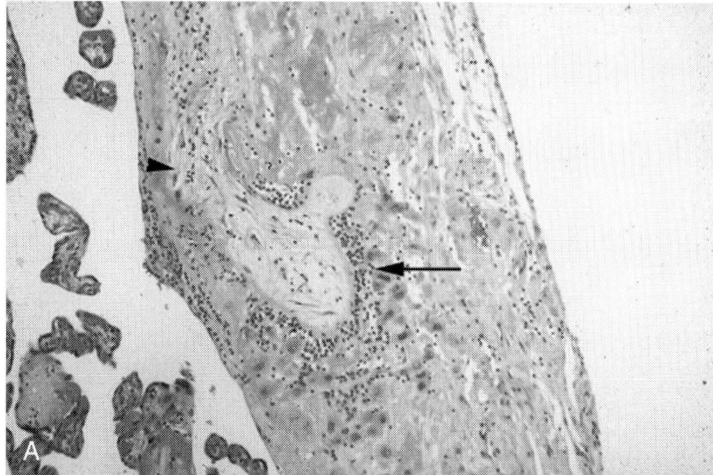

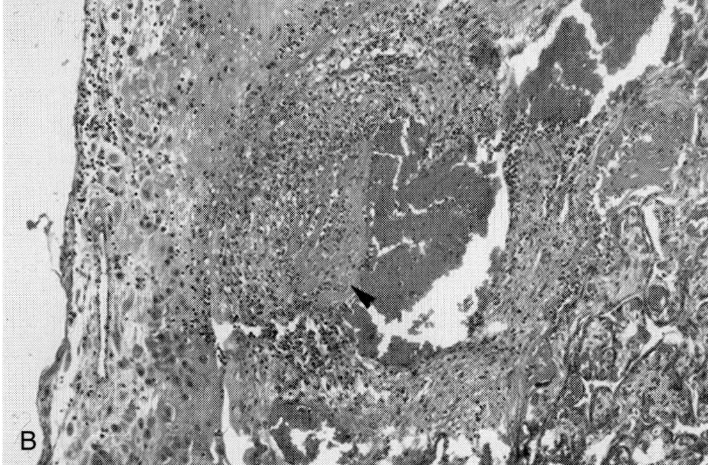

Figure 8–11. **A,** Basal plate, delivered placenta, normal term birth. Note anchoring villus with a peripheral rim of decidual (maternal) leukocytes *(arrow),* and sparse infiltration *(arrowhead).* Note the villous contours are well preserved. (H & E, ×10.) **B**, Basal plate, delivered placenta, spontaneous preterm birth at 29 weeks. Anchoring villus with extensive lymphocytic infiltration. Note loss of villous structure, and mural thrombus *(arrowhead)* in fetoplacental vessel. (H & E, ×10.)

decidual lymphocytes than expected, but also the migration of (maternal) decidual lymphocytes into the (fetal) chorion and amnion. Although this has been associated with chronic bacterial infection such as syphilis, it is more commonly seen in patients with no history of or risk factors for sexually transmitted diseases. Like other chronic inflammatory lesions (e.g., chronic villitis, intervillositis, and chronic uteroplacental vasculitis), it is most likely an autoimmune or alloimmune response of maternal lymphocytes to trophoblast or placental stromal antigens.[107] Chronic marginating choriodeciduitis may accompany the noninflammatory, bandlike death of cells of the chorionic trophoblast at the chorionic-decidual interface ("laminar chorionic necrosis") and may originate from apoptosis of the chorionic cytotrophoblast.

In uncomplicated term deliveries we have found decidual plasma cells to be uncommon, which is reasonable given the potential functions of antibody-forming cells in the basal plate and juxtaposed to fetal placental cells. However, decidual plasma cells in extraplacental membranes and the basal plate accompany a wide range of complications of pregnancy, including severe Rh isoimmunization, antiphospholipid antibody–related pregnancy compromise, cytomegalovirus, herpes, syphilis, attempts to treat intraamniotic bacterial infections by tocolysis, defective trophoblast conversion of uteroplacental arteries, and maternal immunologic disorders. In the basal plate, dense chronic decidual inflammation may accompany uteroplacental vascular lesions. Chronic uteroplacental vasculitis (Fig. 8–5*C*) is significantly more common in early euploid pregnancy loss than aneuploid pregnancy loss[108] and is among the lesions associated with low birth weight infants.[14] Causal relationships among elevated levels of antiphospholipid antibodies, chronic uteroplacental vasculitis, and poor pregnancy outcome have been proposed. It is speculated that antiphospholipid antibodies directly cause pregnancy failure by inducing deleterious cellular immune responses, rather than by initiating coagulation.[109]

Decidual Hemosiderin

Decidual hemosiderin deposition indicates that decidual bleeding has occurred 24 to 48 hours before delivery. In a recent study, decidual hemosiderin, in either extraplacental or basal plate decidua, was found significantly more frequently in preterm than in term deliveries.[110] Decidual hemosiderin was associated with an increased likelihood of preterm delivery because of preeclampsia or nonhypertensive abruption but was not related to clinical bleeding within 72 hours of delivery. Basal plate hemosiderosis was associated with a significantly increased incidence of villous infarct (p <.0001), uteroplacental vessels without physiologic change (p <.003), increased numbers of circulating nucleated erythrocytes (p <.0007), uteroplacental vascular thrombosis (p <.0001), and villous fibrosis and hypovascularity (each p <.0001). Preterm delivery for whatever reason appears to be commonly associated with subclinical decidual bleeding. Such bleeding in the basal plate is related to other histologic evidence of chronic uteroplacental vascular pathology. Decidual hemosiderin has also been described to be more prevalent in cases with numerous avascular villi.[111]

Basal Plate Myofibers

Basal myofibers can be observed in the basal plate of the delivered placenta (Fig. 8–12). Having observed them in association with conditions of abnormal placental separation, and recognizing the greater incidence of abnormal third stage of labor in preterm delivery, we studied the distribution of these histologic features in term and preterm placentas and according to the clinical indication for preterm delivery.[112] Forty-four of 457 preterm placentas (9.6%) had basal plate myofibers, compared with 1 of 108 term control placentas (0.9%) (p <.001). Uteroplacental vessels with abnormal physiologic changes (incomplete or absent conversion) were more frequent and placental weights were lower in cases with basal plate myometrial fibers. In 35 of the 44 cases (80%) a focus of basal myometrial fibers was adjacent to a basal spiral vessel; in 20 of the 35 foci (57%) the spiral artery lacked physiologic changes, and two additional foci showed thrombosed uteroplacental vessels. Therefore in 63% of foci of basal plate

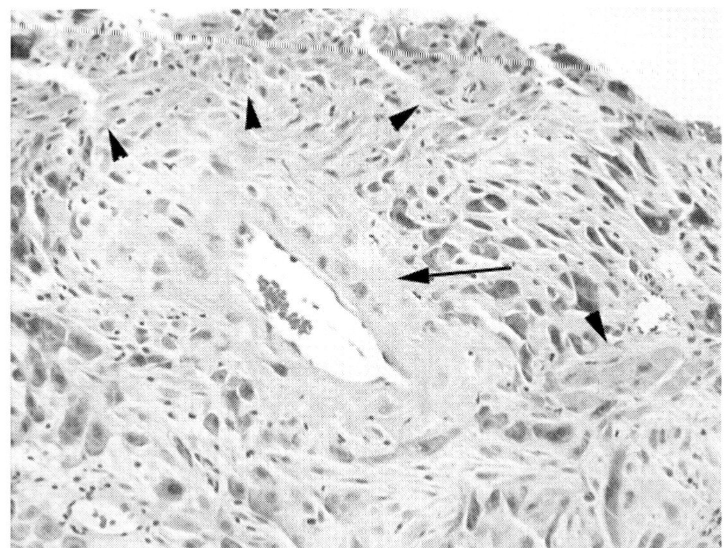

Figure 8–12. Basal plate, preterm delivery. Note myometrial fibers *(arrowheads)* and uteroplacental vessel with normal physiologic conversion but apparent reduced lumen caliber *(arrow)*. Several interstitial trophoblasts are nearby in the decidual stroma. (H & E, ×4.)

myometrial fibers the adjacent basal plate vessel was abnormal. The distribution of basal plate myometrial fibers did not differ among the different causes of preterm delivery represented in the study population (premature rupture of the fetal membranes, preterm labor, preeclampsia, and nonhypertensive abruption). Experimental models have suggested that hypoxia is a cytotrophoblast mitogen[113] and also a tropic factor for cytotrophoblast migration.[114] Zhou and associates [115] have speculated that local uterine hypoxia may stimulate deeper myometrial invasion. We hypothesize that our foci of basal plate myometrial fibers, the majority of which were adjacent to pathologic uteroplacental vessels, represent local abnormalities of depth of cytotrophoblast invasion. Qureshi and co-workers[116] have described this lesion as a minimal form of placenta accreta.

REFERENCES

1. Salafia CM, Starzyk KA, Pezzullo JC, et al: Quantitative differences in arterial morphometry define the placental bed in preeclampsia. Hum Pathol 28:353, 1997.
2. Robertson WB, Manning PJ: Elastic tissue in uterine blood vessels. J Pathol 112:237, 1974.
3. Harris JWS, Ramsey EM: The morphology of human uteroplacental vasculature. Contrib Embryol Carneg Inst 38:43, 1966.
4. Pijnenborg R, Dixon G, Robertson WB, Brosens I: Trophoblastic invasion of human decidua from 8 to 18 weeks of pregnancy. Placenta 1:3–19, 1980.
5. Pijnenborg R, Bland JM, Robertson WB, Brosens I: Uteroplacental arterial changes related to interstitial trophoblast migration in early human pregnancy. Placenta 4:397, 1983.
6. Brosens I, Robertson WB, Dixon HG: The physiological response of the vessels of the placental bed to normal pregnancy. J Pathol Bacteriol 93:569, 1967.
7. Matijevic R, Meekins JW, McFadyen IR, Pijnenborg R: Physiological changes of spiral arteries and blood flow in the placental bed during early pregnancy. Contemp Rev Obstet Gynaecol 8:127, 1996.
8. Boyd JD, Hamilton WJ: Somite stages: the decidua capsularis. In The human placenta. Cambridge, 1970, W Heffer & Sons.
9. Brosens I: The utero-placental vessels at term—the distribution and extent of the physiological changes. Trophoblast Res 3:61, 1988.
10. Loke YW, Butterworth BH: Heterogeneity of human trophoblast populations. In Gill TJ III, Wegmann TG, Nisbet-Brown E (eds): Immunoregulation and fetal survival. Cambridge, 1987, Oxford University Press, p 197.
11. Blankenship TN, Enders AC, King BF: Trophoblastic invasion and modification of uterine veins during placental development in macaques. Cell Tissue Res 274:135, 1993.
12. Pijnenborg R: The placental bed: reflections on the physical forces that direct endovascular trophoblast migration. (In Press).
13. Khong TY, Liddell HS, Robertson WB: Defective hemochorial placentation as a cause of miscarriage: a preliminary study. Br J Obstet Gynaecol 94:649, 1987.
14. Salafia CM, Ernst L, Pezzullo JC, et al: The very low birth weight infant: maternal complications leading to preterm birth, placental lesions, and intrauterine growth. Am J Perinatol 12:106, 1995.
15. Naeye RL: Pregnancy hypertension, placental evidences of low uteroplacental blood flow, and spontaneous premature delivery. Hum Pathol 20:441, 1989.
16. Arias F, Rodriquez L, Rayne SC, Kraus FT: Maternal placental vasculopathy and infection: two distinct subgroups among patients with preterm labor and preterm ruptured membranes. Am J Obstet Gynecol 168:585, 1993.
17. Brosens I, Robertson WB, Dixon HG: The role of the spiral arteries in the pathogenesis of preeclampsia. In Wynn RM (ed): Obstetrics and gynecology annual 1. New York, 1972, Appleton-Century-Crofts, p 177.
18. Robertson WB, Brosens I, Dixon G: Uteroplacental vascular pathology. Eur J Obstet Gynecol Reprod Biol 5:47, 1975.
19. Robertson WB: Discussion: pathology of the uteroplacental bed. In Sharpe F, Symonds EM (eds): Hypertension in pregnancy. New York, 1987, Perinatology Press, p 115.
20. Pijnenborg R: The human decidua as a passageway for trophoblast invasion. Trophoblast Res. (In Press, 1998).
21. Khong TY, De Wolf F, Robertson WB, et al: Inadequate maternal vascular response to placentation in pregnancies complicated by preeclampsia and by small-for-gestational age infants. Br J Obstet Gynaecol 93:1049, 1986.
22. Robertson WB, Brosens I, Dixon HG: The pathological response of the vessels of the placental bed to hypertensive pregnancy. J Pathol Bacteriol 93:581, 1967.
23. Meekins JW, Pijnenborg R, Hanssens M, et al: A

study of placental bed spiral arteries and trophoblast invasion in normal and severe preeclamptic pregnancies using histological and immunohistochemical techniques. Br J Obstet Gynaecol 101:669, 1994.

24. McFadyen IR, Price AB, Geirsson RT: The relation of birthweight to histological appearances in vessels of the placental bed. Br J Obstet Gynaecol 93:476, 1986.
25. Brosens I, Renaer M: On the pathogenesis of placental infarcts in preeclampsia. J Obstet Gynaecol Br Commonw 79:794, 1972.
26. Pijnenborg R, Anthony J, Davey DA, et al: Placental bed spiral arteries in the hypertensive disorders of pregnancy. Br J Obstet Gynaecol 98:648, 1991.
27. Sheppard BL, Bonnar J: The ultrastructure of the arterial supply of the human placenta in pregnancy complicated by fetal growth retardation. Br J Obstet Gynaecol 83:948, 1976.
28. Brosens IA, Robertson WB, Dixon HG: Fetal growth retardation and the arteries of the placental bed. Br J Obstet Gynaecol 84:656, 1977.
29. DeWolf F, Brosens I, Renaer M: Fetal growth retardation and the maternal arterial supply of the human placenta in the absence of sustained hypertension. Br J Obstet Gynaecol 87:678, 1980.
30. Pijnenborg R, Bland JM, Robertson WB, et al: The pattern of interstitial trophoblastic invasion of the myometrium in early pregnancy. Placenta 2:303, 1981.
31. Aplin JD, Charlton AK, Ayad S: An immunohistochemical study of human endometrial extracellular matrix during the menstrual cycle and first trimester of pregnancy. Cell Tissue Res 253:231, 1988.
32. Ballegeer V, Spitz B, Kieckens L, et al: Predictive value of increased plasma levels of fibronectin in gestational hypertension. Am J Obstet Gynecol 161:432, 1989.
33. Lazarchick J, Stubbs TM, Romein L, et al: Predictive value of fibronectin levels in normotensive gravid women destined to become preeclamptic. Am J Obstet Gynecol 154:1050, 1986.
34. Lockwood CJ, Peters JH: Increased plasma levels of $ED1^+$ cellular fibronectin precede the clinical signs of preeclampsia. Am J Obstet Gynecol 162:358, 1990.
35. Ulloa-Aguirre A, August AM, Golos TG, et al: 8-Bromo-adenosine 3′,5′-monophosphate regulates expression of chorionic gonadotropin and fibronectin in human cytotrophoblasts. J Clin Endocr Metab 64:1002, 1987.
36. Pijnenborg R, Vercruysse L, Ballegeer V, et al: The distribution of fibronectin in the placental bed in normotensive and hypertensive human pregnancies. Trophoblast Res 6:343, 1992.
37. Aplin JD: Expression of integrin $\alpha_6\beta_4$ in human trophoblast and its loss from extravillous cells. Placenta 14:203, 1993.
38. Damsky CH, Fitzgerald ML, Fisher SJ: Distribution patterns of extracellular matrix components and adhesion receptors are intricately modulated during first trimester cytotrophoblast differentiation along the invasive pathway, in vivo. J Clin Invest 89:210, 1992.
39. Zhou Y, Damsky CH, Chiu K, et al: Preeclampsia is associated with abnormal expression of adhesion molecules by invasive cytotrophoblasts. J Clin Invest 91:950, 1993.
40. Divers MJ, Bulmer JN, Miller D, Lilford RF: Beta 1 integrins in third trimester human placentae no differential expression in pathological pregnancy. Placenta 16:245, 1995.
41. Pijnenborg R, Luyten C, Vercruysse L, et al: Attachment and differentiation in vitro of trophoblast from normal and preeclamptic human pregnancies. Am J Obstet Gynecol 175:30, 1996.
42. Bischof P, Martelli M: Proteolysis in the penetration phase of the implantation process. Placenta 13:17, 1992.
43. Lala PK, Hamilton GS: Growth factors, proteases and protease inhibitors in the maternal-fetal dialogue. Placenta 17:545, 1996.
44. Moll UM, Lane BL: Proteolytic activity of first trimester human placenta: localization of interstitial collagenase in villous and extravillous trophoblast. Histochemistry 94:555, 1990.
45. Nawrocki B, Polette M, Marchand V, et al: Membrane-type matrix metalloproteinase-1 expression at the site of human placentation. Placenta 17:565, 1996.
46. Polette M, Nawrocki B, Pintiaux A, et al: Expression of gelatinases A and B and their tissue inhibitors by cells of early and term human placenta and gestational endometrium. Lab Invest 71:838, 1994.
47. Graham CH, McCrae KR: Altered expression of gelatinase and surface-associated plasminogen activator activity by trophoblast cells isolated from placentas of preeclamptic patients. Am J Obstet Gynecol 175:555, 1996.
48. Chen HL, Yang Y, Hu XL, et al: Tumor necrosis factor alpha mRNA and protein are present in human placental and uterine cells at early and late stages of gestation. Am J Pathol 139:327, 1991.
49. Hofmann GE, Horowitz G, Scott RT Jr, et al: Transforming growth factor α in human implan-

tation trophoblast: immunohistochemical evidence for autocrine/paracrine function. J Clin Endocr Metab 76:781, 1993.

50. Simon C, Frances A, Piquette G, et al: Interleukin-1 system in the maternotrophoblast unit in human implantation: immunohistochemical evidence for autocrine/paracrine function. J Clin Endocr Metab 78:847, 1994.
51. Selick CE, Horowitz GM, Gratch M, et al: Immunohistochemical localization of transforming growth factor-beta in human implantation sites. J Clin Endocr Metab 78:592, 1994.
52. Lysiak JJ, Hunt J, Pringle GA, et al: Localization of transforming growth factor β and its natural inhibitor decorin in the human placenta and decidua throughout gestation. Placenta 16:221, 1995.
53. Jokhi PP, Chumbley G, King A, et al: Expression of the colony stimulating factor 1 receptor (c-fms product) by cells at the human uteroplacental interface. Lab Invest 68:308, 1993.
54. Jokhi PP, King A, Loke YW: Reciprocal expression of epidermal growth factor receptor (EGF-R) and c-erbB2 by non-invasive and invasive human trophoblast populations. Cytokine 6:433, 1994.
55. Hara N, Fujii T, Okai T, et al: Histochemical demonstration of interleukin-2 in decidual cells of patients with preeclampsia. Am J Reprod Immunol 34:44, 1995.
56. Keith JC Jr, Pijnenborg R, Spitz B, et al: Assessment of differential serum cytotoxicity in gestational hypertension using a fibrosarcoma cell line and the MTT assay. Hypertens Pregnancy 14:81, 1995.
57. Keith JC Jr, Rowles TK, Dilorenzo K, et al: Preeclampsia. J Perinatol 13:417, 1993.
58. Meekins JW, McLaughlin PJ, West DC, et al: Endothelial cell activation by tumour necrosis factor-alpha (TNF-α) and the development of preeclampsia. Clin Exp Immunol 98:110, 1994.
59. Visser W, Beckmann I, Bremer HA, et al: Bioactive tumor necrosis factor-α in preeclamptic patients with and without the HELLP syndrome. Br J Obstet Gynaecol 101:1081, 1994.
60. Pijnenborg R, McLaughlin PJ, Vercruysse L, et al: Immunolocalization of tumor necrosis factor-α (TNF-α) in the placental bed of normotensive and hypertensive human pregnancies. Unpublished.
61. Hunt JS, Chen HL, Miller L: Tumor necrosis factors: pivotal components of pregnancy? Biol Reprod 54:554, 1996.
62. Khong TY, Chambers HM: Alternative methods of sampling placentas for the assessment of uteroplacental vasculature. J Clin Pathol 45:925, 1992.
63. Cusick W, Salafia CM, Ernst L, et al: Low dose aspirin therapy and placental pathology in women with poor prior pregnancy outcomes. Am J Reprod Immunol 34:141, 1995.
64. Trudinger BJ, Giles WB, Cook CM: Uteroplacental blood flow velocity–time waveforms in normal and complicated pregnancy. Br J Obstet Gynaecol 92:39, 1985.
65. Lunell NO, Lewander R, Mamoun I, et al: Uteroplacental blood flow in pregnancy induced hypertension. Scand J Clin Lab Invest Suppl 169:1984.
66. Redline RW, Patterson P: Pre-eclampsia is associated with an excess of proliferative immature intermediate trophoblast. Hum Pathol 26:594, 1995.
67. Salafia CM, Starzyk KA, Lage JM, et al: Lipoprotein(a) deposition in the uteroplacental bed and in basal plate uteroplacental arteries: atherosclerosis-associated processes in normal and complicated pregnancies. Trophoblast Res. (In Press, 1998).
68. Bukovsky A, Labarrere CA, Haag B, et al: Tissue factor in normal and transplanted human kidneys. Transplant 54:644, 1992.
69. Torry RJ, Labarrere CA, Gargiulo P, Faulk WP: Natural anticoagulant and fibrinolytic pathways in renal allograft failure. Transplant 58(8):926, 1994.
70. Silver RK, Peaceman AM, Adams DM: Understanding prostaglandin metabolites and platelet-activating factor in the pathophysiology and treatment of the antiphospholipid syndrome. Clin Perinatol 22:357, 1995.
71. Wallenburg HC: Low-dose aspirin therapy in obstetrics. Curr Opin Obstet Gynecol 7:135, 1995.
72. DeWolf F, Carreras LO, Moerman P, et al: Decidual vasculopathy and extensive placental infarction in a patient with repeated thromboembolic accidents, recurrent fetal, and a lupus anticoagulant. Am J Obstet Gynecol 142:829, 1982.
73. Khong TY, Sawyer IH, Heryet AR: An immunohistologic study of endothelialization of uteroplacental vessels in human pregnancy—Evidence that endothelium is focally disrupted by trophoblast in preeclampsia. Am J Obstet Gynecol 167:751, 1992.
74. Salafia CM, Minior VK, Pezzullo JC, et al: Intrauterine growth retardation in infants of less than 32 weeks gestational age: associated placental pathology. Am J Obstet Gynecol 173:1049, 1995.
75. Bowie EJW: Lipid-related clotting reactions of clinical significance. Arch Pathol Lab Med 116:1345, 1992.
76. Berg K, Roald B, Sande H: High Lp(a) lipoprotein level in maternal serum may interfere with placental circulation and cause fetal growth retardation. Clin Genet 46:52, 1994.
77. Meekens JW, Pijnenborg R, Hanssens M, et al:

Immunohistochemical detection of lipoprotein(a) in the wall of placental bed spiral arteries in normal and severe preeclamptic pregnancies. Placenta 15:511, 1991.

78. Ross R: The pathogenesis of atherosclerosis—an update. N Engl J Med 314:488, 1986.
79. Rabbani LE, Loscalzo J: Recent observations of the role of hemostatic determinants in the development of the atheromatous plaque. Atherosclerosis 105:1, 1994.
80. Redman CWG: Current topic: preeclampsia and the placenta. Placenta 12:301, 1991.
81. Andrew A, Bulmer JN, Morrison L, et al: Subinvolution of the uteroplacental arteries: an immunohistochemical study. Int J Gynecol Pathol 12:28, 1993.
82. Dekker GA, de Vries JIP, Doelitzsh PM, et al: Underlying disorders associated with severe early onset preeclampsia. Am J Obstet Gynecol 173:1042, 1995.
83. Harpel PC, Borth W: Fibrin, lipoprotein(a), plasmin interactions: a model linking thrombosis and atherogenesis. Ann NY Acad Sci 233, 1992.
84. Hustin J, Schaaps, JP: Echographic and anatomic studies of the maternotrophoblastic border during the first trimester of pregnancy. Am J Obstet Gynecol 157:162, 1987.
85. Hustin J, Schaaps JP, Lambotte R: Anatomical studies of the uteroplacental vascularization in the first trimester of pregnancy. Trophoblast Res 3:49, 1988.
86. Jaffe R: Investigation of abnormal first-trimester gestations by color Doppler imaging. J Clin Ultrasound 21:521, 1993.
87. Moll W: Invited commentary: absence of intervillous blood flow in the first trimester of human pregnancy. Placenta 16:333, 1995.
88. Karimu AL, Burton GJ: Significance of changes in fetal perfusion pressure to factors controlling angiogenesis in the human term placenta. J Reprod Fertil 102:447, 1994.
89. Dommisse J, Tiltman AJ: Placental bed biopsies in placental abruption. Br J Obstet Gynaecol 99:651, 1992.
90. Harris BA: Peripheral placental separation: a review. Obstet Gynecol 43:577, 1988.
91. Wigglesworth S, Singer DB: Textbook of fetal and perinatal pathology. Cambridge, Mass, 1991, Blackwell Scientific Publications.
92. Mooney EE, al Shunnar A, O'Regan M, et al: Chorionic villous haemorrhage is associated with retroplacental haemorrhage. Br J Obstet Gynaecol 101:965, 1994.
93. Batcup G, Tovey LAD, Longster G: Fetomaternal blood group incompatibility studies in placental intervillous thrombosis. Placenta 4:449,1983.
94. Giles WB, Trudinger BJ, Baird PJ: Fetal umbilical artery flow velocity waveforms and placental resistance: pathological correlation. Br J Obstet Gynaecol 92:31, 1985.
95. Los FJ, DeWolf BT, Huisjes HJ: Raised maternal serum-alpha fetoprotein levels and spontaneous fetomaternal transfusion. Lancet 1210, 1979.
96. Myers RA, Fujikura T: Placental changes after experimental abruptio placentae and fetal vessel ligation of rhesus monkey placenta. Am J Obstet Gynecol 100:846, 1968.
97. Groome LJ, Owen J, Neely CL, et al: Oligohydramnios: antepartum fetal urine production and intrapartum fetal distress. Am J Obstet Gynecol 165:1077, 1991.
98. Arabin B, Jimenez E, Vogel M, Weitzel HK: Relationship of utero and fetoplacental blood flow velocity wave forms with pathomorphological placental findings. Fetal Diagn Ther 7:173, 1992.
99. Laurini R, Laurini J, Marsal K: Placental histology and fetal blood flow in intrauterine growth retardation. Acta Obstet Gynecol Scand 73:529, 1994.
100. Read MA, Boura ALA, Walters WAW: Effects of variation in oxygen tension on responses of the human fetoplacental vasculature to vasoactive agents in vitro. Placenta 16:667, 1995.
101. Nelson DM, Swanson PE: Breaks in the syncytial trophoblast layer of human placental villi are due to apoptosis. Placenta 17:387, 1996.
102. Ludwig H, Metzger H: Das uterine Placentarbett post partum in Rasterelektronmikroskop, zugleich ein Beitrag zur Frage der extravasalen Fibrinbildung. Arch Gynecol 210:251, 1971.
103. Labarrere CA, Faulk WP: Anchoring villi in human placental basal plate: lymphocytes, macrophages and coagulation. Placenta 12:173, 1991.
104. Bendon RW, Hommel AB: Maternal floor infarction in autoimmune disease: two cases. Pediatr Pathol Lab Med 16:293, 1996.
105. Frank HG, Malekzadeh F, Kertschanska S, et al: Immunohistochemistry of two different types of placental fibrinoid. Acta Anat 150:55, 1994.
106. Whitelaw PF, Croy BA: Granulated lymphocytes of pregnancy. Placenta 17:533, 1996.
107. Labarrere C, Althabe O, Caletti E, et al: Deficiency of blocking factors in intrauterine growth retardation and its relationship with chronic villitis. Am J Reprod Immunol Microbiol 10:14, 1986.
108. Salafia CM, Maier D, Vogel C, et al: Placental and decidual histology in spontaneous abortion: de-

tailed description and correlations with chromosome number. Obstet Gynecol 82:295, 1993.

109. Erlendsson K, Steinsson K, Johannsson JH, Giersson RT: Relation of antiphospholipid antibody and placental bed inflammatory vascular changes to the outcome of pregnancy in successive pregnancies of 2 women with systemic lupus erythematosus. J Rheumatol 20:1779, 1993.
110. Salafia CM, López-Zeno JA, Sherer DM, et al: Histologic evidence of old intrauterine bleeding is more frequent in prematurity. Am J Obstet Gynecol 173:1065, 1995.
111. Redline RW, Pappin A: Fetal thrombotic vasculopathy: the clinical significance of extensive avascular villi. Hum Pathol 26:80, 1995.
112. Sherer DM, Salafia CM, Minior VK, et al: Histologic evidence of abnormally deep trophoblast invasion: clinical correlations. Obstet Gynecol 87:444, 1996.
113. Fox H: The villous cytotrophoblast as an index of placental ischaemia. J Obstet Gynaecol Br Commonw 71:885, 1967.
114. Tominaga T, Page EW: Accommodation of the human placenta to hypoxia. Am J Obstet Gynecol 94:679, 1966.
115. Zhou Y, Chiu Y, Brescia RJ, et al: Increased depth of trophoblast invasion after chronic constriction of the lower aorta in rhesus monkeys. Am J Obstet Gynecol 169:224, 1993.
116. Jacques SM, Qureshi F, Trent VS, Ramirez NC: Placenta accreta: mild cases diagnosed by placental examination. Int J Gynecol Pathol 15:28, 1996.

9

Placental Pathology and Multiple Gestation

Virginia J. Baldwin

Effective examination of placentas from multiple gestation is not technically difficult, but it does require careful consideration of a number of aspects specific to the multiple conception. For most pathologists the biggest challenge with placentas from multiple gestation is remembering to make all the observations needed for complete evaluation. The reward for the extra time expended can be essential pathoanatomic data that cannot be obtained any other way. Multiple gestations are high-risk pregnancies, and thoughtful and methodical assessment of the placentas can produce information necessary for the interpretation of gestational events and fetal outcome.

This chapter provides a framework for the general pathologist who may not have the opportunity to examine many placentas from multiple gestations. Clinicians who manage and deliver multiple gestations will find information they can use in counseling their patients and guidelines for handling the delivered placenta so the pathologist can provide as much information as possible. The majority of the discussion refers to twin placentas, with a brief section on applying the principles to higher multiples. Readers interested in additional details are referred to more extensive presentations.[1–4]

Pathologic examination of tissues is a Socratic process of question and answer. The questions may relate to clinical events, clinical findings, or clinical outcomes and may be posed by clinicians or patients. There may be questions in the literature from physiologists, biochemists, other basic science researchers, or the clinical medical community at large. The appearance of the tissues may raise questions, and the pathologist may have questions about pathophysiology and clinicopathologic correlations. The most useful answers are possible when clinicians and pathologists have a close and cooperative working relationship, and the patient and medical science also benefit from their collaboration.

A number of steps should be followed to achieve the best answers possible. The specimens must be submitted for examination in the proper fashion and with the proper information. The examination must be undertaken with a thoughtful understanding of the questions being asked and the kinds of information that can be obtained (Table 9–1). The findings have to be correlated with the clinical details to determine the significance. Any outstanding questions or unexplained findings must be coded in such a way as to be accessible for future review.

PRELIMINARY CONSIDERATIONS

Selection of Twin Placentas for Laboratory Examination

In an age of cost containment and outcome analysis, it is a fair question to ask which placentas should be submitted for laboratory examination. Because multiple gestations are a priori high-risk pregnancies, an argument exists for examining all multiple gestation placentas. The only possible exception might be clinically normal, equally grown, unlike-sex, term twins with separate and equally grown placentas. Even in that case, the gross features of the placentas should be recorded in the mother's chart and the placentas should be held for a week before discard in case neonatal or postpartum problems become evident. The placentas should be stored at 4° C instead of frozen.

All placentas from complicated twin pregnancies should be examined in detail in the laboratory.

Table 9–1. Heuristic Method for Effective Pathologic Examination of Placentas from Multiple Gestation

The following questions are designed to help you focus your examination of placentas from multiple gestations, and they are in an approximate order of consideration. Especially important are comparisons between the placental portions of the infants and determinations of the relationship of these findings to any discordancies of the infants themselves. These questions apply to twins and higher multiples.

1. Do you have the whole specimen, including the umbilical cord, and how do you know?
2. What is the gestational age, and how do you know?
3. What is the mother's reproductive history? If not given, how will you find out?
4. Have any previous relevant specimens from this patient been examined in your laboratory, such as embryos, fetuses, or placentas? Do you need to review them before you examine or complete the current specimen? Have you?
5. Was this a spontaneous or assisted multiple conception. If assisted, how? Were there any interventions during the pregnancy related to the numbers of embryos developing? What do you need to look for in the specimen related to that information?
6. What were the significant general medical or obstetrical clinical events during the pregnancy, such as maternal illness, vaginal bleeding, hypertension, or drug exposure, and what should you be looking for in the specimen that might reflect that history?
7. What were the results of antenatal investigations, such as ultrasound examinations, Doppler studies, amniocenteses, and cordocenteses? Can you relate the results to the indicated birth order of the infants? If not, what do you need to do to be able to do so? What do you need to look for in the specimen to provide quality control follow-up of the results?
8. Were there any complications of the pregnancy related to the multiple nature of the gestation? What was done about them? Were interventions such as decompression amniocentesis or feticide used? What do you need to look for in the specimen related to these procedures?
9. What was the course of labor and delivery? Were there any events that might suggest a search for specific placental findings?
10. What was the sex, birthweight, and condition of each infant at birth? Is there any other neonatal information you need about the infants? If that information is not provided, what do you need to do to get it? Have you? Can you relate that information to the birth order of the infants? If not, what do you need to do to be able to do so? Have you? What do you need to look for in the placenta to explain any discordancies?
11. What is the overall pattern of the placentation: number of disks, patterns of membranes, location and nature of septum, and so on? How does this relate to the reported sex of the infants regarding zygosity determination?
12. Which cord belongs to which infant? How do you know? How will you identify them if they have not been marked or have been marked but not assigned. *This is **very** important!*
13. How appropriately developed, by linear measurement of the cord and weight of the fresh trimmed placenta(s), is the specimen for the gestational age and size of the infants? How did you assess that?
14. How do the placental portions for each infant compare in volume? How did you assess that? How does that relate to the development of the respective infants? How do you explain your findings?
15. Are there any special procedures, such as taking specimens for microbiology, cytogenetics, electron microscopy, or metabolic studies, that you should do before sectioning the tissues? How did you decide what to do? What are the results? What do they mean?
16. Should the specimen be photographed before dissection? Why? What do you want to show?
17. Should the placenta be injected to identify fetofetal anastomoses? How have you decided that? How will you do it? How will you record your findings? How will you interpret your results?
18. How will you label the placenta to display the results of your injection studies to best advantage in a photograph? Would a diagram be better? How will you draw it as you go along?
19. How far apart are the umbilical cord insertions? Do the insertion patterns differ? In what way? What does that mean? Are there any abnormalities of the umbilical cords that could have affected fetal perfusion? How extensive? How significant do you think it was? How did you decide?
20. Is there any abnormality of the reflected membranes or their attachment that can be related to clinical events or neonatal findings, and what were your criteria?
21. What is the pattern of attachment of the septal walls between the infants? What are the components of each septum? How have you decided that?
22. How would you describe the respective chorionic vascular territories? How do you explain any differences? Have you identified any anastomoses? How? What is the significance of your findings?
23. Are there any differences in the appearance of the maternal surfaces of each infant's portion of the placenta? How do you explain your findings? Is the surface fragmented? If so, why? How are you assessing possible causes?
24. How does the appearance of serial sections of the parenchyma compare to the norm for age? What focal lesions are there? How extensive are the changes, if any? How does the parenchyma of each infant compare? What are the differences? How extensive are they? How do you interpret your findings? Should the slices be photographed? If so, what are you planning to show?
25. What sections do you submit for microscopy, and why? How will you assess the intertwin septa? Do you need to use any special stains? What for?
26. What are the microscopic findings? How does villous maturity compare to the norm for age? How do you assess villous abnormalities, and how do you explain them? Are there any microscopic differences between the portions from each infant? How do you explain them? How important are they?
27. How do you correlate your findings with the clinical course of the pregnancy, the results of special procedures, and the specifics of each infant?
28. Do you need to talk to the maternal or neonatal clinician? Why? What does that add to your interpretation?
29. What additional reading or literature review is needed for final clinicopathologic interpretation? Who will do it? When?

Table 9–1. Heuristic Method for Effective Pathologic Examination of Placentas from Multiple Gestation ***Continued***

30. How will you report your findings? To whom? When?
31. Do your interpretations have significance for the further counseling or management of the infants or the family? What? What are you doing about it?
32. How will you code your findings for future retrieval?
33. Is this a case for permanent storage of blocks or selected wet tissues? Why?
34. Are there any teaching aspects of the case? How do you plan to make use of them?
35. Is the case worth reporting to colleagues, either on its own or as part of a broader review? Why? Who will do it? When?

When one or more of the fetuses of a multiple gestation is stillborn, the following questions may be helpful:

- What evidence exists on the placenta for the mode of fetal death? What are your criteria?
- What evidence for the timing of fetal death is on the placenta? What are your criteria? Can you differentiate timing of fetal death if more than one fetus died in utero?
- Should the placenta and fetus be photographed together? What do you want to show?
- How do you relate microscopic findings to the clinical interval of fetal death and possible contribution to fetal death? What are your criteria?
- Do the placental findings relate to the cause of fetal death? How? What is the sequence and mechanism? If two or more of the fetuses are stillborn, do your placental findings suggest a relationship of the deaths? If so, what, and what is your evidence for that?
- Do your findings suggest an explanation for possible fetal or neonatal complications in a surviving multiple? What?

If the twins have survived, the placentas are processed as routine surgical specimens. If one or both of the twins have died, either before or around the time of delivery, the placenta is examined as part of the autopsy. If one or both twins die after the placenta has been prosected, the placental details are located and included in the autopsy report and interpretation. If no autopsy is performed on the deceased twins, the placenta is processed with as much information about the twins as possible.

Preparation for Sending Placentas to Laboratory

All twin placentas must be sent to the laboratory with the cords clearly identified as to twin of origin. Identification must be done by the delivery physician in the delivery room and can be marked with sutures, clamps, safety pins, or whatever method is convenient. There must be some notation on the specimen or the requisition as to what the cord identifiers indicate. The pathologist can make some observations that suggest the birth order, but the only certain identification is at the time of delivery. Without clear identification of the portions of the placenta, any pathologic condition noted cannot be properly assigned to the affected twin and clinicopathologic interpretation is incomplete. Identification may have medicolegal implications as well.

All twin placentas should be sent to the laboratory without fixative. This requires more care in handling, but fresh tissues are essential for many of the examinations that may be needed depending on the nature of the problems in the individual case. Specifically, cytogenetic, microbiologic, and vascular injection studies are impossible in fixed placentas. However, some information can still be obtained relevant to zygosity and morphology, so examination of fixed placentas is better than no examination at all.

All twin placentas must be accompanied by a completely filled-out requisition that includes particularly the sex of the twins and their birth weights, in addition to the usual information about the pregnancy, labor and delivery, and neonatal outcome. Results of prenatal investigations such as ultrasound findings and cytogenetic studies may be helpful as well. When correlating pathology findings with prenatal findings the pathologist must keep in mind that birth order does not necessarily coincide with recorded order of fetal presentation in utero with ultrasound. The pathologist may need to review this with the ultrasonographer depending on the findings.

Information to be Obtained from the Pathologist's Examination of Twin Placentas

Three main categories of findings are obtainable from twin placentas: patterns of placentation and zygosity assessment, lesions of monochorionic placentation, and distribution patterns of singleton lesions.

The patterns of placentation, specifically the number of disks and the nature of the intertwin septum, may have significance for zygosity determination. In addition, discordant variations in the pattern of placentation for each twin, such as anomalies of the umbilical cord, may have clinical significance with discordant growth or development of the twins.

The majority of clinical complications in twin pregnancies occur when the pattern of placentation is monochorionic (i.e., a common outer layer with one or two inner sacs). This is the group of twins with the highest rate of all the complications, including malformations, morbidity, and mortality. Careful examination of these placentas may be the only source of information about complex clinical events during pregnancy.

All the lesions described elsewhere in this volume, as identified in singleton placentas, can be seen in the placentas from multiple pregnancy, and they look the same grossly and microscopically. The key observation to be made when they are found in twin placentas is the relative distribution in the two placental portions. In twin placentas the two portions must not only be analyzed as individual units but also compared and contrasted, and the findings correlated with the history and clinical situation of each twin.

The information obtained from examination of twin placentas may be needed in a number of situations. The report of the placental examination becomes part of the maternal record *and* part of the record of *each* twin. The placental findings may be a key part of discussions at morbidity and mortality rounds, and the information is incorporated into any autopsy examination and interpretation of deceased twins. The well-documented report of placental findings in twins may play an important role in settling disputes over the quality of obstetric care.

EXAMINATION

Twin placentas are readily examined with little additional special equipment as part of the routine processing of singleton placentas. The extra time required for prosecting twin placentas can be fitted into the daily schedule of placenta cutting.

Facilities and Equipment

As in all placenta prosection stations, blood precautions are required and using a cutting surface by a sink is preferable. An overhead light with a magnifying lens is often helpful, and a nearby photography setup is valuable. The following equipment and tools are all that is needed for most cases:

- Sharp medium-length straight scissors
- Medium-sized nontoothed forceps
- Scalpel with #22 blade
- Long bladed sharp knife
- Long metal ruler
- Direct weight scale with a dish, such as a metal pie plate, large enough for a placenta
- 50 ml syringe and #20, #18, and #25 needles

Specific cases require x-ray facilities such as a small countertop unit, cytogenetics culture materials, microbiology specimen containers, electron microscopy fixative, and deep-freeze containers.

Hands-free dictation systems facilitate recording of findings as the specimens are prosected, and taking of fresh blocks of tissue is feasible for most cases. The routine blocks taken on our service are described with the prosection details discussed below, and the slides are routinely stained with hematoxylin and eosin. Portions of the placenta, appropriately identified as to twin of origin, should be saved in formalin until the case is signed out or should be saved permanently, depending on the case and the storage facilities of the individual laboratory.

Procedure

Twin placentas can consist of two separate disks and gestational sacs, two distinct disks with shared or overlapping sac membranes, creating a distinct shared septum, or one disk with various membrane patterns (Fig. 9–1). The pathologist should take a few moments to orient the placenta, determine the pattern, and clarify the identification of the umbilical cords. This information should be part of the initial description in the pathology report.

If the placenta consists of *two separate disks,* each with its own cord and membranes, each can be processed in turn, usually in order of birth. Each placenta should be examined in the way a singleton placenta would be, as detailed in the initial chapters in this text, with attention to the need to compare and contrast findings in the two portions and correlate them with the size and condition of the twins. Any anomalies of the cords and cord insertions and the relative sizes, weights, and parenchymal appearances of the disks should be recorded. The following routine sections should be taken, with any lesions as additional blocks:

- A: two cross sections of umbilical cord (placental end and fetal end) and a roll of reflected membranes from twin A
- B: specific section of the fetal surface to include several chorionic vessels, and specific section of the maternal surface, from twin A
- C, D, E: three full-thickness blocks of the placental disk, taken randomly but away from the placental margins, from twin A
- F: cord and membranes from twin B
- G: fetal and maternal surfaces from twin B
- H, I, J: full-thickness sections from twin B

When the *disks are separate but have partially fused or overlapping membranes* (Fig. 9–1*A*), the appearance and proportion of overlap are described and a section of a roll of the shared septum is submitted. If the septum is attached on the surface of one of the disks, a section of the attachment site, the so-called T section, is included. These sections can be submitted in block K or as block F between the two sets of blocks (my preference). The rest of the examination is the same as for the completely separate twin portions as in the first situation.

The *single disk or fused placenta* can be oriented on the prosection surface with the first delivered twin's portion on the right. It may take a moment to manipulate (gently) the specimen so that the disk, membranes, and cords are oriented as near as possible to the intrauterine position, but this will clarify the overall arrangement of the specimen and make the subsequent examination easier.

Ascertainment of Birth Order if the Cords Are Not Identified

If the cords are not identified as to twin of origin, or if the cords are marked in some way but the significance of the indicators is not clear, some clues may be found in the specimen. Features in the umbilical cords, in the pattern of membrane rupture, or in the gross appearances of the placentas may be correlated with clinical information to suggest birth order.

If there is a marked discrepancy in the birth weight of the twins and a marked difference in the thickness of the umbilical cords, the thicker cord may belong to the heavier infant. If one twin died in utero, its cord may appear macerated. Clinical observations on the requisition such as a two-vessel cord or other features seen at the time of delivery may help in assigning an unmarked cord.

When the specimen is oriented, the delivery rupture site in the membranes for each twin should be identified. Sometimes it is obvious that one twin was delivered through the reflected membranes of its sac and the other through the inter-twin septum. It is reasonable to suspect that the twin delivered through the septum was the second twin.

If clinical information on the requisition suggests that one twin was meconium stained, might be infected, or had oligohydramnios because of absent urine output, corroborating pathologic evidence in the placenta may help suggest a birth order.

If making an assignment of birth order based on any of these features, the pathologist should include his or her reasoning and interpretation in the report. If a birth order cannot be assigned to the placental portions, an arbitrary assignment should be made for purposes of prosection, and that information recorded in the report.

Examination of the Single-disk Twin Placenta

The single-disk twin placenta is potentially the most complex twin placenta pattern to examine,

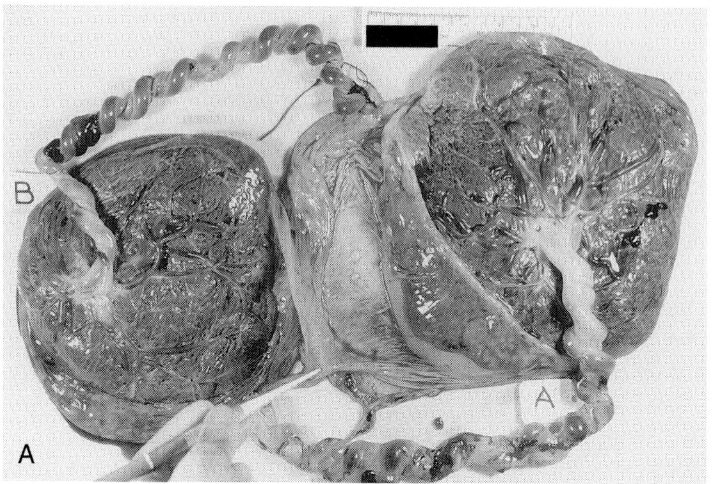

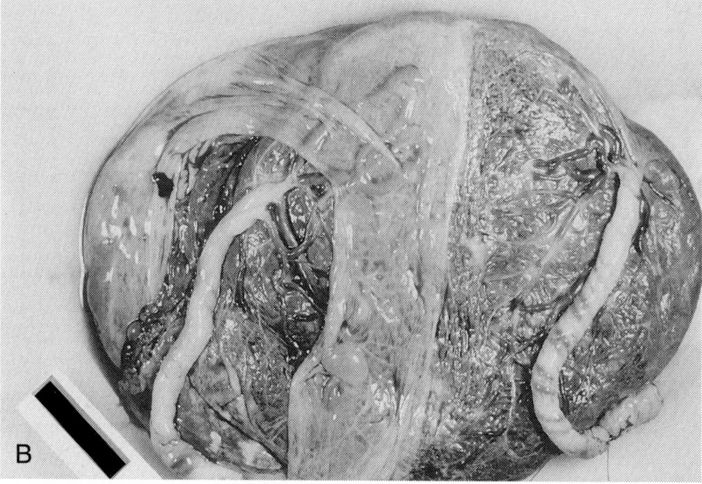

Figure 9–1. Possible patterns of placentation with twins. **A**, Dichorionic diamnionic placentation with separate disks but shared and partially overlapping septal membranes. **B**, Dichorionic diamnionic fused single-disk placenta with septal attachment across the chorionic surface between the circulation territories of each twin.

but a specific order of procedure can help with the details. It is simpler to examine the components from both twins in each segment of the examination in turn, rather than try to do all the observations for one twin and then the other. As the cords and membranes are trimmed off and examination of the disk is begun, the pathologist will need to keep track of which side is which, especially when examining the maternal surface and sectioning the parenchyma. A habitual approach should be followed so that inevitable interruptions do not lead to forgotten data.

Cords and Membranes

First, the pathologist examines the cord of twin A as usual, describing the cord itself and the insertion site, before removing the cord from the placenta and submitting the usual sections. If the insertion is velamentous, the distance from the insertion point in the membranes to the placental margin is noted and the intramembranous vessels are described with comments as to their type, intactness, and final insertion onto the placenta. The insertion may be into the intertwin septum, with vessels passing in the septum to the placental surface. When the septum is dichorionic diamnionic, this is analogous to velamentous insertion and can be described as such, indicating that it is a septal insertion. Next the outer free reflected membranes or chorion laeve of the sac of the same twin is examined in the usual fashion, noting the rupture site if the membranes are not too extensively torn. They are removed to the point of origin of the septum to make the usual membrane roll.

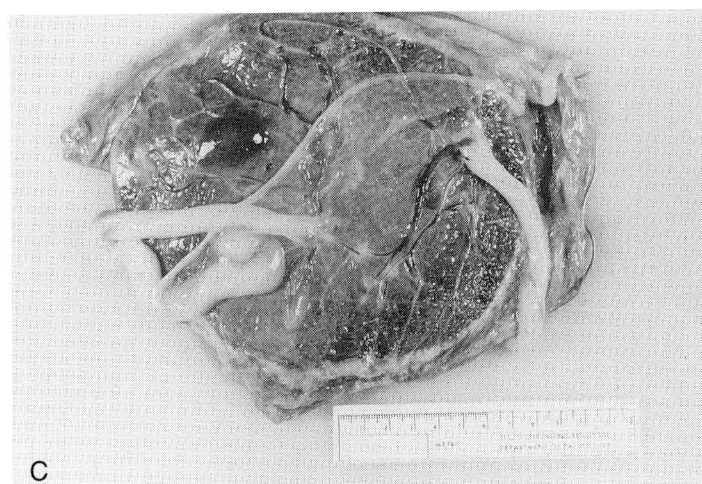

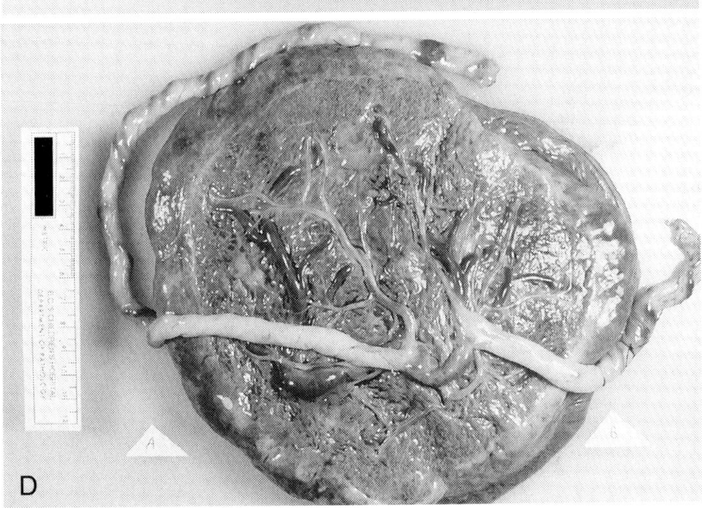

Figure 9–1 *Continued* **C**, Monochorionic diamnionic placenta with more delicate intertwin septum whose orientation can be independent of the vascular pattern of the chorionic surface. **D**, Monochorionic monoamnionic placenta with no septum between the (usually) closely inserted cords.

The cord and membranes of twin B are examined in the same fashion, taking the same sections. The additional observation of the distance between the insertion sites of the two cords is recorded.

The umbilical cord in term twins tends to be about 8 cm shorter than in singletons.[5] Concordance in monochorionic pairs suggests a possible genetic influence on cord length.[6] Interesting observations related to the concept of fetal activity as a factor in cord length include a cluster of unusually long cords[1] and an increased incidence of cords without spiraling.[7]

Septum

Single-disk twin placentas usually have an identifiable wall or septum demarcating the two sides of the disk (Fig. 9–1*B* and *C*). If no septal tissues are found, the fetal surface of the placenta should be examined between the cord insertion sites (Fig. 9–1*D*). The amnionic lining of the gestational sac tends to separate from the underlying chorionic surface more readily in later pregnancy, and it may be completely separated in the delivered third-trimester placenta. An apparent single sac that is actually due to complete separation of the amnion is more common than a truly single sac. However, if the cords insert within a few centimeters of each other and it is certain that the amnion layer is complete and intact between the insertions with no sign of a membrane fold, there is probably a monochorionic monoamniotic pattern of placentation with both twins in the same sac.

The nature of the membrane wall or septum between most twins who share a single placental disk is essential information, based on observations of the thickness and attachment site (Fig. 9–2). This wall may be intact, may contain the delivery opening for the second twin, or may be widely torn. Depending on the pattern of placentation, the septum contains two layers of amnion with varying amounts of interposed chorionic tissue, or two layers of amnion only. In the former, the septum is thick and tends to be opaque (Fig. 9–2*A*). Sometimes four layers can be separated with careful dissection, although this may be difficult if the chorionic layers are thin or have fused. The chorionic component is an extension of the chorionic tissue of the underlying placenta, with the septum firmly anchored to the fetal surface of the disk. There may be a triangular wedge of chorion and fibrin along the attachment, the so-called ultrasound lambda sign.[8] This dichorionic diamniotic pattern of placentation in most cases represents two distinct gestational sacs intimately apposed because of physical proximity during implantation and growth. Therefore the attachment of the septum is also the border between the fetal surfaces of the two placental portions and indicates a zone called the vascular equator between the chorionic circulations of the twins. The diamniotic septum tends to be thin and translucent (Fig. 9–2*B*). Because it contains only the amnionic layers simply reflected from the fetal surface of the disk, it is not actually anchored to the fetal surface and the site of attachment is highly variable. The septum can be lifted from the placental sur-

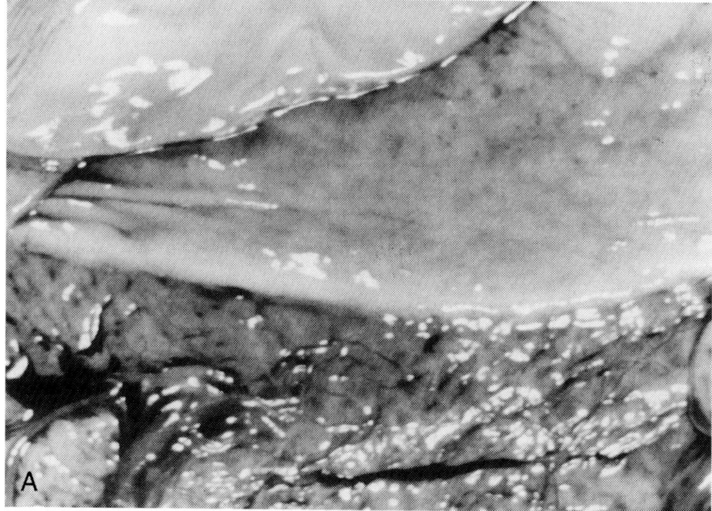

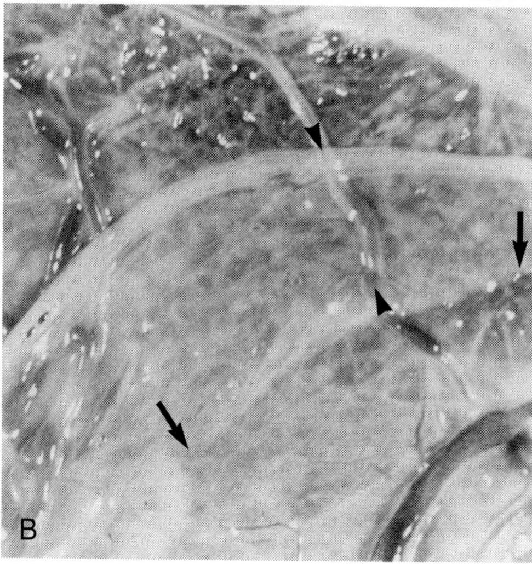

Figure 9–2. Gross appearances of possible intertwin septal membranes. The four-layer dichorionic diamnionic septum is usually opaque and thick (**A**) compared with the two-layer diamnionic septum (**B**) in which the vessel can be followed even through the overlying septal membrane (between *short arrows,* with *long arrows* indicating septal base on chorionic plate).

face and may be oriented at any angle to the vascular equator between the twins' chorionic circulations (Fig. 9–3*A*).

After the details of the septum are described, most of it should be cut off, leaving a small amount on the placental surface. A section of the membrane roll of the septum is then submitted along with a vertical section of the attachment site, which should look like an inverted T.

Chorionic Vessels and Injection Studies

The pattern of the chorionic fetal surface vessels and details of intertwin vascular anastomoses are key observations to record from twin placentas. The borderline or vascular equator is located, and the relative proportion of the fetal surface of the placenta occupied by vessels from each twin is recorded. Unequal vascular development can be a factor in discordant twins and can be observed in all patterns of single-disk twin placentas. The degree of vascularization of each side and the patency of the vessels should be noted. The fetal surface sections should not be taken until injection studies have been completed, if these are indicated.

Intertwin vascular anastomoses are almost universal in monochorionic single-disk twin placentas, probably occur in all cases with no septum, and are present in 90% to 95% of cases with a diamniotic septum. With very rare exceptions anastomoses are not found in single-disk placentas with a chorionic layer in the septum. The individual placenta may contain up to a dozen demonstrable vascular connections (counting a compound anastomosis as one), but 50% of placentas with anastomoses have only one or two connections, and another 25% have three.[1]

Single-connection intertwin vascular anastomoses occur as fetal surface artery-to-artery (arterial) or vein-to-vein (venous) connections or as artery-capillary-vein (arteriovenous or parenchymal) connections, in either direction, via the capillary circulation of the deep villous tissue (Fig. 9–3). There are also complex anastomoses with combinations of connections from a number of small branches from the same terminal vessel, which may have both surface and parenchymal connections (compound). The frequencies of the different types are related to the clinical outcomes, but overall the most common patterns are a combination of arterial and parenchymal anastomoses (25% to 40% of placentas with anastomoses) and only arterial or only parenchymal anastomoses (20% each). Other combinations of the possible connections are seen in less than 10% each.

Possible anastomotic sites should be located by examining the vascular equator between the fetal surface circulations of the twins. Removing the amnionic layer from this region may make it easier to see small connections. In the normal situation, fetal artery and vein branches are paired on the fetal surface, the artery passing above the vein when they cross, and the vessels penetrate the chorionic plate side by side. Possible anastomosing vessels can be found by looking for arteries and veins that are unpaired and apparently heading toward the circulation territory of the other twin. Surface vessel anastomoses, arterial or venous, can be seen relatively easily because the vessels can be followed visually from one cord to the other on the fetal surface (Fig. 9–3*B*). These anastomoses can be confirmed with injection, especially if they are fairly small or part of a compound group. The parenchymal artery-capillary-venous or "third-circulation" connections can be suspected from the surface appearance but must be confirmed with injection. These connections are suggested by finding an unpaired artery from one twin that penetrates the chorionic plate within a few millimeters of a penetrating unpaired vein from the other twin (Fig. 9–3*C*).

There are many methods of injecting the chorionic vessels to demonstrate anastomoses, and each has advantages and drawbacks. Research protocols use a number of sophisticated systems, but in a busy surgical pathology laboratory air injection is a satisfactory compromise. Injection is not possible if the placenta has been fixed in formalin, and problems may occur if the placenta has been fragmented during delivery. In the latter case the pathologist can only record the visible surface connections and indicate suspect but unproven deep connections.

When a potential anastomotic site is located, a 50 ml syringe with a needle of appropriate size for the vessel is inserted into the vessel parallel to the fetal surface and near the suspected connection to avoid artifactual filling of nearby branches (Fig.

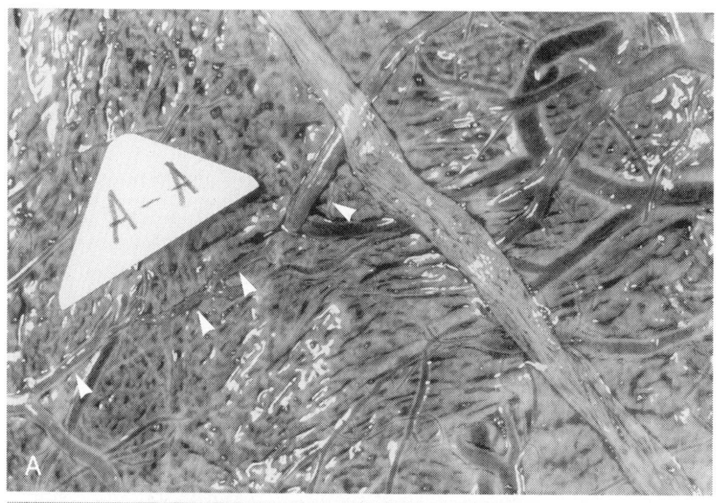

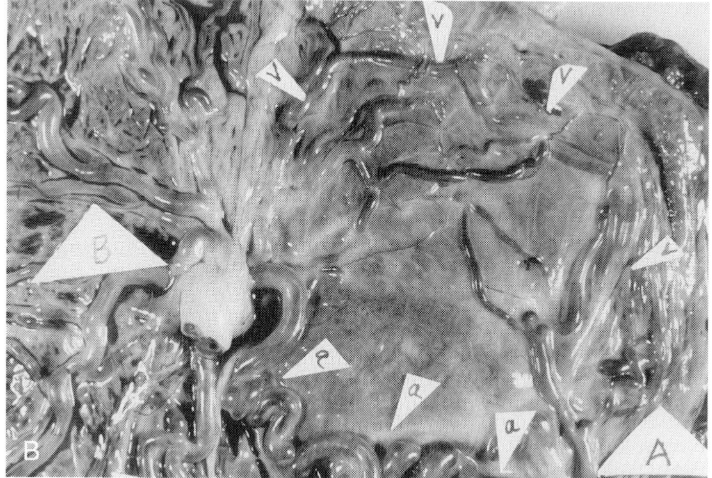

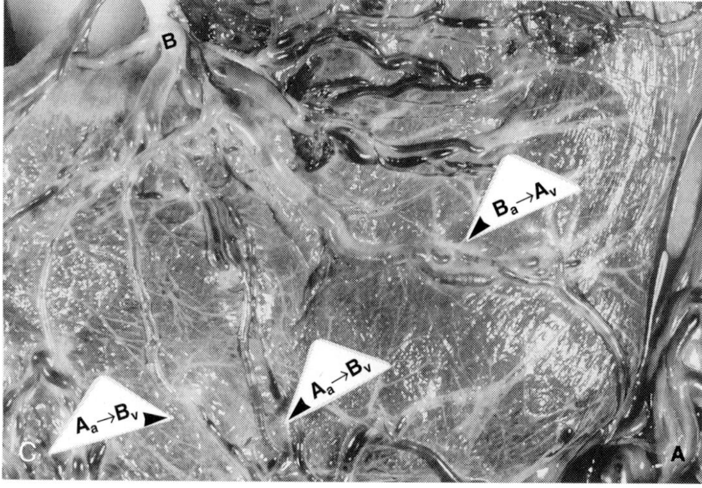

Figure 9–3. Most common patterns of fetofetal chorionic vessel anastomoses in monochorionic placentas. **A**, The artery-to-artery anastomosis *(arrows)* is partially filled with air and can be seen passing under the apparent "attachment" of the diamnionic intertwin septum, here rolled to make its location more visible. This shared vessel also connected with venous branches in both directions in a complex compound pattern. **B**, Tortuous artery-to-artery and vein-to-vein anastomoses are labeled as *a,a,a* and *v,v,v* respectively. **C**, Three parenchymal anastomoses were demonstrated by air injection, two from *A* to *B* and one from *B* to *A*. Note the close proximity of the ends of the vessels in each pair, which is especially easily seen in the left anastomosis.

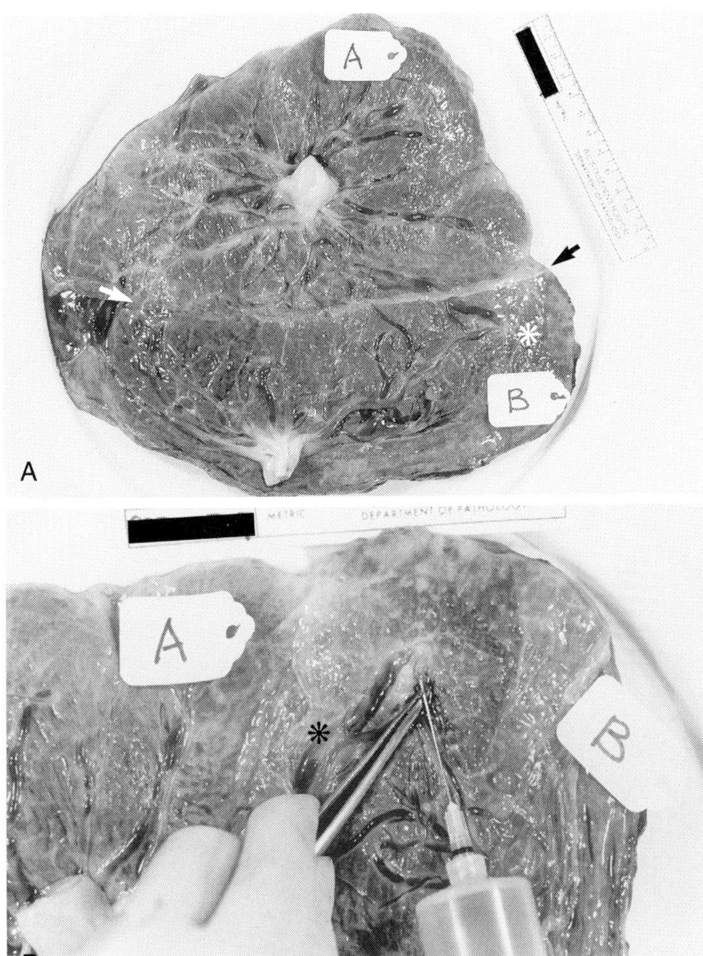

Figure 9–4. Injection technique for the demonstration of parenchymal fetofetal anastomoses. **A**, Overview of the placenta of monochorionic twins. Note the line of "attachment" of the delicate diamnionic septum (between *arrows*), which clearly bears no relation to the vascular equator between the twins' vascular territories. The possible site of a parenchymal anastomosis can be seen just above the label *B (star)*. **B**, The tip of the injection needle has been inserted into the arterial component of the suspect anastomosis, the forceps has blocked return flow in the artery, and air has been injected. The air bubble in the vein *(star)* confirms the parenchymal connection.

9–4). The needle is pointed toward the anastomosis and the vessel behind the needle is blocked with forceps to prevent backflow of air. The injection is made with slow and steady pressure to allow the air to flow through the tissues without rupturing the vessels. The airflow is quickly obvious in surface connections but may take a moment to work through the villous parenchyma and appear in the other surface vessel of deep connections. Parenchymal connections can be demonstrated from either the arterial or the venous side. The size of the vessel connection that can be demonstrated is limited only by the skill of the examiner. The pathologist new to this procedure may find it helpful to practice demonstrating parenchymal connections on singleton placentas, using the normal artery-to-vein anatomy.

The details of any anastomoses identified, including the size and type of vessels involved, are described. The record should indicate the twin of origin for arterial or venous connections of different-sized vessels and for arteries and veins of parenchymal and compound connections. The verbal description can be supplemented with photographs, and in complex cases a line drawing that becomes part of the report may be particularly helpful (Fig. 9–5).

Placental Disk

The overall shape and size of the placental disk are recorded. The maximum diameter, the width at right angles, and the average or range of thick-

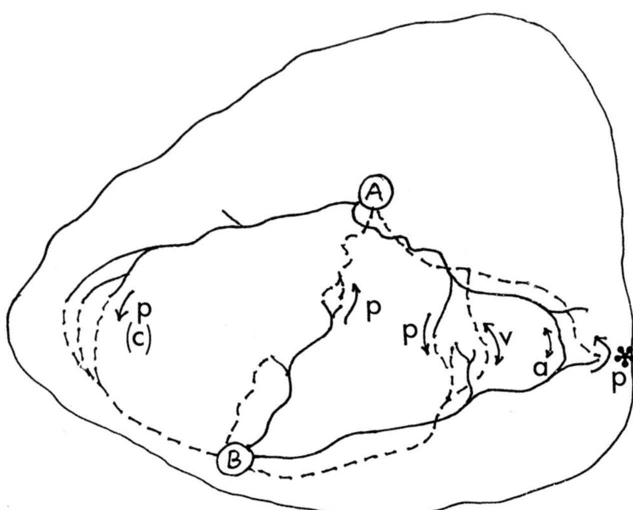

Figure 9–5. Results of injection studies of monochorionic twin placenta. This drawing, copied from the one made at the prosection bench after completion of the injection studies, is of the same placenta shown in Figure 9–4 with the injection site starred. Arteries are indicated with a solid line, veins with a dotted line, and the direction of blood flow with arrows. Such visual documentation of fetofetal anastomoses can become part of the mother's and infants' charts. Even from a rough drawing such as this it is readily apparent that there are two parenchymal anastomoses from *A* to *B,* two from *B* to *A,* and one each surface arterial and venous connection. These twin girls were delivered at 37 weeks. Twin *A* weighed 2300 g, and twin *B* 2600 g, a differential of 11%. The contributing factors are mild asymmetry of chorionic volume, favoring twin *A,* and an unknowable hemodynamic effect of the multiple anastomoses.

ness are measured to the nearest 0.5 cm, and the intact placenta trimmed of cords and membranes is weighed to the nearest 5 g. In markedly asymmetric dichorionic single-disk placentas, the sides of the parenchyma can be separated by cutting through the disk at the line of attachment of the septum, and the respective portions can be weighed separately.

Reported twin placental weights suggest that dichorionic separate placentas grow less well than singletons, with the twin placenta weights at or slightly below the lowest weight in the normal range for gestational age-matched singletons.[9–11]

The respective fetal and maternal surfaces of the placenta are examined in the usual fashion, and the routine sections are taken. The disk is serially sliced at 1 cm intervals from the maternal to the fetal surface, parallel to the axis between the cords if possible. The appearances of the parenchyma is recorded as usual, noting any differences in the appearances of the two portions. Shared cotyledons from parenchymal anastomoses may be evident because the injected air will have forced out the fetal blood, the villous tissue will be pale but normally textured. The size of any such areas should be recorded. The random parenchymal full-thickness sections are taken as usual.

Special Studies

Additional studies may be needed depending on the history and gross findings. Many of these are the same as encountered with examination of singleton placentas and are done for the same reasons and with the same techniques. These studies include subamniotic bacterial cultures and parenchymal viral cultures, amnion and chorion for cytogenetics, amnion and villous tissue for electron microscopy, and villous tissue for metabolic analysis. The possible role of confined placental mosaicism in growth-restricted twins has not been assessed and could be considered, especially with dichorionic twins.

X-ray examination of twin placentas is indicated when there is a history of early gestational

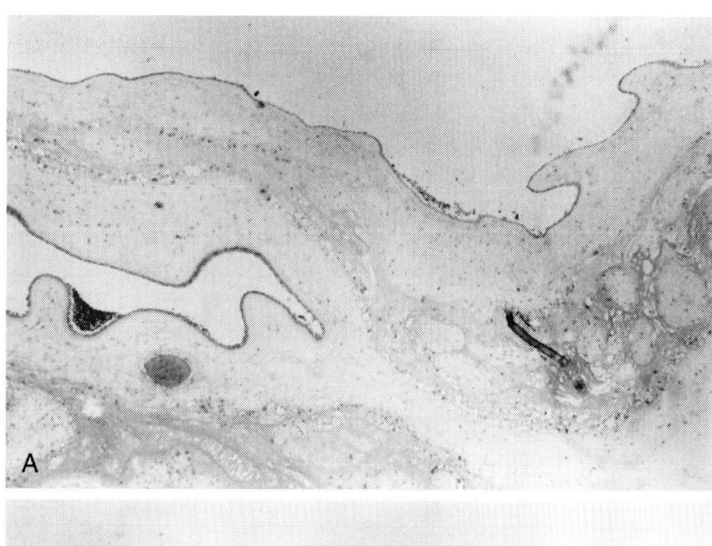

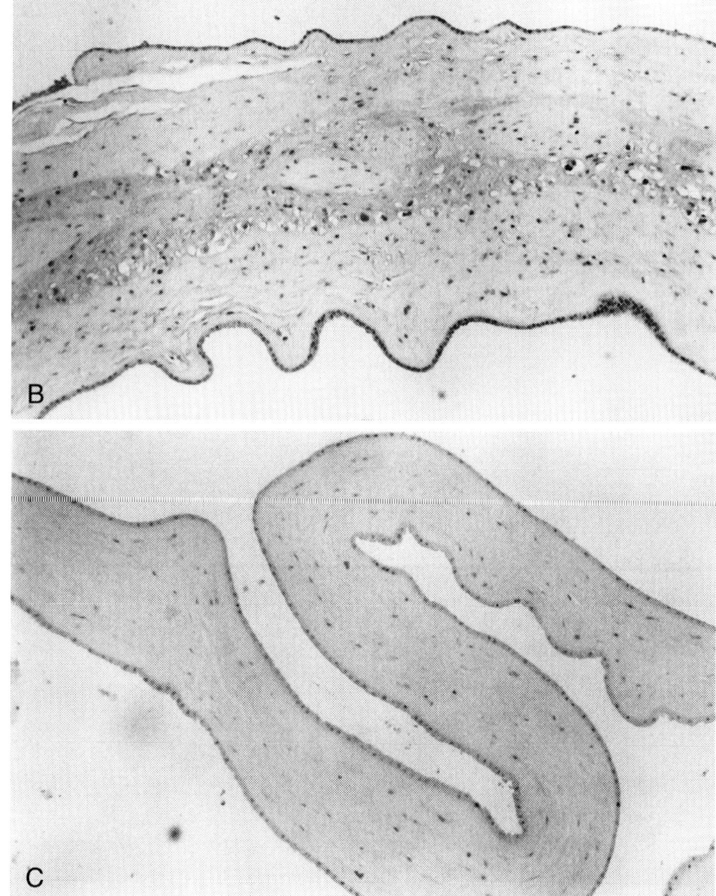

Figure 9–6. Histologic patterns of intertwin septal membranes. Dichorionic diamnionic septum is shown as the T section in **A** and part of the membrane roll at higher power in **B**. **A**, The fetal surfaces of each twin's side of the septum can be seen, as can the manner in which the chorionic tissue penetrates the septum from the underlying placenta. **B**, Two atrophic villi and apparent fusion of the two chorionic components are visible. **C**, Part of the membrane roll of a diamnionic septum with only two layers of amnion back to back. (A T section of a diamnionic septum is difficult to obtain because the septum is not attached to the placental surface.) (H&E; **A** $\times 3$; **B** and **C** $\times 6$.)

fetal loss, whether spontaneous or induced. This procedure confirms the presence of embryonic and fetal remnants, which may be nondescript on gross examination, and allows dating of the deceased conceptus based on bone age criteria. Countertop equipment such as a Faxitron unit is convenient and produces satisfactory films (Fig. 9–16*F*).

In occasional cases, there are unusual features that are difficult to section properly in fresh tissue. Cysts, unusual masses or hematomas, and unusual membrane relationships, for example, may be easier to section if the tissues are fixed in formalin for a few hours. The added quality of the sections is worth the wait.

Histology Reporting

The routine histologic sections can be supplemented with special stains if indicated by the findings, as with singleton placentas. The histologic reporting of twin placentas is the same as for singleton placentas with two additional important items: documentation of the components of the septum and comparison of the findings in the tissues between the twins.

The gross appearance of the intertwin septum may suggest the number of contained layers, but this should be confirmed histologically (Fig. 9–6). When there is chorion between the amnionic layers, the zone of chorionic tissue may vary in thickness. In some cases the two layers of chorion are obvious, but in others the chorionic layers are scant and it may seem that there is only one layer. The presence of *any* chorionic tissue in the septum is consistent with the dichorionic interpretation. The term "monochorionic" is reserved for placentas having only one common outer layer of chorion surrounding both twins, with one or two inner sacs of amnion only.

The tissues from each side of a twin placenta can have quite different features. Even monochorionic twin placentas can have considerably discordant microscopic findings, and these may be clinically significant.

PLACENTATION AND ZYGOSITY

The patterns of twin placentas seem to depend on three variables: the number of eggs fertilized, the timing of the twinning process in single-egg twins, and the relative location of the implantation sites in the wall of the uterus when there are two separate developing blastocysts. Determination of zygosity from the placenta includes knowledge of the sex of the infants (Table 9–2). Knowing the pattern of placentation and the sex of the twins, the pathologist can interpret zygosity in about 50% to 55% of cases in North America.

When the twins come from separate ova, they are called polyovular or dizygotic. They can be the same or opposite sex, but each will have both amnion and chorion layers in their gestational sacs. Whether the placentas are fused or not seems to depend on how close together they implant in the wall of the uterus. The gestational sacs may be completely distinct, share overlapping membranes, or become sufficiently apposed that they become a single disk with an intertwin septum. These are all dichorionic diamniotic (DCDA) (and also referred to as DiDi) placentas. When the twins are not the same sex, they have come from separately fertilized eggs. The very rare exceptions to this dictum are heterokaryotic monozygotic twins and dispermic monovular twinning (see the later section on unusual lesions).

When twins come from a single egg that undergoes a twinning process at some point after fertilization, they are called monovular or monozy-

Table 9–2. Patterns of Placental Disks and Membranes Related to Zygosity

	Number of Disks					
	Two Disks		One Disk			
Septum	Chorion and amnion ± overlap of parts of the chorionic surfaces		Chorion and amnion		Amnion only	No septum
Sex of infants	Unlike	Like	Unlike	Like	Like	Like
Zygosity	Dizygotic	?	Dizygotic	?	Monozygotic	Monozygotic

gotic. With the very rare exceptions already noted, these twins are the same sex. The impetus for and the mechanism of this twinning process of the single zygote are unknown, but it has been suggested that the event can occur at different times in the 2 weeks after fertilization and that this timing determines the pattern of placentation.[2] The later the twinning in the development of the components of the gestational sac, the fewer the layers around each twin. Thus single-egg twins can have all the possible patterns of placentation: dichorionic diamniotic with separate or fused placental masses and a four-layer septum, single-disk monochorionic with a two-layer diamniotic septum (MCDA) (also referred to as DiMo), or single-disk monochorionic monoamniotic (MCMA) (also referred to as MoMo) with no septum. Because monochorionic placental patterns come only from later twinning of single zygotes, a single disk with a common outer layer of chorion implies monozygosity of the twins.

The problem of determining zygosity from the placenta occurs with like-sex twins who have a dichorionic placenta. This pattern can be seen with either polyovular or monovular twinning. Whether the placental portions are separate or fused has *no* implications for zygosity determination. Zygosity determination in like-sex twins with dichorionic placentas requires other studies such as blood group or DNA analysis.[12]

The frequency of the different patterns of placentation depends on the population base, and the variation is mainly in the frequency of dizygotic twinning, the type of twinning most affected by maternal, genetic, and environmental factors. In North America, with its mixed population group, a spontaneous twin pregnancy occurs in every 80 to 100 pregnancies. Of these twins, about two thirds have dichorionic placentas and one third are monochorionic, with the proportion of diamniotic and monoamniotic about 10:1.

Importance of Zygosity Determination

There are several reasons to determine the zygosity of twins, not the least of which is that the parents want to know. There are also medical and scientific reasons to determine zygosity.

The extensive literature on twin studies has arisen from one basic premise: that by comparing a feature in so-called identical and fraternal twins, the different degrees of genetic and environmental influences on that feature can be determined. Unfortunately, real life is not so simple, and many variables can confound such studies, variables that are too often disregarded.[1] One of the most important is zygosity determination. One of the problems is that determining zygosity in later life is expensive and time consuming, although a number of techniques are available.[1] Adequate placental examination at birth could reduce by half the sets of twins who require additional studies—an important contribution. Cord blood taken at birth could be used for the rest.[12]

Determining zygosity in some cases of anomalies, diseases, or malignancies affecting twins may have implications for investigation and management of the co-twin, for genetic counseling of unaffected siblings, and for further reproductive plans of the parents.

DISCORDANT DEVELOPMENT OF THE TWIN PLACENTA

Developmental variations in twin placentas can have clinical significance. These involve the umbilical cord, fetal chorionic vascularization, and chorionic volume (Fig. 9–7). Discordant development involving intertwin vascular anastomoses and cord complications in monoamniotic twins are discussed in the next section.

Anomalies of the Umbilical Cord and Fetal Chorionic Vascularization

Anomalies of the umbilical cord are more frequent in twin placentas and include aberrant insertions and absence of one umbilical artery. Also, the frequency of cord anomalies increases with increasing proximity of the twins, from separate dichorionic placentas to monochorionic disks.[1] Marginal and velamentous insertions, including insertions into a dichorionic septum, may occur as a function of intrauterine crowding, with secondarily distorted placental growth.[13] In other cases they are associated with additional abnormalities of placental vascularization and may represent more complex developmental errors. Similarly, the absence of one umbilical artery may be

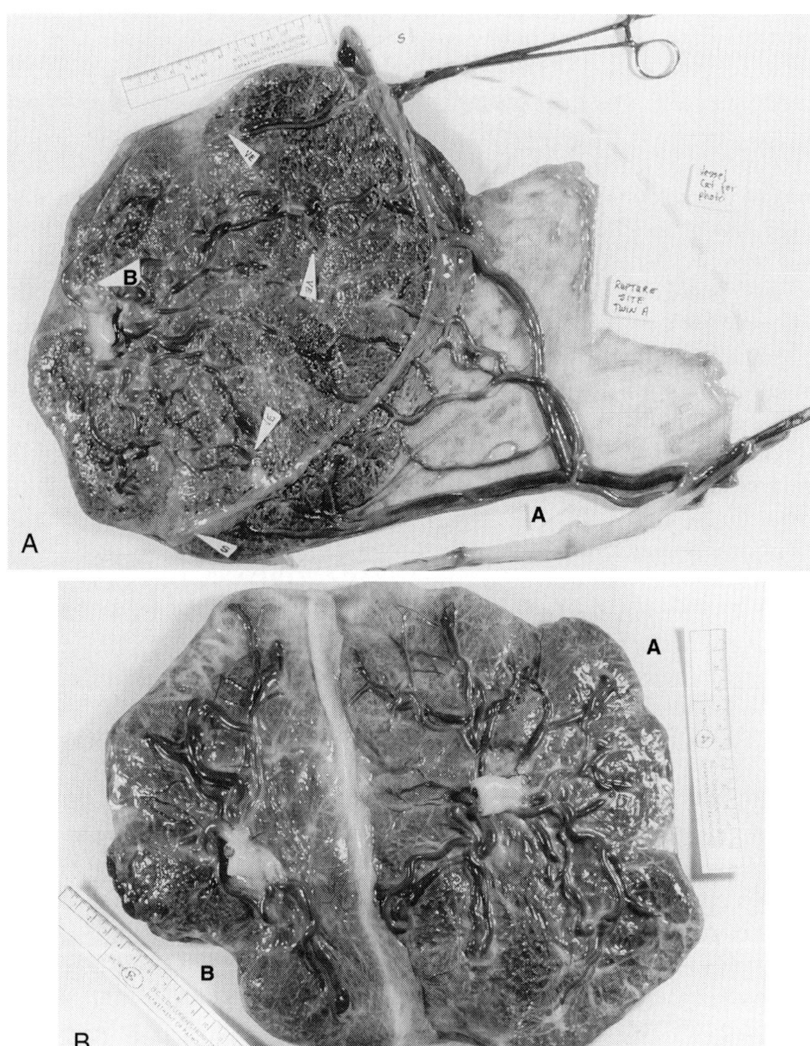

Figure 9–7. Discordant placental development and possible fetal effects. **A**, Monochorionic male twins that differed in weight by 17%. The smaller twin, *A*, had a marked velamentous insertion of the cord (the two hemostats indicate the ends of a vessel that had to be cut to take the picture, with the rupture site of twin *A's* membranes between velamentous vessels), and only 40% of the chorionic surface (the vascular equator indicated by the three small white triangles). The base of the diamnionic septum is indicated by the two pointers on either side of the disk. The effect of these developmental discordancies may have been modified by the number of bidirectional intertwin anastomoses also documented in this case. **B**, Dichorionic female twins that differed by 15% in weight, with the smaller twin on the side with the smaller chorionic volume and fewer fetal surface vessels.

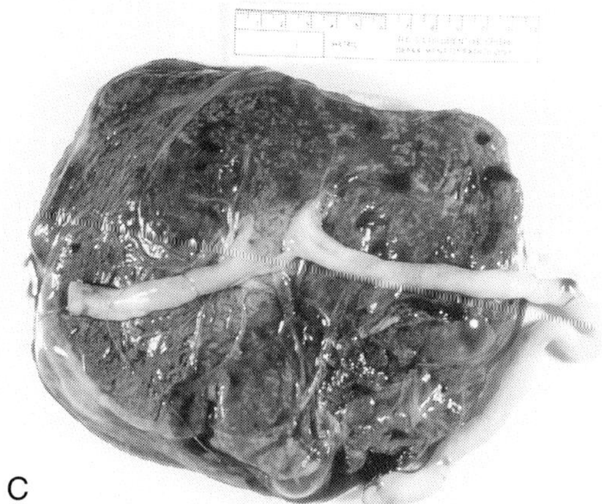

C

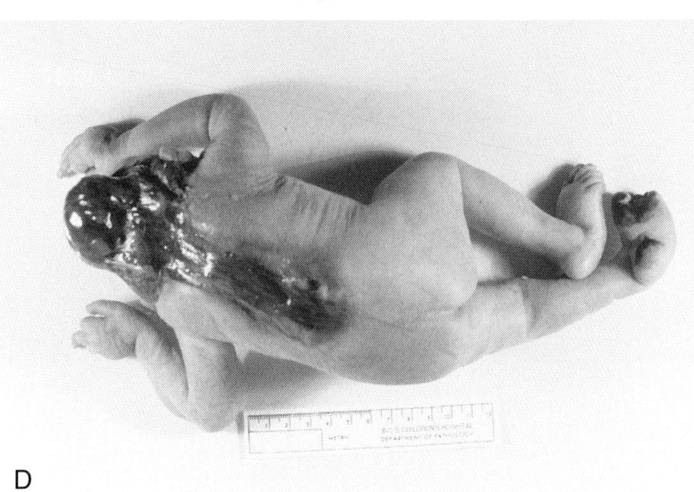

D

Figure 9–7 *Continued* **C** and **D,** A monochorionic monoamnionic placenta (**C**) and the discordantly affected male twin with severe craniospinal rachischisis (**D**). The male co-twin was normal. The only difference in the placenta was that the anomalous twin had a two-vessel umbilical cord.

an isolated finding or may be part of a malformation complex in the affected twin. In some cases the anomalous cord has a combination of lesions, such as only one umbilical artery and a velamentous insertion. In other cases both twins have anomalous cords with the same (concordant) or different (discordant) lesions.

The pattern of cord insertions and the number of cord vessels have significance beyond descriptive completeness. There is a greater association of fetal malformations with anomalously inserted umbilical cords, although it is not clear whether the anomalous cord provides a threshold for manifestation of the fetal anomaly or whether both are the effect of a common teratogenic influence.[14] Velamentous cord insertions are also associated with increased perinatal complications, including fetal death and decreased fetal weight.[15] Similarly, the absence of one umbilical artery is associated with abnormal development (Fig. 9–7*C* and *D*) and perinatal complications, including a significant effect on fetal growth.[16] Anomalous cords are more frequent with perinatal mortality of twins, especially in monochorionic twin sets.[1] The majority of concordant cord anomalies are in monochorionic twin sets. When cord anomalies are discordant, the affected twin is more often the smaller twin, particularly in association with velamentous insertions (Fig. 9–7*A*) or single-artery cords.[1,16]

Chorionic Volumes

Discordant placental development consisting of discordant volumes of placental tissue for each twin can be associated with discordant growth of the twins. With dichorionic placentas asymmetries of chorionic volume may reflect differences in implantation sites, possibly resulting from regional variations in maternal perfusion (Fig. 9–7*B*). With monozygotic twins different chorionic volumes may reflect asymmetric twinning at a somewhat more subtle level than is seen with the gross anomalies of monozygotic duplication discussed in the next section. Weight discordance of twins greater than 15% has been associated with discordance of placental weights ranging from 17% to 50%, with the smaller twin attached to the smaller placental portion.

Abnormalities of the umbilical cord can be seen combined with asymmetric development of chorionic volume and decreased fetal vascularization of the chorionic surface (Fig. 9–7*A* and *B*). These combinations are associated with discordant problems in fetal development, especially greater degrees of growth discordance.[1,17] As with all the associations of developmental abnormalities of the placenta with problems of fetal growth and development, it is not clear whether the primary problem is in the placenta with consequences for the fetus, whether that is a more general problem with the entire conceptus, reflected in both the fetus and placenta, or whether both mechanisms are operative. Systematic analysis of growth restriction of twins and possible confined placental mosaicism is a study waiting to be done.

SIGNIFICANCE OF A MONOCHORIONIC PLACENTA

The various theories of single-egg or monozygotic twinning suggest that it is an anomalous embryonic process and thus itself a malformation. This concept is supported by observations that monozygotic twins are at greater risk than dizygotic twins for almost all bad outcomes.[1] Monozygotic twins are more likely to be delivered prematurely, be significantly growth discordant, or have developmental anomalies. Also, they are overrepresented in all patterns of twin mortality throughout gestation. However, when this excess of monozygotic twins in complications of twinning is examined in greater detail, twins with monochorionic placentation account for almost all of it. For example, in one review, 37% of 1160 twin placentas were monochorionic, but 32% of surviving twin sets had monochorionic placentas compared with 51% of sets in which one or both twins died.[1] In this same review, when a cause of death could be assigned in cases of twin mortality, complications of monochorionic monozygosity accounted for 20% to 45% of stillbirth, perinatal, and later mortality.

The contribution of monochorionic monozygosity to twin morbidity and mortality is associated with three potential complications of this pattern of twinning: consequences of intertwin vascular communications, monoamniotic twins, and anomalies of monozygotic duplication.[18]

The importance of the placental findings in monozygotic twins cannot be overstated. Some of the twins in this category are so discordant that teratogenic or hereditary influences may be invoked. Identifying the affected pregnancy as monozygotic by confirming that the placenta is monochorionic and recording the vascular and other variations inherent in monochorionic placentations explain the abnormalities of the twins as an aberration in the process of twinning in the affected pregnancy, with no known increased recurrence risk or implications for siblings. The value of this interpretation for the family has to be experienced to be believed.

Consequences of Intertwin Vascular Connections

The presence of intertwin vascular connections creates the possibility of a net imbalance of blood flow across those connections, and thereby the varieties of twin transfusion syndrome (TTS) (Fig. 9–8).[1,4] Whether these connections are clinically significant probably depends on the number and pattern of the connections, especially the type, and therefore the possible directions of blood flow. Correlations of vascular anatomy with functional blood flow are still conjectural, although we can make reasonable suggestions.

Fetal blood flow through intertwin vascular anastomoses probably is dynamically variable, depending on fluctuating fetal flow dynamics such as fetal blood pressure, cardiac rates, and body movements. These effects may be compounded by additional complications of anomalies of cord insertion, vascular development, and chorionic asymmetry. It is likely that flow in the surface ar-

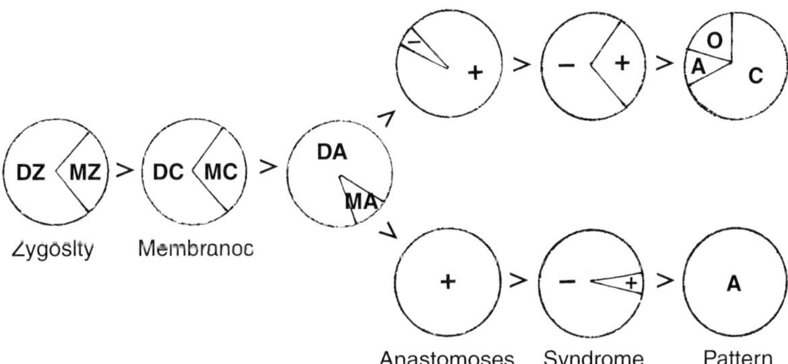

Figure 9–8. Relationships of patterns of placentation and twin transfusion syndromes. This flow chart depicts the relative relationships of patterns of placentation, fetofetal anastomoses, and twin transfusion syndromes. The proportions shown are approximate averages from the widely varied data available.[1] *DZ,* Dizygous; *MS,* monozygous; *DC,* dichorionic; *MC,* monochorionic; *DA,* diamnionic; *MA,* monoamnionic; +, present; −, absent; *A,* acute; *C,* chronic; *O,* other patterns, including acute complicating chronic and fluctuating chronic twin transfusion syndrome.

terial or venous connections fluctuates in either direction. Flow through parenchymal arteriovenous connections is probably unidirectional, from the artery to the vein. Flow patterns in compound anastomoses depend on the components and are often complex.

TTS is not a common complication of twin pregnancies, but it is important because of the high intrauterine and perinatal mortality and morbidity. The clinical and counseling value of careful and complete pathologic documentation of the placenta in these cases cannot be overstated. Unfortunately, the perinatal morbidity encountered in survivors may be the basis of a medicolegal dispute over care and the pathologist's report of the placental findings may be pivotal evidence.

TTS occurs in three main patterns: acute, chronic, and combinations of acute on chronic. The clinical diagnosis of TTS in infants is usually based on physical examination of the twins and tests of hemoglobin levels. Pathologic examination of the placenta with confirmation of monochorionicity and documentation of the presence of supportive anastomoses is essential in these cases. If no anastomoses are present in the placenta, other explanations for the clinical findings must be sought.[1] Some features of TTS have been reported in up to one third of monochorionic twin pairs.[19] Clinically significant TTS is more commonly encountered with diamniotic than monoamniotic twins, although the reasons for this difference in the face of universal anastomoses in monoamniotic placentas are unknown.

Chronic Twin Transfusion Syndrome

Chronic TTS is the most common pattern of TTS, encountered in up to 25% of placentas having anastomoses. The syndrome results from a combination of vascular connections and flow patterns that leads to an imperfectly compensated flow in one direction and thus a slow net transfusion from one twin to the other. It can be detected antenatally by ultrasound examination as early as 14 weeks.[20] The intragestational manifestations are variable in pattern, degree, and time of identification. Diagnosis of chronic transfusion is suggested by discordant fetal growth and fluid volumes, particularly a stuck twin, in the second trimester, and a number of other assessments are possible. The findings may progress, fluctuate, or reverse unpredictably, but earlier and more pronounced abnormalities seem to equate with fatal outcome. Classically the twins are premature. The chronic donor is undergrown, pale, and anemic, and the chronic recipient is large, plethoric, and polycythemic. Additional discussions of the obstetric and neonatal considerations are available, including the findings with intervention techniques.[1–4] Discussion of the findings with the clinicians concerned is often very helpful for the pathologist and obstetric attendant.

Evaluation of the placenta in cases of TTS is easier if the pathologist can determine the results of intragestational and neonatal investigations and some details about the appearance and condition of the infants at birth. It is absolutely essential that

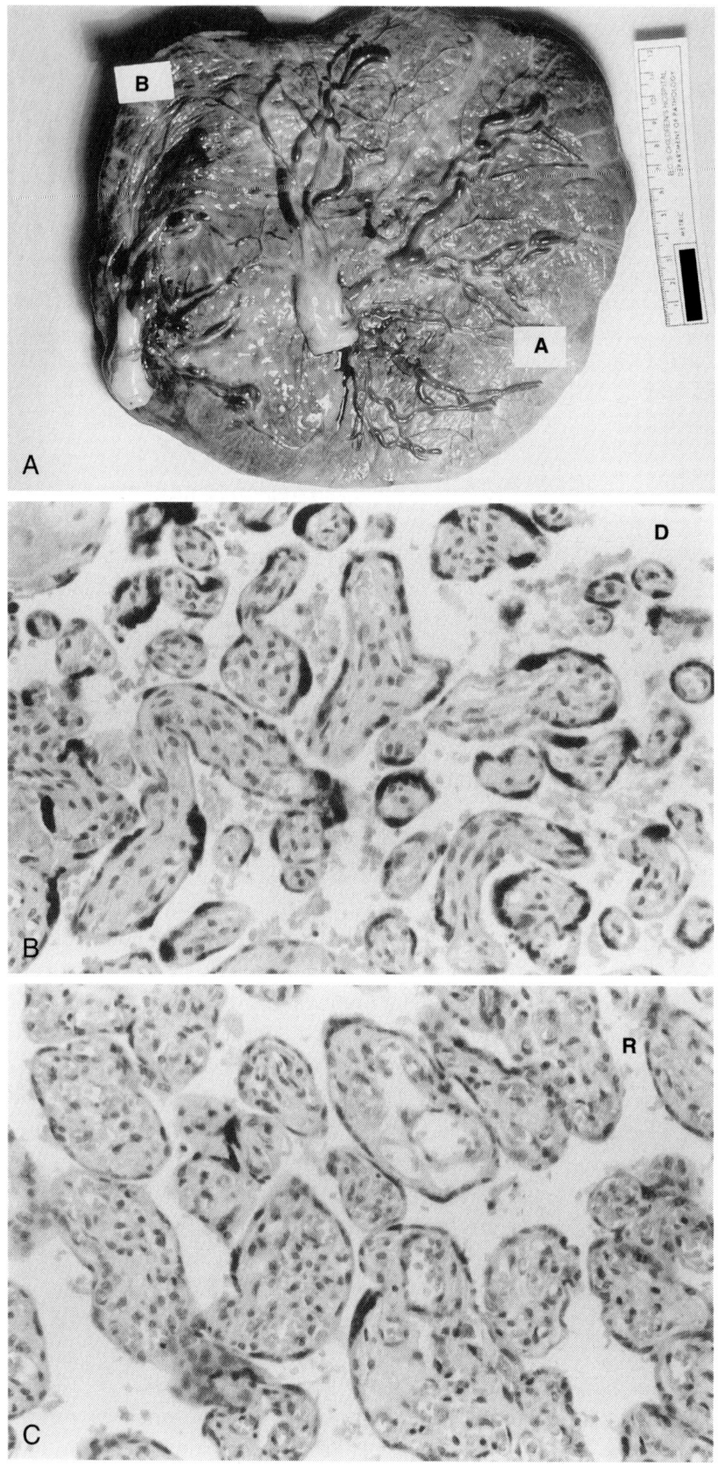

Figure 9–9. Placental findings in chronic twin transfusion syndrome. **A**, Placenta of male twins who differed by 33% in weight; the smaller twin, *B,* was growth retarded and had been a stuck twin. In addition to a smaller chorionic volume and decreased fetal vascular units on the chorionic plate, there were five large parenchymal anastomoses from *B* to *A,* a small one from *A* to *B,* and one venous surface shunt. **B**, The donor villous tissue was more variable in maturation with many ischemic areas *(D).* **C**, The recipient tissue was more uniform, slightly immature, and generally congested *(R)* (H&E; ×15).

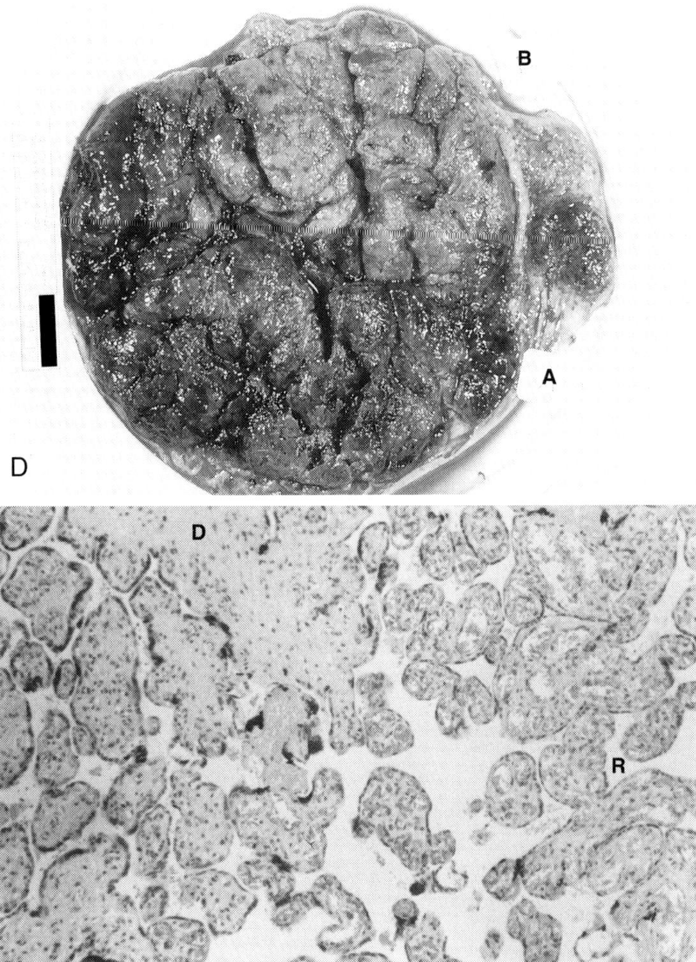

Figure 9–9 *Continued* **D**, Placenta of female twins who differed by only 7.5% in weight after birth. **E**, The smaller twin, however, was in heart failure, as can be seen from the differential appearances of the maternal surface of the placenta and the junctional zone of the villous tissues from the donor *(D)* and recipient *(R)* (H&E, ×6.)

the cords be identified as to the twin of origin at the time of delivery. An educated guess can be made based on observations described previously in the chapter, but this choice and the reasons for it must be noted in the report (Fig. 9–7*A*).

The placental findings include general observations of twin placentas, details of the fetal vasculature, and morphology of the villous tissue.

Placentas from twins with chronic TTS have more anomalous cord insertions, and asymmetries of chorionic volume and vascularization are encountered, with the donor twin's portion more commonly affected. The importance of these observations is that when discordant or abnormal chorionic development is present in addition to intertwin vascular anastomoses, both factors must be considered in any discussion of the cause of fetal growth abnormalities or pathologic conditions.

The pattern of vascular anastomoses in cases of chronic TTS varies from the usual pattern in monochorionic placentas. In one review 37% of placentas from twins with chronic TTS severe enough to lead to death of one or both twins had parenchymal anastomoses only while 16% had arterial-parenchymal combinations and 10% had arterial anastomoses only.[1] In comparison, of monochorionic placentas when both twins survived, 8% had parenchymal anastomoses only but nearly 40% had arterial-parenchymal combinations and 20% had arterial anastomoses only. In all, nearly 80% of placentas in chronic TTS cases at autopsy had parenchymal anastomoses and two thirds of the anastomoses documented were parenchymal. This skewing of distribution is not surprising because unbalanced blood flow is the pathophysiologic basis of chronic TTS and flow in parenchymal anastomoses probably is unidirectional and fluctuates less than flow in surface connections. When twins survived but were reported to have some signs of chronic TTS, two thirds of the placentas had potentially compensating additional anastomotic arterial, venous, or compound channels.

The appearance of the villous tissue depends in part on the condition of the infants at birth, and a uniform pattern is not always encountered (Fig. 9–9).[1] The donor territory has been variously described as immature and hydropic or atrophied and ischemic, possibly varying with severity and stage of the syndrome. The recipient's territory is usually more uniform and congested.

Because of the high mortality of TTS a number of treatment options have been used, including selective fetocide or actual removal of one fetus, decompression amniocenteses, fetal therapy, and interruption of the anastomoses.[1] Depending on the pattern of the anastomoses in the individual case, these methods have met with varying success. The placental findings depend on the method used, and the fetal vasculature must be documented carefully as usual. The most direct therapeutic approach is interruption of the anastomoses with laser photocoagulation, and the success of this procedure also depends on the anatomy and the severity and stage of the process at the time of the procedure. In these cases it is important to document the sites of laser ablation, confirm interruption of anastomoses, and identify any residual unablated anastomoses (Fig. 9–10).[21]

Acute Twin Transfusion Syndrome

Purely acute TTS is the simplest but least common (5%) of the hemodynamic imbalances across intertwin anastomoses. In the classic case no abnormalities have been noted during gestation and the condition is diagnosed at birth, usually in the third trimester. The twins have little or no growth discordance, but the recipient is plethoric and the donor pale. Until compensatory fluid shifts have taken place, the infants' hemoglobin concentrations are normal, attesting to the acuteness of the transfusion. The placenta is monochorionic with at least one surface anastomosis of arterial or venous type. The basis for the syndrome is the rapid shift of a large volume of blood from one twin to the other across one or more surface anastomoses.

As with chronic TTS the pathologist should document the monochorionic pattern of placentation and the pattern of intertwin anastomoses, correlating the findings with the information about the infants based on clear identification of the cords as to twin of origin. The congestion of the villous tissue parallels the plethora and pallor of the respective infants.

Acute TTS can occur in more complex situations, for example, as a complication of intervention procedures in cases of chronic TTS, as a natural terminal event in established cases of chronic TTS, and between twins with discordant growth for reasons other than chronic TTS. The placental findings depend on the situation. In these cases particularly, reviewing the case with the clinicians can be useful in sorting out the events and correlating them with the placental findings.

Acute-on-Chronic Twin Transfusion Syndrome

The presence of acute-on-chronic TTS is suspected when the smaller twin is plethoric and the larger twin is pale. This syndrome was identified in 45% of the chronic TTS cases in one review.[1] These cases imply that some acute event has occurred to upset the previously stable, albeit imbalanced, flow, and that surface anastomoses are present to allow a large volume of blood to shift rapidly. In many cases the upsetting event seems to be the demise of the donor twin, although the reasons for the death may not be evident. With the appropriate anastomoses the survivor can bleed across into the no-pressure vascular sink of the dead twin, and the blood loss may be enough to lead to the remaining twin's death in turn.

The mechanism of an acute shift in the hemodynamic situation in cases of chronic TTS is important because less severe shifts may explain discordant visceral and cerebral damage in surviving twins. The importance of pathologic examination of the placenta in these cases is unquestioned. Making a diagnosis of damage resulting from complications of intertwin anastomoses has major implications for family counseling and for management and prognosis of the affected infant.

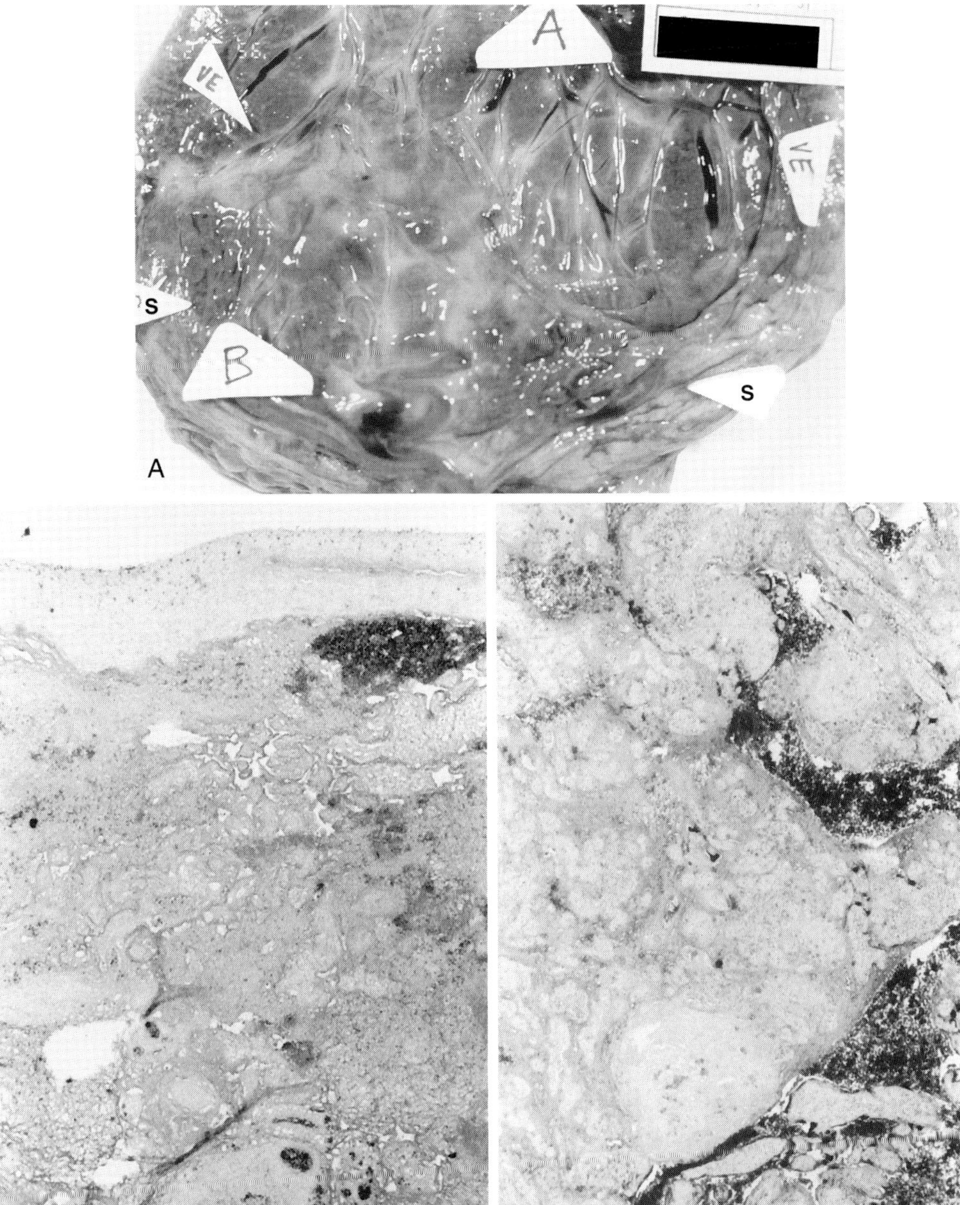

Figure 9–10. Placental features after laser ablation of fetofetal anastomoses. Laser ablation of anastomoses was performed at 24 weeks' gestation because of severe chronic twin transfusion syndrome. This is case 33 in De Lia's report.[21] The situation improved, but the smaller twin stopped growing again and had reverse end-diastolic flow, so the twins were delivered by section at 32 weeks. Twin *B* was 54% smaller than twin *A* at birth. Part of the persistent growth failure was attributed to the marked asymmetry of the chorionic volume, (one third to the smaller twin [VE–VE]) and pronounced ischemic changes of twin *B's* villous territory compared with twin *A's*. The septal base (S–S) was located so that only one eighth of the chorionic surface was in sac *B*. Note the pale areas on the chorionic plate along the vessels in the region of the vascular equator. These were the laser "hits." The microscopic appearance of the tissues beneath these "hit" zones was altered focally with **(B)** the chorionic and subchorionic region and **(C)** the tissues just distal to **B.** The changes consisted of bland coagulative necrosis of amniochorial connective tissues with occluded vessels on the surface, subchorial thrombosis and fibrin deposition, distal villous vessel obliteration, and segmental avascular villi focally embedded in perivillous fibrin. (H&E; ×3.)

Significance of Possible Placental Findings in Monoamniotic Placentas

The important placental observations in monoamniotic twins include all those already described for monochorionic placentas plus the possibility of cord entanglements because the twins are in the same inner sac. In the diagnosis of monoamnioticity the pathologist must make sure that the amnion is intact and complete between the cord insertions with no evidence of a septum between the cords (Fig. 9–1*D*). Confirmation of monoamnioticity may need to be correlated with prenatal ultrasound diagnosis because management of the pregnancy and delivery may have depended on that diagnosis.

A number of individual reports suggest that discordant anomalies in monoamniotic twins may be related to discordant developmental abnormalities in the umbilical cord, such as unusually long cords and two vessel cords on the affected side (Fig. 9–7*C*). Whether the cord anomaly represents an additional threshold phenomenon for discordant manifestation of the fetal anomaly in theoretically genetically identically predisposed fetuses or is simply an additional manifestation of discordant anomalous development remains to be determined.

In truly monoamniotic placentas the cords usually insert close to each other, sometimes within 1 or 2 cm. There are virtually always large surface anastomoses between the cord insertions, and the circulations of the twins may overlap extensively on the chorionic plate. Despite this, chronic TTS is uncommon in monoamniotic twins, with rates of about 5% reported.[22] Somewhat surprisingly, simple acute TTS is not reported except in case reports of cutting the wrong cord.[23] However, acute TTS may explain damage in a survivor following fetal death of one twin, analogous to the mechanism discussed for acute-on-chronic TTS. Careful documentation of the intertwin circulations is essential in all such cases.

Entanglement of the cords is a problem unique to monoamniotic twins. Fetal entanglement of the cord around the neck or other parts of the body, often of the other twin, has been reported in up to 22% of cases of monoamniotic twins.[22] Contralateral entanglements are important not only because of cord compression, but also because the wrong cord may be cut when the first infant is delivered.[23]

Much of the interest in monoamniotic twins has been the potential for entanglements of the two cords together and resultant fetal morbidity and mortality (Fig. 9–11). Identifying the tangled cords is easier than assessing the significance to the fetuses. Entangled cords may be longer than usual, and the complexity of the entanglements may be remarkable, with near Gordian knot proportions in some cases.[24] Two main patterns of entanglement are seen. Equally entwined or knotted cords may have varying sites of compression in both. Alternatively one cord is variably wound around the second cord, which passes through the loops of the first cord with no alteration except possibly sites of compression along the portion contained within the loops of the second cord.

The potential significance of these cord entanglements is difficult to assess. When fetal death is associated with a pathologic condition in the cords, cause and effect seems a reasonable suggestion. Fetal death with cord entanglements is often associated with retention in utero and maceration of the affected twin.[1] Entanglement of cords has been reported in up to 72% of monoamniotic twin sets with associated mortality of up to 68% of the affected twins, usually before birth and many concordant. In a review of monoamniotic twin mortality, 47% of the monoamniotic twins died.[1] Just over 55% of the deaths were attributable to cord entanglements, but 44% were due to other causes, such as multiple anomalies or prematurity, or were of undetermined cause.

In cases of perinatal morbidity or mortality the contribution of tangled cords to fetal distress or perinatal asphyxia is more difficult to assess. The interpretive problem is analogous to assessment of the significance of true knots in singleton cords, discussed elsewhere in this text. Doppler studies of cord vessel blood flow are promising,[25] but the clinical results must be correlated with the details of the cord entanglements.

Cord entanglements are unquestionably a risk factor for monoamniotic twins, but the magnitude of that risk for mortality and morbidity must be examined carefully in each case. Documentation of the cord relationships is an important component of that analysis. In these cases delivery suite

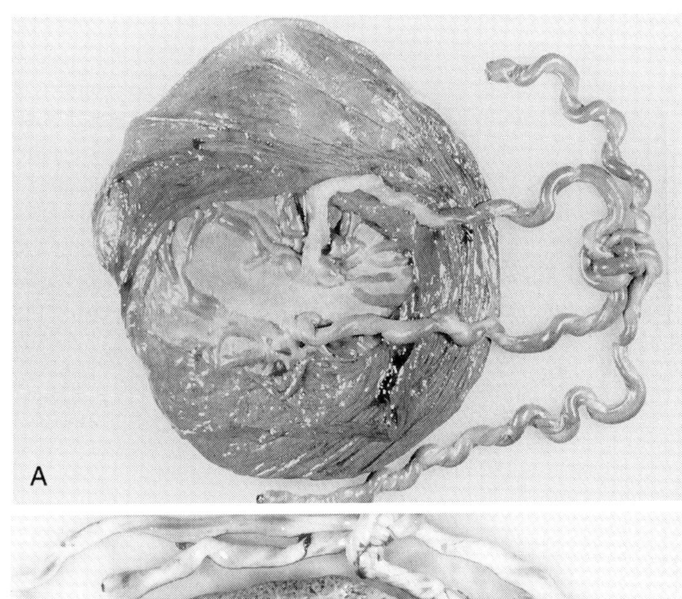

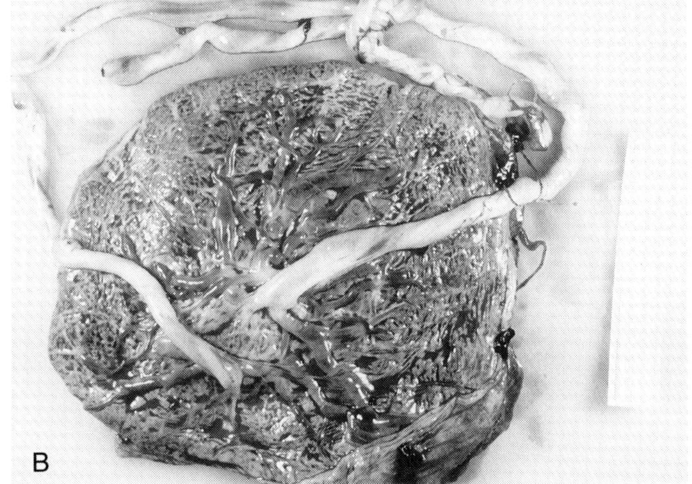

Figure 9–11. Cord entanglements in monochorionic twins. The complex entanglement in **A** was associated with asphyxia of the second-born twin, who died at 2 days of age (case 33 in reference 1). Careful examination of the entanglement revealed that one cord went straight through while the other wound around itself and the through-passing cord. Unfortunately, the cords had not been identified in the case room, so it could not be determined which part of the entanglement was more significant. In another case, **B,** the second twin (suture on cord) did well but the first twin was stillborn despite resuscitation. The cords were wrapped around each other, but details were not available. A possible complicating feature was the presence of two venous anastomoses.

identification of the twin of origin, if that is possible, is even more important because the other clues to birth order based on membrane rupture are not available.

Placental Findings in Anomalies of Monozygotic Duplication

Anomalies of monozygotic duplication consist of symmetric and asymmetric duplications. These are rare defects but among the most bizarre of human malformations, and being able to identify them as anomalies of twinning with no other reproductive significance for future pregnancies is extremely important to the families. The placental findings are more associated observations than pathophysiologically significant in these cases, with one key exception: the external pattern of asymmetric twinning, the chorangiopagus parasiticus or so-called acardiac twin.

Symmetric Duplication Anomalies

All the patterns of conjoined twins are symmetric duplication anomalies, and the varieties are well documented.[1,26,27] The placentas are always monochorionic monoamniotic. The major placental findings depend on the number of umbilical regions and therefore the pattern of conjunction, and they are mainly concerned with the number of umbilical cords and the number of vessels in the cord(s). A single cord from the placental surface may divide before inserting into the twins, or two cords may originate separately and fuse closer to the infant(s). The total number of umbilical vessels ranges from three to six.

Asymmetric Duplication Anomalies

In the asymmetric group of abnormalities of monozygotic duplication, one of the twins is so abnormal that the only way it can survive is by parasitizing the more normal twin. There are three patterns of attachment of the abnormal twin: internal, superficial, or external. None of the abnormal twins has a placenta of its own, although some have their own umbilical cord.

The internal twin is the so-called fetus-in-fetu or *endoparasitic twin.* The details of the attachment of these twins to the host twin are not well described in most case reports, although some reports refer to a pedicle of sorts attached to a cyst wall. Some reported cases raise the question of differentiation of these twins from teratomas.[1] Endoparasitic twins are rare but deserve careful investigation, including DNA analysis.

The superficially attached or *ectoparasitic twin* is the rarest pattern of asymmetric twinning and consists primarily of portions of redundant fetal anatomy attached to the host twin at various midline locations.[1] There are no particular features in the placenta of the host twin, and no placental structures of any sort have been described with the aberrant tissues.

The pattern of asymmetric twinning with the most important placental findings is the externally connected acardiac or *chorangiopagus parasiticus twin* (CAPP). In these cases the placental anatomy allows the abnormal twin to survive but also plays a major role in the development of the malformations. The abnormal twin can have a variety of primary developmental defects, which are modified by superimposed hypoxic-ischemic damage caused by the vascular anatomy of the placenta.

The umbilical cord of the abnormal twin in CAPP twinning can contain one or two arteries, or two arteries can fuse partway along the cord. The placentas are all monochorionic and can be monoamnionic or diamnionic. The key to the placental anatomy is contained in the name; the chorionic vessels of the normal twin connect directly with the cord vessels of the abnormal twin (Fig. 9–12). The connections are direct artery to artery and vein to vein and can be at the level of the umbilical cords, on the chorionic plate of the normal twin, or a combination. The abnormal twin has no villous tissues of its own, and the placenta and chorionic circulation of the normal or pump twin supplies both twins. Because the vascular connections are direct, the blood flow in the vessels of the abnormal twin is the reverse of normal, into the twin via the arteries and out of the twin via the vein. This pattern has led to one of the names for this pattern of twinning, twin reversed arterial perfusion (TRAP) sequence. Because of this reversed pattern of flow, and because the blood going into the abnormal twin is the used de-

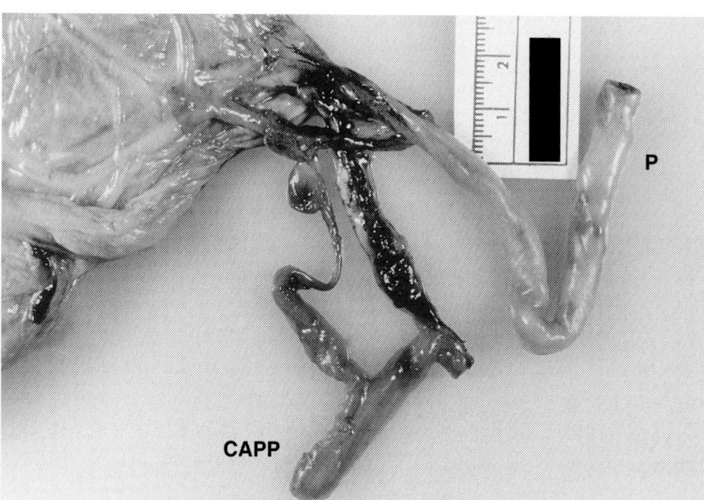

Figure 9–12. Chorangiopagus parasiticus—example of anastomoses. In this case the diamnionic intertwin septum "attached" at the cord insertion but the details could not be determined because of tearing of the specimen. One cord arose marginally, and 1 cm from the margin it divided into two with a three-vessel cord proceeding to the normal pump twin *(P)* and a two-vessel cord (damaged at delivery) to the *CAPP* twin. Many of the chorionic surface vessels contained mural thrombi. The twins died in utero, but autopsy of the pump twin was declined.

oxygenated blood coming directly from the arteries of the normal or pump twin, the abnormal twin sustains acquired hypoxic-ischemic damage to the already aberrant tissues.

The pathologic delineation of the vascular anatomy in CAPP twins has three potentially important clinical aspects.[1] First, these anatomic features of the fetofetal vascular connection define this group of anomalous twins and confirm that these often dramatically bizarre fetuses are an aberration of development of this pregnancy alone with no known consequences for future pregnancies—an important consideration when counseling these families. Second, complications of intervention procedures may be explained by variations in the anatomy of the cords and connections. Third, damage to the surviving twin, whether intervention procedures have been performed or not, may be determined by the fetofetal connections. If any concerns exist about the case, photographic documentation or drawings of the connections may be helpful additions to the pathology report.

SIGNIFICANCE OF DISCORDANT PLACENTAL PATHOLOGY

Discordant developmental variations and the effects of discordant blood flows are discussed above. In this section the focus is on acquired discordant pathology and what that might mean for the twins. Infections and acquired villous lesions are the main concerns, and clinicopathologic correlation with the condition of the twins is essential. The gross and microscopic pathologic features of these conditions and the significance for the affected fetus are the same in twins as in singletons. The important consideration is the degree of concordance or discordance of involvement of the placenta and how that correlates with involvement of the twins (Fig. 9–13).

INFECTIONS

Most fetal infections manifest in the placenta ascend into the amniotic cavity from the cervix or vagina or arrive in the villous tissue from the maternal blood, but the manifestations do not always fit with the usual concepts of pathophysiology.[1] Genetically based differences in fetal resistance or in the placental barrier to infection might explain some of the differences, but others remain unclear. Unfortunately, the literature makes little reference to the placental pattern or specific histologic characteristics, so the pathologist is left to explain the exceptions as best as is possible. Infection is an area of twin pathology that needs detailed contributions from careful pathologists.

With ascending infections the usual pattern is that the lowest or first-presenting twin is the only one infected or is the more severely involved if both are infected (Fig. 9–13*A* and *B*).[28] Probably the second twin is infected by transmembrane spread of the organisms, but there is not necessarily a direct relation to the severity of the inflammation in the first sac and reported cases of transmembrane infection have not yet been correlated with the histology of the septum.

Infections reaching the uterus in intervillous blood would theoretically be the same risk to the placental portion of both twins regardless of the pattern of placentation. However, there are well-recognized cases in which only one twin is affected or in which both are infected but only one twin has clinical disease.[1] Unfortunately, the reports of discordant transplacental fetal infections give no details of placental histology, so the degree of concordance of placental infection is unknown. Complete descriptions of patterns of placentation correlated with histologic evidence of placental infection and clinical evidence of fetal infection are clearly needed.

PARENCHYMAL PATHOLOGY

Discordant parenchymal pathology is particularly relevant to asymmetric growth of twins, and the incidence increases with increasing degrees of discordant growth. It is tempting to attribute differential growth to the discordant involvement of the placenta, but lesser degrees of these same parenchymal lesions can be seen with normally grown twins. Also, interpretation of the importance of the parenchymal lesion may be made more difficult if there are additional discordant developmental abnormalities such as asymmetries of chorionic volume or anomalies of the umbilical cord (Fig. 9–13*C* to *F*).

A number of discordant villous lesions have been seen with twins, including evidence of villous ischemia, perivillous fibrin deposition, evidence of problems with fetal blood flow, nonspecific villitis, and villous hydrops.[1] Explaining discordance on the basis of genetic differences in the fetuses and hence their placentas seems reasonable when the twins are of unlike sex and dichorionic, but is not so helpful when the same discordance is seen in monochorionic placentas. The problem becomes especially difficult for lesions of unknown etiology. This is another area of the placental pathology of multiple pregnancy that needs careful evaluation and clear descriptions of the findings correlated with the condition and outcome of the twins.

Discordant ischemic changes might be expected with separately implanted placentas, suggesting that one was less advantageously implanted, but in a reported series of cases more than three fourths of the affected twin placentas were single disks and 7% of the affected sets were monochorionic.[1] Discordant excessive perivillous fibrin was more frequently seen with fused than separate dichorionic placentas, and in nearly 15% of discordantly affected cases the placentas were monochorionic. Discordant nonspecific villitis was not common in this series of cases of discordant parenchymal pathology, but in 87% the placentas were monochorionic. Discordance of fetal vascular pathology and hydrops is not yet well described in the literature.

Although interpretation of the discordance may be open to question, the finding of lesions parallel to the fetal discordance is important for clinical explanation and evaluation.

OTHER CLINICOPATHOLOGIC CORRELATIONS OF TWIN PLACENTAS

In some fetal anomalies the placental findings are helpful. For example, dichorionic twins discordant for renal agenesis had a placenta with unilateral amnion nodosum (Fig. 9–14).[1] Unfortunately, the renal defect was not known before delivery, this discordant placental finding was not noted at the time of delivery, and there was great clinical concern about the difficulty ventilating the lungs of one of the twins. Part of the problem was undoubtedly that the external phenotype of oligohydramnios was minimal, attributed by the autopsist to a possible cushioning effect of the sac of the other, normal twin.

Amniotic bands and fetal disruptions are described with twins who may be discordantly affected. The placental findings are the key to the diagnosis in such cases.[1]

PLACENTAL FINDINGS WITH FETAL DEATH OF TWINS

The placental findings of fetal death of twins are no different than with singletons except that the potential causes are increased when the placentation is monochorionic. In those cases it is worthwhile to look carefully at the chorionic circulations, even if the vessels are collapsed, to see whether intertwin anastomoses might have been important.

Pathologically more complex are cases of discordant twin death in utero with continuation of the pregnancy. A pregnancy that starts as a multiple gestation may not continue as such because one of the fetuses dies in utero. Fetal death has different causes and can be spontaneous or induced. Fetal death takes different forms at different times of the pregnancy, although the distinction becomes less clear as the dead fetus is retained for a prolonged time. With the routine use of ultrasound in prenatal assessment, most cases of fetal loss in utero are known clinically and these findings can be documented for quality assurance purposes. However, there are still cases in which the pathologist will be the one to identify the fetal death. In cases of spontaneous fetal death, the efforts are directed to identifying the pattern of placentation and the probable cause of fetal death.

Some pathologists and clinicians may question the value of detailing the pathologic anatomy of fetal death of twins in utero. This information has three important uses. First, prenatal diagnosis of twins and twin demise should be confirmed and an attempt made to determine the cause for purposes of quality assurance monitoring of the accuracy of prenatal investigations. Second, if the surviving twin has any abnormality, the presence of a deceased twin may explain the lesions, depending on the details of the septum and other findings. This

Text continued on page 247

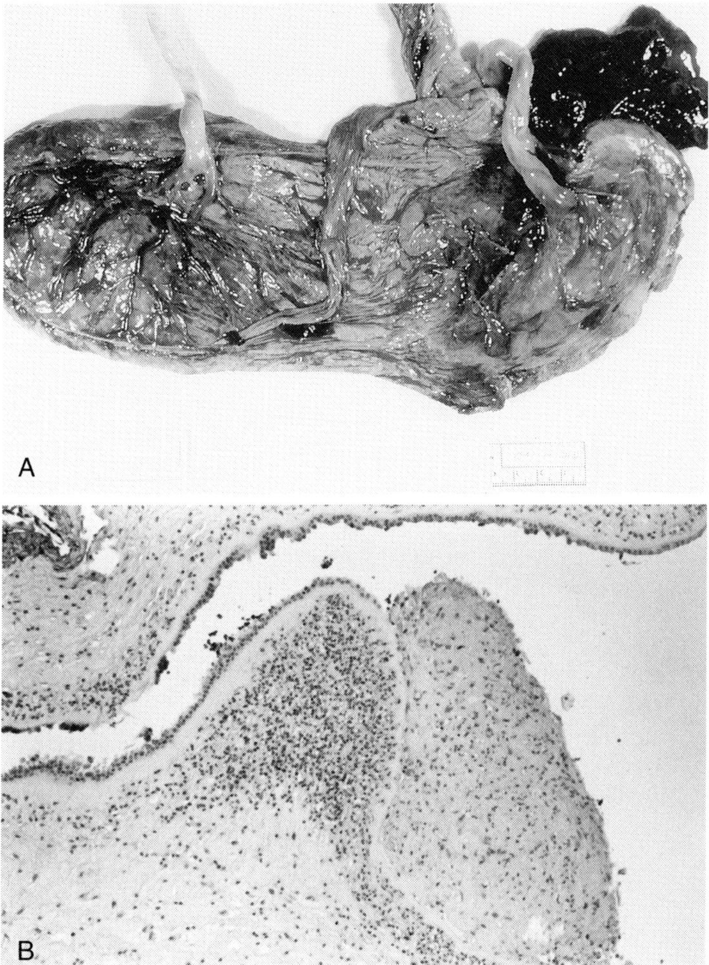

Figure 9–13. Examples of discordant placental pathology with twins. **A**, Ascending infection. In this pregnancy there had been chronic leakage of amniotic fluid from 15 weeks. Spontaneous delivery of dichorionic male twins at 22 weeks was associated with maternal clinical signs of ascending infection. Both twins died within minutes of birth. The placenta had separate disks but shared overlapping membranes with greater opacity on side *A*. At birth both sides were inflamed as seen on histologic examination, but side *A* was more severely affected. The organism was *Escherichia coli*. **B**, Ascending infection in twin *B*. In this pregnancy of female dichorionic twins the fragmented but labeled placenta consisted of separate disks. There had been leakage of amniotic fluid for 11 weeks before section delivery at 30 weeks. In this case, twin *B's* side had the greater inflammation with involvement of amnion nodosum. This observation was contrary to the usual patterns of ascending infection, so the ultrasound findings were reviewed. The twins were side by side in the uterus, rather than one above the other, and identified as *A* and *B* based on side. It was twin *B's* sac that had been leaking. Amnion nodosum with leakage oligohydramnios is unusual, as is the presence of inflammatory cells in the nodule (H&E; ×6).

Illustration continued on following page

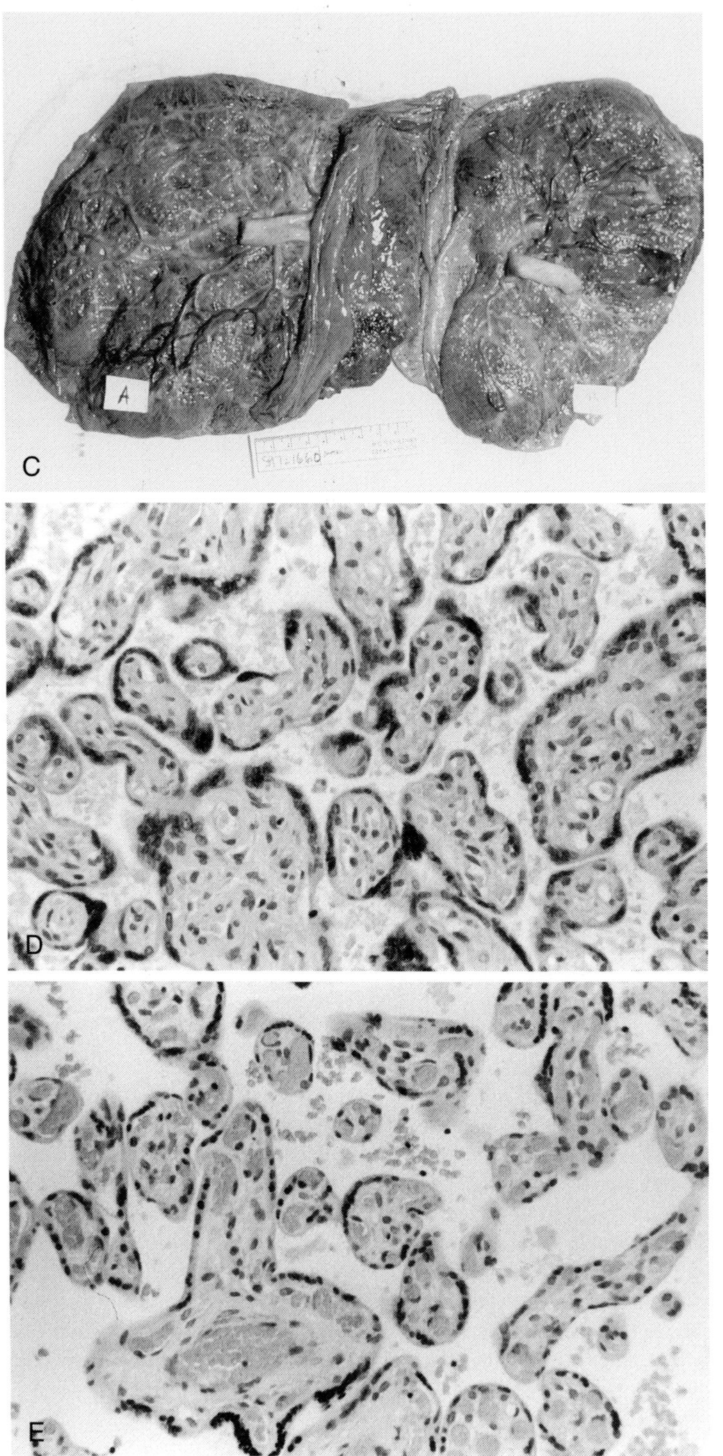

Figure 9–13 *Continued* **C**, **D**, and **E**, Villous ischemia. These were term dichorionic dizygotic twins who differed in weight by 26% at birth. Both did well. The placenta was separate disks with shared membranes. The weight of the disks differed concordantly by 37%. There was greater ischemic change in the basal villi of the smaller female twin *B* than the larger male twin *A*. The explanation for the apparent perfusion discrepancy is unknown. (H&E; ×15.)

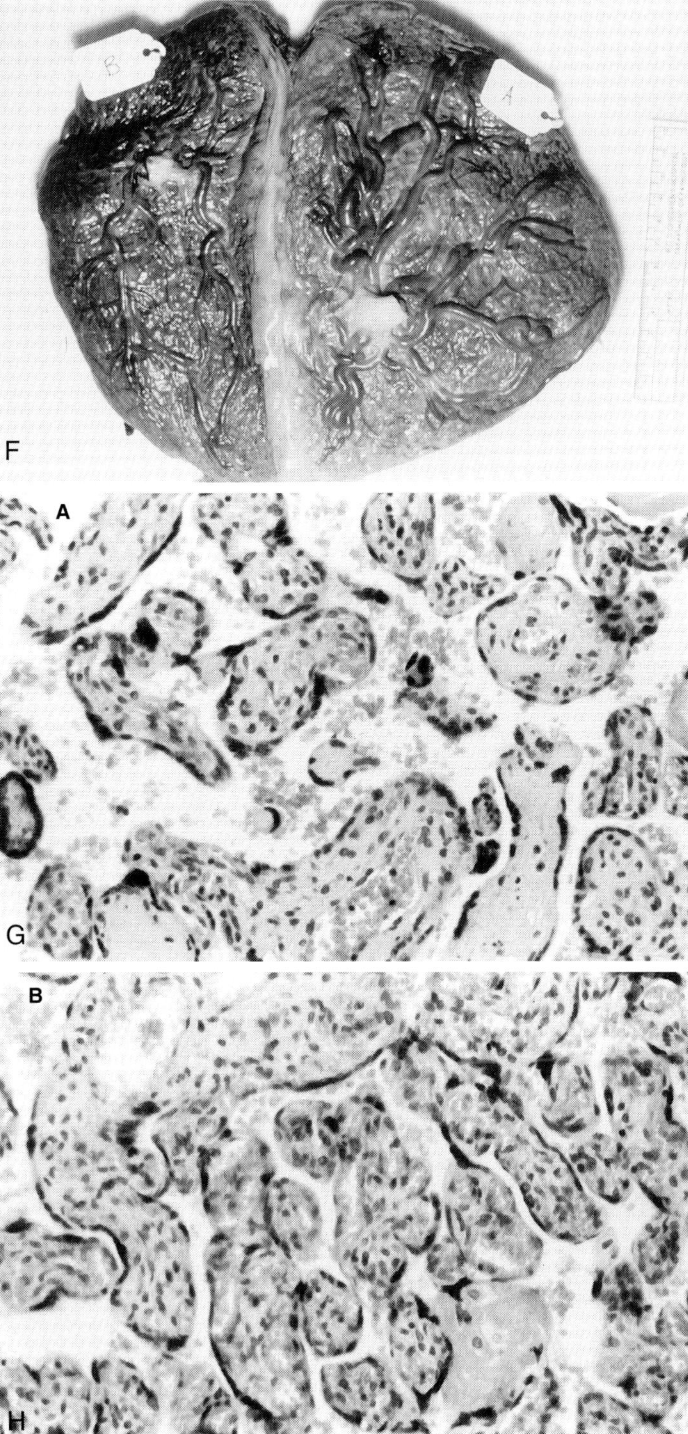

Figure 9–13 *Continued* **F**, **G**, and **H**, Avascular villi and villitis. These were term dizygotic dichorionic twins who differed in weight by 30%. The respective placental portions of the asymmetric single-disk placenta differed by 39%, but in the opposite direction, with the larger portion identified with the smaller female twin *A*. This apparent discrepancy seemed to have been offset by the presence of nonspecific villitis and extensive villous sclerosis on side *A* compared with side *B*, as well as increased perivillous fibrin. The differences seemed greater than might be attributed to zygosity differences, but additional explanations are unknown (H&E; ×15).

Illustration continued on following page

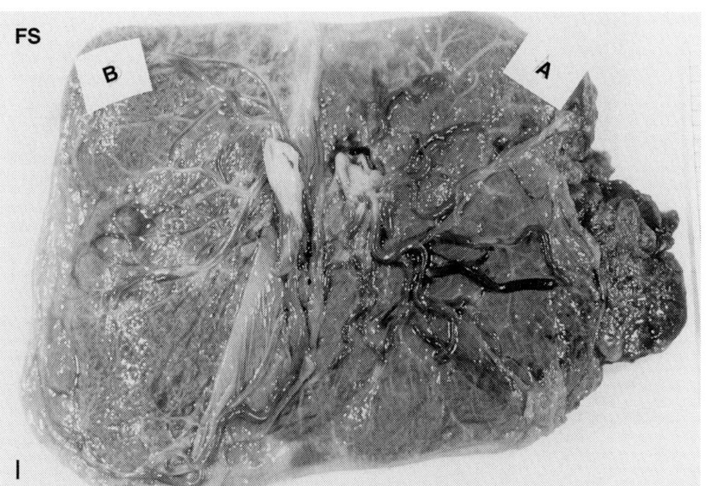

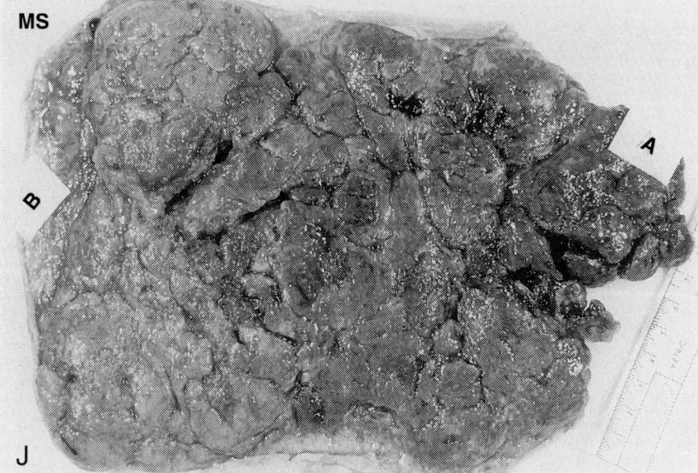

Figure 9–13 *Continued* **I**, **J**, **K**, and **L**, Ischemia and edema, zygosity unknown. These were dichorionic male twins delivered electively at 32 weeks because of persistent growth arrest of twin *B*. The twins differed by 25% with twin *B* small for gestational age. Both did well. There was mild asymmetry of the chorionic volume favoring the larger twin, and twin *B's* cord had a velamentous insertion into the dichorionic septum *(FS)*. The villous tissue on side *B* was paler *(MS)* and was edematous and ischemic *(B)* compared with the more appropriate but congested tissues of twin *A* *(A)*. No explanation for the differential pathology is apparent (H&E; ×15).

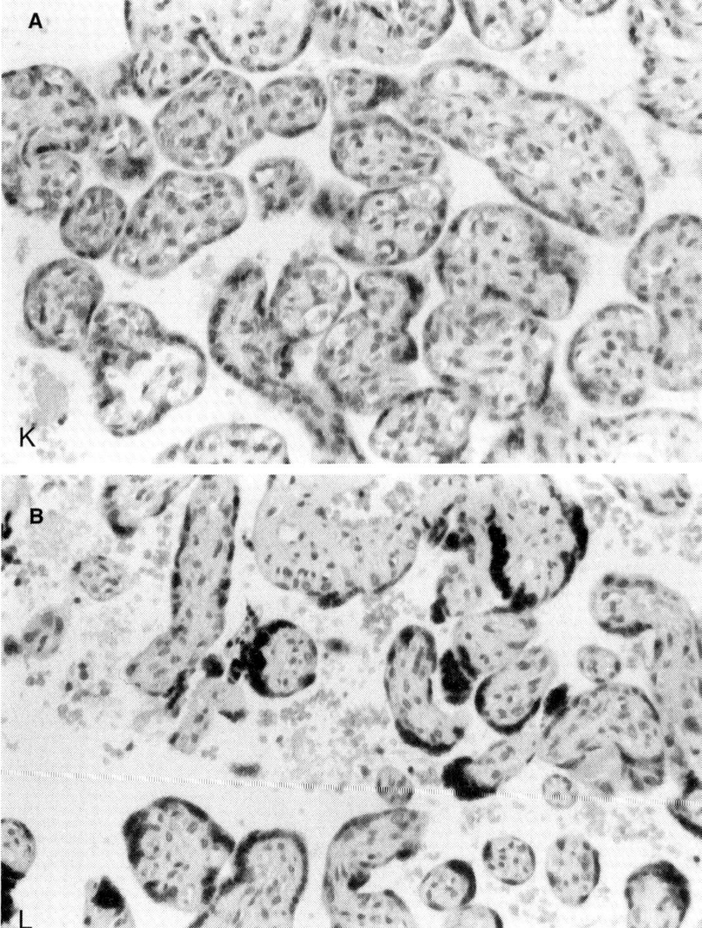

Figure 9–13 *Continued.* See legend on opposite page

Illustration continued on following page

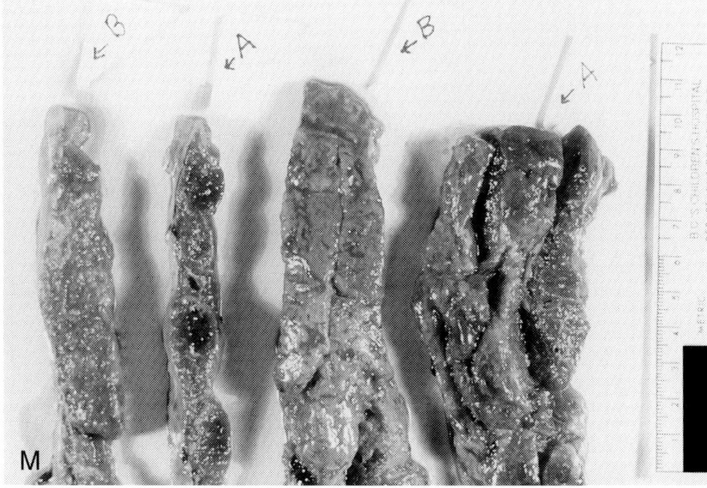

Figure 9–13 *Continued* **M**, Fetal vasculopathy. These were dichorionic male twins delivered at 33 weeks by emergency section for fetal distress (which twin was affected is uncertain). They differed in weight by 20% with concordant 3:2 asymmetry of the placenta. The smaller side *B* was paler and microscopically marked by relative villous immaturity, fetal vessel mural thrombi, hemorrhagic endovasculopathy, and villous sclerosis. Twin *B* died at 8 days of age and was determined to have a trisomy 21, while the co-twin was chromosomally normal. The zygosity of the twins was not assessed, so dispermic monovular or heterokaryotic monozygotic twinning cannot be ruled out. The explanation for the differential fetal vascular pathology remains unknown. These lesions are not a recognized part of trisomy 21.

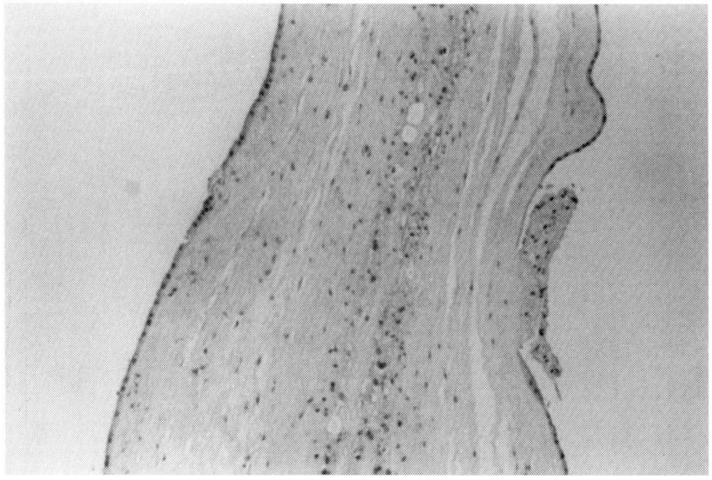

Figure 9–14. Discordant anomalies and placental findings. These were dizygotic twins with prostatic and anorectal aplasia in the male twin *B*. In the fused dichorionic placenta there was prominent amnion nodosum on side *B* only, as seen on this section of the septum (H&E; ×6).

information is vital for reproductive counseling of the family and for management and prognosis of the surviving twin. An occasional corollary is the importance of this kind of information in disputes over quality of care. Third, the death of an expected twin, even if early in the pregnancy, is still a loss for the family, and they often grieve as deeply as if the twin had been liveborn. These families need and deserve as full an explanation as possible to get on with their lives. The psychosocial value of this use of the pathology information cannot be overstated.

Vanishing Twin

A vanishing twin is one that is identified in the first 10 weeks of pregnancy but then collapses or disappears. Ultrasound studies suggest that overall rates of early multiple pregnancy loss may be as high as 78% depending on the patient population, the timing of the ultrasonography, and the number of scans performed.[29] Before ultrasound examination these were found as unexpected residues on the delivered placenta and were identified by the pathologist. Two additional patterns are seen now, an identifiable residue compatible with the early loss or no discernible residue despite a positive clinical history.[1]

When a residue is identified, it is usually an initially unimpressive, nondescript, irregular plaque of thickened tissue in the membranes adjacent to or actually part of the survivor's disk (Fig. 9–15). When these masses are dissected carefully, the second sac is found containing more or less identifiable embryonic residues. Radiographs may identify bony remnants in what otherwise seems an amorphous mass. Histologic examination of the plaque may identify the membrane pattern of the placentation and thereby provide a clue as to the etiology of the embryonic demise. Microscopic evidence of a diamniotic intertwin septum suggests that complications of monozygotic twinning might be important in the embryonic death, but other than that possibility the cause of death of these early embryos is conjectural.

Fetus Papyraceus

The fetus papyraceus results from fetal death in the second trimester with retention of the dead fetus until its delivery with the survivor. The fetal remnant is usually attached to part of the placenta of the survivor and is a gray-brown compressed mass with variably identifiable anatomy (Fig. 9–16). Radiographs help with definition of the residue, including an estimate of bone age at the time of death. Unless there are extensive intertwin vascular communications so the survivor can recruit the dead twin's placental portion, the collapse of the fetal circulation leads to gradual reduction of maternal circulation through that villous territory, creating a firm, pale mass of avascular sclerotic villi embedded in fibrin. The dead twin's placental portion may be a separate mass or a residual portion of the survivor's disk, depending on the original pattern of placentation. Careful sectioning of the junction zone may identify the nature of the intertwin septum.

The cause of death in most cases of fetus papyraceus cannot be determined from the placental findings. However, identification of the pattern of placentation and details of the cord of the dead twin are important because monochorionic twins may die of severe twin transfusion syndrome and anomalies of the umbilical cord have been implicated in these cases.

Much of the literature on fetus papyraceus has dealt with implications for the surviving twin. Although most survivors are normal, a number of lesions suggesting a vascular-ischemic complication have been reported.[1] Any suggestion of a clinicopathologic correlation of the death of the twin with the lesions in the survivor is not warranted unless a monochorionic placenta with possible intertwin anastomoses has been documented. This is key information for management of the survivor and counseling of the family.

Lesions That Cause Spontaneous Loss of Twins in Middle to Late Gestation

Other than the patterns of fetal compromise already described with monochorionic placentations, the placental lesions potentially causing death of twins in middle to late gestation are the same as for singletons and have the same appearances grossly and microscopically. As always, accurate identification of the twin of origin of the placental portions is essential for valid clinicopathologic correlations.

Text continued on page 253

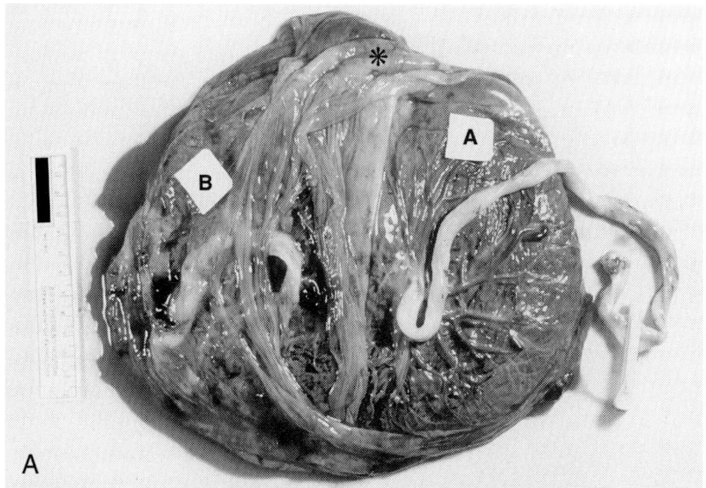

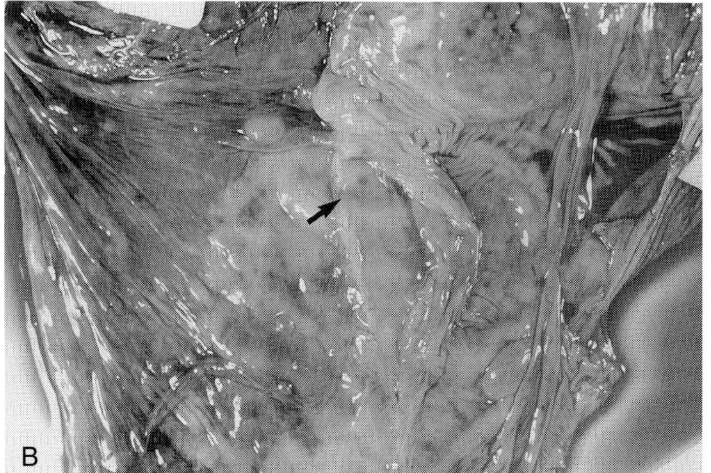

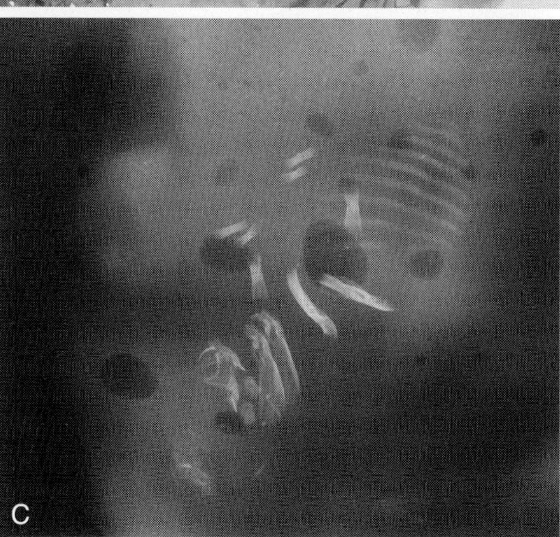

Figure 9–15. First-trimester fetal death in multiple gestation—vanishing twin. This apparently dichorionic fused twin placenta came from spontaneous normal male term twins of undetermined zygosity. **A**, The reflected membranes at one side of the septum seemed oddly thickened *(star)*. **B**, Closer inspection revealed a mass with optic pigment *(arrow)*. **C**, A radiograph of this mass confirmed an embryonic residue of 8 to 10 weeks' size.

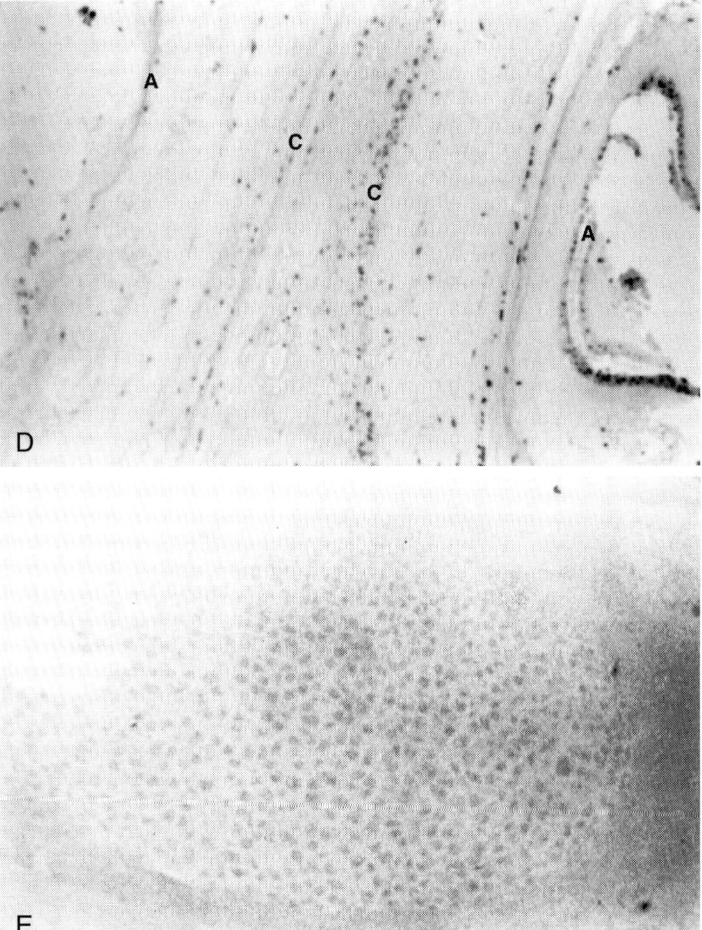

Figure 9–15 *Continued* The septum **(D)** around this embryo was dichorionic *(c,c)* diamnionic *(a,a)*, with degeneration of the amnion on the side of the embryo compared with the live triplet's side. The only histologically recognizable embryonic tissue was an island of cartilage **(E).** The cause of death of this unsuspected member of a trichorionic triamnionic triplet set could not be established (H&E; **D** ×6; **E** ×15).

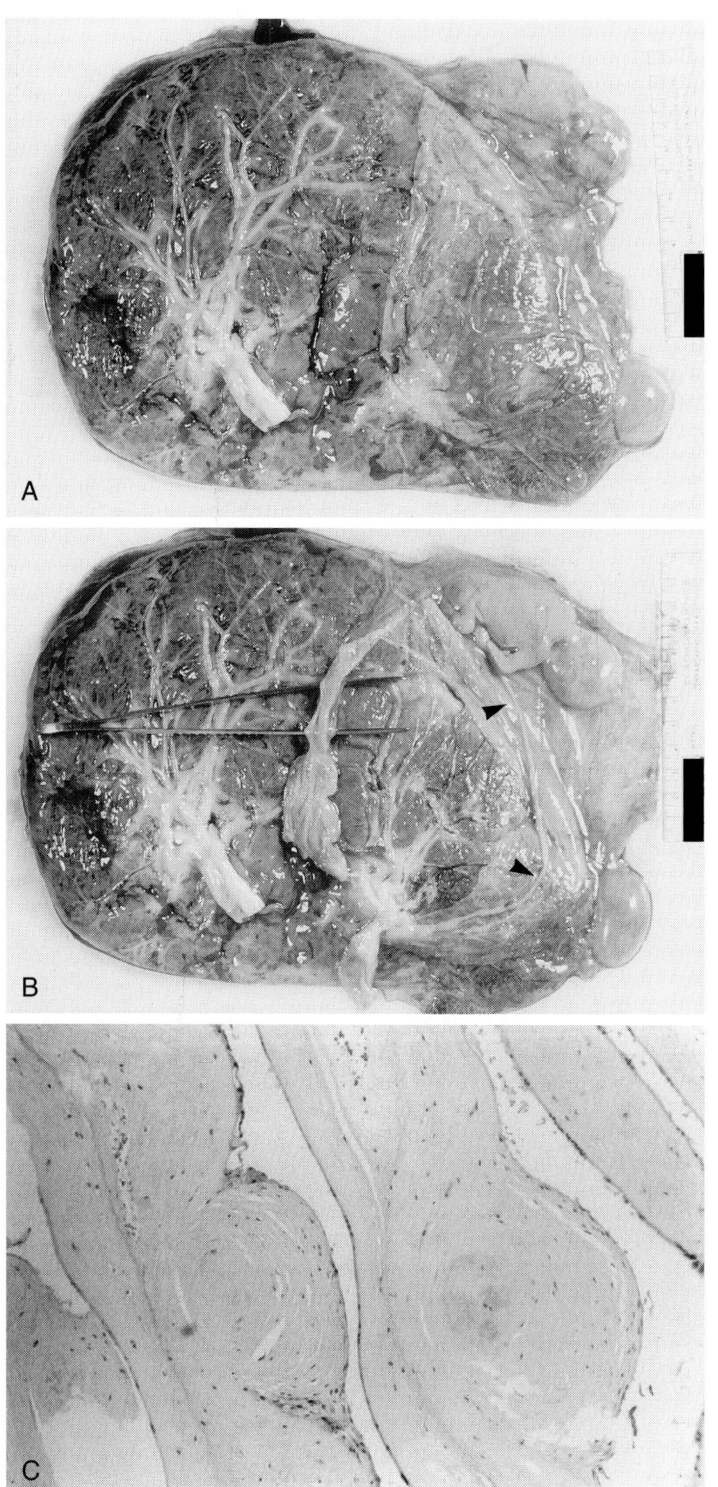

Figure 9–16. Second-trimester fetal death in multiple gestation—fetus papyraceus. This placenta was submitted with a history of early fetal demise with a normal surviving male co-twin at term. **A**, About one third of the chorionic surface was occupied by a collapsed sac containing a fetal shape. **B**, When this sac was opened, a fetus papyraceus was seen with a thin umbilical cord *(arrows),* which seemed to insert adjacent to the cord of the survivor. No identifiable area of sclerotic placenta that might have represented parenchyma from the dead twin was found, and this was because it was a monochorionic diamnionic placenta, confirmed histologically **(C),** with an unusual nodular degeneration on the dead twin's side. (H&E; ×6.)

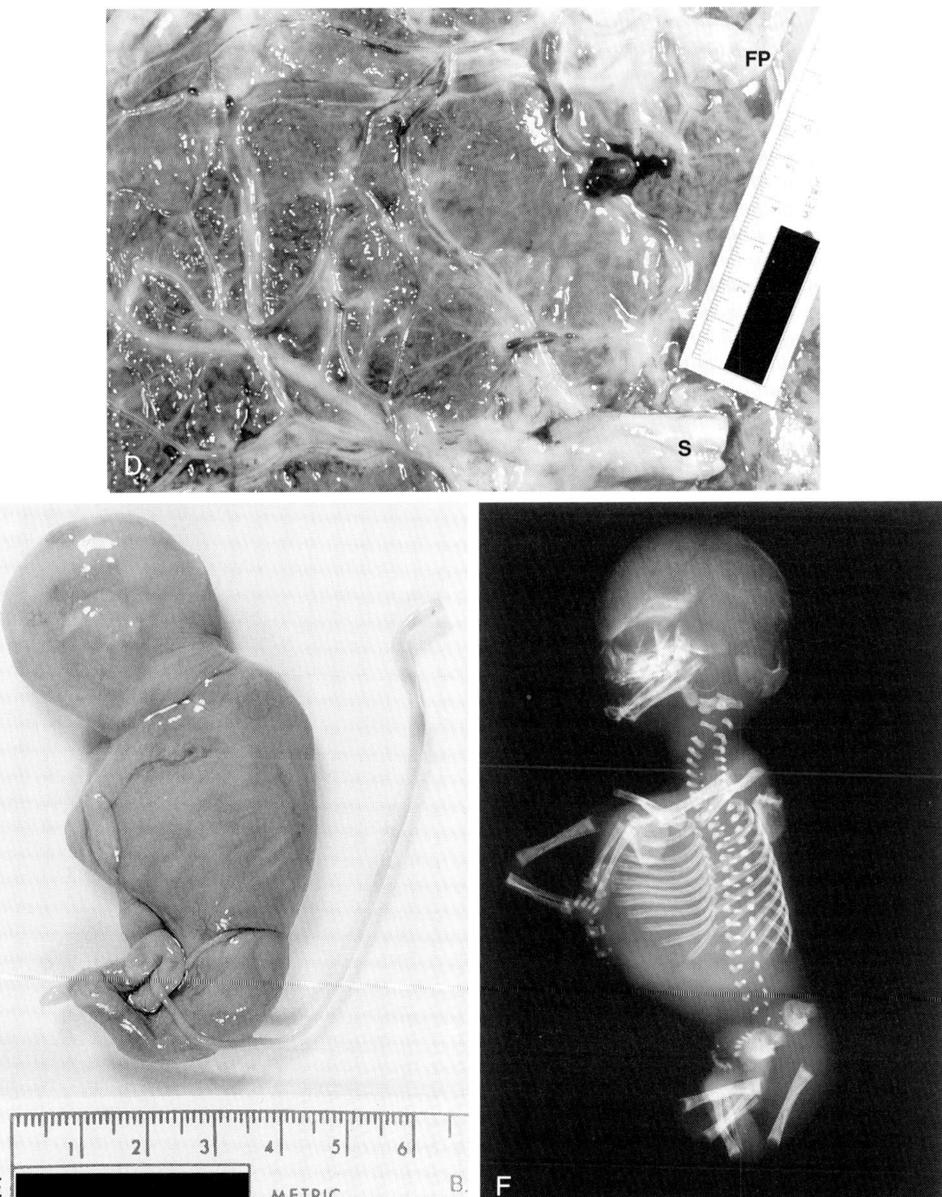

Figure 9–16 *Continued* **D**, A number of anastomoses were found, and the survivor (cord *S*) was able to recruit the dead (cord *FP*) twin's vascular territory through these connections. The cause of death was cord compression with loops of cord entangling the legs and abdomen of the fetus papyraceus **(E)**. The crown-rump length of the fetus papyraceus was compatible with 13 weeks' gestation, but the bone age (*F*) was more appropriate for 15 to 16 weeks, suggesting growth retardation before fetal death. The suggestion in this case was early twin transfusion syndrome with death of the donor caused by cord entanglement as oligohydramnios developed. To date, the survivor is normal.

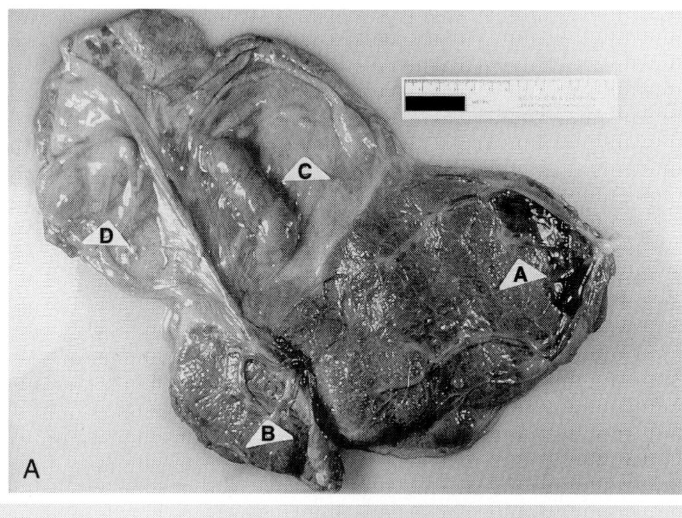

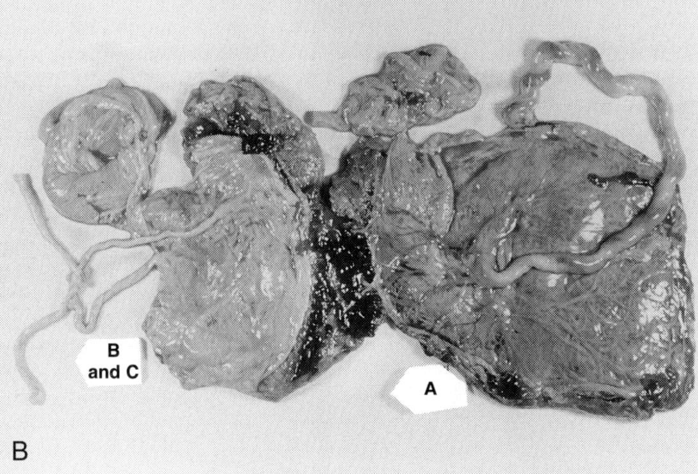

Figure 9–17. Placental findings after elective embryo-fetal terminations during pregnancy. **A**, Embryonic termination. This was a set of induced quadruplets reduced to twins at 13 weeks' gestation. Normal twin girls were delivered at 31 weeks because of vaginal bleeding from placenta previa. The placenta was quadrichorionic quadriamnionic with a shared disk for the surviving fetuses, *A* and *B,* and separate disks for each of the terminated fetuses, *C* and *D.* The terminated embryos can be seen as fetoform masses contained in their collapsed gestational sacs, each a fetus papyraceus. The survivors had decreased vascularization of the chorionic surface and velamentous insertions of the cords, and there was a single artery in the cord of the larger quadruplet *A.* Quadruplet *B* was 26% smaller and had a smaller chorionic volume with villous ischemia. Zygosity has not been determined. **B,** Fetal termination. In this spontaneous triplet set, triplets *B* and *C* were seen to be anencephalic and monoamnionic with a normal triplet *A.* Elective termination of *B* and *C* by means of intracardiac injection of potassium chloride was done at 19 weeks. Within the week, ascending infection developed in the mother and the triplets were delivered at 21 weeks. Triplet *A* died shortly after birth. The triplet girls were proved monozygous with DNA studies. The monoamnionic triplets had fusion defects of the spine in addition to anencephaly and had a complex entanglement of their cords. Triplet *A* was developmentally normal. This discordance of anomalies with monozygosity and entanglement of the cords of the affected fetuses raises the interesting question of the possible threshold effect of vascular forces on the manifestation of a defect. The placenta was dichorionic diamnionic. The fetal surfaces are cloudy in both sacs, but much more so in the sac for *B* and *C,* suggesting a complication of the termination procedure. Gram-positive cocci were seen in the fetal tissues of *B* and *C,* suggesting contamination just before the termination injection or contamination of the injected material. Interestingly, no organisms were identified in the necrotizing chorioamnionitis.

Placental Findings with Induced Embryonic or Fetal Death

The residues of elective embryo reduction in high multiple pregnancies are similar to the spontaneous vanishing twin, and documentation of these cases should be a mandatory quality assurance procedure (Fig. 9–17*A*).[1]

Elective midtrimester fetal death has been undertaken in twin pregnancies with discordant fetal abnormalities as an intermediate management option between terminating the pregnancy, including the normal twin, or continuing the pregnancy with maternal and fetal risks from the abnormal twin.[1,30] The indications have been either discordant metabolic, structural, and cytogenetic abnormalities or cases with severe twin transfusion syndrome. The methods used are focused on the abnormal twin, and the placental features are analogous to the fetus papyraceus if the pregnancy continues for at least 10 weeks.[31] In cases of failure of the procedure, examination of the placenta may provide an explanation such as complications of monochorionicity and vascular anastomoses or procedural complications such as infection, bleeding, or villous damage (Fig. 9–17*B*).

Placental Features of Interval Delivery in Multiple Gestation

Occasionally the fetuses of a multiple pregnancy are delivered days or even months apart, with retention of the placental portion of the delivered fetus.[1,32] The pathophysiology of interval delivery is not understood. The affected sets are

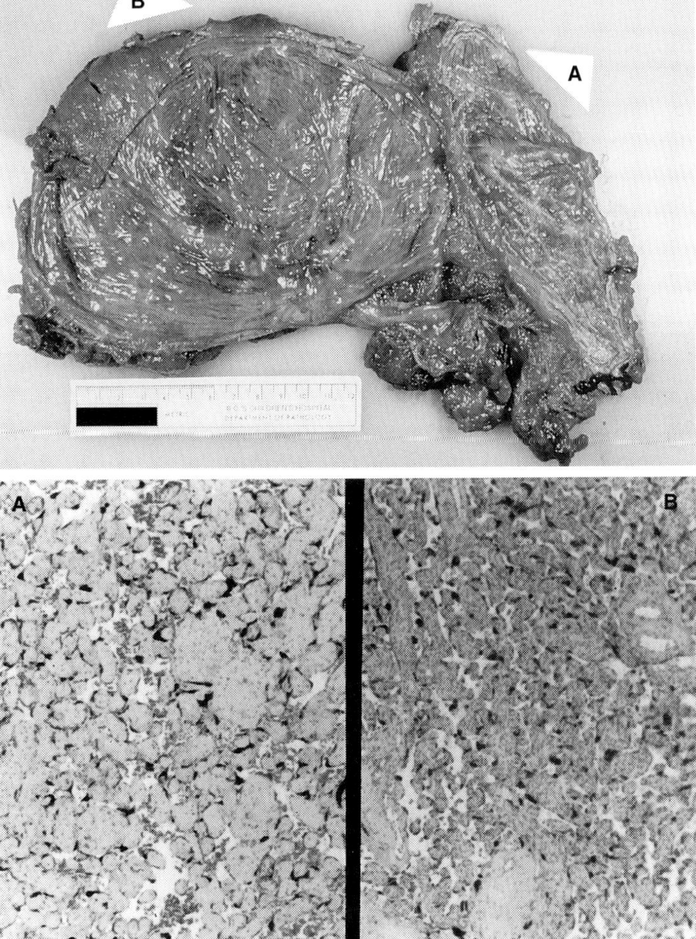

Figure 9–18. Placental features of interval delivery. This dichorionic diamnionic placenta was delivered at 27 weeks with a viable male twin *B* who did well. Twin *A*, sex unknown, was delivered spontaneously at 22 weeks, followed by arrest of labor. There was ascending infection, with chorioamnionitis more marked on side *A*. The villous tissue of twin *A* was uniformly sclerosed, compatible with 5 weeks of cessation of fetal circulation. Twin *B's* tissues were moderately ischemic but with no villous sclerosis (H&E; ×3).

almost all dichorionic, and the placental portions of the first twin are uniformly involuted and without distinguishing features (Fig. 9–18). The appearance of the placental portion of the surviving twin depends on the gestational age of its delivery and any lesions that might accompany delivery.

OTHER UNUSUAL LESIONS OF TWIN PLACENTAS

Almost any variation, permutation, or combination is possible in biologic systems, and multiple gestation is no exception.[1] The patterns of placentation can be quite bizarre and tax the pathologist's powers of observation and interpretation, for example, one twin apparently totally included within the sac of another, monochorionic but apparently separate disks, or intertwin septa that are only partly dichorionic. Some patterns of insertion of the umbilical cord defy embryologic explanation, such as at the apex of the free membranes. Some of these anomalies are developmental morphologic curiosities that do not seem to have specific clinical significance, but two conditions deserve further discussion, twins with trophoblastic disease and unlike-sex monochorionic twins.

Molar Twins

An interesting aspect of placental pathology in twins is the occurrence of gestational trophoblastic disease, so-called molar twins. Five patterns of concurrent fetus and molar placental tissue were described before sophisticated genetic analysis was possible.[33] The most convincing molar twin is the occurrence of an apparently normal fetus and placenta with a separate molar placental mass. This appears to represent a dizygotic conception with one zygote developing as an androgenetic diploid chorioma or complete mole (Fig. 9–19).[34] A second pattern of normal fetus and molar twin has been identified with the abnormal placental portion more closely similar to the appearance of the partial mole, although with a diploid set of chromosomes.[35] Possibly these cases are examples of abnormally developing dispermic monovular twins with the molar component arising from the fertilized polar body or are the result of uniparental disomy for an undetermined chromosome. Clarification of the genetic basis awaits application of available techniques to new cases. By developing a close working relationship with the prenatal diagnosticians and obstetricians, the pathologist can be made aware of these rare cases and can request that tissues be sent to the laboratory fresh and as soon as possible for best results.

Monochorionic Twins of Different Sex

In the discussion above on determination of zygosity, it was noted that the sex of the infants was an important observation in cases of dichorionic placentas. The implication was that unlike-sex twins implied dizygosity, reducing the number of sets of dichorionic twins for which other studies would be needed to like-sex sets, which could be either monozygotic or dizygotic. It was also indicated that monochorionic placentas implied monozygosity and the twins would be expected to be the same sex. The cases of monochorionic twins of different sex are rare but provide an opportunity to look at some remarkable variations in development of twins. Detailed discussion of the genetic complexities are beyond the scope of this chapter, but it is helpful to be aware that these possibilities exist.

Postzygotic numerical and structural chromosomal aberrations have been reported with discordant manifestations in apparently monozygotic twins, referred to as monozygotic heterokaryotic twins. The most common reported abnormality is discordance for phenotype sex with a variety of chromosomal combinations, although discordance for autosomal disorders is also recognized.[36]

Fertilization of a polar body as well as the oocyte from the same egg, leading to twins, was suspected for almost a century before it could be proved with DNA studies.[37] This pattern is referred to as dispermic monovular twinning. Fertilization at the second meiotic division could be the source of diploid sexually different embryos from the same egg, with one sperm fertilizing the secondary oocyte and a second sperm fertilizing the second polar body. The placentas in the identified cases have been monochorionic, which seems at odds with such early creation of separate zygotes.

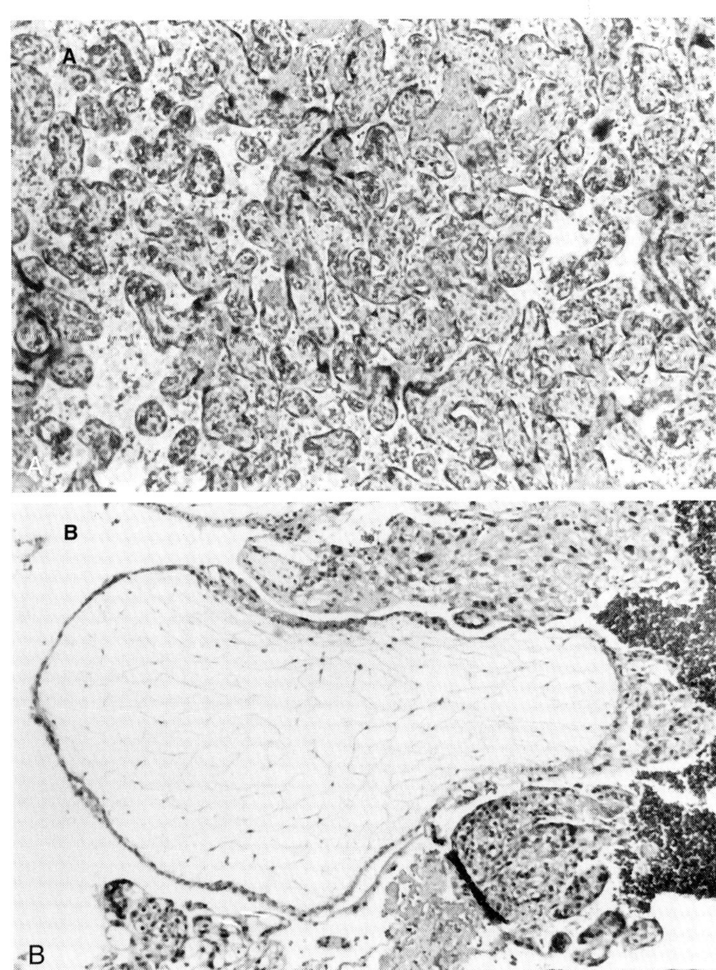

Figure 9–19. Molar twins. This was a known molar twin pregnancy with spontaneous delivery at 24 weeks because of abruption of the molar portion of the placenta. The normal male *A* infant (**A**) died at 3 months of age from complications of prematurity. The molar "placenta" (**B**) weighed nearly three times the placental disk of twin *A* and was a distinct and totally molar mass with the largest cystic villus 1.5 cm. Histologic examination showed that placenta *A* was within normal limits for age with no evidence of molar transformation in the sections taken. The appearance of sections of "placenta" *B* was that of a classic mole or chorioma, but unfortunately the specimens taken for cytogenetics study were not analyzed (H&E; ×6).

However, it is unlikely that unlike-sex twins with a dichorionic placenta would be considered a problem to be investigated, so the true incidence of this pattern of twinning remains unknown.

The message from these admittedly rare examples of twinning variations and complications is that they occur. When the placental features and clinical details do not fit with recognized patterns, the pathologist should take a moment to consider whether an unusual but important biologic principle is involved.

CONSIDERATIONS FOR SUPERTWIN PLACENTAS

All the aspects of twin placentas described in this chapter apply equally to triplets and higher multiples, although the permutations and combinations increase with greater numbers of infants. Virtually any combination of single- or multiple-egg origins of the fetuses can be represented when there are three or more. Therefore the patterns of placentation are potentially as complex as the discussion of twin placentas might suggest. Careful identification of the fetus of origin of the different portions of the placenta(s) is essential for any useful interpretation of the findings. A measured stepwise approach with accurately labeled diagrams simplifies the description. Zygosity determination becomes more complex, although the means used are the same.

All the complications of twin pregnancies with their associated placental features are encountered in supertwin gestations.[1] The situation of elective early embryonic reduction has become more common in cases of high fetal in vitro fertilizations, and the findings are mentioned above in the section on fetal death. Complications of monochorionic placentations are important with supertwins. In fact, the incidence of the asymmetric twinning anomaly described above as the external chorangiopagus parasiticus twin is more common in triplet sets than would be expected on the basis of the relative rates of twins and triplets.[38]

Sorting out the placental features of complex triplets and higher multiples is a fascinating process and worthy of the extra time and attention required.

REFERENCES

1. Baldwin VJ: Pathology of multiple pregnancy. New York, 1994, Springer-Verlag.
2. Benirschke K, Kaufmann P: Multiple pregnancy. In Pathology of the human placenta, 3rd ed. New York, 1995, Springer-Verlag, p 719.
3. Derom R, Derom C, Vlietinck R: Placentation. In Keith LG, Papiernik E, Keith DM, et al (eds): Multiple pregnancy. New York, 1995, Parthenon, p 113.
4. Machin GA, Still K: The twin-twin transfusion syndrome: vascular anatomy of monochorionic placentas and their clinical outcomes. In Keith LG, Papiernik E, Keith DM, et al (eds): Multiple pregnancy. New York, 1995, Parthenon, p 367.
5. Soernes T, Bakke T: The length of the human umbilical cord in twin pregnancies. Am J Obstet Gynecol 157:1229, 1987.
6. De Silva N: Zygosity and umbilical cord length. J Reprod Med 37:850, 1992.
7. Lacro RV, Jones KL, Benirschke K: The umbilical cord twist: origin, direction and relevance. Am J Obstet Gynecol 157:833, 1987.
8. Wood SL, St. Onge R, Connors G, Elliot PD: Evaluation of the twin peak or lambda sign in determining chorionicity in multiple pregnancy. Obstet Gynecol 88:6, 1996.
9. Ward BS: Cellular growth of the placenta in twin pregnancy late in gestation. Placenta 6:107, 1985.
10. Naeye RL: Do placental weights have clinical significance? Hum Pathol 18:387, 1987.
11. Pinar H, Sung CJ, Oyer CE, Singer DB: Reference values for singleton and twin placental weights. Pediatr Pathol Lab Med 16:901, 1996.
12. Derom R, Vlietinck RF, Derom C, et al: Zygosity determination at birth: a plea to the obstetrician. J Perinat Med 19:234, 1991.
13. Benirschke K: Placental morphogenesis. In Wynn RM (ed): Fetal hemostasis. Vol. 1. Proceedings of the First Conference. New York, 1965, New York Academy of Sciences, p 217.
14. Robinson LK, Jones KL, Benirschke K: The nature of structural defects associated with velamentous and marginal insertion of the umbilical cord. Am J Obstet Gynecol 146:191, 1983.
15. Ottolenghi-Preti GF: Sopra un rarissimo caso di gravidanza gemellare con un feto papiraceo e con inserzione velamentosa del funiculo del feto vivo. An Ostet Ginecol Med Perinat 93:173, 1972.
16. Heifetz SA: Single umbilical artery: a statistical analysis of 237 autopsy cases and review of the literature. Perspect Pediatr Pathol 8:345, 1984.
17. Potter EL, Craig JM: Pathology of the fetus and the infant, 3rd ed. Chicago, 1975, Year Book.
18. Baldwin VJ: Anomalies of monozygotic duplication. In Ward RH, Whittle M (ed): Multiple pregnancy. London, 1995, RCOG Press, p 100.
19. Boyd JD, Hamilton WJ: The human placenta. Cambridge, 1970, W Heffer & Sons.
20. Bebbington MW, Wittmann BK: Fetal transfusion syndrome: antenatal factors predicting outcome. Am J Obstet Gynecol 160:913, 1989.
21. De Lia JE: Surgery of the placenta and umbilical cord. Clin Obstet Gynecol 39:607, 1996.
22. Lumme RH, Saarikoski SV: Monoamniotic twin pregnancy. Acta Genet Med Gemellol 35:99, 1986.
23. McLeod F, McCoy DR: Monoamniotic twins with unusual cord complication (case report). Br J Obstet Gynaecol 88:774, 1981.
24. Quigley JK: Monoamniotic twin pregnancy: a case record with review of the literature. Am J Obstet Gynecol 29:354, 1935.
25. Abuhamad AZ, Mari G, Copel JA, et al: Umbilical artery flow velocity waveforms in monoamniotic twins with cord entanglement. Obstet Gynecol 86:674, 1995.
26. Potter EL, Craig JM: Pathology of the fetus and the infant, 3rd ed. Chicago, 1975, Year Book.
27. Guttmacher AF, Nichols BL: Teratology of conjoined twins. Birth Defects 3(1):3, 1967.
28. Benirschke K: Routes and types of infection in the fetus and the newborn. J Dis Child 99:28, 1960.
29. Landy HJ, Weiner S, Corson SL, et al: The "vanishing twin"; ultrasonographic assessment of fetal disappearance in the first trimester. Am J Obstet Gynecol 155:14, 1986.
30. Redwine FO, Hayes PM: Selective birth. Semin Perinatol 10:73, 1986.
31. Saier F, Burden L, Cavanagh D: Fetus papyraceus: an unusual case with congenital anomaly of the surviving fetus. Obstet Gynecol 45:217, 1975.
32. Wittmann BK, Farquharson D, Wong GP, et al: De-

layed delivery of second twin: report of four cases and review of the literature. Obstet Gynecol 79:260, 1992.

33. Beischer NA: Hydatiform mole with coexistent foetus. Aust NZ J Obstet Gynecol 6:127, 1966.
34. Fisher RA, Sheppard DM, Lawler SD: Twin pregnancy with complete hydatidiform mole (46,XX) and fetus (46,XY): genetic origin proved by analysis of chromosome polymorphisms. Br Med J 284:1218, 1982.
35. Deaton JL, Hoffman JS, Saal H, et al: Molar pregnancy coexisting with a normal fetus: a case report. Gynecol Oncol 32:394, 1989.
36. Perlman EJ, Stetten G, Tuck-Muller CM, et al: Sexual discordance in monozygotic twins. Am J Med Genet 37:551, 1990.
37. Bieber FR, Nance WE, Morton CC, et al: Genetic studies of an acardiac monster: evidence of polar body twinning in man. Science 213:775, 1981.
38. James WH: A note on the epidemiology of acardiac monsters. Teratology 16:211, 1978.

10

Trophoblastic Diseases: Complete and Partial Hydatidiform Moles

Aron E. Szulman

The term "gestational trophoblastic diseases" encompasses two pathologic conceptuses (the complete and partial hydatidiform moles) and two neoplasms (the malignant choriocarcinoma and the placental site trophoblastic tumor, of which there are benign and malignant versions).[1] Fundamental advances in the understanding of hydatidiform moles were made in the past two decades through the application of comparative cytogenetics (variously aided by studies of enzyme and human leukocyte antigen [HL-A] polymorphisms) that determined the different genomic individuality and parental derivation of the two conceptuses.[2–7] At the same time the correlation of results of such studies with the phenotype of the conceptuses led to the delineation of the two separate entities: (1) the familiar classic syndrome of the diploid diandric complete hydatidiform mole (CHM), without an ascertainable embryo (which dies early in its development) and with pronounced trophoblastic hyperplasia and rapidly progressing villous hydrops, and (2) the triploid diandric partial hydatidiform model (PHM), with an ascertainable embryo or fetus, only focal (syncytio)trophoblastic hyperplasia, and focal villous hydrops.[3,4,8,9]

Rare cases are encountered among hydatidiform moles that do not fit completely within the above model, for example, those described as CHMs of biparental origin,[3,5,10] those of androgenetic origin that include a young surviving embryo,[11,12] or the rare "PHMs" that turn out to be of nontriploid (e.g., trisomic) constitution.

The pathology of trophoblastic diseases still suffers from inconsistencies of approach among the numerous contributors and is handicapped by lack of a common terminology and sometimes even of a shared definition of CHM and PHM. The definition I accept follows the view of W.W. Park[13] that hyperplasia of the villous trophoblast is the fundamental attribute of a mole. The edema of placental villi, although useful in drawing attention to the specimen, is a secondary phenomenon associated with a variety of conditions, such as the so-called hydropic abortus (HA). No residual trophoblastic diseases, including chorionic cancer, are related to villous waterlogging, whereas their relationship to trophoblastic dyscrasias remains firmly established.

The two types of hydatidiform mole each present a pathologic conceptus best understood in terms of embryology[14,15] and genetics.[2,9] Each consists of an embryo and a placenta whose phenotypes and fates differ markedly between the two, since they are programmed by their distinct, respective genomes. Neither molar conceptus is a neoplasm or a tumor, and such terms are best avoided in discussing these diseases. CHM and PHM can be diagnosed by the pathologist on morphologic grounds alone in the vast majority of cases,[16,17] and the application of flow or image cytometry or of more elaborate techniques is seldom required. This chapter presents the two principal clinicopathologic syndromes with detailed gross and microscopic descriptions that will facilitate the differential diagnosis among the various entities facing the pathologist.

TROPHOBLAST: A UNIQUE TISSUE

The trophoblast is the first organ of the implanting embryo derived from the outer cell mass of the blastula. It is responsible for anchorage of the blastula and the secretion of human chorionic gonadotropin (hCG), which is essential in the maintenance of pregnancy. The placental villi are formed in the third postfertilization week through evagination of the trophoblastic outermost layer by the extraembryonic mesenchyme.[18] Thus the organ from the start has its characteristic permanent configuration. The trophoblast clothing the villi settles at once into the basic cambium-like cytolayer from which arises a superficial continuous ribbon of syncytial cells formed by the fusion of several subjacent cells. The main, anchoring villi give rise to trophoblastic columns consisting of an orderly honeycomb-like sheet of intermediate trophoblast[14–16] covered by syncytial cells and pointing toward the maternal decidua (Fig. 10–1). On reaching the decidua the trophoblast forms a shell from which further, single-cell penetration of the decidua (and later of the connective tissue of the myometrium) is effected. The important function of the extravillous intermediate trophoblast is substitution for the mural elements of the decidual arterioles to regulate the blood supply to the conceptus.[19] According to recent investigations a temporary blockage of the arteriolar lumina by the

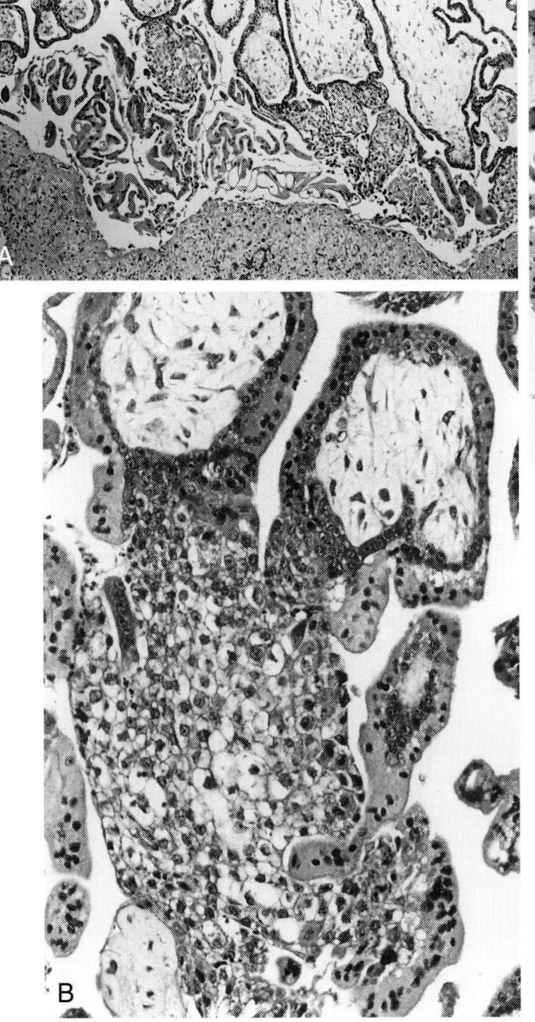

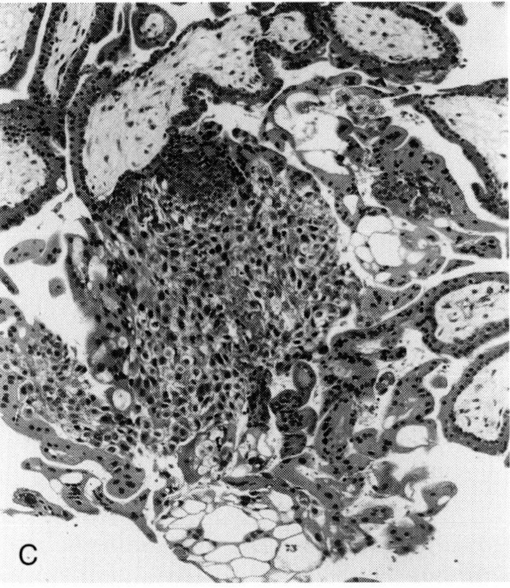

Figure 10–1. A, Normal placenta at implantation site; 6 weeks MA. A confluence of trophoblastic columns appears at the right; gross activity of syncytium can be seen in the center and left. Note the light texture and moderate cellularity of the villous stroma; no erythrocytes are present yet. The decidua is strewn with intermediate cytotrophoblastic cells; Nitabuch's line is visible over the left one third. **B,** Normal placenta; 7½ weeks MA. Two villi with a high-power view of fusing trophoblastic columns. Note the enclosure of syncytial cells and the regular, honeycomb-like character of the intermediate cytotrophoblast. The vessels in the right villus are distended with embryonic blood. **C,** Normal placenta: trophoblast at implantation site, 7 weeks MA. Note fusing trophoblastic columns and syncytial accumulation: hyperplasia within physiologic limits, as seen at the implantation site.

trophoblast may cause the intervillous space to be bathed by a maternal blood transudate rather than by whole blood.[20] The trophoblastic invasion is a physiologic process, and the active appearance of the trophoblast, including the focal widening of the syncytium layer and the vacuolation of its cells on contact with the decidua, does not signify a pathologic process (Fig. 10–1). Another area of intimate contact of trophoblast with maternal tissues results from trophoblast's slight, usually subclinical embolization into the pulmonary circulation. The cells' subsequent passage into the systemic circulation is being investigated because both trophoblast and embryonic nucleated erythrocytes may serve as a source of DNA for prenatal diagnosis.[21]

The direct contact of the trophoblast with maternal blood and tissues is made possible by its antigenic neutrality as the perivillous and extravillous trophoblast is devoid of both the HL-A[22] and blood group A, B, and H[23] polymorphic antigens. The HL-A-G antigen present on the extravillous intermediate cells is a class 1 monomorphic dimer molecule that evokes no immune reaction.[24] Absent also are cell surface molecules that would constitute targets for natural killer (NK) cells,[25] while the complement-negating protein CD46[26] helps to protect all trophoblastic cells from humoral maternal immunity. The tissue seems accordingly invulnerable to maternal rejection and thus capable of protecting the total conceptus.[27,28] Nevertheless, the molecular profile of the trophoblastic cell surfaces is not fixed but rather changes on decidual invasion with respect to adhesion receptors and extracellular matrix ligands. Such alterations point to the controls of tro phoblastic behavior and their failure, as in invasive CHM and cancer.[29]

COMPLETE HYDATIDIFORM MOLE

Clinical Aspects

CHM is a rare disease in Western nations, occurring in 1 of 1500 to 2000 pregnancies. It is much more common in Asia.[30,31] The existence of a racial component is strongly suggested by an investigation conducted in Hawaii that demonstrated a high incidence of CHMs among Asian women irrespective of whether they were born in the Far East or in Hawaii, whereas the incidence among whites and Hawaiians was low.[32] Further suggestions as to the presence of a genetic element stem from cases of familial incidence including identical twins. Recurrence is rare, but its chances increase steeply after each repeat. Maternal age plays a role; incidence is high before 20 and after 35 to 40 years. Neither paternal race nor age seems to be significant.[32–34]

The first symptom[35–37] of CHM is vaginal bleeding, which may be accompanied by tell-tale molar vesicles. Later signs and symptoms are uterine enlargement (beyond that warranted by the duration of amenorrhea), hyperemesis, and preeclampsia associated with high levels of hCG, which also is likely to cause ovarian theca-lutein cysts. Respiratory insufficiency from massive embolization of placental elements to the lungs and thyroid storm are rare complications. Many of the above clinical signs and symptoms are becoming less frequent thanks to the availability of early ultrasound[38] and the accurate measurement of maternal hCG levels.[39,40] Thus first-trimester diagnosis based on the absence of heart movements and presence of high hCG levels can result in nearly 90% accuracy.[41] Early diagnosis allows treatment to be applied at a mean gestational age of 12 weeks, a month earlier than in the past.[42] Nevertheless, the high hCG levels that characterize the early moles remain associated with a frequency of residual trophoblastic disease (RTD) unchanged by early evacuation.[42]

The most important aspect of CHM is the propensity for trophoblastic villous invasion beyond the decidual placental site and for trophoblastic malignant transformation to choriocarcinoma or (much less frequently) to a placental site trophoblastic tumor. The first two conditions are heralded clinically by persistently high hCG levels and irregular behavior of the hCG recession curves after evacuation of the mole.[43] Since either the biologically nonmalignant invasive mole or choriocarcinoma is eminently curable by modern chemotherapy, the clinical entity RTD[1,16,35–37] covers both conditions usually without pathologic diagnosis. The diagnosis of choriocarcinoma accordingly is clinically obvious in the presence of a uterine neoplasm or of a systemic metastasis (e.g., to brain, kidney, or liver).[44] It should be remembered that molar emboli to lungs or retrograde venous spread of molar elements to adnexa and vulvo-vagina are likely to be noncancerous and do not determine a diagnosis of malignancy.[16,45–47] Mischief may be caused by massive pulmonary embolization[48] or by vulvar implants, which are notoriously difficult to treat[49]; neglected cases in the past were known to culminate in uterine rupture with hemorrhage and sepsis, but these phenomena are referable to the embolizing and invasive properties of normal trophoblast and its faculty for "tapping" vessels and causing hemorrhage. The biologically nonmalignant character of the invasive CHM was borne out by experiments in nude mice and immunologically inert hamsters, which survived well the transplant of CHM tissues from both invasive and noninvasive moles and died only of choriocarcinoma.[50]

The incidence of choriocarcinoma is said to be unrelated to invasive mole. Modern imaging techniques (computed tomography, nuclear magnetic resonance, and color flow Doppler) confirm the earlier notion that subclinical degrees of myometrial invasion and lung embolization[51] can occur in CHM and are apt to resolve spontaneously.

Embryology and Pathologic Anatomy

CHM arises through an abnormal fertilization and gross genomic abnormality (referred to below) that lead to early loss of the embryo proper and to a highly characteristic metamorphosis of the placenta. For pregnancy to take place, the earliest postfertilization development must adhere to a near-normal pattern because the stages of morula, blastula, and implantation have to be achieved. The formation of the placenta presumably starts in the usual way with the appearance of the first generation of chorionic villi during the third postfertilization week (fifth week menstrual age [MA]).[18] The molar phenotype begins to assert itself soon after as the trophoblastic hyperplasia overwhelms attempts at formation of the orderly bilayer of perivillous trophoblast and of the trophoblastic columns (Fig. 10–2*A* and *B*). The configuration of the villous tree seems also modified; as seen in early molar specimens[17,52] most of the villi are stubby polygonal structures with a cauliflower-like appearance when cut across (Fig. 10–2*A*), instead of the usual less cellular, fingerlike branching villi. The stroma is unusually cellular with a mucoid appearance of the ground substance, which soon becomes dominated by the growing edema. Starting at the preedematous stages there is often a striking random necrobiosis of stromal cells, a phenomenon unique for the CHM (Fig. 10–2*A*).[3,17] In both the normal and molar villous stroma numerous capillary vessels are formed in situ, but in the case of CHM they remain empty of blood and undergo early degeneration,[3,4] much as they would in nonmolar placentas in cases of early (before 6½ weeks MA) embryonic demise.[53,54]

Edema appears early in the CHM villi and leads to eventual cistern formation.[4] The steadily accumulating fluid collects in a few stromal loculi, but these soon coalesce into a central cavity with a simultaneous compression and recession to the periphery of the now slowly maturing stromal mesenchyme (Fig. 10–2*C*). The process finishes with a large, grapelike villus much expanded by fluid contained by a wall of avascular, poorly cellular connective tissue. The inner edge of the cisternal wall becomes sharply demarcated halfway through the process; devoid of a specific lining epithelium, it is reminiscent of the edge of synovial membranes (Fig. 10–2*D*). Cisterns characteristically appear only in CHM and PHM; they are rare indeed in trisomies, where they involve only an occasional villus. The molar fluid contains hormones secreted by the syncytiotrophoblast[55] and procoagulant substances that are most likely capable of promoting clotting when spilled into the intervillous blood space. It seems legitimate to speculate that the clotting process may cause local villous infarction and that it may spread to the decidual vessels, producing local necrosis and thus (late) uterine bleeding.[56]

The trophoblast is by definition hyperplastic, the two layers actively participating; they cover the villous surface more or less completely, probably as a function of time. The degree of hyperplasia differs among specimens and within a single specimen (Fig. 10–2*E*). The molar trophoblast physiologically resembles that of the early normal gestation, since it sustains active growth and a continuous secretion of hCG with low levels of human placental lactogen (hPL) and placental alkaline phosphatase (PLAP).[57] The antigenic correspondence between the normal and the molar trophoblastic populations is equally striking because the phenotype of the HL-A antigens is similar in both cases, including the invasive mole.[58–60] The HL-A antibodies encountered in women carrying a CHM seem to be engendered by the antigens of the villous mesenchymal elements as in normal gestations.[61] Important differences between the normal and molar trophoblast include an increased proliferation rate, high genomic polyploidization rate (referred to below), and chromosomal instability, all in the CHM, where the frequency of chromosomal breaks, losses, and translocations is also much higher.[62]

Diagnosis

Staging is an important element in the diagnosis of hydatidiform moles. It has become obvious that both CHM and PHM undergo a gradual morphologic evolution[4,17] discernible from the earliest phases as a staggered process in a growing placenta. The villi of a CHM, accordingly, are represented on a pathologist's slide as in a stationary snapshot showing each villus in its own stage of the developmental sequence. The staggered nature of the process is most obvious in the first few gestational weeks, whereas the end stages easily predominate in the older placentas. Since until recently uterine evacuation of a CHM, whether spontaneous or surgical, tended to be relatively late, the standard descriptions of its pathologic anatomy have been based on the fully developed stages, the minuscule autolyzed embryo and its membranes are lost in the bulky specimen, which consists of grossly expanded, closely packed vesicles 1 to 3 cm in diameter that give the classic macroscopic appearance of a bunch of grapes (Fig. 10–2*F*). The hyperplastic trophoblast surrounds the circumference of the villi, with the initially attempted normal two-layer pattern replaced by an exuberant, multilayered, focally anaplastic cytotrophoblast and syncytiotrophoblast (Fig. 10–2*E*).

With the advent of sonography uterine evacuation has been taking place at increasingly early stages of gestation. Although the ultrasound diagnosis of a snowstorm appearance has to wait until the end of the first trimester, a diagnosis of embryonic death alone (missed abortion) warrants surgical uterine emptying, often performed as early as 6 to 8 weeks MA. A presumptive gross pathologic diagnosis cannot usually be made at these early stages, but microscopic examination can distinguish between a CHM and a nonmolar abortus. The former shows a probably still focal trophoblastic hyperplasia overtaking the villi, accompanied by cellular stroma with primitive-looking fibroblasts, receding empty capillaries, and incipient, perhaps still focal, edema. Stromal spotty necrobiosis and endothelial degeneration in the capillaries may already be present; the two should be regarded as separate processes. It is specimens from these stages that must be knowledgeably examined, since the presence of early preedematous, seemingly unaffected villi in addition to early molar ones may suggest a partial mole.[16,17,52] In cases of nonmolar abortus associated with early embryonic demise (before 6 to 7 weeks MA),[53,54] the placenta is apt to show uniform generalized edema without trophoblastic hyperplasia and without cistern formation (Fig. 10–3). The stromal vessels may still be present but remain empty of (nucleated) erythrocytes if the embryo dies before their normal appearance.[53] The trophoblastic columns and the cytotrophoblastic shell remain normally prominent and retain much of their structure, as described in the section on the trophoblast.

Examination of the placental site is relevant to the diagnosis of hydatidiform moles. CHMs in this location are frequently associated with diffuse and marked trophoblastic atypia manifest as nuclear irregularity, enlargement, and hyperchromasia; such atypia is only infrequently seen in PHMs. In neither case is the atypia of prognostic significance.[63] Placental site nodules of intermediate trophoblast[64] have been described as following CHM, but the incidence must be rare.

Embryo in Complete Hydatidiform Moles

As already stated, the embryo dies early in development, presumably between days 15 and 31 fertilization age (4 to 6½ weeks MA), when crown-rump length is less than 5.5 mm.[65] This proposed time-frame is based on the obligatory survival of the embryonic disk until day 14, when it provides the extraembryonic mesenchyme that organizes

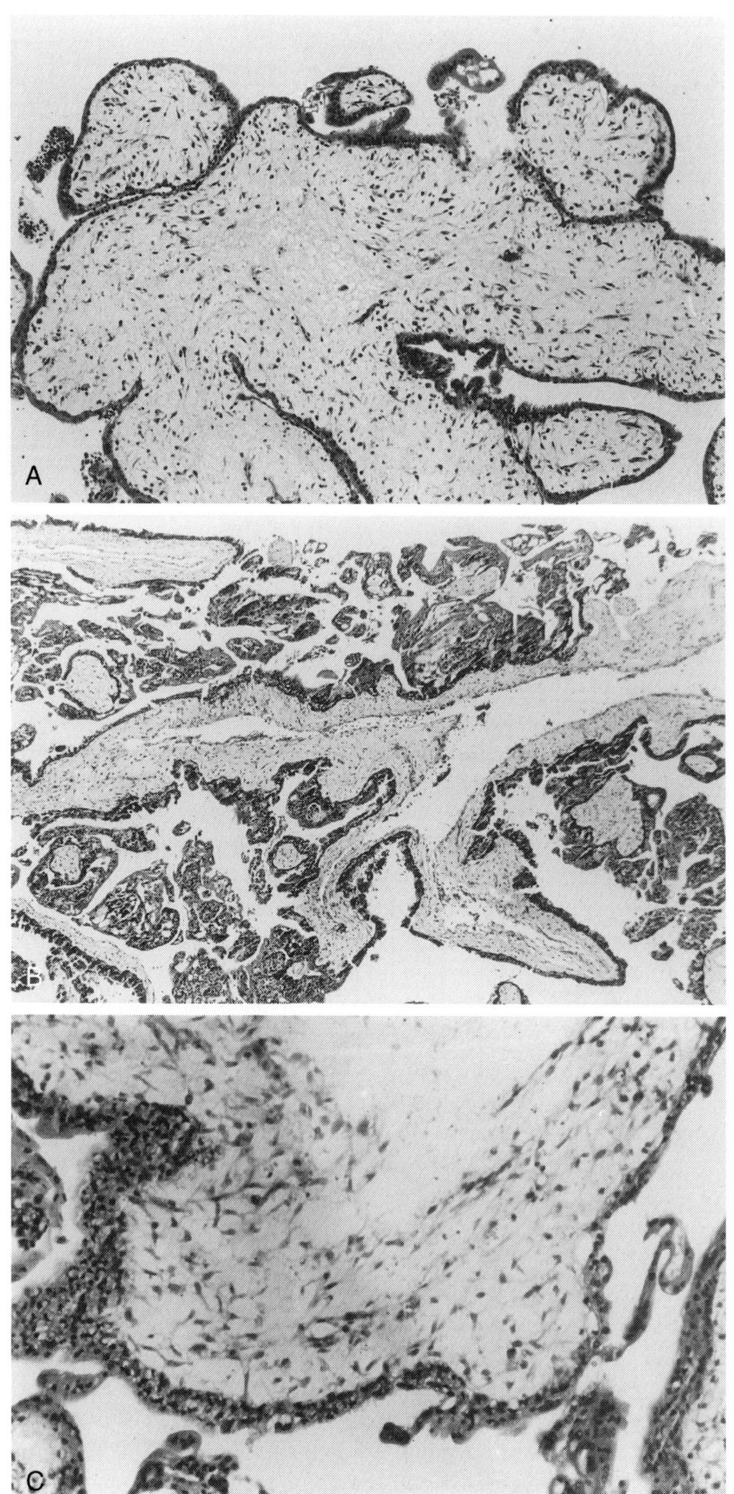

Figure 10–2. A, Early complete hydatidiform mole (CHM), 7 weeks MA. Short bulbous villi with rich cellular, vasculogenic stroma; focal necrobiosis of fibroblasts (seen as eosinophilia of a whole cell and as karyorrhexic dust). Incipient slight trophoblastic hyperplasia. Early edema visible in the center of this cauliflower-like complex.[52] **B,** Very early CHM, 8 weeks MA. Chorion and few early villi with marked but still focal trophoblastic hyperplasia. Note its exuberant character and the surprising size of numerous tufts projecting into the perivillous maternal blood space (which possibly are liable to embolization). **C,** Cistern formation in progress. CHM, 12 weeks MA. A "young" villus showing a rapidly accumulated centrally located fluid pushing the stroma to the periphery. The stroma is still edematous and quite cellular; several well-formed capillaries, empty of blood, can be seen. Inner edge of wall is not yet well demarcated. Trophoblast is mostly in stage of "normal" bilayer in this field. (*A:* slide courtesy R.W. Redline, M.D., Institute of Pathology, Case Western Reserve University, Cleveland, Ohio.)

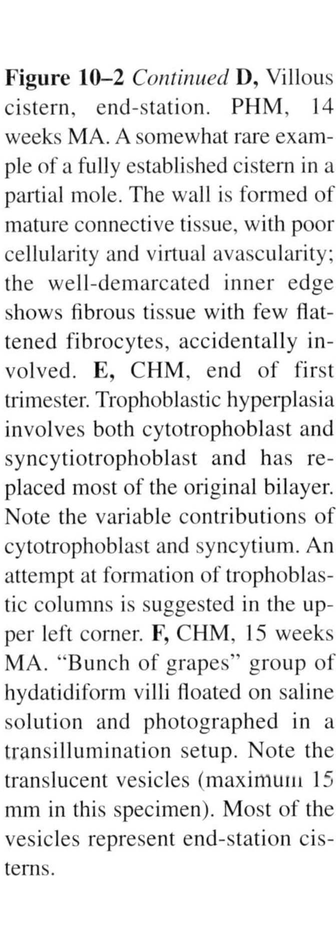

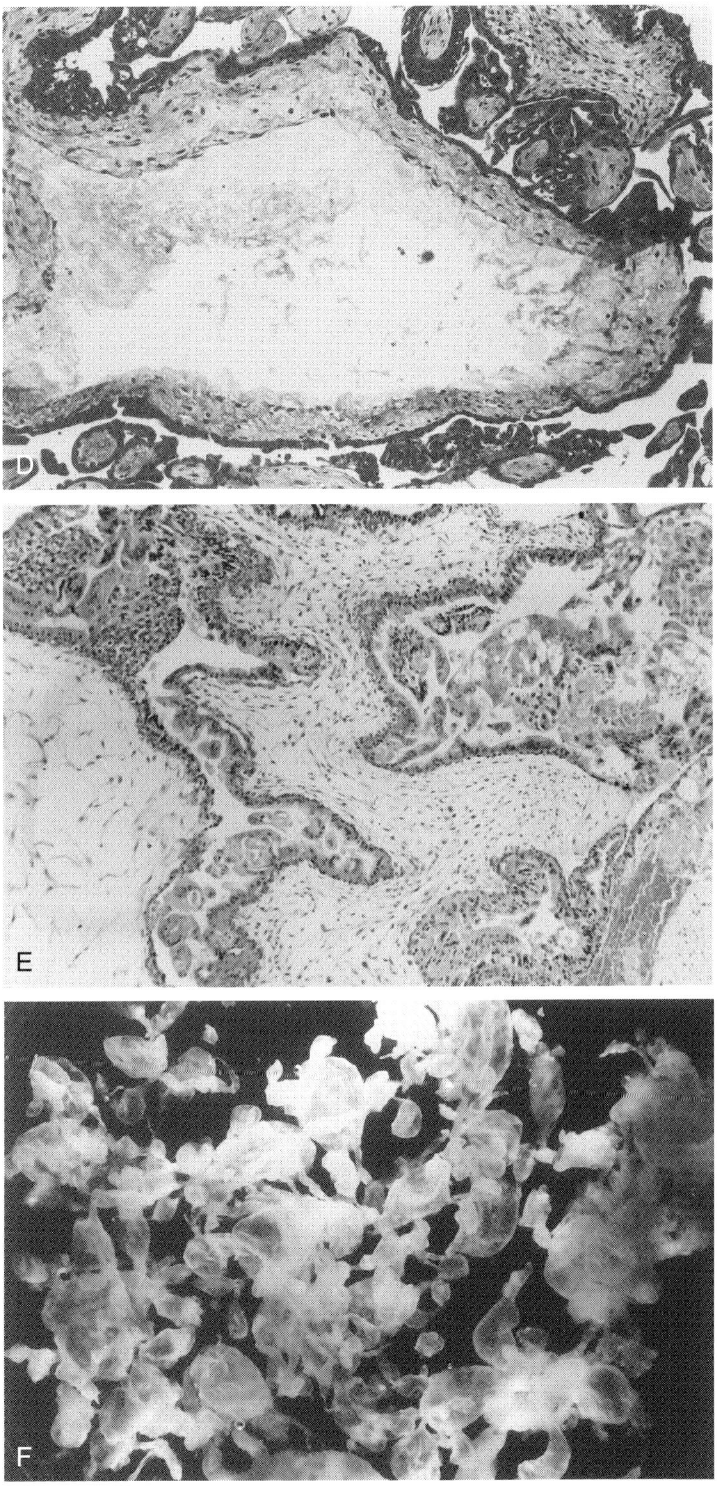

Figure 10–2 *Continued* **D,** Villous cistern, end-station. PHM, 14 weeks MA. A somewhat rare example of a fully established cistern in a partial mole. The wall is formed of mature connective tissue, with poor cellularity and virtual avascularity; the well-demarcated inner edge shows fibrous tissue with few flattened fibrocytes, accidentally involved. **E,** CHM, end of first trimester. Trophoblastic hyperplasia involves both cytotrophoblast and syncytiotrophoblast and has replaced most of the original bilayer. Note the variable contributions of cytotrophoblast and syncytium. An attempt at formation of trophoblastic columns is suggested in the upper left corner. **F,** CHM, 15 weeks MA. "Bunch of grapes" group of hydatidiform villi floated on saline solution and photographed in a transillumination setup. Note the translucent vesicles (maximum 15 mm in this specimen). Most of the vesicles represent end-station cisterns.

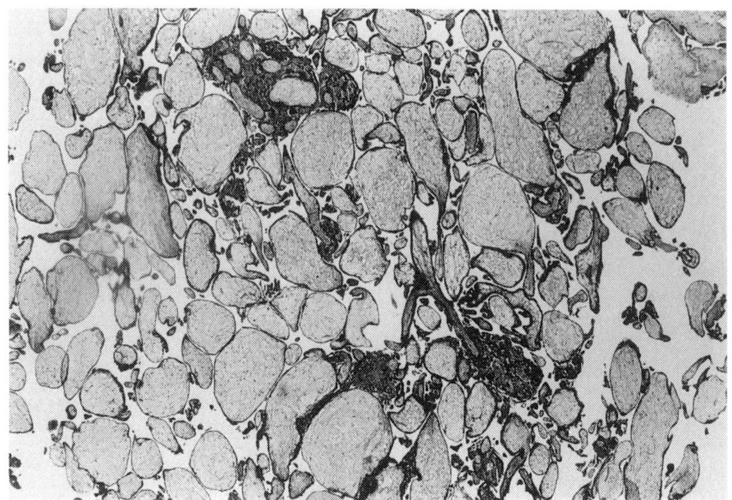

Figure 10–3. Hydropic abortus, placenta; "blighted ovum," 10 weeks MA. Uniform villous edema, without trophoblastic hyperplasia and without cistern formation. An occasional trophoblastic column must not be misinterpreted as expressing hyperplasia.

the placenta,[18] and the consistent appearance of nucleated, yolk sac–derived erythrocytes in normal placentas on day 31 or 32,[53] while they are conspicuously absent in CHMs. Rare exceptions to the latter rule have been noted.[11,12,66] In such genetically verified cases the embryo apparently survives long enough to produce and circulate its blood through the placenta. This finding should not contradict the diagnosis; several cases of residual disease following an early CHM with villous embryonic erythrocytes or embryonal tissues such as yolk sac or amnion are on record.[11,66]

Twins: Complete Hydatidiform Mole and Normal Conceptus

Twin conceptuses of a CHM and a normal fetus are rare (estimated incidence 1 in 22,000 to 100,000 pregnancies[67]) but are important because they are difficult to diagnose clinically and pose problems related to the twin nature of the pregnancy, salvaging of the normal fetus, and a propensity of the CHM twin to lead to residual trophoblastic disease.[67,68]

Multiple conceptions are common in patients treated with gonadotropin (e.g., in in vitro fertilization and embryo transplants), and twins, triplets, and other multiple pregnancies have been encountered in which one of the conceptuses is a CHM. First-trimester and even later ultrasound examination may fail to diagnose the condition correctly, and pathologic specimens from the early cases are liable to be misinterpreted because signs of villous molar change are not yet clear; the separate placentas and the fetus can be more readily distinguished in later stages. Appropriate tissues can be sampled for chromosomal, imaging, or DNA analysis to confirm the diagnosis.[69–71] Occasionally the molar placenta appears compressed and degenerated, most likely because of damage wrought by the normal twin, but generous sampling will make microscopic diagnosis possible. In some cases intimate interdigitations of the two placentas produce a deceptive microscopic appearance of commingled molar and normal elements, leading to an erroneous diagnosis of diploid PHM[71,72] with a normal fetus, a dubious entity. Obviously, attention in cases of twins with a mole focuses on allowing the fetus to reach viability. Although the danger of RTD is not much greater in cases diagnosed late in gestation, the fate of the fetus is precarious and only a small proportion survive into extrauterine life.[67,68]

Twinning is more common than meets the eye, for mortality of one or both individuals seen early in the first trimester by ultrasound is surprisingly high.[73,74] Accordingly, the pathologist needs to be aware of the possibility of two separate populations of villi, however intimately intermixed, since the possibility of an unsuspected lurking twin does exist, especially in early products of conception curettage specimens. Ultrasound has introduced the entity of the vanishing twin.[73,74] Such a twin dies in the first few weeks of gestation and becomes invisible on the sonography screen within the first trimester, but it may add an inconspicuous amount of placental tissue to the placenta of the surviving partner. Accordingly, a nonmolar vanishing twin may contribute its placental remnant to the molar placenta, creating a spurious mosaic because of the appearance of an incongruous clone on genetic (chromosome, DNA) analysis. If it survives beyond 6½ weeks MA,[53,54] it may add a number of villi still bearing its (nucleated) erythrocytes and confuse the diagnosis.[11,12,66]

Prognosis

Prognosis of CHM continues to depend on multiple items of the patient's clinical profile,[1,75] preeminent among which are undue uterine enlargement, high preevacuation hCG levels and their subsequent anomalies, and promptness of instituting therapy. The pathologist has less to contribute, since no information as to prognosis is lent by the degree of anaplasia of the trophoblast[76]; the number of molar cells in the G2/M phase (or the level of tetraploidy) as given by DNA flow cytometry[77]; the trophoblastic proliferation rate as given by the proliferative cell nuclear antigen (PCNA)[78] or the cell proliferation marker,[79] both visualized by immunohistology; the zygosity of the molar conceptus[80,81]; or the level of aneuploidy as determined by DNA cell imaging or in situ hybridization,[82] although trophoblastic aneuploidy has been claimed to have some value.[83]

The hCG extinction curve is the sole reliable instrument of prognosis and control of chemotherapy. Such treatment—it must be emphasized—does not imply malignancy, since most patients are in effect being treated for an invasive or embolic mole. Although chemotherapy cures more than 90% of patients and permits subsequent successful reproduction, some drug combinations do increase the risk of late-onset cancer.[84]

Choriocarcinoma is the most important sequela of CHM, but the underlying genetic change remains unknown. Since this cancer often strikes during or shortly after pregnancy, it is possible that the homozygosity for a recessive inherited gene[2] is in operation. The inherited gene may be a mutated tumor suppressor that becomes associated with an activated protooncogene. Such activation would have a step-limiting function that delays the final, full phenotypic change, thus accounting for the delayed clinical manifestations.[40,43–45]

PARTIAL HYDATIDIFORM MOLE

Clinical Aspects

The approximate incidence of PHM is that of triploidy in human pregnancy, estimated to be 1% to 2%.[85] Because the majority of triploids have a diandric origin, PHM is the most common gestational trophoblastic disease. Since most diandric triploid conceptuses come to early abortion, the following approximations are relevant: of the 50% of early abortuses with chromosomal anomalies, 15% are triploid,[86] of which in turn 80% are diandric.[8,9] The resultant figure of 6.6% for PHMs in the abortus population has not been met, however, making PHM an often missed condition.[16,17,87,88] The predominance of diandric over digynic triploids has been questioned,[89] but since this seems likely to apply to triploids that survive into the second and third trimesters, it would be unlikely to much modify the above calculation for early abortuses. It certainly does not detract from the consensus that a large proportion of first-trimester PHMs escape identification.

The partial mole appears to have no significant association with maternal age, race, or geographic location.[90,91] Its significance lies in the fact that even though it echoes many of the features of the complete mole, it is usually a bland condition, free of untoward sequelae and without effect on future reproductive performance. Apart from the trophoblastic hyperplasia and hydatidiform villous swelling, the clinicopathologic features that may be shared—however infrequently—by the two syndromes include early embryonic death, undue uterine enlargement, high hCG levels, hyperemesis and preeclampsia, and residual disease.[3,16] However, the signs and symptoms in the vast majority of patients with PHM are mild: the uterus tends to be small or normal for dates, and the hCG level is seldom greater than 100,000 mIU/ml. Only in a small proportion of cases, usually those with drawn-out gestations, does a high hCG concentration prove troublesome.[90,91] Thus pre-

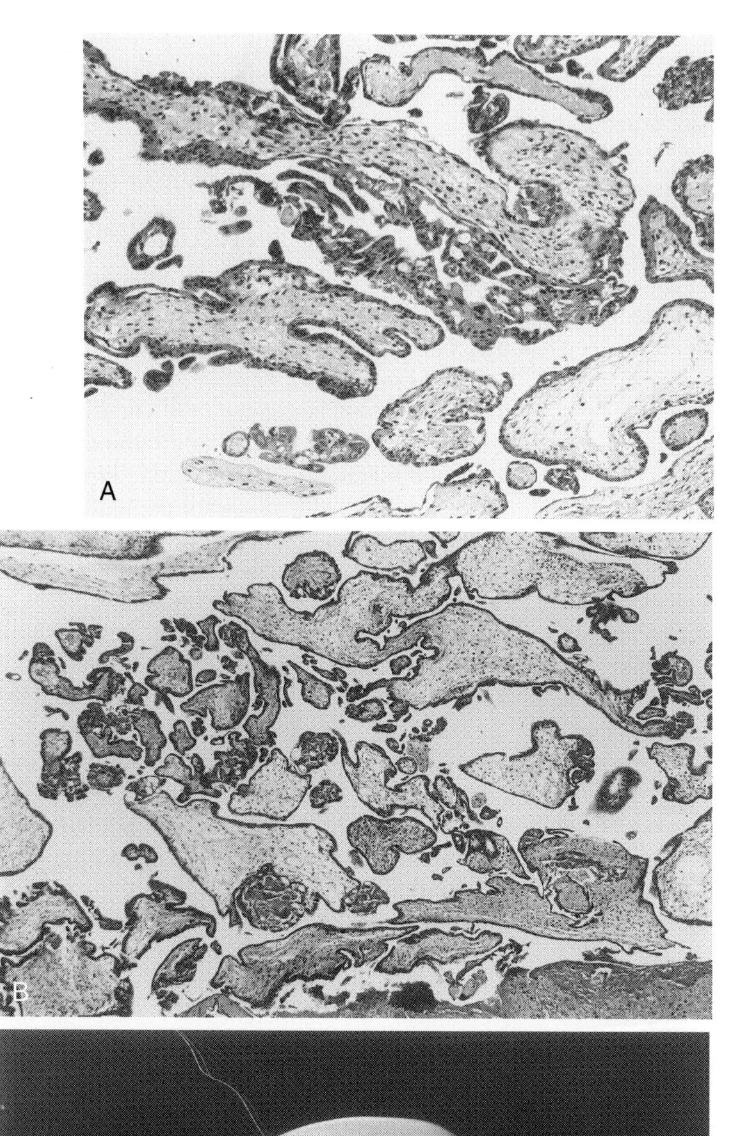

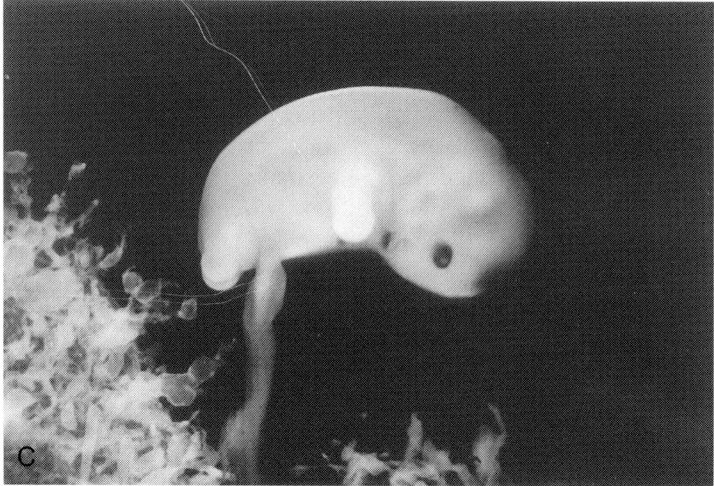

Figure 10–4. A, Partial hydatidiform mole (PHM), 11 weeks MA, trophoblastic hyperplasia. Note the all-syncytial character of the hyperplastic layer. Also shown are clear edema of a villus *(right lower corner)* and mild fibrosis elsewhere. Embryonic death occurred 3 weeks before. **B,** PHM, 11 weeks MA, panoramic view. Note the presence of "small villi"; larger villi with hydrops, fluid loculating in one (right lower corner). Focal trophoblastic hyperplasia, favoring locations inside villous surface concavities. Fibrosis, mainly in small villi—in wake of embryonic death 3 weeks before. **C,** PHM, 9 weeks MA. Malformed, slightly macerated embryo, about 8 weeks MA, retained for 1 week post mortem.

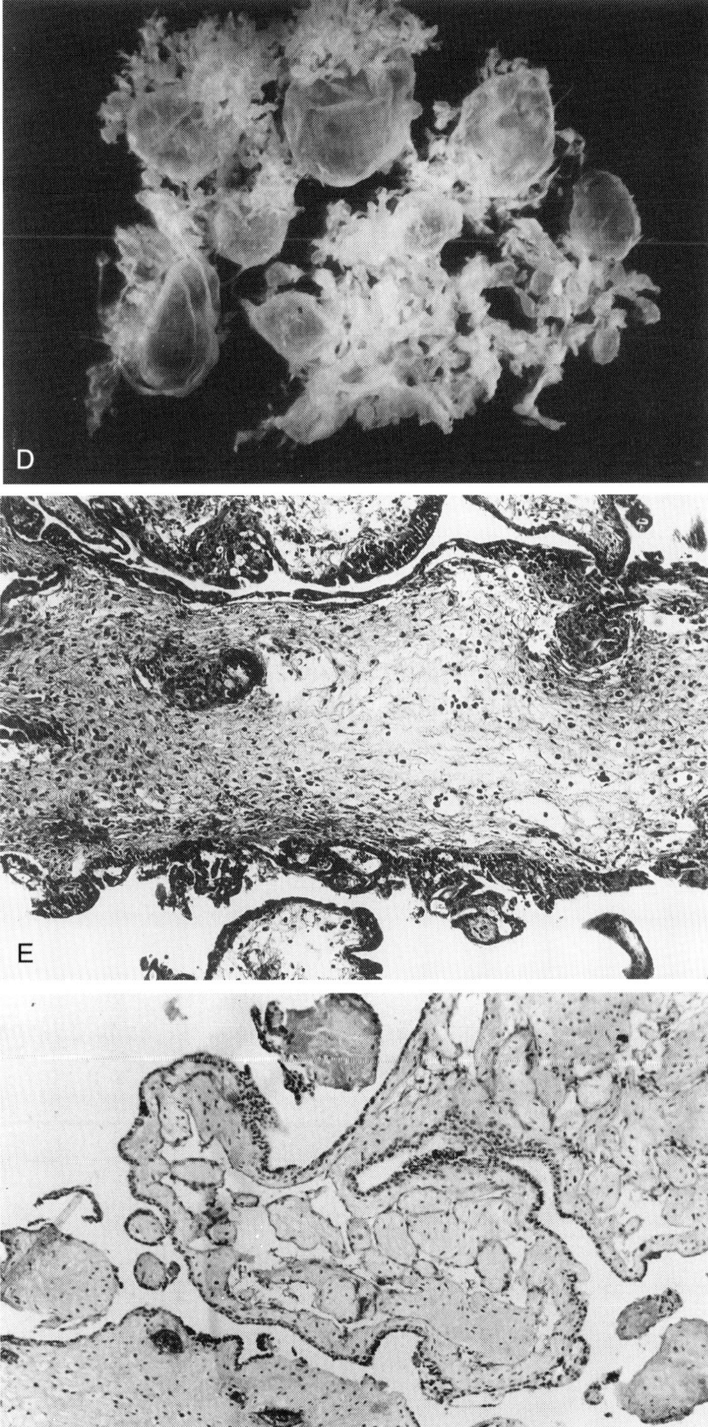

Figure 10–4 *Continued* **D,** PHM, 13 weeks MA. Well-developed villous vesicles up to 15 mm diameter, against a background of smaller vesicles and nonexpanded villi. **E,** PHM, 10 weeks MA. A villus showing two inclusions, formed by incursions of both layers of surface trophoblast into the subjacent stroma. (The one on the right seems to have just started on its journey from the surface.) The inclusions are lumenless; the lucent areas in the center are produced by syncytial cytoplasmic vacuolation. **F,** PHM, 18 weeks MA. Mazelike, ectatic vessel(s). This is a rare finding in PHMs and is usually past the first trimester. The endothelium is positive for factor VIII; erythrocytes are only rarely encountered in the lumen.

eclampsia and thyrotoxicosis can occur in the second trimester. Several affected patients were reported as carrying a live fetus with the stigmata of triploidy.[92] Such patients have high levels of hCG and are prone to RTD; it has been suggested that they have a rare but important syndrome coming to a head at midpregnancy.[93] The commonly encountered PHMs, however, present no distinguishing clinical or pathologic features that bear on their future course and ultimate prognosis.

The pathologic substrate of residual disease after uterine evacuation is an invasive partial mole. This is detected by an anomalous hCG return curve and has been visualized by ultrasound and nuclear magnetic resonance imaging. It is a rare sequela not accompanied by venous embolization,[94,95] although finer tomography techniques have demonstrated minute trophoblastic pulmonary foci, which apparently have little clinical import. These conditions respond well to chemotherapy.[37]

The incidence of invasive PHMs is low. In hospital populations it is stated as rather less than 5% of cases,[90,91] but this is likely to be an overestimate because the denominator of this ratio would be much larger if the total PHM population of nonhospitalized and missed cases were included. The high incidence of PHM has not been so far reflected in a correspondingly increased number of reported PHMs with a normal twin, and only a few sporadic cases are on record[96]; it remains to be seen whether the RTD incidence is high in such cases.

The association of partial moles with choriocarcinoma has not been proved. No chorionic cancer has been reported in the numerous published hospital series, including the two cited above,[94,95] which encompassed 590 patients. Several authors have reported single cases, in which the cancer followed a PHM after prolonged, unsurveyed intervals.[97] Two of these cancers had a diploid constitution[98] (one with a miniscule questionable additional triploid peak[99]) on flow cytometry; a few other reports described a PHM placenta with a small, in situ, anaplastic, noninvasive trophoblastic area that was not further investigated. Such cases will certainly be studied in the future by molecular DNA techniques, both retrospectively and prospectively. To date no fully authenticated case of cancer derived from a PHM is on record.

Embryology, Pathologic Anatomy, and Diagnosis

As with CHM, in the earliest stages the PHM placenta most likely develops along normal lines. The pathologic modifications take place after initial formation of the villi in the third postfertilization week (fifth week MA). The pathognomonic placental features become ascertainable later than those of the CHM, and the embryo survives much longer. Specimens of PHM before 6 to 7 weeks MA are rarely seen by pathologists and may be difficult to appreciate: the placenta may seem normal because villous edema and syncytiotrophoblastic hyperplasia are inconspicuous and the embryo may still be alive. Our experience of early cases remains virtually limited to PHMs that come to the pathologist after 7 to 8 weeks MA in the guise of spontaneous or missed abortions, the latter quite common because ultrasonography easily spots a dead or absent embryo or fetus but is slow to perceive small-diameter, scattered villous vesicles. Probably some of the undiagnosed PHMs reside in these early populations.

The morphologic attributes of a partial mole are focal trophoblastic hyperplasia (Fig. 10–4*A*), focal, most often mild to moderate, hydatidiform villous change (Fig. 10–4*B*), and prolonged survival of the embryo (Fig. 10–4*C*) or less often the fetus.[3,4,8,16,17] The trophoblastic hyperplasia rarely becomes pronounced; it is usually confined to the syncytiotrophoblast, which often displays cytoplasmic vacuolation. The villous fluid accumulation follows the same morphologic steps as those in the complete mole (Figs. 10–2*D* and 10–4*D*). The process, however, is much slower, and the end-station cisterns appear much later. Their numbers therefore are likely to be small, and diagnosis may have to rely on other features. Interspersed among the groups of villi with hydatidiform changes are groups of small villi that are seemingly normal or covered by hyperplastic trophoblast (Fig. 10–4*B*). Whether they are destined to engage in the slow hydatidiform evolution is a moot point; it seems, however, that their fibrosis (following death of the embryo or fetus) would preclude such a process.[53,54] In either case the morphologic checkerboard pattern provides an important diagnostic point virtually unique for the partial mole.[3,8,17]

In addition to the hydatidiform change and the trophoblastic hyperplasia, characteristics shared with the complete mole, the partial syndrome is characterized by several morphologic features of its own.[8] Chief among these is the pronounced sharp-angled scalloping of the villous outlines (Fig. 10–4*A* and *B*), found even in the younger specimens and apt to become more pronounced with villous fibrosis. Close in frequency and of some diagnostic usefulness are the so-called trophoblastic inclusions, in reality narrow, *lumenless* incursions of the surface trophoblastic bilayer into the villous stroma (Fig. 10–4*E*). Although seen in some cases of trisomic and normal-appearing placentas, they can occur in profusion in the triploid moles beginning in early stages; occasionally, however, they are absent. Another form of incursion of trophoblast into the stroma results in the presence of single-cell intermediate trophoblast that is positive for hPL; its diagnostic value is slight, since it occurs in villi of placentas with other chromosomal errors.

A peculiar form of a vascular malformation, lined by endothelium that is positive for factor VIII and having a complex, mazelike outline, is seen infrequently in specimens past 16 weeks MA (Fig. 10–4*F*). Such vessels are usually empty of erythrocytes, suggesting a lack of connection to the general circulation or, more likely, an origin after death of the embryo or fetus. They are of diagnostic significance, since they occur only exceptionally in other conditions, such as CHM.[17]

The pathologist is not likely to see an invasive PHM. Only two cases have been described, and these show a histologically unremarkable incursion of trophoblast-plus-villi into the myometrium underlying the placental site decidua.[100,101] They probably will be more frequently visualized by ultrasound and other noninvasive imaging means.

Early Demise of the Embryo or Fetus

The embryo in PHM is apt to die in the first trimester, and survival beyond 8 to 9 weeks MA is infrequent.[8] Most often only fragmented autolyzed remnants of the embryo are found. The rare larger or better preserved specimens are of interest because they show typical congenital anomalies, further corroborating the triploid status of the conceptus.[92] As long as the embryo or fetus remains alive, it maintains a normal placental villous circulation: the capillaries in both the hydatidiform and the small villi are distended with erythrocytes that often remain nucleated beyond the usual limit of 11½ weeks MA. After embryonic or fetal demise the villous capillaries retain their erythrocytes and remain identifiable for several weeks, incomparably longer than the ephemeral empty capillaries of the complete moles. This difference is associated with the relatively long preservation of the embryonic or fetal erythrocytes that provide a useful footprint of the dead and missing embryo. Consequent on the cessation of the intravillous circulation, fibrosis of the mesenchyme develops in villi not yet affected by edema.[53,54] This does not detract from the diagnostic hallmarks of PHM; the majority of partial moles past the first trimester are in fact seen in this state. Since edema is often slight to moderate, the fibrosis relatively prominent, and the dead embryo encased in a small, no longer enlarging gestational sac, the uterus tends to be small for dates, a common finding in the PHM syndrome.[90]

DIFFERENTIAL DIAGNOSIS OF COMPLETE HYDATIDIFORM MOLE, PARTIAL HYDATIDIFORM MOLE, AND HYDROPIC ABORTUS

As hinted above, aside from trophoblastic hyperplasia, no single morphologic feature can be used to diagnose a complete or a partial mole, since many of these features can be found elsewhere and pathologic diagnosis depends on their agglomeration in one placenta. Of importance here is the availability of adequate material (optimally more than five placental blocks), especially with PHM in which pathologic changes are disposed in a checkerboard fashion and are often inconspicuous. Familiarity with the embryologic development of the early conceptus and with the progressive and staggered character of molar development will help in distinguishing between CHM and PHM and keep the so-called hydropic abortus (HA) in its place. HA is a vague entity, its name derived from more or less generalized villous hydrops, that follows embryonic death before 8 weeks MA[53,54] and whose vesicles do not usually reach beyond 5 mm in diameter. Trophoblastic hyperplasia is absent; it must not be confused with the growth of trophoblastic columns and their confluence to form the trophoblastic shell or with focal trophoblastic exuberance at the implantation site (Fig. 10–1).

The microscopic differentiation between CHM and PHM is helped by consideration of the placental general landscape: the closely packed, cistern-containing hydatidiform villi in CHM (Fig. 10–2*E*) versus the patchy two-tone disposition of the villi, only some of which seem to be undergoing hydatidiform change in PHM (Fig. 10–4*B*). The composition of the trophoblast and its degree of hyperplasia, as well as the distinct features of villous mesenchymal edema and vasculature in CHM and PHM, have already been described (see Table 10–1). Since the embryo dies early in CHM, there is no villous fibrosis, whereas in PHM the relatively late embryonic or fetal demise allows stromal fibrosis of villi not yet taken over by edema.[53,54] While the preceding description applies to the end-picture of CHM and PHM, attention is drawn to their respective early stages, especially to the preedema villi in CHM (Fig. 10–2) and the inconspicuous state of the characteristic features in PHM. With either type of early mole the diagnosis hinges on the nature of the trophoblast; in my experience hyperplasia is diagnosable in CHM even in its earliest stages available,[16,17,52] while it remains hard to locate at similar stages of PHM.

Several authors have reported a facilitation, and sometimes a reversal, of diagnosis of CHMs or PHMs when ploidy of the tissues was established.[102] The easiest way has been an analysis by flow cytometry, but other techniques are gaining ground, notably DNA in situ hybridization and DNA image cytometry (see below).

GENETICS

Complete Hydatidiform Mole

CHM results from a compound error of fertilization: an "empty egg" that has lost its chromosome set of 23,X (possibly by extrusion of both haploid sets in the first or second polar body) is fertilized by a sperm carrying a haploid set of 23,X. The latter doubles without the usual cytokinesis to give the requisite 46 chromosomes, resulting in a homozygous CHM (diandric diploidy).[2] The sperm brings an X-containing set that gives a female karyotype; one with an Y chromosome would give a nonviable 46,YY zygote. Dispermic fertilizations can also occur; they give 46,XX or XY heterozygous conceptuses that account for 20% to 25% of CHMs.[103] Fertilization by a diploid sperm remains a theoretical possibility that is difficult to prove. In any case such conceptuses constitute a total allograft in the maternal body. The fertilization process leaves the egg cytoplasm intact, and the maternal mitochondria are preserved, attesting to the egg's identity; their relationship to the paternal chromosomes awaits interpretation.[104]

The genomic homozygosity of the CHM (reduced by one half in heterozygous moles) is likely to bring forth the expression of recessive lethal genes that may cause an early, clinically occult liquidation of some molar zygotes; it may also contribute to the characteristically early demise of the embryo proper. The latter and other phenotypic phenomena, however, are thought to result from the exclusively paternal source of molar chromosomes and the absence of maternal ones, a doctrine based on classic micromanipulation experiments involving an exchange of pronuclei among freshly fertilized murine eggs.[105,106] In these experiments the zygotes containing a male and a female pronucleus developed normally; those with two female pronuclei had a moderately long-surviving embryo but a poor trophoblast, while those with two male pronuclei mimicked the CHM by giving rise to an exuberant trophoblast with an embryo that died early in organogenesis. Clearly the parental chromosomes are differentially imprinted during the respective gametogenetic processes. In the case of CHM the double dose of paternal chromosomes is responsible for the trophoblastic hyperplasia, while the absence of a maternal set does not allow for the embryo's survival. The picture is reversed in digyny, in which the embryo fares much better because of the presence of maternal chromosomes whose imprinting pattern favors its development. These findings are also relevant to the interpretation of PHM.

Table 10–1. Clinicopathologic Features of Complete and Partial Hydatidiform Mole

Karyotype	Trophoblastic Hyperplasia	Hydatidiform Change	Villous Vessels	Embryo/Fetus	Clinical Presentation	Ultrasound	hCG	Sequelae
CHM 46,XX 46,XY Diandric diploidy	Both cytotrophoblast and syncytiotrophoblast Early superimposition of hyperplasia on normal-looking trophoblast bilayer	Early, generalized villous hydrops with rapid cistern formation; "bunch of grapes" gross appearance	Very early in situ formation, empty of blood; short lived Exceptional early cases with nucleated red blood cells	Early demise of embryo; alive until formation of extraembryonic mesenchyme	Late first trimester; bleeding, large uterus, high hCG, toxemia	"Snowstorm" appearance in late first trimester Early embryonic demise plus high hCG levels	High levels, $>10^5$ mIU/ml	RTD in ±20%, includes invasive/embolizing mole and choriocarcinoma (2% –5%)
PHM 69,XXY XXX XYY Diandric triploidy	Mild-moderate hyperplasia, virtually all syncytial Focal, often inconspicuous; many tissue blocks warranted.	Focal, slowly progressing with sparse cistern formation	Well formed, possibly ectatic, filled with blood Slow involution after embryo/fetal death	Well in evidence; lives till 8–9 weeks MA or longer Stigmata of triploidy, very occasionally of seemingly normal anatomy	Late, often second trimester; uterus small or normal; toxemia after 18 weeks MA; hCG above normal	First trimester: "missed abortion" Second trimester: focal hydrops; absent embryo or malformed fetus	Mildly to moderately raised levels $< 10^5$ mIU/ml	RTD very infrequent (invasive mole; no embolization) No choriocarcinoma cases authenticated

hCG, Human chorionic gonadotropin; *MA,* menstrual age; *US,* ultrasound; *RTD,* residual trophoblastic disease.

PARTIAL HYDATIDIFORM MOLE

The PHM is the result of a fertilization error in which two instead of one sperm penetrate the egg, imparting two independently drawn paternal haploid sets to give a triploid zygote of 69 chromosomes.[3,6,9] A minority of such triploids may arise through a fertilization by a diploid sperm (a product of error of meiosis, M1 or M2). The sex chromosome constitution of the digynic triploids bears on their survival, for the expected ratio of 1:2:1 for XXX:XXY:XYY is disturbed by the great paucity of the XYY cases.[8] The XYY triploids encountered present an early embryonic demise with the usual secondary placental changes. There are no other discernible clinicopathologic differences among the triploid PHMs.

Several cases are on record in which a PHM phenotype was associated with triandric tetraploidy presumed to result from fertilization by three sperm or by two, one of which was diploid.[107] These unique cases are of theoretical significance because they allow the generalization that the molar phenotype is brought about by the dominance of the molar genome by paternal DNA (Table 10–2): total dominance brings forth a CHM phenotype, whereas partial dominance—in the presence of a maternal contribution—is associated with a "diluted" one of a PHM.[107]

The preceding considerations imply that the phenotype of CHM and PHM could be brought about by disturbances in the balance between the normally imprinted parental DNA contributions to the zygote. The doctrine of genomic imprinting may help to account for CHMs or PHMs that do not fit the accepted model. Thus there can be an addition or loss of whole or parts of paternal or maternal chromosomes that are normally connected respectively with trophoblastic hyperplasia (and perhaps other features of CHM) or with embryonic and fetal development. Relevant examples are nontriploid PHMs whose phenotype is explicable by a disomy for a sector of paternal DNA that programs for molar phenotype[10,12,16] or by DNA imparted to the genome through somatic crossing over.[108] Another proposition is that disturbances of genomic balance are due to failure of initial imprinting or failure of its maintenance.[109] The answers to such questions seem resolvable on a molecular level and may be expected in the foreseeable future.

MOLECULAR INVESTIGATIONS

FLOW CYTOMETRY

The technical principle underlying flow cytometry (FCM) is the electronic, automated measurement of fluorochrome-conjugated DNA in individual cell nuclei as they pass through a laser beam.[110] Each DNA package excites a proportional level of fluorescence relayed by the computerized cytometry system to produce a histogram, previously or simultaneously calibrated by diploid cells. Flow cytometry analyzes the DNA contents of interphase cells counted in tens of thousands and presents them according to their DNA ploidy. It is efficient in giving relative estimates of diploid, triploid, and higher polyploidy cell populations and less efficient in documenting the (usually minor) aneuploid populations that fall

Table 10–2. Parental Chromosome Origin and Placental Phenotype

Chromosome Number	Origin of Haploid Sets Paternal/Maternal	Placental Phenotype
46: Biparental diploidy	1:1	Normal
69: Digynic triploidy	1:2	Nonmolar
69: Diandric triploidy	2:1	Partial hydatidiform mole
69: Triandric triploidy	3:0	Complete hydatidiform mole
92: Biparental tetraploidy	2:2	Nonmolar
92: Triandric tetraploidy	3:1	Partial hydatidiform mole

Placental complete molar phenotype appears where the paternal chromosomes dominate the genome in the absence of the maternal component; when present the latter "dilutes" the phenotype to one of partial hydatidiform mole. Note that statements of ploidy alone are insufficient and should include the parental origin of chromosomal sets.

between the euploid peaks. Given the requisite apparatus the method is rapid and inexpensive and provides information about the essential genomic character of the placental tissue examined.[111] It helps to discriminate between CHM (diploid) and PHM (triploid) and between PHM and a hydropic abortus (diploid or near-diploid), with the limitation that no information is given as to the parental genomic origin of the cells' ploidy status (see Table 10–2). FCM has revealed a surprisingly high heterogeneity of ploidy in the CHM trophoblast. The G2/M peak is frequently high, which poses a problem because premitotic cells are indistinguishable from those with genuine tetraploidy. An arbitrary figure of 20% to 25% is adopted by various investigators as a diagnostic threshold for tetraploidy,[88,111,112] and the presence of an octoploid peak helps the latter assumption. However, true tetraploid CHMs seem to be rare; as disclosed by in situ DNA ploidy and hybridization studies (see below), tetraploidy affects only some parts of the trophoblast. At all events "tetraploidy" in CHMs remains without influence upon their morphology or clinical behavior, even if they tend to be associated with higher hCG levels.[111]

Image Cytometry[113] and In Situ DNA Hybridization[114]

Image cytometry (ICM) measures the DNA content of individual nuclei examined in situ in tissue sections[115,116] or of nuclei obtained from fresh tissue or from known histologic areas of paraffin-embedded tissue specimens. Spread on a slide (cytospin),[117,118] either preparation is stained by Feulgen reagent, and the DNA content of each nucleus is read in terms of optical density measured by a video-based image cytometer (e.g., CAS100 or CAS200 image analyzing system) with the appropriate software.[113] Calibration is effected by measuring the signal given by cells of known DNA content. Each nucleus can at the same time be characterized as to its morphologic characteristics, and in tissue slide preparations the cells can be studied in their pristine surroundings.

In situ hybridization (ISH) is performed on tissue sections by use of DNA probes that anneal specifically to DNA targets in interphase nuclei. The chromosome-specific probes are directed to specific genes, pericentromeric or telomeric tandem repeats, or longer DNA stretches that may involve painting of whole chromosomes. The probes are either fluorescein labeled or visualized by the biotin-avidin method. They are used for studies of cell ploidy or of chromosomal abnormalities in individual cells, which are examined in their natural tissue context. The sex chromosome status can be ascertained by using probes specific for the X or Y chromosome.[117]

Archival paraffin-embedded tissues are suitable for ISH studies. Examination of thin tissue sections presents special problems (e.g., truncation of nuclei), but the development of rapid, automatic scoring by digital microscopy promises to make ISH a powerful method of coordinating genomic and phenotypic parameters.[114]

Applied to trophoblastic diseases ICH and ISH disclose the basic ploidy of a placenta, information useful in the differential diagnosis among CHM, PHM, and hydropic abortus. ICH and ISH have also demonstrated the heterogeneity of ploidy in the trophoblast as it grows beyond the perivillous situation. This is most pronounced in CHM in which tetraploidy arises by endoreduplication or endomitosis[119] and dominates the extravillous trophoblast.[116,117] The villous mesenchyme and perivillous trophoblast, on the other hand, stay within diploid (or triploid) limits, bearing witness to the original genomic constitution.[120] Polyploidy and aneuploidy are reflected in nuclear enlargement and atypia easily seen in extravillous areas, including the implantation site.[63,117,118] As in other investigations none of the changes detected so far by the above studies bear significantly on the clinical behavior and prognosis of CHM or PHM.[82]

Genomic Molecular Studies

Genomic molecular studies, employed mainly in identification of the parental origins of moles of either type and in the establishment of origins of chorionic cancers, depend on the comparison of DNAs from the relevant sources made possible by the existence of extensive DNA polymorphisms. The basic method makes use of the restriction fragment length polymorphisms (RFLPs). It hinges on the polymorphisms of cleavage spots for bacterial endonucleases, whose disposition in an individual genome is inherited (except de novo mutations) according to Mendelian rules. Multiple restriction fragments of DNA cut by a nuclease of choice are separated according to size by electrophoresis and visualized on a Southern blot[121] by labeled probes that pick up the fragments suitable for comparison.[122] The newer methods take advantage of heritable, high-degree DNA polymorphisms associated with variable number tandem repeats (VNTRs). These are composed of short, less than 50 base-pair (bp) cores whose allelic variations depend on different numbers of the core units arranged in a row. Multifocal VNTRs of the same basic unit are strewn throughout the genome and can be visualized by a specific probe that anneals with the tandem repeats to give a highly individual DNA fingerprint in a Southern blot.[123] More convenient is the use of a unique, single-locus, high-heterozygosity, hypervariable minisatellite genomic stretch, usually within 10 kilobases in length, that can be similarly traced by a specific probe.[124] More recently, thanks to the Human Genome Mapping Project, increasing numbers of single-locus hypervariable minisatellite and microsatellite[125] (units of few, e.g., 2, 3, or 4 bp) regions and their framing sequences have become known and can be amplified by polymerase chain reaction (PCR).[126] This allows the simplest method of DNA comparison to date, since it dispenses with the Southern blotting procedures and requires only a juxtaposition and comparison of PCR products after gel electrophoresis.

The patterns of DNA fragments in RFLP studies or of single-locus allelic variations permit a comparison among the DNAs of the parents and the moles. CHMs reflect their diandric origins, and PHMs reveal their two paternal and one maternal alleles.[127] In addition, monospermic and dispermic origins of CHM can be elucidated.[103] Many of the investigations are carried out on DNA extracted from archival paraffin-embedded tissues, and CHM may be tentatively diagnosed without examining the paternal DNA if maternal DNA can be proved to be absent. Absence of paternal alleles from DNA excludes a gestational event, as found in nongestational tumors of trophoblastic morphology.[128,129] Gestational choriocarcinoma and PSTT may be assigned their origin in previous pregnancies[130]; the surprising finding here is the origin of some cancers from conceptuses of pregnancies antedating the one immediately preceding the clinical manifestation of neoplasia.[131,132] Thus, while both CHM and PHM yield no conceptual surprises, gestational trophoblastic cancers have been found to originate, often unexpectedly, in trophoblast of past, unsuspected pregnancies and at times in nonfertilized ova or other tissues, giving a homozygous or heterozygous genome derived from that of the patient herself.

CONCLUSION

The basic concepts of GTD remain within the established paradigm originally based on pathologic anatomy and cytogenetics. Although sophisticated new molecular techniques are clarifying the parental genomic derivation of CHM and PHM and the varied origins of malignant trophoblastic neoplasms, the actual genes or gene complexes responsible for the individual phenotypes associated with the diverse trophoblastic syndromes remain to be elucidated. High-resolution molecular studies will provide further insights into the mechanisms governing the origin and prognosis of CHM and PHM, especially the mechanisms of transition to invasive moles, the development of trophoblastic cancers from the complete mole and the biparental placenta, and the apparent freedom of PHM from trophoblastic cancer.

The currently employed techniques now aimed mainly at comparative chromosomal and DNA analyses are likely to gain in sophistication and scope. They need to be wedded to the high diagnostic acumen of the tissue pathologist, since he or she remains in charge of the basic field of operations.

Clinicopathologic similarities notwithstanding, complete and partial hydatidiform moles are separate disease entities. Little is to be gained by viewing them as members of a spectrum.

A plea implicit in this chapter concerns definitions and terminology. Their standardization and acceptance would do much for communication among workers and institutions dealing with trophoblastic diseases. One version, available in a World Health Organization Technical Report,[1] can serve as a common basis for continuing discussion in that area.

REFERENCES

1. World Health Organization Scientific Group: Gestational trophoblastic diseases. In Technical Report Series No. 692. Geneva, 1983, WHO.
2. Kajii T, Ohama K: Androgenetic origin of hydatidiform mole. Nature 268:633, 1977.
3. Szulman AE, Surti U: The syndromes of hydatidiform mole. I. Cytogenetic and morphologic correlations. Am J Obstet Gynecol 131:665, 1978.
4. Szulman AE, Surti U: The syndromes of hydatidiform mole. II. Morphologic evolution of the complete and partial mole. Am J Obstet Gynecol 132:20, 1978.
5. Jacobs PA, Wilson CM, Sprenkle JA, et al: Mechanism of origin of complete hydatidiform moles. Nature 286:714, 1980.
6. Lawler SD, Fisher RA, Pickthall J, et al: Genetic studies on hydatidiform moles. I. The origin of partial moles. Cancer Genet Cytogenet 5:309, 1982.
7. Lawler D, Povey T, Fisher A, Pickthall J: Genetic studies on hydatidiform mole. II. The origin of complete moles. Ann Hum Genet 46:232, 1982.
8. Szulman AE, Philippe E, Boue JG, et al: Human triploidy: association with partial hydatidiform moles and nonmolar conceptuses. Hum Pathol 12:1016, 1981.
9. Jacobs PA, Szulman AE, Funkhouser J, et al: Human triploidy: relationship between parental origin of the additional haploid complement and development of partial hydatidiform mole. Ann Hum Genet 46:223, 1982.
10. Sunde L, Vejerslev LO, Jensen MP, et al: Genetic analysis of repeated, biparental, diploid, hydatidiform moles. Cancer Genet Cytogenet 66:16, 1993.
11. Paradinas FJ, Fisher RA, Brown P, Newlands ES: Diploid hydatidiform moles with fetal red blood cells in molar villi. 1. Pathology, incidence and prognosis. J Pathol 181:183, 1997.
12. Fisher RA, Paradinas FJ, Soteriou BA, et al: Diploid hydatidiform moles with fetal red blood cells in molar villi. 2. Genetics. J Pathol 181:189, 1997.
13. Park WW, Lees JC: Choriocarcinoma (a general review with an analysis of 516 cases). Arch Pathol 49:73 and 205, 1950.

13a. Park WW: Choriocarcinoma—a study of its pathology. Philadelphia, 1971, FA Davis.

14. Boyd JD, Hamilton WJ: The human placenta. Cambridge, 1970, Heffer.
15. O'Rahilly R, Muller F: Human embryology and teratology, 2nd ed. New York, 1996, John Wiley & Sons.
16. Szulman AE: Trophoblastic disease: pathology of complete and partial hydatidiform moles. In Reed GB, Claireaux AE, Cockbrun F (eds). Disease of the fetus and newborn: pathology, imaging, genetics, and management, 2nd ed. New York, 1995, Chapman & Hall.
17. Paradinas FJ: The histological diagnosis of hydatidiform moles. Curr Diagn Pathol 1:24, 1994.
18. Luckett WP: Origin and differentiation of the yolk sac and extraembryonic mesoderm in presomite human and rhesus monkey embryos. Am J Anat 152:59, 1978.
19. Pijnenborg R, Robertston WB, Brosens I, et al: Trophoblast invasion and the establishment of haemochorial placentation in man and laboratory animals. Placenta 2:71, 1981.
20. Jauniaux E, Jurkovic D, Campbell S: Current topic: in vivo investigation of the placental circulations by Doppler echography. Placenta 16:323, 1995.
21. Simpson JZ, Elias S: Fetal cells in maternal blood (prospects for noninvasive prenatal diagnosis). New York, 1994, New York Academy of Sciences.
22. Bulmer JW, Johnson PM: Antigen expression by trophoblast populations in human placenta and their possible immuno-biologic relevance. Placenta 6:127, 1985.
23. Szulman AE: The A, B, and H blood-group antigens in human placenta. N Engl J Med 286:1028, 1972.
24. Kovats S, Main EK, Librach C, et al: A class I antigen, HLA-G, expressed in human trophoblasts. Science 248:220, 1990.
25. King A, Kalra P, Loke YW: Human trophoblast cell resistance to decidual NK lysis is due to lack of NK target structure. Cell Immunol 127:230, 1990.
26. Atkinson JP, Farries TF: Separation of self from non-self in the complement system. Immunol Today 8:212, 1987.
27. Medawar PB: Some immunological and endocrinological problems raised by the evolution of viviparity in vertebrates. Symp Soc Exp Biol 7:320, 1953.
28. Redman CWG: The fetal allograft. Fetal Med Rev 2:21, 1990.
29. Damsky CH, Fitzgerald ML, Fisher SJ: Distribution patterns of extracellular matrix components and adhesion receptors are intricately modulated during first trimester cytotrophoblast differentiation along the invasive pathway, in vivo. J Clin Invest 89:210, 1992.
30. Buckley J: Epidemiology of gestational trophoblastic disease. In Szulman AE, Buchsbaum

HJ (eds): Gestational trophoblastic disease. New York, 1987, Springer-Verlag, p 8.

31. Palmer JR: Advances in the epidemiology of gestational trophoblastic disease. J Reprod Med 39:155, 1994.
32. Matsuura J, Chiu D, Jacobs PA, Szulman AE: Complete hydatidiform mole in Hawaii: an epidemiological study. Genet Epidemiol 1:271, 1984.
33. Parazzini F, La Vecchia C, Pampallona S: Parental age and risk of complete and partial hydatidiform mole. Br J Obstet Gynaecol 93:583, 1986.
34. Parazzini F, Mangili G, La Vecchia C, et al: Risk factors for gestational trophoblastic disease: a separate analysis of complete and partial hydatidiform moles. Obstet Gynecol 78:1039, 1991.
35. Curry SL, Hammon CB, Tyrey L, et al: Hydatidiform mole: diagnosis management and long term follow up. Obstet Gynecol 45:1, 1975.
36. Kohorn EL: Molar pregnancy: presentation and diagnosis. Clin Obstet Gynecol 27:181, 1984.
37. Berkowitz RS, Goldstein DP: Medical progress: chorionic tumors. N Engl J Med 335:1740, 1996.
38. Jurkovic D, Jauniaux E (eds): Ultrasound and early pregnancy. New York, 1996, Parthenon.
39. Tyrey L: HCG: properties and assay methods. Semin Oncol 22:121, 1995.
40. Bagshawe KD: Choriocarcinoma: a model for tumour markers. Acta Oncol 31:99, 1992.
41. Romero R, Horgan JG, Kohorn EI, et al: New criteria for the diagnosis of gestational trophoblastic disease. Obstet Gynecol 66:553, 1985.
42. Soto-Wright V, Bernstein M, Goldstein DP, Berkowitz RS: The changing clinical presentation of complete molar pregnancy. Obstet Gynecol 86:775, 1995.
43. Lurain JR, Brewer JI, Torok EE, Halpern B: Natural history of hydatidiform mole after primary evacuation. Am J Obstet Gynecol 145:591, 1983.
44. Buckley JD, Henderson BE, Morrow CP, et al: Case-control study of gestational choriocarcinoma. Cancer Res 48:1004, 1988.
45. Szulman AE: Trophoblastic disease: clinical pathology of hydatidiform moles. Obstet Gynecol Clin North Am 15:443, 1988.
46. Jackson TJ, Enzer N: Hydatidiform mole with benign metastasis to the lung: histologic evidence of regression lesions in the lung. Am J Obstet Gynecol 78:868, 1959.
47. Ring AM: The concept of benign metastasizing hydatidiform moles. Am J Clin Pathol 58:111, 1972.
48. Kohorn ET: Clinical management and neoplastic sequelae of trophoblastic embolization associated with hydatidiform mole. Obstet Gynecol Surv 42:484, 1987.
49. Goldberg GL, Yon DA, Block B, Levin W: Gestational trophoblastic disease: significance of vaginal metastases. Gynecol Oncol 24:155, 1986.
50. Kato M, Tanaka K, Takeuchi S: The nature of trophoblastic disease initiated by transplantation into immunosuppressed animals. Am J Obstet Gynecol 142:497, 1982.
51. Mutch DG, Soper JT, Baker ME, et al: Role of computed axial tomography of the chest in staging patients with nonmetastatic gestational trophoblastic disease. Obstet Gynecol 68:348, 1986.
52. Keep D, Zaragoza MV, Hassold T, Redline RW: Very early complete hydatidiform mole. Hum Pathol 27:708, 1996.
53. Szulman AE: Examination of the early conceptus. Arch Pathol Lab Med 116:696, 1991.
54. Szulman AE: Embryonic death: pathology and forensic implications. In Dimmic JE, Singer D (eds): Perspectives in pediatric pathology: forensic aspects in pediatric pathology, vol 19. Basel, 1995, Karger, p 43.
55. Chew PCT, Ratnam SS, Goh HH: Testosterone in major vesicle fluid and theca-lutein cyst fluid. Br J Obstet Gynaecol 85:218, 1978.
56. Kaplan SS, Szulman AE, Surti U: Effect of hydatidiform molar vesicular fluid on blood coagulation. Am J Obstet Gynecol 153:703, 1985.
57. Brescia RJ, Kurman RJ, Main CS, et al: Immunocytochemical localization of chorionic gonadotropin, placental lactogen, and placental alkaline phosphatase in the diagnosis of complete and partial hydatidiform moles. Int J Gynecol Pathol 6:213, 1987.
58. Sunderland CA, Redman CWG, Stirrat GM: Characterization and localization of HLA antigens on hydatidiform mole. Am J Obstet Gynecol 151:130, 1985.
59. Bulmer JN, Johnson PM, Sasagawa M, Takeuchi S: Immunohistochemical studies of fetal trophoblast and maternal decidua in hydatidiform mole and choriocarcinoma. Placenta 9:183, 1988.
60. Sasagawa M, Ohmomo Y, Kanazawa K, Takeuchi S: HLA expression by trophoblast of invasive moles. Placenta 8:111, 1987.
61. Lawler SD, Fisher RA: Immunogenicity of hydatidiform mole. Placenta 8:195, 1987.
62. Habibian R, Surti U: Cytogenetics of trophoblasts from complete hydatidiform moles. Cancer Genet Cytogenet 29:271, 1987.
63. Montes M, Roberts D, Berkowitz RS, Genest DR: Prevalence and significance of implantation site trophoblastic atypia in hydatidiform moles and spontaneous abortions. Am J Clin Pathol 105:411, 1996.
64. Silva E, Tornos C, Lage J, et al: Multiple nodules

of intermediate trophoblast following hydatidiform moles. Int J Gynecol Pathol 12:324, 1993.
65. Dickey RP, Gasser RF, Olar TT, et al: The relationship of initial embryo crown-rump length to pregnancy outcome and abortus karyotype based on new growth curves for the 2-31 mm embryo. Hum Reprod 9:373, 1994.
66. Van de Kaa CA, Poddighe PJ, Nillesen WN, et al: Early embryonal tissues do not exclude a diagnosis of complete hydatidiform mole. (In Press.)
67. Stellar MA, Genest DR, Bernstein MR, et al: The natural history of twin pregnancy with complete hydatidiform mole and coexisting fetus. Obstet Gynecol 83:35, 1994.
68. Bristow RE, Shumway JB, Khouzami AN, et al: Complete hydatidiform mole and surviving coexistent twin. Obstet Gynecol Surv 51:705, 1996.
69. Azuma C, Saji F, Takemura M, et al: Triplet pregnancy involving complete hydatidiform mole and two fetuses: genetic analysis by deoxyribonucleic acid fingerprint. Am J Obstet Gynecol 166:664, 1992.
70. Osada H, Iitsuka Y, Matsui H, Sekiya S: A complete hydatidiform mole coexisting with a normal fetus was confirmed by variable number tandem repeat (VNTR) polymorphism analysis using polymerase chain reaction. Gynecol Oncol 56:90, 1995.
71. Van de Kaa CA, Robben JCM, Hopman AHN, et al: Complete hydatidiform mole in twin pregnancy: differentiation from partial mole with interphase cytogenetic and DNA cytometric analysis on paraffin embedded tissue. Histopatholy 26:123, 1995.
72. Szulman AE, Surti U: Strict clinicopathologic criteria in the diagnosis of partial hydatidiform mole: a plea renewed. Am J Obstet Gynecol 152:1107, 1985.
73. Jauniaux E, Elkhazen N, Leroy F, et al: Clinical and morphologic aspects of the vanishing twin phenomenon. Obstet Gynecol 72:577, 1988.
74. Sampson A, de Crespigny LC: Vanishing twins: the frequency of spontaneous fetal reduction of a twin pregnancy. Ultrasound Obstet Gynecol 2:107, 1992.
75. Bagshawe KD: Risk and prognostic factors in trophoblastic neoplasia. Cancer 38:1373, 1976.
76. Genest DR, Laborde O, Berkowitz RS, et al: A clinicopathologic study of 153 cases of complete hydatidiform mole (1980-1990): histologic grade lacks prognostic significance. Obstet Gynecol 78:402, 1991.
77. Fukunaga M, Endo Y, Ushigome S: Clinicopathologic study of tetraploid hydropic villous tissues. Arch Pathol Lab Med 120:569, 1996.
78. Cheung ANY, Ngan HYS, Chen WZ, et al: The significance of proliferating cell nuclear antigen in human trophoblastic disease: an immunohistochemical study. Histopathology 22:565, 1993.
79. Jeffers MD, Richmond JA, Smith R: Trophoblast proliferation rate does not predict progression to persistent gestational trophoblastic disease in complete hydatidiform mole. Int J Gynecol Pathol 15:34, 1996.
80. Lawler SD, Fisher RA, Dent J: A prospective genetic study of complete and partial hydatidiform moles. Am J Obstet Gynecol 164:1270, 1991.
81. Mutter GL, Pomponio RJ, Berkowitz RS, Genest DR: Sex chromosome composition of complete hydatidiform moles: relationship to metastasis. Am J Obstet Gynecol 168:1547, 1993.
82. Van de Kaa CA, Schijf CPT, de Wilde PCM, et al: Persistent gestational trophoblastic disease: DNA image cytometry and interphase cytogenetics have limited predictive value. Mod Pathol 9:1007, 1996.
83. Martin DA, Sutton GP, Ulbright TM, et al: DNA content as a prognostic index in gestational trophoblastic neoplasia. Gynecol Oncol 34:383, 1989.
84. Rustin GJ, Newlands ES, Lutz JM, et al: Combination but not single-agent methotrexate chemotherapy for gestational trophoblastic tumors increases the incidence of second tumors. J Clin Oncol 14:2769, 1996.
85. Jacobs PA, Angell RR, Buchanan IM, et al: The origin of human triploids. Ann Hum Genet 42:49, 1978.
86. Boue A, Boue J: Cytogenetics of pregnancy wastage. In Harris H, Hirschborn K (eds): Advances in human genetics, vol 15. New York, 1985, Plenum Press.
87. Jeffers MD, O'Dwyer P, Curran B, et al: Partial hydatidiform mole: a common underdiagnosed condition; a 3-year retrospective clinicopathological and DNA flow cytometric analysis. Int J Gynecol Pathol 12:315, 1993.
88. Fukunaga M, Ushigome S, Endo Y: Incidence of hydatidiform mole in a Tokyo hospital: a 5-year (1989 to 1993) prospective, morphological, and flow cytometric study. Hum Pathol 26:758, 1995.
89. McFadden DE, Panzar JT: Placental pathology of triploidy. Hum Pathol 27:1018, 1996.
90. Szulman AE, Surti U: The clinicopathologic profile of the partial hydatidiform mole. Obstet Gynecol 59:597, 1982.
91. Berkowitz RS, Goldstein DP, Bernstein MR: Natural history of partial molar pregnancy. Obstet Gynecol 66:677, 1985.

92. Doshi N, Surti U, Szulman AE: Morphologic anomalies in triploid liveborn fetuses. Hum Pathol 14:716, 1983.
93. Lewis PE, Cefalo RC: Triploidy syndrome with theca lutein cysts and severe pre-eclampsia. Am J Obstet Gynecol 133:100, 1979.
94. Rice LW, Berkowitz RS, Lage JM, et al: Persistent gestational trophoblastic tumor after partial hydatidiform mole. Gynecol Oncol 36:358, 1990.
95. Goto S, Yamada A, Ishizuka T, et al: Development of post-molar trophoblastic disease after partial molar pregnancy. Gynecol Oncol 48:165, 1993.
96. Nwosu EC, Ferriman E, McCormack MJ, et al: Partial hydatidiform mole and hypertension associated with a live fetus—variable presentation in two cases. Hum Reprod 10:2459, 1995.
97. Looi LM, Sivanesaratnam V: Malignant evolution with fatal outcome in a patient with partial hydatidiform mole. Aust NZ J Obstet Gynecol 21:51, 1981.
98. Gardner HA, Lage JM: Choriocarcinoma following a partial hydatidiform mole: a case report. Hum Pathol 23:468, 1992.
99. Bagshawe KD, Lawler SD, Paradinas FJ, et al: Gestational trophoblastic tumours following initial diagnosis of partial hydatidiform mole. Lancet 335:1074, 1990.
100. Szulman AE, Ma HK, Wong LC, et al: Residual trophoblastic disease in association with partial hydatidiform mole. Obstet Gynecol 57:392, 1981.
101. Gaber LW, Redline RW, Mostoufi-Zadeh M, et al: Invasive partial mole. Am J Clin Pathol 85:722, 1986.
102. Conran RM, Hitchcock CL, Popek EJ, et al: Diagnostic considerations in molar gestations. Hum Pathol 24:41, 1993.
103. Fisher RA, Povey S, Jeffreys AJ, et al: Frequency of heterozygous complete hydatidiform moles, estimated by locus-specific minisatellite and Y chromosome–specific probes. Hum Genet 82:259, 1989.
104. Wallace DC, Surti U, Adams CW, Szulman AE: Complete moles have paternal chromosomes but maternal mitochondrial DNA. Hum Genet 61:145, 1982.
105. Barton SC, Surani MAH, Norris ML: Role of paternal and maternal genomes in mouse development. Nature 311:374, 1984.
106. Surani MAH, Barton SC, Norris ML: Nuclear transplantation in the mouse: heritable differences between parental genomes after activation of the embryonic genome. Cell 45:127, 1986.
107. Surti U, Szulman AE, Wagner K, et al: Tetraploid partial hydatidiform moles: two cases with a triple paternal contribution and a 92,XXXY karyotype. Hum Genet 72:15, 1986.
108. Groden J, Nakamura Y, German J: Molecular evidence that homologous recombination occurs in proliferating human somatic cells. Proc Natl Acad Sci USA 87:4315, 1990.
109. Marazzo DP: Mole/chorion genomic imprinting. In Jauniaux E, Barnea ER, Edwards R (eds): Embryonic medicine and therapy. New York, 1997, Oxford University Press.
110. Lage JM: Flow cytometric analysis of nuclear DNA content in gestational trophoblastic disease. J Reprod Med 36:31, 1991.
111. Lage JM, Mark SD, Roberts DJ, et al: A flow cytometric study of 137 fresh hydropic placentas: correlation between types of hydatidiform moles and nuclear DNA ploidy. Obstet Gynecol 79:403, 1992.
112. Fukunaga M, Ushigome S, Fukunaga M, Sugishita M: Application of flow cytometry in diagnosis of hydatidiform moles. Mod Pathol 6:353, 1993.
113. Cohen C: Image cytometric analysis in pathology. Hum Pathol 27:482, 1996.
114. Waldman FM, Sauter G, Sudar D, et al: Molecular cytometry of cancer. Hum Pathol 27:441, 1996.
115. Carey FA: Measurement of nuclear DNA content in histological and cytological specimens: principles and applications. J Pathol 172:307, 1994.
116. Barclay IDR, Dabbagh L, Babiak J, Poppema S: DNA analysis (ploidy) of molar pregnancies with image analysis on paraffin tissue sections. Am J Clin Pathol 100:451, 1993.
117. Van de Kaa CA, Hanselaar AG, Hopman AH, et al: DNA cytometric and interphase cytogenetic analysis of paraffin-embedded hydatidiform moles and hydropic abortions. J Pathol 170:229, 1993.
118. Jeffers MD, Michie BA, Oakes SJ, et al: Comparison of ploidy analysis by flow cytometry and image analysis in hydatidiform mole and non-molar abortion. Histopathology 27:415, 1995.
119. Sarto GE, Stubblefield PA, Lurain J, et al: Mechanisms of growth in hydatidiform moles. Am J Obstet Gynecol 148:1014, 1984.
120. Berezowsky J, Zbieranowski I, Demers J, et al: DNA ploidy of hydatidiform moles and non-molar conceptuses: a study using flow and tissue-section image cytometry. Mod Pathol 8:775, 1995.
121. Southern EM: Application of DNA analysis to mapping the human genome. Cytogenet Cell Genet 32:52, 1982.
122. Ko T-M, Hsieh C-Y, Ho H-N, et al: Restriction fragment length polymorphism analysis to study the genetic origin of hydatidiform mole. Am J Obstet Gynecol 164:901, 1991.
123. Saji F, Tokugawa Y, Kimura T, et al: A new approach using DNA fingerprinting for the determination of androgenesis as a cause of hydatidiform mole. Placenta 10:399, 1989.

124. Wong Z, Wilson V, Patel I, et al: Characterization of a panel of highly variable minisatellites cloned from human DNA. Ann Hum Genet 51: 269, 1987.
125. Weber JL, May PE: Abundant class of human DNA polymorphisms which can be typed using the polymerase chain reaction. Am J Hum Genet 44:388, 1989.
126. Saiki RK, Gelfand DH, Stoffel DH, et al: Primer-directed enzymatic amplification of DNA with a thermostable DNA polymerase. Science 239:487, 1988.
127. Fisher RA, Newlands ES: Rapid diagnosis and classification of hydatidiform moles with polymerase chain reaction. Am J Obstet Gynecol 168:563, 1993.
128. Fisher RA, Newlands ES, Jeffreys AJ, et al: Gestational and non-gestational trophoblastic tumours distinguished by DNA analysis. Cancer 69:839, 1992.
129. Arima T, Imamura T, Sakuragi N, et al: Malignant trophoblastic neoplasms with different modes of origin. Cancer Genet Cytogenet 85:5, 1995.
130. Fisher RA, Paradinas FJ, Newlands ES, Boxer GM: Genetic evidence that placental site trophoblastic tumours can originate from a hydatidiform mole or a normal conceptus. Br J Cancer 65:355, 1992.
131. Fisher RA, Soteriou B, Meredith L, et al: Previous hydatidiform mole identified as the causative pregnancy of choriocarcinoma following birth of normal twins. Int J Gynecol Cancer 5:64, 1995.
132. Osada H, Kawata M, Yamada M, et al: Genetic identification of pregnancies responsible for choriocarcinomas after multiple pregnancies by restriction fragment length polymorphism analysis. Am J Obstet Gynecol 165:682, 1991.

COMPREHENSIVE REVIEW ARTICLES

Freedman RS, Tortolero-Luna G, Pandey DK, et al: Gestational trophoblastic disease. Obstet Gynecol Clin North Am 23:545, 1996.

Lage JM, Wolfe NG: Gestational trophoblastic disease: new approaches to diagnosis. Clin Lab Med 15:631, 1995.

Paradinas FJ, Browne P, Fisher RA, et al: A clinical, histopathological and flow cytometric study of 149 complete moles, 146 partial moles and 107 non-molar hydropic abortions. Histopathology 28:101, 1996.

Redline RW, Abdul-Karim F: Pathology of gestational trophoblastic disease. Semin Oncol 22:96, 1995.

Szulman AE: Gestational trophoblastic diseases. In Coulam CB, Faulk WP, McIntyre JA (eds): Immunological obstetrics. New York, 1992, WW Norton.

Szulman AE: The natural history of early human spontaneous abortion. In Barnea ER, Check JH, Grudzinskas TG, et al (eds): Implantation and early pregnancy in humans. New York, 1995, Parthenon.

TEXTBOOKS ON GESTATIONAL TROPHOBLASTIC DISEASES

Hancock BW, Newlands RS, Berkowitz RS: Gestational trophoblastic disease. London, 1997, Chapman & Hall.

Ishizuka N, Tomoda Y: Gestational trophoblastic disease. Japan, 1990, University of Nagoya Press.

Silverberg SG, Kurman RJ: Tumors of the uterine corpus and gestational trophoblastic disease. In Rosai J, Sobin LH (eds): Atlas of tumor pathology. Washington, DC, 1992. Armed Forces Institute of Pathology.

Szulman AE, Buchsbaum HJ: Gestational trophoblastic diseases. New York, 1987, Springer-Verlag.

11

Gestational Trophoblastic Disease

Debra S. Heller

Gestational trophoblastic disease (GTD) can be viewed in two ways. From the pathologist's point of view, GTD is classified according to well-defined histopathologic criteria. It should be recognized, however, that tissue for histopathologic diagnosis is not always available and that treatment plans rely predominantly on clinical criteria. Clinical classifications of GTD are based on prognostic implications rather than histology. This chapter first reviews the histopathology of GTD and then presents the clinical point of view.

HISTOPATHOLOGIC CRITERIA

The World Health Organization histopathologic classification of GTD is given in Table 11–1. Hydatidiform moles are discussed in Chapter 10 and are not further considered here.

Invasive Mole

In invasive mole confined to the uterus, molar tissue invades the myometrium (Fig. 11–1*A*). The histologic criteria for a mole are applicable: hydropic, avascular villi with trophoblast proliferation (Fig. 11–1*B*), although edema may be less than in hydatidiform mole. It is the presence of chorionic villi that distinguishes invasive mole from choriocarcinoma. When persistent GTD occurs outside of the uterus, it is usually choriocarcinoma; however, invasive mole can spread to extrauterine locations such as lung and brain.[1] Invasive mole outside of the uterus is usually confined to blood vessels rather than invading surrounding tissue. Although chemotherapy is the mainstay of treatment for persistent GTD, at times a uterine focus of invasive mole persists, and the patient undergoes hysterectomy. Hysterectomy is generally necessary to confirm a histologic diagnosis of invasive mole, so that many of these lesions are classified clinically as GTD without being distinguished from choriocarcinoma.

The differential diagnosis of invasive mole includes placenta increta, placenta percreta, and choriocarcinoma. In hysterectomy specimens this is usually not a difficult distinction. The villi of placenta increta and percreta do not show hydropic change or trophoblast proliferation. There are no chorionic villi in choriocarcinoma. The diagnosis of the presence and the type of GTD can be difficult on curettage samples, however, where the tissue may be scant and it may not be possible to evaluate the presence or absence of chorionic villi or myometrial invasion. Small amounts of proliferating trophoblast on a curettage specimen may represent a portion of an incomplete abortion, a hydatidiform mole, an invasive mole, or a cho-

Table 11–1. World Health Organization Histopathological Classification of Gestational Trophoblastic Disease

Hydatidiform mole
Partial hydatidiform mole
Complete hydatidiform mole
Invasive mole
Choriocarcinoma
Placental site trophoblastic tumor
Miscellaneous trophoblastic lesions
Exaggerated placental site
Placental site nodules and plaques
Unclassified lesions

From Silverberg S, Kurman R: Classification and pathology of gestational trophoblastic disease. In Atlas of tumor pathology, tumors of the uterine corpus and gestational trophoblastic disease. Washington, DC, 1992, Armed Forces Institute of Pathology.

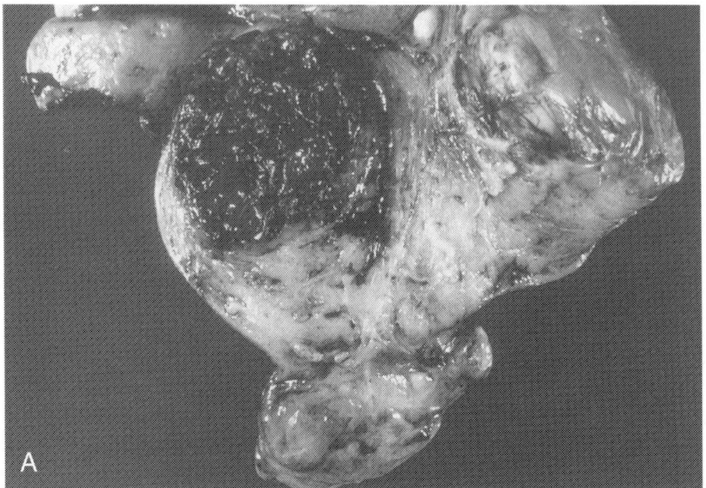

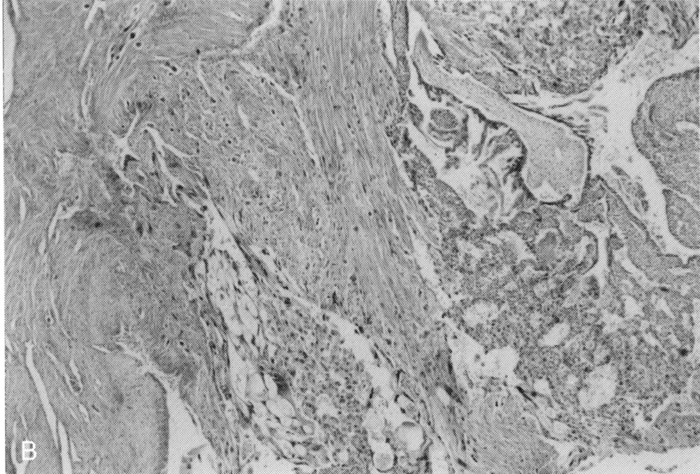

Figure 11–1. Invasive mole. **A,** Large hemorrhagic nodule is present within the myometrium. **B,** Hydropic molar villus with proliferating trophoblast within the myometrium.

riocarcinoma. Trophoblast in a normal gestation should be small in amount and lack atypia. A suspicion of GTD is greater if there is a known antecedent mole. Clinical history, human chorionic gonadotropin (hCG) titers, imaging studies, and repeat sampling may be required to establish a diagnosis of GTD.

Choriocarcinoma

The incidence of choriocarcinoma in the United States has been estimated at 1 in 24,096 pregnancies and 1 in 19,920 live births, with much higher rates in Asia, in the order of 1 in 6000 to 8000 pregnancies.[2] The most important risk factor for choriocarcinoma is a recent history of a hydatidiform mole, which is reported in 29% to 83% of gestational choriocarcinomas.[3] Other risk factors include maternal age of 40 years or greater or 19 years or less. Other, less well-established risk factors include race, with a greater risk in nonwhite populations, pregnancies resulting from the combination of blood groups A and O parentage, diet, endogenous estrogen, and environmental toxins.[4] Although most choriocarcinomas are preceded by moles, any type of pregnancy may precede choriocarcinoma. Choriocarcinomas have also rarely been reported to arise within a term placenta.[5]

The presenting symptoms of choriocarcinoma are protean and depend on the site of the tumor. Often choriocarcinoma initially presents at a metastatic site, and the diagnosis should always be considered in the workup of patients of reproductive age for a mass lesion.

On gross examination choriocarcinoma is extremely hemorrhagic and often extensively necrotic. Because of the elevated serum β-hCG levels, the ovaries may be enlarged and contain theca lutein cysts (Fig. 11–2). Histologic examination shows a biphasic population of cytotrophoblast or intermediate trophoblast and syncytiotrophoblast (Fig. 11–3). There are no chorionic villi, except in the rare case arising when the disease is identified within a mature placenta. Infiltration of surrounding tissues is extensive and often accompanied by extensive necrosis and hemorrhage. Mitotic activity is brisk. Currently no standard histopathologic grading system is in use. The tumors generally stain strongly for hCG and less so for human placental lactogen (hPL), reflecting the syncytiotrophoblast component of these neoplasms. Monomorphic choriocarcinomas have rarely been reported. These may be confused with a placental site trophoblastic tumor (PSTT) but are more atypical, with higher nuclear/cytoplasmic ratios, and patients have higher serum hCG levels than those with PSTT.[6]

The most common metastatic sites for choriocarcinoma in the autopsy series of Tang, Liu, and Song[1] were lung, brain, and vagina, but metastases to the kidney, spleen, liver, and pelvis were also found. Since 100% of the 61 patients with choriocarcinoma in this study had lung metastases, the authors postulated that lung was the first site of spread, with subsequent hematogenous dissemination.

Choriocarcinomas are generally diploid. Neither ploidy nor S-phase fraction has been found to correlate with outcome.[7] Genetic analysis may help determine whether a choriocarcinoma is of gestational or nongestational origin and can be used to pinpoint the antecedent pregnancy. For example, a tumor containing both maternal and paternal chromosomal material has more likely arisen from a normal gestation, whereas one purely composed of paternal material more likely originated from a mole. In addition, genetic analysis may be useful in distinguishing poorly differentiated neoplasms from GTD by revealing their lack of paternal component.[8]

Placental Site Trophoblastic Tumor

PSTT is a rare form of GTD first described in 1976.[9] Because of the usually benign behavior of these lesions, PSTT was originally thought to be a dramatic form of "syncytial endometritis" or an exaggerated placental site.[10] PSTT can occur after any form of antecedent pregnancy, although most follow term gestations[6] and may be manifested many years later. PSTTs have been reported across the entire reproductive age range. The most common symptom is irregular bleeding. Rarely, nephrotic syndrome, disseminated intravascular coagulopathy, amenorrhea, or virilization develops. Serum hCG levels at presentation are usually low. Although most reported cases of PSTT have behaved in a benign fashion, aggressive metastatic disease has been reported in 10% to 15% of cases.[7,11]

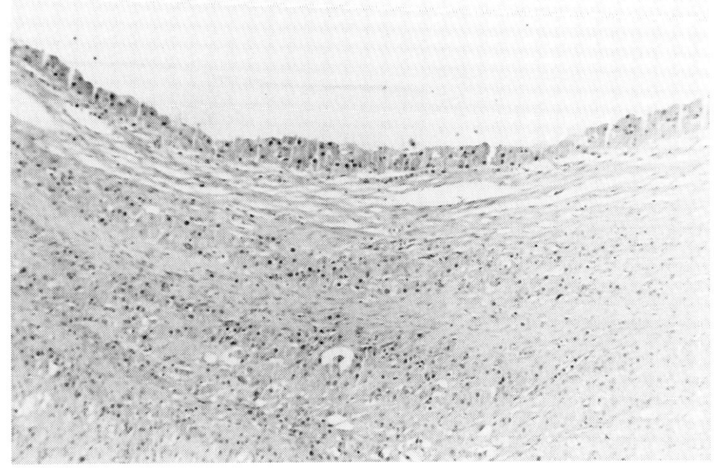

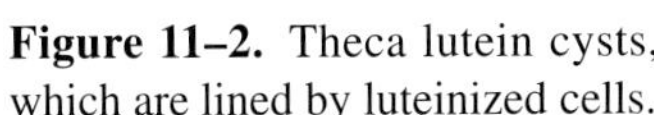

Figure 11–2. Theca lutein cysts, which are lined by luteinized cells.

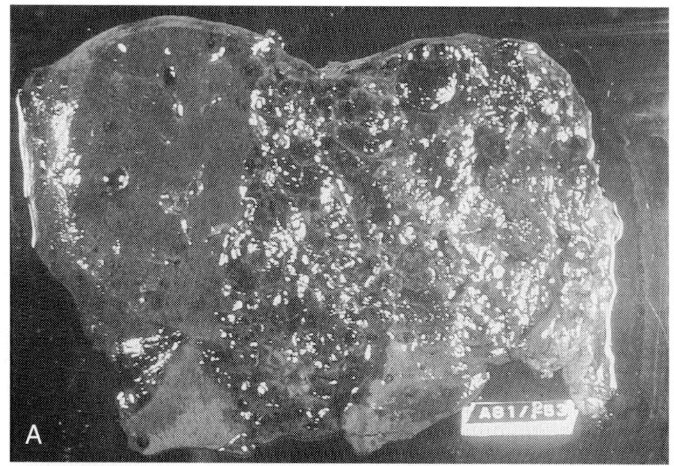

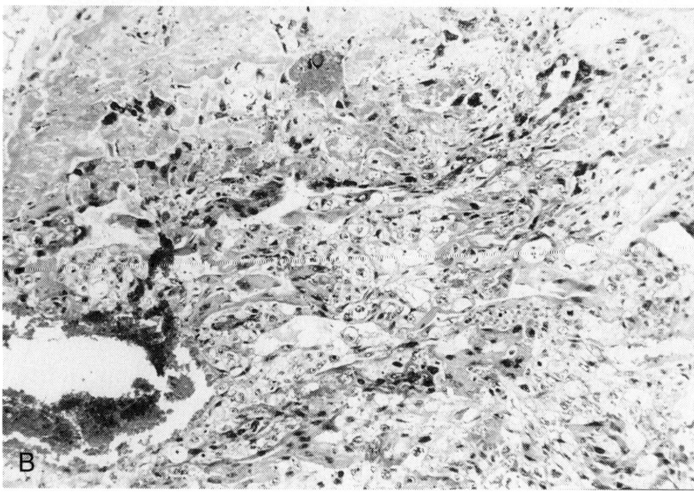

Figure 11–3. Choriocarcinoma. **A,** Markedly hemorrhagic tumor metastatic to liver. **B,** The tumor shows hemorrhage and necrosis.

PSTTs have three distinct growth patterns. The tumors may grow as polyps into the endometrial cavity, may be found as an intermyometrial mass, or may diffusely infiltrate myometrium.[6] Histologic examination of the neoplasm shows mononuclear and occasional multinuclear giant cells with abundant clear or eosinophilic cytoplasm that infiltrate between bundles of myometrial smooth muscle (Fig. 11–4). In contrast to the characteristic pattern of choriocarcinoma, which obliterates small vessels with adjacent hemorrhage, PSTTs surround and infiltrate vessels with abundant fibrinoid deposition, mimicking a normal implantation site.[6] Necrosis and hemorrhage are not characteristic features. Mitotic activity is variable.

hPL staining is usually stronger than hCG staining, reflecting the intermediate trophoblast origin of the lesion; however, a choriocarcinoma-like pattern of greater hCG than hPL staining has been reported.[12] The intermediate trophoblast of PSTT also stains for cytokeratin and placental alkaline phosphatase (PLAP).[12,13]

There are no well-established criteria for prediction of aggressive behavior. Mitotic counts have been found to be poor predictors of outcome,[14,15] although more than 5 mitoses per 10 high-power fields, clear rather than eosinophilic cytoplasm, and necrosis are reported to be more common in the more aggressive lesions.[6] Confounding the issue, mitotic counts may differ in curettage and hysterectomy specimens as well as in foci of metastatic disease.[15]

Most PSTTs are diploid.[8] In one study all evalu-

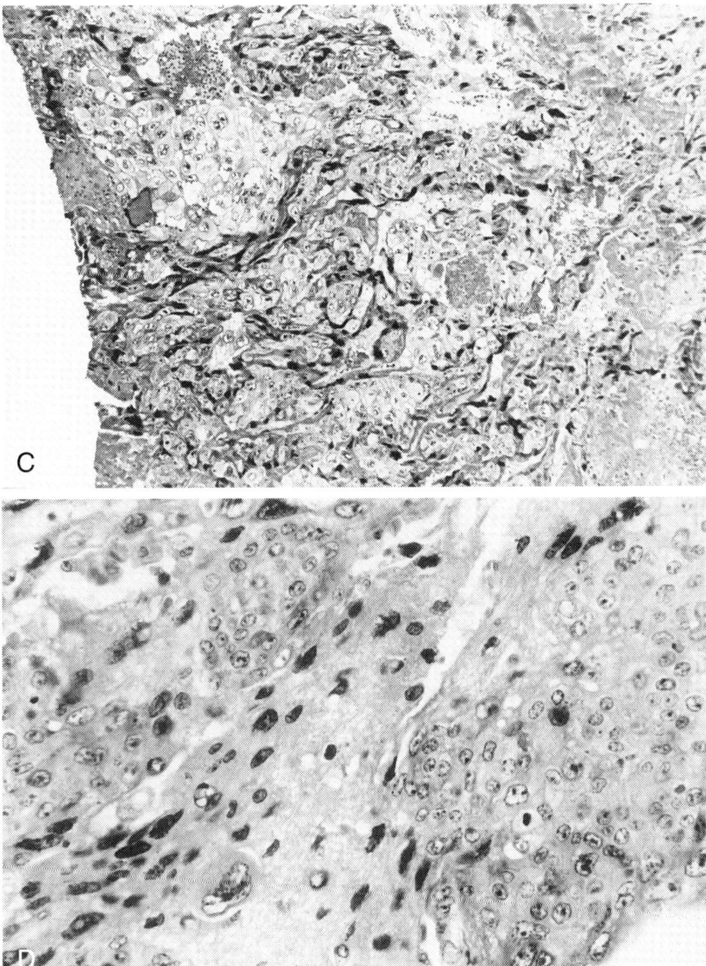

Figure 11–3 *Continued* **C** and **D,** The tumor is biphasic, and no chorionic villi are present.

ated PSTTs were diploid and no correlation was found between histopathology, immunohistochemistry, ploidy, or S-phase fraction and outcome.[7]

Some patients have been cured with a simple curettage, while others have died of metastatic disease despite aggressive therapy. In general, a hysterectomy is the treatment of choice. The most common metastatic site is the lungs, but metastases to lymph nodes, brain, liver, kidney, vagina, stomach, and spleen have also been reported. Metastases are relatively resistant to chemotherapy.[14,15]

The diagnosis of PSTT can be difficult on a curettage specimen. The differential diagnosis of PSTT includes normal implantation site, exaggerated placental site, and placental site nodule. hCG and hPL measurements, repeat curettage, and imaging studies may be necessary to arrive at the correct diagnosis, although the tissue from a second procedure may be negative even in the presence of PSTT. PSTTs are rare after early pregnancy as opposed to normal and exaggerated placental sites. Normal and exaggerated placental sites also are more likely to be detected soon after the preceding pregnancy. Exaggerated placental sites show no confluency and contain bland cells with few or no mitoses. In one study the authors noted that the intermediate trophoblast of PSTT had cells with cytoplasmic vacuoles and spindled cells more often than that of exaggerated placental sites.[12] Placental site nodules are well circumscribed, eosinophilic, paucicellular lesions. Histologic impression of a mass lesion, increased nuclear size, atypia, and abundant or atypical mitoses favor PSTT.[6]

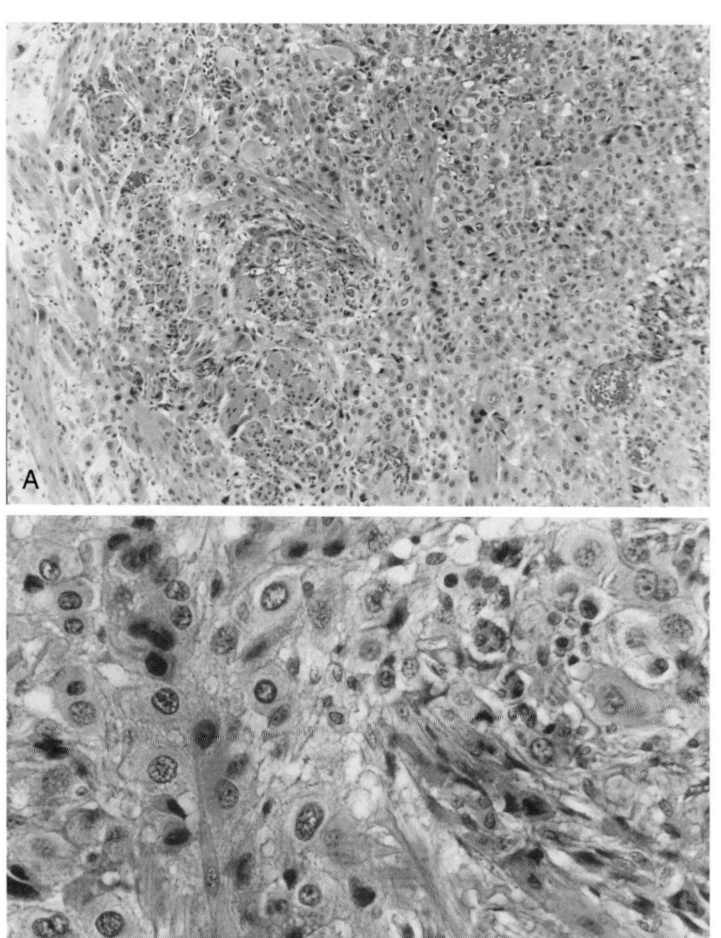

Figure 11–4. Placental site trophoblastic tumor. **A,** Intermediate trophoblastic cells splaying myometrial bundles. **B,** The tumor is composed of a monomorphic population of intermediate trophoblastic cells.

Exaggerated Placental Site

Exaggerated placental sites are usually seen within a short time of an antecedent pregnancy, either normal or molar. They are composed of intermediate trophoblastic cells that infiltrate the decidua and myometrium (Fig. 11–5). They have no clinical significance but may be mistaken for PSTT on a curettage specimen. With exaggerated placental sites the other characteristic findings of pregnancy, such as villi and decidua, should be sought. The intermediate trophoblastic cells in an exaggerated placental site stain with hPL and cytokeratin.[12]

Placental Site Nodule or Plaque

Placental site nodules and plaques represent incompletely involuted implantation sites. They are usually incidental findings but may cause irregular vaginal bleeding. These nodules are composed of benign proliferations of intermediate trophoblastic cells in the endometrium or endocervix and can be present many years after a pregnancy. They are usually well circumscribed, although they may extend into adjacent tissue, mimicking invasion.[16] Placental site nodules are minimally cellular, composed predominantly of amorphous eosinophilic material made up of fibrinoid and collagen.[6] The

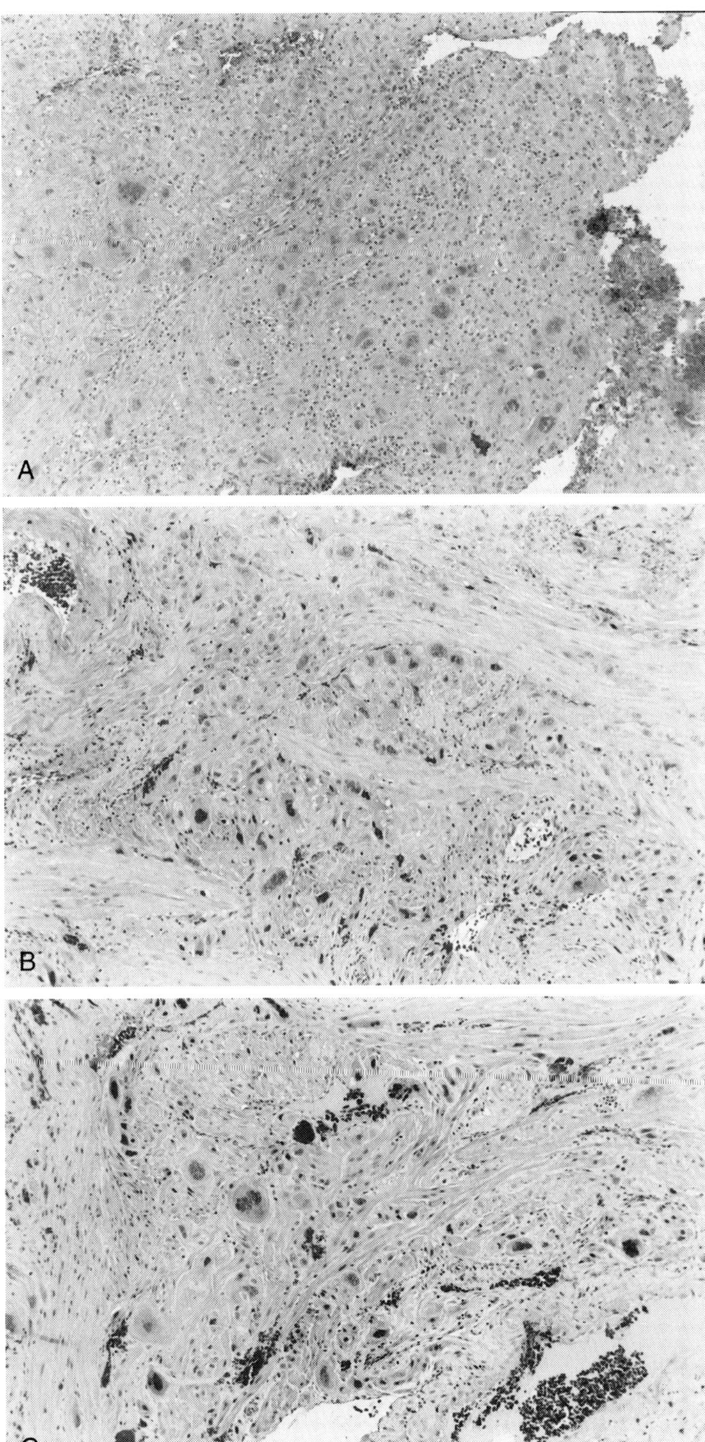

Figure 11–5. Exaggerated placental site. Numerous intermediate trophoblastic cells are seen infiltrating decidua (**A**) and myometrium (**B** and **C**).

Illustration continued on following page

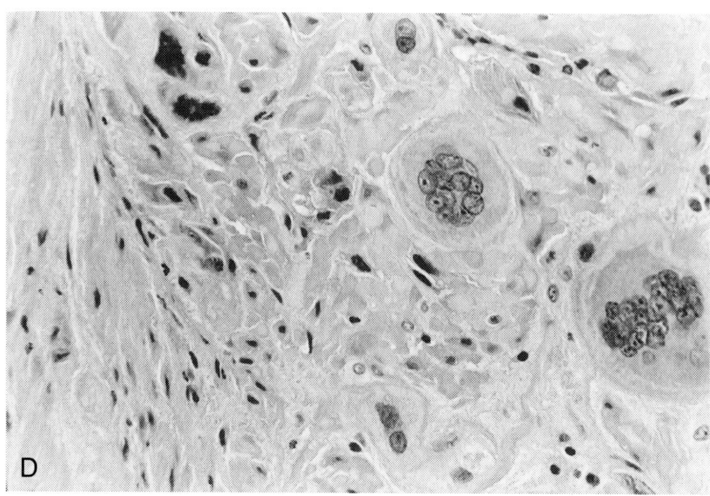

Figure 11–5 *Continued* Multinucleation of intermediate trophoblastic cells is seen (**D**).

few intermediate trophoblastic cells are scattered within the nodules (Fig. 11–6). These cells may show increased nuclear size with hyperchromatism, but the changes are degenerative and mitoses are rare or absent. Plasma cells may be seen surrounding the nodules for up to 9 months after delivery.[6]

In an immunohistochemical study of placental site nodules, Heuttner and Gersell[16] found strong staining with PLAP, cytokeratins AE1 and AE3, and epithelial membrane antigen. hPL and hCG were of lesser intensity, and vimentin was focally positive. Placental site nodules also stain for pregnancy specific β-1 glycoprotein.[17]

Although generally accepted as benign lesions, multiple placental site nodules occurring after a molar pregnancy with mildly elevated hCG levels have been described.[18]

The differential diagnosis of placental site nodule includes decidua, placental polyp, exaggerated placental site, PSTT, and epithelial lesions. Decidual cells have smaller nuclei without hyperchromasia. Placental polyps are composed of hyalinized chorionic villi. Exaggerated placental site has intermediate trophoblastic cells infiltrating decidua and myometrium rather than forming nodules or plaques, is not hyalinized, and is associated with a recent pregnancy. PSTTs usually involve large areas and are infiltrative. Epithelial lesions can be distinguished by immunohistochemistry (see below).

Nontrophoblastic Tumors That Can Be Confused with Gestational Trophoblastic Disease

Immunohistochemistry can be most helpful in distinguishing GTD from some possible lookalikes. Although overlap exists in the immunohistochemical staining patterns of the various types of GTD, the combination of hCG, hPL, and PLAP can be useful in separating GTD from an undifferentiated carcinoma. Desmin and muscle-specific actin positivity distinguish a leiomyosarcoma from PSTT.[6] Nongestational choriocarcinoma is exceedingly rare and usually is admixed with other germ cell tumor elements. A variety of nontrophoblastic tumors may contain syncytiotrophoblast-like giant cells, but careful evaluation usually shows the primary pattern of the tumor.

CLINICAL CRITERIA

The diagnosis of persistent GTD is most often based on serial serum hCG titers after evacuation of a molar pregnancy. Persistent GTD follows hydatidiform moles in 45% of cases, term gestations in 25%, spontaneous abortions in 25%, and ectopic pregnancies in 5%.[6] In a recent study persistent GTD developed in 38% of patients treated conservatively for complete hydatidiform mole.[19] The most important clinical predictors of persis-

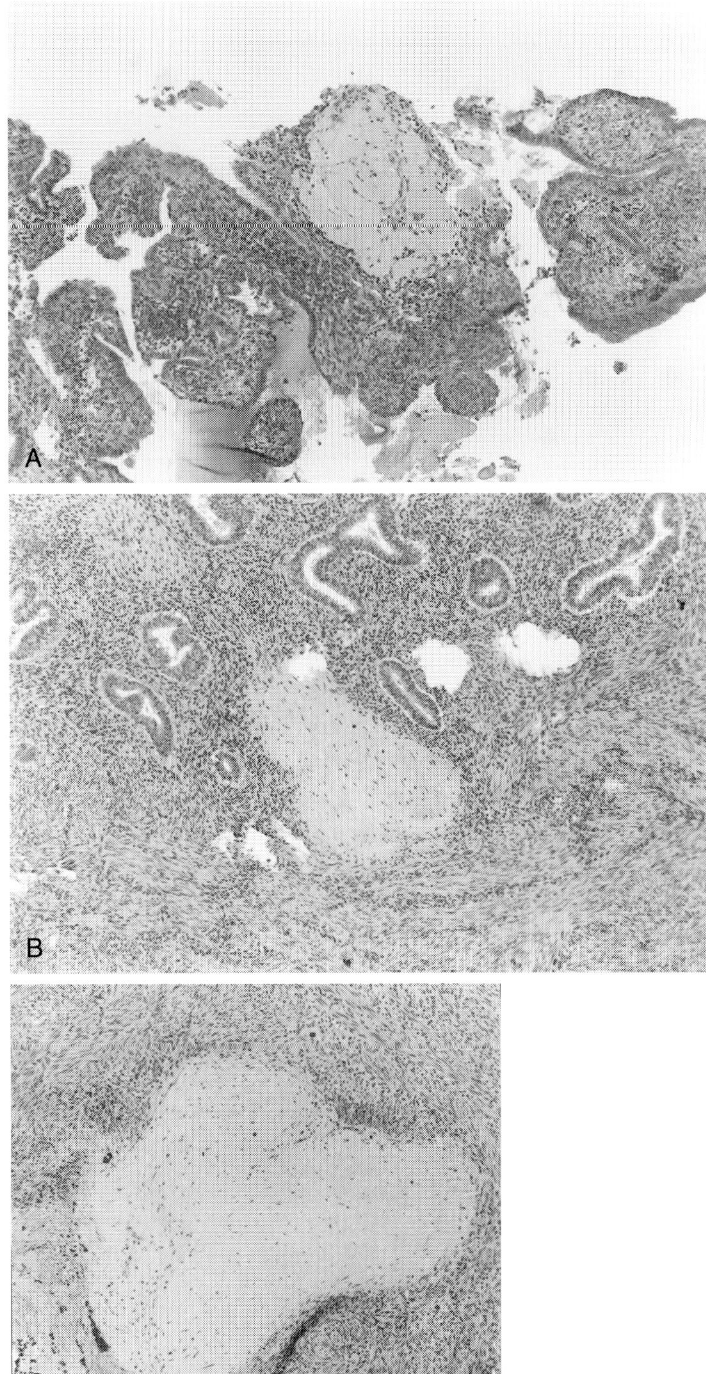

Figure 11–6. Placental site nodule. **A,** Nodule seen on curettage specimen. **B,** Nodule seen at hysterectomy. **C,** The nodule is well circumscribed. It is composed predominantly of eosinophilic acellular material, with occasional intermediate trophoblastic cells.

Table 11–2. National Cancer Institute Classification of Metastatic Gestational Trophoblastic Disease

- Nonmetastatic gestational trophoblastic disease
- Good-prognosis metastatic disease
  - Duration less than 4 months
  - Low pretherapy hCG (<100,000 IU/24-hour urine or <40,000 mIU/ml serum)
  - No brain or liver metastases
  - No antecedent term pregnancy
  - No prior chemotherapy
- Poor-prognosis metastatic disease
  - Duration greater than 4 months
  - High pretherapy hCG (>100,000 IU/24-hour urine or >40,000 mIU/ml serum)
  - Brain or liver metastases
  - Antecedent term pregnancy
  - Prior chemotherapy

From Hammond CB, Borchert LG, Tyrey L, et al: Am J Obstet Gynecol 115:451, 1973.

Table 11–3. International Federation of Obstetrics and Gynecology Staging System for Gestational Trophoblastic Disease

- I. Disease confined to the uterus
  - IA. No risk factors
  - IB. One risk factor
  - IC. Two risk factors
- II. Disease outside the uterus but limited to genital structures
  - IIA. No risk factors
  - IIB. One risk factor
  - IIC. Two risk factors
- III. Disease extends to lungs with or without known genital tract disease
  - IIIA. No risk factors
  - IIIB. One risk factor
  - IIIC. Two risk factors
- IV. All other metastatic disease
  - IVA. No risk factors
  - IVB. One risk factor
  - IVC. Two risk factors

Risk factors: hCG >100,000 mIU/ml, disease duration >6 months since antecedent pregnancy.
Prior chemotherapy should be noted in reporting
Placental site trophoblastic tumors should be reported separately
Histologic verification of disease not required

From Pettersson F: Acta Obstet Gynecol Scand 71:224, 1992. © 1992 Munksgaard International Publishers Ltd., Copenhagen, Denmark.

Table 11–4. World Health Organization Scoring System for Gestational Trophoblastic Disease

Prognostic factor	0 point	1 point	2 points	3 points
Age	≤39 years	>39 years	—	—
Antecedent pregnancy	Hydatidiform mole	Abortion	Term	—
Interval from end of antecedent pregnancy to start of chemotherapy	4 months	4–6 months	7–12 months	>12 months
β-hCG (IU/L)	$<10^3$	10^3–10^4	10^4–10^5	$>10^5$
ABO blood group (female × male)	—	O × A, A × O	B, AB	—
Largest tumor	—	3–5 cm	>5 cm	—
Site of metastases	—	Spleen, kidney	Gastrointestinal tract, liver	Brain
Number of metastases	—	1–4	4–8	>8
Prior chemotherapy	—	—	Single drug	Two or more drugs

Low risk = 0 to 4 points, intermediate risk = 5 to 7 points; high risk = 8 or more points.
From Gestational trophoblastic diseases: report of a WHO scientific group. (WHO technical report series #692.) Geneva, 1983, World Health Organization.

tent disease in this study were preevacuation hCG levels greater than 100,000 mIU/ml, age greater than 35 years, and history of a previous molar pregnancy.

Because chemotherapy rather than surgery is the mainstay of therapy, clinical criteria for the diagnosis of GTD are most often applied. There is frequently no histologic confirmation of the diagnosis, although most extrauterine GTD is actually choriocarcinoma. The extent of disease is evaluated with a metastatic workup that includes imaging studies of the chest, brain, abdomen, and pelvis, serum hCG, complete blood cell count, and baseline liver and renal function tests. Clinical classifications attempt to identify low- and high-risk disease. A variety of classifications and modifications of these classifications are used to plan treatment and evaluate prognosis. The most common systems are the National Cancer Institute (NCI), World Health Organization (WHO), and International Federation of Obstetrics and Gynecology (FIGO) systems (Tables 11–2 to 11–4). While some authors have attempted to evaluate the usefulness of one system over the other,[20] Ayhan and associates[21] found that a combination of the various criteria was most reliable in predicting treatment failures.

Low-risk metastatic GTD can usually be cured with single-agent chemotherapy with preservation of fertility.[22] Multiagent chemotherapy with selective use of adjuvant radiation therapy and surgery cures most patients with high-risk metastatic GTD.[23] Procedures such as hysterectomy, craniotomy, and thoracotomy also have a place in the management of GTD.[24] Radiation therapy is used as an adjunct principally for intracranial and hepatic disease, in which it can be palliative for drug-resistant disease, decrease pain, improve hemostasis, and decrease mass effect.[25] Even in patients with brain metastases, survival has been reported to be as high as 80%.[25]

REFERENCES

1. Tang M, Liu T, Song H: Choriocarcinoma and invasive mole—clinicopathologic study of 65 autopsied cases. Chinese Med J 101:890, 1988.
2. Brinton L, Bracken M, Connelly R: Choriocarcinoma incidence in the United States. Am J Epidemiol 123:1094, 1986.
3. Semer D, Macfee M: Gestational trophoblastic disease: epidemiology. Semin Oncol 22:109, 1995.
4. Palmer J: Advances in the epidemiology of gestational trophoblastic disease. J Reprod Med 39:155, 1994.
5. Lage J, Roberts D: Choriocarcinoma in a term placenta: pathologic diagnosis of tumor in an asymptomatic patient with metastatic disease. Int J Gynecol Pathol 12:80, 1993.
6. Redline R, Abdul-Karim F: Pathology of gestational trophoblastic disease. Semin Oncol 22:96, 1995.
7. Fukunaga M, Ushigome S: Metastasizing placental site trophoblastic tumor—an immunohistochemical and flow cytometric study of two cases. Am J Surg Pathol 17:1003, 1993.
8. Wolf N, Lage J: Genetic analysis of gestational trophoblastic disease: a review. Semin Oncol 22:113, 1995.
9. Kurman RJ, Scully RE, Norris HJ: Trophoblastic pseudotumor of the uterus: an exaggerated form of "syncytial endometritis" simulating a malignant tumor. Cancer 38:1214, 1976.
10. Young RH, Clement PB: Malignant lesions of the female genital tract and peritoneum that may be underdiagnosed. Semin Diagn Pathol 12:14, 1995.
11. Denny L, Dehaeck K, Nevin J, et al: Placental site trophoblastic tumor: three case reports and literature review. Gynecol Oncol 59:300, 1995.
12. Motoyama T, Ohta T, Ajioka Y, et al: Neoplastic and non-neoplastic intermediate trophoblasts: an immunohistochemical and ultrastructural study. Pathol Int 44:57, 1994.
13. Fukunaga M, Ushigome S: Malignant trophoblastic tumors: immunohistochemical and flow cytometric comparison of choriocarcinoma and placental site trophoblastic tumors. Hum Pathol 24:1098, 1993.
14. Finkler N: Placental site trophoblastic tumor—diagnosis, clinical behavior, and treatments. J Reprod Med 36:27, 1991.
15. Hoffman JS, Silverman A, Gelber J, et al: Placental site trophoblastic tumor: a report of radiologic, surgical and pathologic methods of evaluating extent of disease. Gynecol Oncol 50:110, 1993.
16. Huettner P, Gersell D: Placental site nodule: a clinicopathologic study of 38 cases. Int J Gynecol Pathol 13:191, 1994.
17. Shitabata P, Rutgers J: The placental site nodule: an immunohistochemical study. Hum Pathol 25:1295, 1994.
18. Silva E, Tornos C, Lage J, et al: Multiple nodules of

intermediate trophoblast following hydatidiform moles. Int J Gynecol Pathol 12:324, 1993.

19. Ayhan A, Tuncer Z, Halilzede H, et al: Predictors of persistent disease in women with complete hydatidiform moles. J Reprod Med 41:591, 1996.
20. Smith DB, Newlands E, Bagshawe KD: Correlation between clinical staging (FIGO) and prognostic groups with gestational trophoblastic disease. Br J Obstet Gynaecol 100:157, 1993.
21. Ayhan A, Yapar E, Deren O, et al: Remission rates and significance of prognostic factors in gestation trophoblastic tumors. J Reprod Med 37:461, 1992.
22. Feldman S, Goldstein D, Berkowitz RS: Low-risk metastatic gestational trophoblastic tumors. Semin Oncol 22:166, 1995.
23. Lurain J: High-risk metastatic gestational trophoblastic tumors—current management. J Reprod Med 39:217, 1994.
24. Soper J: Surgical therapy for gestational trophoblastic disease. J Reprod Med 39:168, 1994.
25. Herrington S: Enhancing cure and palliation: radiation therapy in the treatment of metastatic gestational trophoblastic neoplasia. Semin Oncol 22:185, 1995.

12

Chorangiomas and Other Tumors

Douglas R. Shanklin

The repertoire of nonchoriomatous tumors of the human placenta is limited, for primary tumors, by two factors: the types of cells that arise during early histogenesis and the short natural life span of the placenta itself. Nonchoriomatous primary tumors are enhanced by metastatic lesions, which in turn are limited by the relative infrequency of malignant disease in women during the usual ages of childbearing and the natural history of those malignancies. The result of collision of primary uterine leiomyoma with placental morphogenesis is a form of inclusion tumor, which is discussed in this chapter as the archetype of all potential forms of incorporation of uterine neoplasms during placental growth and maturation.

TUMORS OF PLACENTAL MESENCHYME

The chorangioma is the most common nonchoriomatous neoplasm of the placenta, with an average incidence of 1:1194.[1] Every chorionic villus is a potential chorangioma through dysplastic conversion of the principal growth balance between the vessels and the stroma. Various terms have been applied to these lesions: hemangioma, placental angioma, chorangioma, mesenchymoma, chorionangioma, vascular hamartoma of the placenta, chorangiofibroma, fibroma, myxoma, and even, implausibly, chorioma. Of these, chorangioma is clearly the best overall term, based on the unique relationship of the vascular and stromal development of villi to the trophoblast. This term is also favored by Benirschke and Driscoll.[2] Fox[3,4] has used the term "placental hemangioma" based on the observation that vascular tumors of the umbilical cord (stalk) have amniotic mesoblast as the tissue of origin rather than chorionic mesoblast. This is correct after delamination of the amnion from the chorion at about 12 days after conception, as shown by Hertig,[5,6] but ignores the earlier commonality of all placental mesoblast. The use of this distinction is less important than recognition of the umbilical cord as a separate compartment of the mature placenta.

The chorangiomas of the placenta may be classified as follows:

1. Vascular tumors of the discoid or parenchymal placenta
   a. Chorangiomas
   b. Mixed cell mesenchymomas
2. Vascular tumors of the umbilical cord

Several of the terms listed above are fundamentally descriptive phrases based on the range of tissue found in individual cases reported from time to time.

The three-part classification of Marchetti[7] in 1939 has some similarities to the above. Chorangiomas are approximately the tumors he placed under "mature vascular tumors," and mixed cell mesenchymomas would include his relatively avascular "immature tumors." The degenerative type is not a distinctive form of tumor, since infarction and hyalinization can occur in all tissue combinations. This class of tumors has been known for 200 years.[8] The number of reports during the nineteenth century is limited, and the modern literature is not voluminous. My recent account[9] is the most comprehensive among other fairly recent reviews.[10] Somewhat earlier reviews are those of Siddall,[11] Kuhnel,[12] DeCosta and associates,[13] and Wallenberg.[14]

Location

Chorangiomas are found in several locations within the mature placenta:

1. In the deeper parenchyma of cotyledons or lobules within cotyledons, the *parenchymal* location; they tend to be near the middle, but this is partly an artifact of giving a different descriptive term to type 2
2. At the lateral edge of the placenta, filling the marginal lake zone and extending back toward the central part of the placenta, the *marginal* location (Fig. 12–1*A*)
3. Within the sheaves of the discord chorion itself, sometimes with only an attenuated amnion between the tumor and the amniotic cavity, the *littoral* location (Fig. 12–1*B*)
4. As a variant of location 3 but beyond the lateral rim of the discoid chorion, the *membranous* location; these presumably arise from remnants of chorion laeve, since pedicles are not seen leading to them from the main placental mass

Chorangiomas are found in two loci of the umbilical cord:

1. Within the substance of the cord itself, the *funicular* location
2. Attached to the umbilical cord by a vascular pedicle at or above the point of cord insertion itself, the *pedicular* location

The possibility of vascular migration with tumor growth might mean, eventually, the finding of a pedicle attached to the surface of the discoid chorion rather than the umbilical cord. In addition to discrete, usually single masses in the locations noted above, larger collections of angiomatous ramuli and villi have been observed to spread across much of the placenta (a condition termed chorangiomatosis) (Fig. 12–1*C*).[15]

Incidence

The nature of case reports has an effect on considerations of incidence, and the techniques used may alter the number of smaller tumors actually found. Incidence values ranging from 1:77[16] to 1:9000[12] have been reported. Wentworth's study involved slicing placentas at intervals of 400 μm.[16] Shaw-Dunn[17] cut specimens at intervals of 3 mm. Both techniques were more precise than was necessary to identify 87% (13:15) of the cases included in the two reports. All of Wentworth's chorangiomas (8:8) were at least 1 cm in diameter, and Shaw-Dunn found two smaller than the coarser method would likely have identified.

Most chorangiomas are found by palpation of the placental specimen, but a few are identified on review of routine histopathologic sections or study of grossly evident lesions of various types. These exercises have been done, with a yield of 1.13% putative microchorangiomas after close review of 1099 lesions subjected to microscopic review,[18] a frequency roughly 13 times that of grossly evident lesions, which was 0.084% of more than 16,700 specimens. This difference suggests that more vigorous sampling of lesions not obviously chorangiomas would yield more cases, but the clinical significance of these smaller lesions is doubtful.

Natural History

A careful review of 2000 first-trimester specimens found no chorangiomas,[19] but with the incidence figures noted above, assuming the initial lesion could be found, a series of 2000 cases is too small to be determinative. The recognition of angiogenins as specific stimuli for vascularization, including that of the placenta,[20–22] and the growth rate of the vasculature generally and of small chorangiomas in particular, which are not known with precision, surely beg the question of whether cases can be clearly identified before midterm gestation. The earliest example with good clinical evidence, by sonography, is that reported by Nahmanovici and co-workers[23] at 19 weeks. This was correlated later with two lesions found at delivery at 39 weeks' gestation. The growth rate of the earliest chorangioma found by pathologic examination, at 21 weeks,[24] is unknown; these authors failed to report the size of their eight tumors from the second trimester. Growth rates, presumptively during the second half of gestation, are often considerable,[25–28] although static images have been described.[29] I have described several reports of

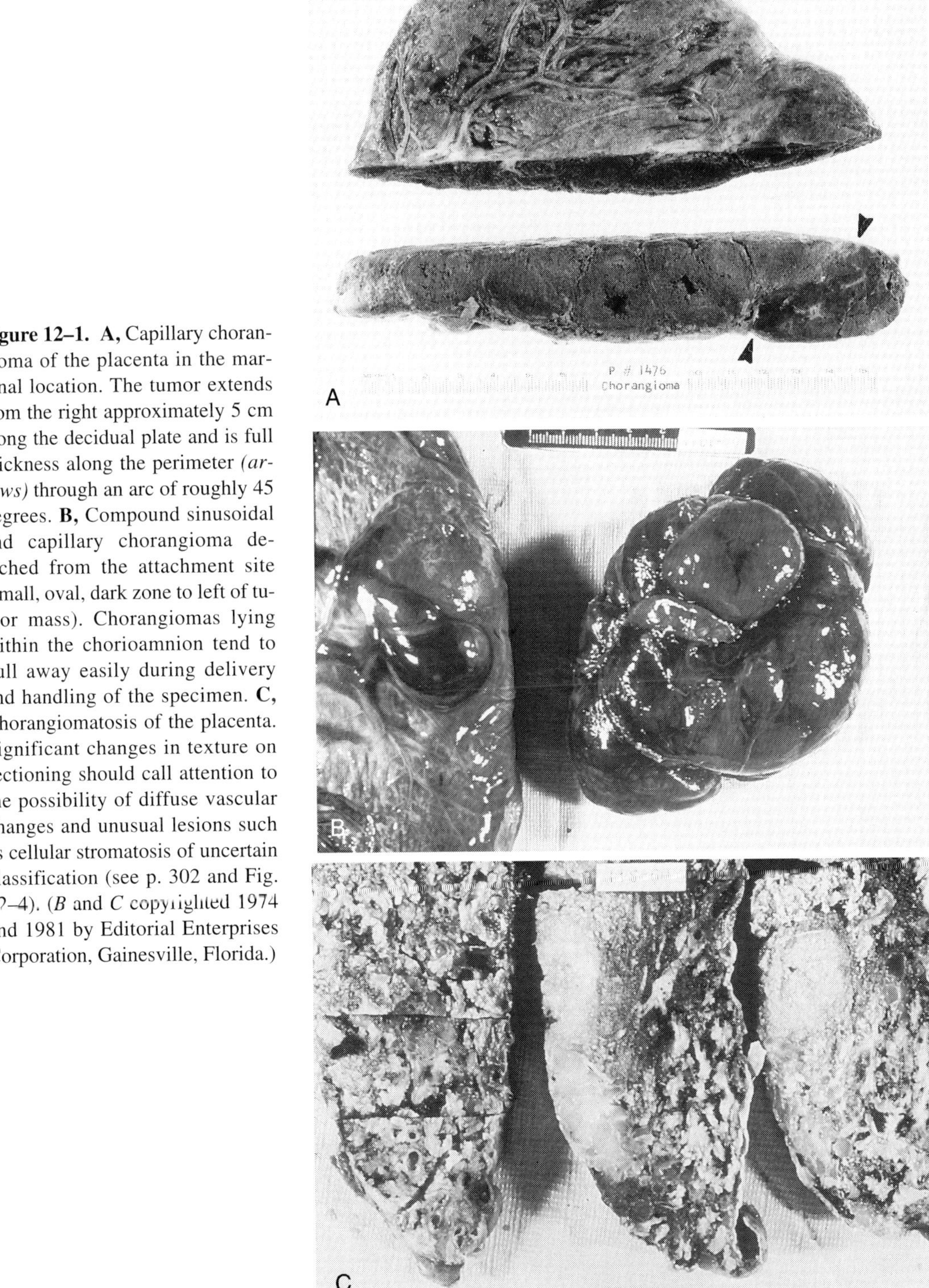

Figure 12–1. A, Capillary chorangioma of the placenta in the marginal location. The tumor extends from the right approximately 5 cm along the decidual plate and is full thickness along the perimeter *(arrows)* through an arc of roughly 45 degrees. **B,** Compound sinusoidal and capillary chorangioma detached from the attachment site (small, oval, dark zone to left of tumor mass). Chorangiomas lying within the chorioamnion tend to pull away easily during delivery and handling of the specimen. **C,** Chorangiomatosis of the placenta. Significant changes in texture on sectioning should call attention to the possibility of diffuse vascular changes and unusual lesions such as cellular stromatosis of uncertain classification (see p. 302 and Fig. 12–4). (*B* and *C* copyrighted 1974 and 1981 by Editorial Enterprises Corporation, Gainesville, Florida.)

masses from 258 to 780 g, sizes that rival the growth of the placenta itself.[30]

Chorangiomas may progress into various types of self-ablation with infarction and slow fibrosis as intrinsic outcomes. Larger tumors can have an obstetric effect with obstruction of labor, especially if the tumor is pedunculated. I have seen a large marginal chorangioma that was the focus for a placental abruption near term.

The principal clinical effect of chorangiomas is fetal and neonatal. This effect is mediated through shunting of fetal blood, bypassing the vascular bed of the villi chorii, which is related to the proportion of sinusoidal vessels and the overall size of the tumor. These two factors translate into a rapid runoff of umbilical arterial blood, and many specimens show enhancement of the umbilical and placental veins. An account by Storch in 1878 described clearly the dilation of the vein on the surface of the mass leading back to the umbilical insertion.[31]

CHORANGIOMA

Definition

Chorangiomas are vascular tumors of the placenta with a dominant network of channels against a background of connective tissue. They can be mainly capillary, sinusoidal, or cavernous. The pattern of villi making up the tumor is either unusual or absent for the level of arborization at which the tumor appears. Chorangiomas are usually solid but can be lobular or serpentine. Clustered aggregates are found rarely and are properly referred to as diffuse chorangiomatosis. Chorangiomas are the principal type of mesenchymal tumor of the human placenta. Most chorangiomas are capillary tumors with a few larger vessels. The pattern in multifocal tumors is usually similar throughout, although strict reproduction of the relative ratio of vessels to connective tissue and the ratio of vessels by size is not seen.

Small, often linear deposits of calcium salts are found at the boundaries of tumor lobules. The lobules may be loosely arrayed or more closely packed. Sectioned surfaces have a uniform texture and color except when infarction is a feature. The infarcted zones resemble other placental infarctions by age of process, and as noted above, careful microscopic study of a grossly apparent infarction occasionally reveals chorangioma as part of the lesion complex. Hemorrhage into the stroma is rare but is difficult to assess because of the intense vascularity.

Capillary Hemangiomas

Capillary hemangiomas are chorangiomas in which almost all vessels are of placental capillary size (Fig. 12–2*A*). It should be noted that capillaries in normal villi are larger than capillaries in adult tissues and seem readily expansile. A few vessels up to two or three times the average diameter of the remainder are acceptable with this definition (Fig. 12–2*B*). Some tumors have complexes of larger vessels, often the size of dilated ramular veins. Occasionally, capillary and mixed sinusoidal patterns occur in adjacent lobules (Fig. 12–2*C*). About 80% of chorangiomas are essentially pure capillary tumors. These have little or no effect on fetal development or neonatal adaptation, even when quite large.

Chorangiosis

Developmental tissues often show distinct or recognizable intermediate forms of neoplasms or paraneoplastic lesions. This occurs in chorangiomas, and despite use of the term for a different lesion by one author, "chorangiosis" is the proper term. This takes the form of (1) increased numbers of vessels per unit area, (2) increased cellularity of vessels, sometimes shown as thickened walls, and (3) the likelihood of distorted vascular profiles. Both Potter[32] and Hörmann[33] illustrated this concept. Potter used the term "placental hypertrophy" to describe the presence of as many as 6 to 10 times the number of vessels expected. Foci of chorangiosis occur occasionally at the edges of overt chorangiomas. We have not found the relation of chorangiosis to fetal distress reported by Altshuler.[34]

True Chorangiomatous Tumors

True chorangiomatous tumors are space-occupying lesions in the ordinary sense. A few show

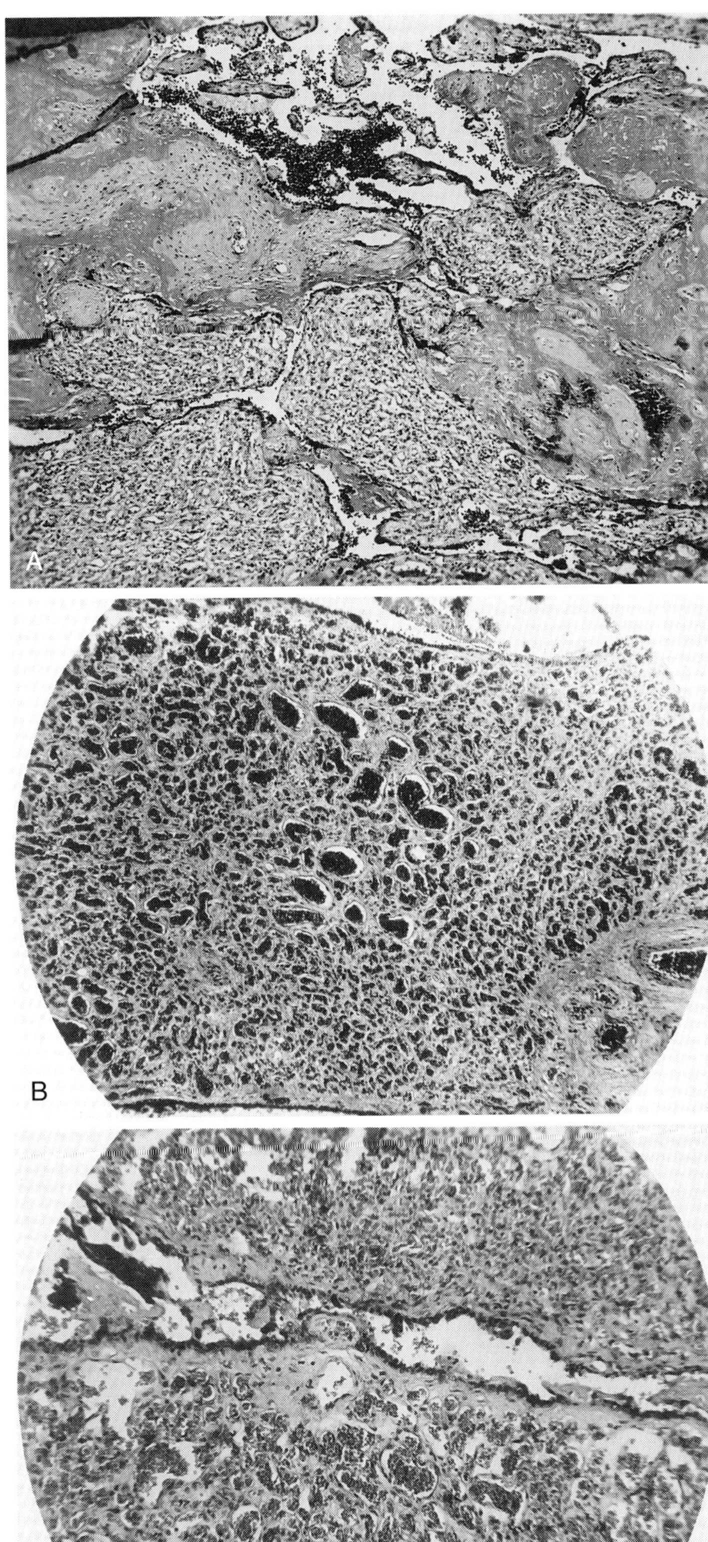

Figure 12–2. **A,** Multiple small lobules of nearly pure capillary chorangioma in a placental field of ramuli and villi chorii partially fused by fibrinoid deposit. Similar small and isolated lobules can be found from time to time in fulfillment of the potential for each villus to become a chorangioma (H&E, ×90). **B,** Capillary chorangioma with a moderate number of small sinusoidal vessels (center of field) and a prominent nutrient or hilar vessel (lower right) (Masson trichrome, ×125). **C,** Adjacent lobules of chorangioma; one lobule has only capillary vessels *(upper)* and the other many larger sinusoids *(lower)*. Note thin layers of syncytiotrophoblast along the lobular edges (Masson trichrome, ×125).

displacement of adjacent tissue even though compression is difficult to express within the open villous pattern of the cotyledons. Their relatively slow rate of growth while the placenta is enlarging mitigates centrifugal displacement of tissues in the manner often seen in adult tumors such as uterine leiomyomas. Hilar or nutrient vessels are inconspicuous. The smaller tumors are usually compact and distinct without lobules. They are single in 85% of cases; two to four nodules of different sizes is the expected pattern when multiple.

Differential Diagnosis

Differential diagnosis of chorangiomas is based mainly on infarction and thrombosis. The extremely rare hemangioma of the maternal decidua is not readily confused with capillary chorangioma, partly because of the location of decidual lesions and partly because of the cavernous and thrombotic appearance of decidual hemangioma.[35] Microscopic study is the only effective method for fully distinguishing between these lesions.

Appearance

The size range for capillary chorangioma in my series is wide: 0.8 cm to 11.5 × 9 × 6 cm. The latter tumor weighed 258 g. Other large tumors have been reported by Dupin and Chabaud,[36] Benson and Joseph,[37] and Fisher.[38] Their color is variable: black-red to purple or brown. Infarct zones are yellow to gray and sometimes have areas of hemorrhage. Dry or granular nonreflective surfaces denote infarction. Generally these lesions are easily sectioned unless considerable lobular calcium is present.

Sinusoidal Hemangiomas

Sinusoidal hemangiomas have a relatively large number of areas of sinus formation. Some are distinctively cavernous. This subclass of chorangioma is pathogenetically related to fetal and neonatal effects based on the extent or proportion of sinusoidal vessels. Reiner and Fries[39] demonstrated a direct surface vessel arteriovenous shunt. Tumors with a prominent surface vein are probably true sinusoidal or cavernous chorangiomas.[31]

Natural History. Sinusoidal hemangiomas arise in recognizable pattern and form during midgestation, the same as the capillary tumors. Some large tumors have not appeared to affect the fetus or newborn.[38,40–42] However, in my series of 251 cases[35] the perinatal mortality was almost 29%. Most of the perinatal deaths in my review and among my cases occurred in the early years. Awareness of the potential significance of these tumors has favorably influenced care of the newborn.[43]

No recent evidence has been presented that chorangiomas can become malignant. Although a spate of reports have appeared over the past 20 years, the time of first diagnosis remains at midgestation, 19 to 21 weeks, despite a few sonograms performed before the diagnosis was actually made. If something unique or critical to placental vascularization culminates at that time, it remains unidentified. The sole candidate that comes to mind is the onset of significant and progressive migration of villous paracapillaries, seen focally during weeks 16 to 18 and progressively after 20 weeks. Whether the angiogenins of Folkman[20–22] are operative in paracapillary migration is unknown, but if they are, they may be related to the growth of chorangiomas in the latter half of gestation.

Fetal Effects. The principal effects of shunting across sinusoidal chorangiomas are gestational prematurity, low birth weight for gestational age, hydramnios, fetal cardiac hypertrophy, fetal cardiac failure, hydrops fetalis, placental hydrops, neonatal cardiac failure, massive fetomaternal hemorrhage, disseminated intravascular coagulation, platelet sequestration syndromes, and neonatal hypoalbuminemia. These findings, alone or in combination, have been described with large tumors,[13,37,44,45] with those of average size, 4 to 7 cm maximum diameter,[13,46,47] and with multiple smaller tumors.[14,38,47,48] Overt fetal distress[26] and fetal death[49] have been reported. A case of chorangioma, neonatal thrombocytopenia, and intracranial hemorrhage was reported from Spain in 1983.[50] Wallenberg's study placed a threshold limit for hydramnios: tumors have a diameter of 5 cm or more,[14] although more recent reports have shown the same effect from multiple tumors individually smaller than 5 cm.[15,47,48] None of my sequential cases have shown hydramnios.

Questions of gestational prematurity and intrauterine growth retardation are less readily answered. Few case reports have provided the essential data on which to base useful assessments. A limited review of data available from 26 cases showed a skew toward low birth weights, although there were several examples of very high weights, a possible reflection of occult fetal hydrops, occasionally superimposed on a low true birth weight.[51] Reinforcing this view is the singular case reported by Sweet and associates[45] in which a markedly hydropic infant lost 940 g of edema fluid at 35 weeks, resulting in a weight of 2120 g, which is a low base weight for the gestational age.

The estimation of gestational prematurity as a result of chorangioma is harder to establish, again because of a lack of cases. The best figure available was a 17.9% rate, 10 examples of 56.[7,14,16,17,41] The problem is finding the proper comparative base; some centers during the years covered by these reports had prematurity rates of 12% to 15%, making 17.9% a point of interest but not sufficiently different to rely on.[52] Two mechanisms related to chorangiomas might lead to premature onset of labor: the effect of hydramnios, especially rapid-onset hydramnios, and abruption caused by a chorangioma at the decidua or at the far angle of the placenta. Both effects are unusual and may also occur at term, so they are not exclusive inducers of premature labor.

Recurrent Chorangiomas

An isolated reported by Chan and Leung[53] raises the prospect of chorangiomas in subsequent pregnancies. Their case involved multiple chorangiomas in both of the patient's pregnancies. Both fetuses were macerated stillborns, and no genetic studies were attempted.

Dysgenetic States and Chorangioma

Multiple chorangiomas and translocational chromosomal abnormalities in one of dizygous twins with nonfused dichorionic placentation were reported by Wurster and co-workers[54] in another isolated account. The general lack of syndromic features in infants whose placentas contain chorangiomas is against any regular pathogenetic relationship, but the technique has not been applied often, if at all. A possible approach to identifying chorangiomatous pregnancies comes from the observation that markedly elevated α-fetoprotein (AFP) levels have been found in maternal serum in several such cases, with[28,55] and without[27] AFP elevations in the amniotic fluid.

An unusual aspect was reported by Stiller and Skafish: the mother had a sudden passage of brown urine at 39 weeks that was found to be hemoglobinuria caused by fetomaternal transfusion.[56] The mother was blood type O, Rh negative, and received anti-Rh globulin at 28 weeks. The placenta had eight clustered nodules of chorangioma up to 5 cm in diameter.

Mesenchymomas of the Mixed Cell Type

Mixed cell mesenchymomas are fibrovascular tumors of the placenta with a dominance of connective tissue over vasculature. The vessels are mostly capillaries or small sinusoids. The density of the connective tissue varies considerably. There can be loose, possibly immature collagen, dense hypermature collagen, and various subpatterns of myxoid tissue. The stromal cells are mostly small, dense, solid nuclei with little or poorly defined cytoplasm, but a few are larger with vesicular nuclei. Stellate nuclei are sometimes found in zones of myxoid stroma.

The mixed cell mesenchymoma is much less common than the overt chorangioma (probable maximal ratio of about 1:13); a review series found mixed cell mesenchymomas to represent just 2% of all placental vascular tumors.[57] Discrete tumors of small or medium size could be confused on gross examination with fibrosis or late-stage infarction.

Mesenchymosis

As noted above, developmental tumors often have identifiable patterns intermediate between normal histogenesis and neoplasia. The abnormal villous pattern of mesenchymosis allows explicit identification by microscopy. These lesions show an expanded cluster of enlarged but distinct villi with pale stroma that contains few vessels of any size. Those present are usually very small. The overlying syncytiotrophoblast is peglike. A few cytotrophoblastic cells are found immediately subjacent to the syncytium and about as often as in normal placentas of the same gestational age as the specimen. Some fields show a few prominent syncytial buds. An interesting and as yet unexplained feature in some cases of mesenchymosis is the presence of plasmacytoid stromal cells. Plasmacytic villitis is an important diagnostic feature of cytomegalovirus placentitis, so it is known that plasma cells can form in the placenta under appropriate conditions. At present there is nothing to associate the plasmacytoid cells of mesenchymosis with cytomegalovirus or any other infective agent. The stroma in mesenchymosis is delicate and loosely fibrillar, lacking the central cisterns of chorioma and the lacunar pockets of hydrops placentalis. Protolumina in angiogenetic cords are sometimes found when the section is cut on a longitudinal line of the cords. This lesion is zonal or segmental; in my series none filled a cotyledon.

True Mesenchymomas

Mesenchymomas are usually smaller than chorangiomas. One possible explanation for this lies in the growth potential of the cell components of both tumors. Vessels with fairly direct connections to the fetal circulation have blood flow as a further stimulus to their molding and growth. Dysplastic villi that are largely connective tissue are likely to grow at the rate of placental stroma, which is modest in normal placentas. I[58] reported a noteworthy example measuring 3 × 3 × 2.5 cm. This was a firm, pale, gray-white nodule deeply embedded in a central cotyledon (Fig. 12–3*A* and *B*). The placenta was a 360-degree circumvallate type of placenta extrachorialis. The mother was a 24-year-old primigravida with borderline hypothyroidism. The infant weighed 3900 g and was normal in all respects. The placental/fetal weight ratio (P/F) was 0.147, nearly average for term. Other examples have a closer balance between the fibrillar stroma and the vessels, which tend to be small (Fig. 12–3*C*).

Although rare, an extensive plexiform mesenchymoma was seen after delivery at 33 weeks with an estimated P/F ratio of 0.252, which is in the normal range for 33 weeks. The child had mild respiratory distress syndrome. A few dilated vessels were found on the surface of the tumors, suggestive of either shunting of blood or vascular pooling. Microscopic examination showed zones of transition between mesenchymosis and overt mesenchymoma. This is the mesenchymal variant of chorangiomatosis (Fig. 12–1*C*).

Only a few predominantly fibrous mesenchymomas have been reported.[3,4,7,13,17] Delivery ranged from 32 to 40 weeks and birth weights were 1886 to 3500 g; in all four cited cases the infant survived without significant incident. The tumors were all solitary, ranging from 1.5 × 1.5 × 1.5 to 10.5 × 8.5 × 1.5 cm.

The pathologist may see a case in which the balance between vessels and stroma causes difficulty in classification. Such cases warrant the taking of additional sections (if not total blocking of the tumor) to assess the full range of histogenesis. Given the rarity of fibrous mesenchymomas, perhaps the final criterion is whether they have any demonstrable circulatory effect on the fetus or newborn. This will require close and detailed communication with the staff of the newborn center.

Lobulation of mesenchymomas and chorangiomas results in an irregular surface or interface with the intervillous space, which causes turbulent maternal flow. Intervillous thrombosis is occasionally found adjacent to or intertwined with lobules of these tumors.

Cellular Stromatosis of Uncertain Classification

Since the publication of my monograph on placental tumors in 1990 an extremely challenging placenta was recorded at Crump Hospital in Memphis (Fig. 12–4). This was the second pregnancy of a 27-year-old woman at 35 weeks. Oligohydramnios was identified. Electronic fetal monitoring suggested fetal cardiac distress; an abdominal section was performed, and the newborn was easily resuscitated. The placenta weighed 983 g. There were multiple old and recent subchorial thrombi. On sectioning, conspicuous enlarged villi with a tendency to form clusters were seen in

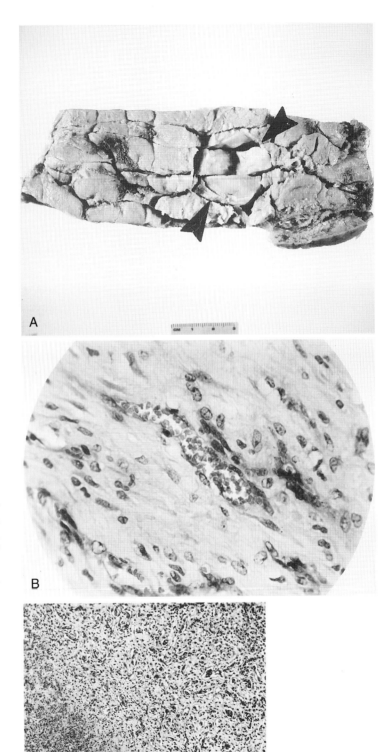

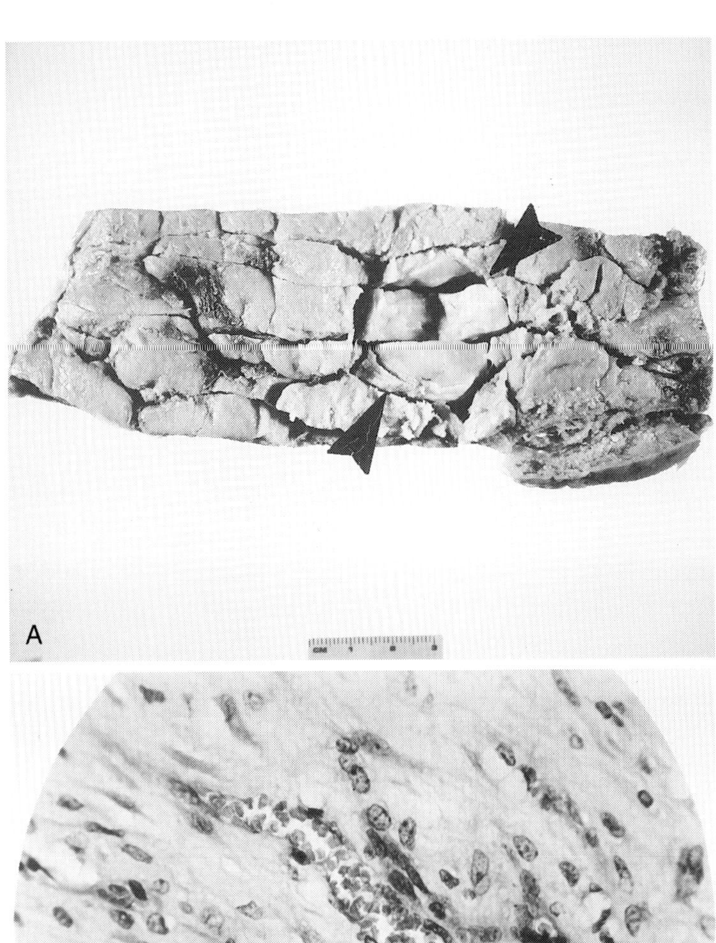

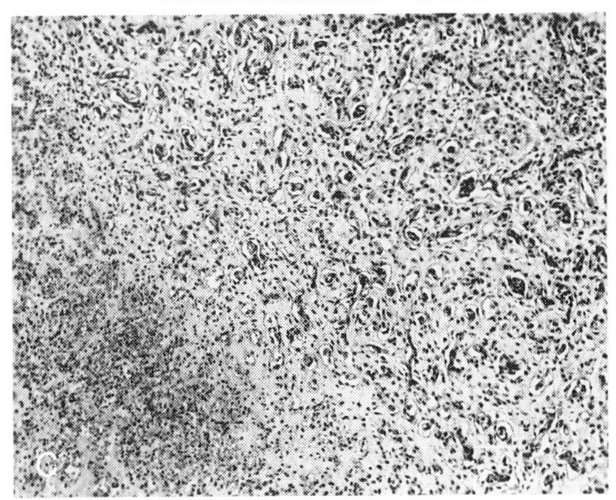

Figure 12–3. A, Mesenchymoma of near-term placenta, approximately 3 cm across. This was palpated during examination of a placenta extrachorialis. The tumor *(arrows)* was quite firm from the high content of fibrous tissue (see *B*). **B,** Representative field of mesenchymoma shown in *A*. A pattern of stroma runs diagonally across the field parallel to the principal vessel shown centrally. A smaller vessel can be seen near the left lower corner (H&E, ×250). **C,** Mesenchymoma with a balance of stromal and vascular development. A different case from that shown in **A** and **B** (H&E, ×125).

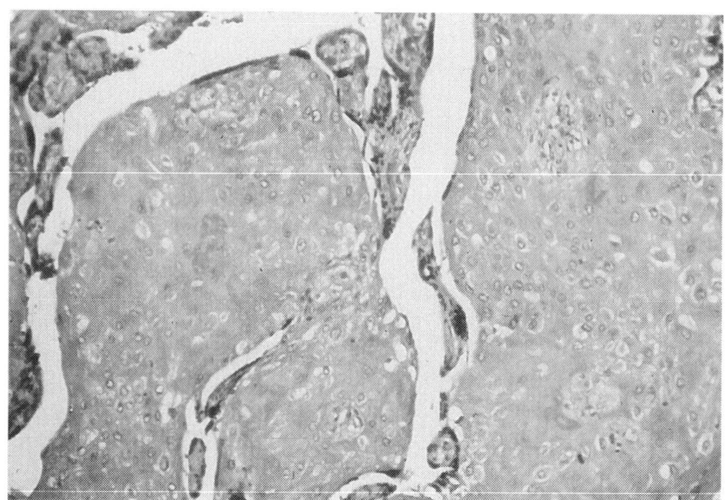

Figure 12–4. Adjacent placental nodules consistent with larger ramuli chorii and showing thin coats of syncytiotrophoblast. The stromal cores are packed with large, pale cells containing vesicular nuclei. These occupy the subsyncytial locus wherein cytotrophoblast is seen normally. About one third of the very enlarged placenta was occupied by these formations (H&E, ×100).

much of the placental parenchyma. These approached 1 to 2 mm in size. The histologic appearance was perplexing. The "villi" had the relative dimensions of ramuli chorii and were generally round or oval, with a thin outer surface of syncytiotrophoblast. The stromal cores were hypovascular to avascular and contained hundreds of large, pale cells with vesicular nuclei that generally filled the entire stromal space with scant fibrillar connective tissue. In fact, since many of these cells occupied the immediately subsyncytial zone characteristic of cytotrophoblast, their evident resemblance to cytotrophoblast became compelling. The cells were clearly not neoplastic in the sense of choriocarcinoma. The ramuli/villi were fairly uniform in size and, despite their intense cellularity, were monotonous in their regularity and general appearance.

MISCELLANEOUS PRIMARY TUMORS OF THE PLACENTA

Mixed Placentoma

Jauniaux and associates[59] reported an astonishing tumor best understood as a form of "coincident" neoplasm rather than a "collision tumor." They described a typical chorangioma surrounded by choriocarcinoma in situ. Since all chorangiomas of the placental mass have trophoblast on their surfaces, the development of such a mixed tumor might be just a matter of chance. Based on the incidence of clinically important chorangiomas noted above, roughly 1:1100 against the frequency of choriocarcinoma, circa 1:40,000, the coincident risk is 1:44 million, an estimate not readily confirmed by the current methods of either obstetric or pathologic practice.

Hepatocellular Adenoma

Chen and associates[60] reported a well-studied case of an intraplacental hepatocellular adenoma. The hepatic cells were reasonably easy to identify, but no distinct sinusoids were found. A number of endothelium-lined spaces contained active erythropoiesis as would be present in the sinusoids of the fetal liver at the 37 weeks of gestation reached by their patient, a 21-year-old gravida 2, para 1. The infant was small for age at 1781 g but did well and was within developmental parameters at 18 months of age.

Nodular Adrenal Cortex

Two reports of adrenocortical nodules within the placenta have appeared.[61,62] Ectopic adrenocortical tissues have been described in a number of unlikely places in the body, including the lung,[63] and in intracranial, extracerebral locations.[64,65] Remarkably, the fetus reported by Wiener and Dallgaard[65] had no adrenal glands in the usual anatomic location superior to the kidneys.

VASCULAR TUMORS OF THE UMBILICAL CORD

The umbilical cord is a tissue compartment distinct from the remainder of the placenta. The gross structure indicates this by the small diameter of contact at the site of cord insertion. Tumors of the umbilical cord are almost always vascular masses either within the cylinder of the cord or attached by a pedicle of varied length. The pedicle usually looks much like the cord. As a rough rule of thumb, cord tumors resemble cellular mesenchymomas when they are diffuse and chorangiomas when they are lobular. Trophoblast is absent from true cord hemangiomas.[66] Primary umbilical cord tumors are among the rarest human neoplasms. As of 1990 approximately eight cases had been reported since 1925, and an intensive Medline search failed to identify any further examples through early 1997. One of these was the case described by the late Edith L. Potter in the first edition of her seminal work *Pathology of the Fetus and the Newborn.*[67] This tumor involved both the cord and the superior surface of the discoid placenta. Unfortunately, Potter did not note whether the surfaces of the lobules had syncytiotrophoblast, so whether the tumor began in the umbilical stalk or from a chorionic base is unknown. I[68] have described a possible precursor nodule of vascularized mesenchyme lacking trophoblast.

Variation in tissue components in cord tumors is high, more so than in chorangiomas and mixed cell mesenchymomas. As obstructions to fetal vascular flow, when the umbilical circulation directly enters the tumor, such cases are likely to cause at minimum poor fetal growth, premature labor, and a difficult neonatal course. I[69] have described one such case in detail. The female infant weighed only 1424 g at 39 weeks. At 3 cm from the placental insertion of the cord was a 4 × 5 × 5 cm bosselated mass (Fig. 12–5). There were no through vessels for either the venous or the arterial arms of the placentofetal circulation. Descriptively this was reported as a fibromyxoangioma of the umbilical cord. Despite the extreme growth retardation the infant survived 8 days. The most striking vascular effect was in very small kidneys with a partial remnant of the glomerulogenetic zone and poorly vascularized glomeruli. There was cardiac hypertrophy and no mass organ lesion of an expressly lethal type. It was concluded that the severity of growth retardation was linked to not otherwise studied organ immaturity despite the well-documented 39 weeks of gestation.

Differential Diagnosis

The differential diagnosis includes cord hematoma and hemorrhagic artifact. Cord hematomas

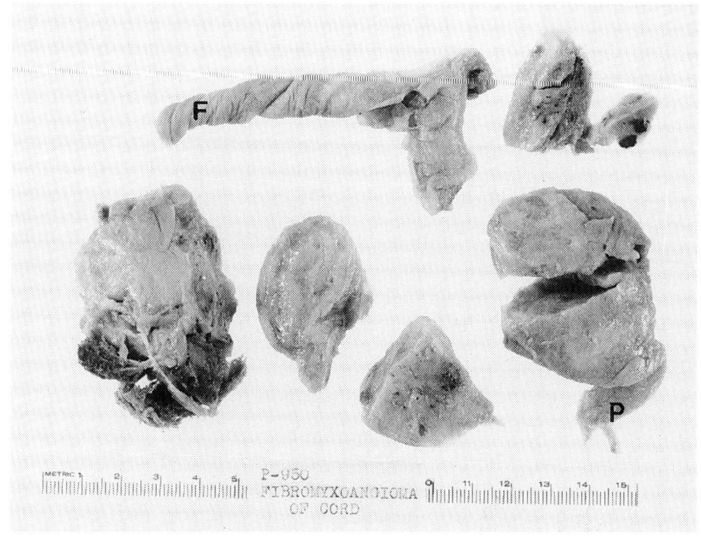

Figure 12–5. Previously sectioned fibromyxoangioma of umbilical cord. The placental end *(P)* is attached to a large bulbous mass; the thin slice, which is second from the left, came from within the cleft in the large bulbous mass. A smaller portion of the tumor is attached to the umbilical cord *(F)* near the fetus. (Copyrighted 1974 and 1981 by Editorial Enterprises Corporation.)

may involve one artery, the vein, or an artery plus the vein. The principal underlying lesions are septic destruction of the wall and hemodynamic rupture, which includes breach of a varix. The vascular dynamics of the umbilical cord has no parallel elsewhere in human anatomy; a large artery and vein with opposing high volume and high pressure can actively rub against each other without the added stability of a strut such as the vertebral column for the aorta and vena cava. Reconstruction of rupture sites by step serial sections has shown thinned fragments of the wall of the vein and artery and telescoping of segments turned inside out, which must have occurred at the time of the incident. This detail is provided so the distinction can be made readily from the tissue pattern of a vascular tumor with interstitial hemorrhage. Hematoma of the cord, in turn, must be distinguished from artifactual tears when the cord is used to remove the placenta forcibly at the end of the third stage of labor. Older hematomas usually show some layering of thrombi, and fresher ones may have a zone of platelet aggregation, events that do not occur in artifactual tears.

MISCELLANEOUS TUMORS AND PARANEOPLASTIC CONDITIONS OF THE CORD

Several rare and distinctive lesions have been described in the human umbilical cord. Tumors in older accounts, reviewed by Haendly in 1923[70] and Browne in 1925,[71] were variously described as teratoma, dermoid, or myxosarcoma telangiectodes, and the distinction of teratoid tumors from pedunculated acardiac fetuses, although discussed, was never entirely clarified as to criteria.[72] An excellent example of teratoma of the umbilical cord is that of Heckmann and associates.[73] Gonzalez-Crussi used this case in his *Fascicle on Extragonadal Teratomas.*[74] Heckmann's case is especially revealing because of the vascular relationships. The tumor was fed by three arteries from the fetal side. The two umbilical arteries were distinct, passing *through* the tumor; the umbilical vein was in a section of the cord outside the tumor.

Teratomas have been described in the extraplacental chorioamnion.[75,76] These pose some problem with classification because of the further finding of a vascular hilum in the tumors, questionably a remnant cord pedicle. The number of cases is small, and the possibility of a totally independent umbilical cord invokes again the possibility of acardiac maldevelopment.[77] The difficulties in interpretation were well summarized by Fox,[4] who listed a number of other reported cases as part of his acceptance of the independent existence of teratomas of the placenta and umbilical cord.

Harris and Wenzel[78] described a vitelline remnant on the cord that was a small nodule containing mainly exocrine pancreas. This was only 4 mm from the dermal reflection at the fetal end of the cord and is best considered an ectopic remnant after retraction of the enteric tube during maturation of the anterior abdominal parieties. Similarly, giant pigmented nevi of the abdomen may involve the cord. Reed and associates[79] described pigmented nevus cells in cord stroma in a case of large pigmented nevus of the anterior abdominal wall. No direct physical connection was noted by the authors.

Large mucoid cysts occasionally form in the cord and displace the vessels. These are unlikely to be confused with hematomas or angiomas, but if a venous varix were to rupture into such a cyst, some effort would be required to make the differential diagnosis by appropriate tissue sections and careful description of the gross findings.

TUMORS METASTATIC TO THE PLACENTA OR A PLACENTAL SITE

Metastasis to the placenta is uncommon in the aggregate and extremely rare for most malignancies. The unique anatomic status of the placenta makes it a potential target for both maternal and fetal tumors. The infrequency of primary malignant tumors of the fetus limits the scope of fetoplacental metastasis. Several of the categories described below have metastatic potential because of their intrinsic aggressiveness, but no reports have come to light in fulfillment of that potential. The scope of metastasis from maternal neoplasms is limited by the difference in age ranges between active childbearing and the so-called cancer ages. The current trend toward later onset of childbearing, in addition to its role in mammary cancer, brings these two age ranges into greater overlap.

One might anticipate a small increment in maternal tumors in pregnancy and then as metastatic lesions within the placenta and allied structures.

Embryonic-Fetal Tumors

Neuroblastoma

Neuroblastoma remains the most common malignancy of early infancy and has been blamed for deaths before birth[80,81] or within minutes after birth.[82] Since the placenta has such a broad role in fetal life, hormone secretion, nutrient absorption, and excretion of metabolic end products and byproducts of protein synthesis, intrafetal metastases can be numerous and large without adversely influencing fetal growth for many weeks. Despite this the number of cases of placental metastasis is few. One likely reason is that the blood flow to the placenta is through small branches of the vesicular arteries, requiring intravascular saturation or bolus transmissions for effective metastasis. Smith and co-workers[83] and Strauss and Driscoll[84] reported intravascular collections of neuroblastic tumor cells in the placental circulation as evidence of this mechanism. I[85] reported stromal metastasis of neuroblastoma in 1990 (Fig. 12–6). In this case the fetus also manifested metastases to skin of the lower extremities and to the liver, suggesting bolus transportation to below the diaphragm from the highly vascularized upper neck and scalp. The tumor arose from the upper cervical sympathetic chain and grew extensively across the scalp. The principal tissue of origin for fetal and neonatal neuroblastoma is the adrenal medulla, which has a different pattern of metastasis. Since relatively few cases have been described, these are speculative mechanisms. It is important that a thorough examination for metastatic sites be conducted in future cases to augment understanding of the behavior of neuroblastoma in fetal life. Generalized hydrops has been described in fetal neuroblastoma[86]; hydrops placentalis would make small placental metastases more difficult to locate.

Giant Pigmented Nevi

Migratory neural crest probably plays no role in the spread of fetal neuroblastoma,[87] but it might do so in the case of giant pigmented nevi, a rare malformation of fetal skin. Once again, the location of giant dermal nevi does not interfere with vital functions of the fetus, so growth can become extensive. Demian and associates[88] reported a case of placental involvement that was not mediated through direct dermal-umbilical spread. The immature nevoid cells filled the stroma of numerous villi and ramuli chorii. Highly pigmented placental structures can be seen grossly, and in such cases ultrastructurally distinctive melanosomes can be identified.[89]

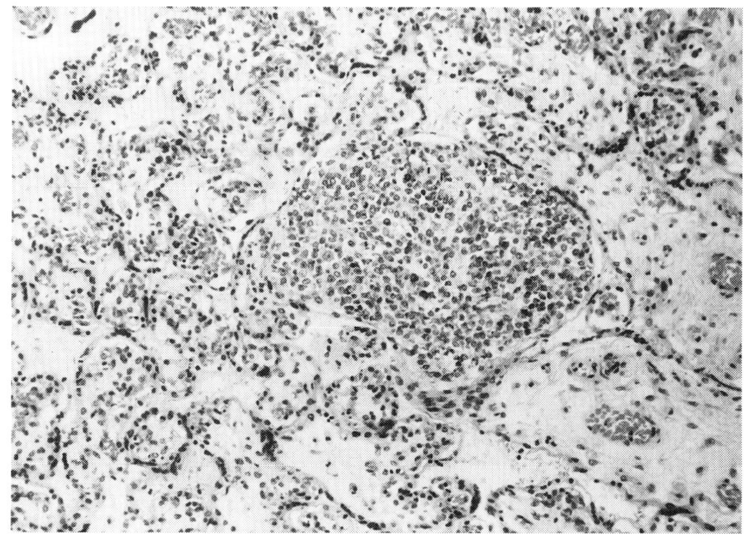

Figure 12–6. Fetal neuroblastoma metastatic to the stromal compartment of an enlarged placental villus. The villi are tightly packed from mild to moderate hydrops, which may be the result of catecholamine secretion by the tumor, a process known to occur in neuroblastoma during infancy (H&E, ×100). (From Shanklin DR: Tumors of the placenta and umbilical cord. Philadelphia, 1990, BC Decker, p 145.)

Congenital Leukemia

Congenital leukemia is a rare condition, and placental involvement is even more rare.[4,90] The differential diagnosis of leukemia of the placenta includes intravascular neuroblastomatosis and severe erythroblastosis fetalis.

Emboli from Intracranial Teratoma

Crump Hospital was the scene for a case of macrocrania and a large, highly vascular cerebral teratoma dominated by ependyma and islands of glial tissue (Fig. 12–7*A*). The obstetric manifestation was cephalopelvic disproportion. The tissue diagnosis in the cerebral mass was not known at the time, but two aspiration decompressions were performed, which sufficiently relieved the obstruction, and delivery followed. Emboli of teratogliomatous tissue were found in both the fetal lung and the placenta (Fig. 12–7*B* and *C*).

Fetal Hepatoblastoma

The important case of placental hepatic adenoma noted above[60] should be contrasted with the recent report of fetal hepatoblastoma metastatic to the placenta and multiple fetal organs.[91]

Sacrococcygeal Teratoma (Potential)

The definitive description of sacrococcygeal teratoma is by Gonzalez-Crussi.[74] These tumors have an impressive variety of tissue types and degrees of dedifferentiation; overt malignant transformation was found in a very large tumor (one third of total fetal mass) at Crump Hospital. This tumor also showed extensive dermal ulceration and anemia from hemorrhage into the amniotic cavity. Hydrops placentalis has been described in sacrococcygeal teratoma and appears to be related to the high content of catecholamine-secreting neuroblastic cells in these tumors. The possibility of arteriovenous shunts through the tumors is realistic, since they have numerous large vascular sinuses.

Fetal Sarcoma (Potential)

The unique report by Semchyshyn and associates[92] is important for the examination of future placentas in cases of unusual fetal tumors. Polyhydramnios and an 18 cm mass along the right lateral fetal body wall were noted during sonography. Section delivery produced a stillborn with a massive tumor described as an undifferentiated congenital sarcoma. Unfortunately, the placenta was not described.

Maternal Tumors

Metastasis to the placenta from visceral organs is unusual in pregnancy[93] and has been reviewed recently by me[94] and by Eltorky and co-workers.[95] The latter group also published comparative data on the relative frequency of malignant tumors in pregnant women; breast and uterine cervical cancers were almost equally represented at 26% each, with leukemia at 15%, lymphoma at 10%, melanoma at 8% and thyroid cancers at 4%. Their review of 56 cases of placental or fetal metastasis from maternal tumors showed a much different profile. Melanoma was the most common primary tumor, 17 of the total (30.4%); when just fetal involvement was considered, 9 of 14 were melanomas (64.3%). Carcinomas of the lung and breast are well represented. Systemic carcinomatosis from several sites, including the ovary, may be manifested in the placenta by intense filling of the intervillous space.[96]

Tumors from Solid Organs

Tumors that spread by the hematogenous route are somewhat more likely to end up in the placenta, especially when metastasis is widespread. This is well illustrated by a mammary angiosarcoma metastatic to the ovary that demonstrated small intervillous metastases.[97] The three most common primary sources are breast cancer, lung cancer (Fig. 12–8*A* and *B*), and dermal melanoma. A recent case report of placental metastasis from a primary ocular melanoma illustrates the intervil-

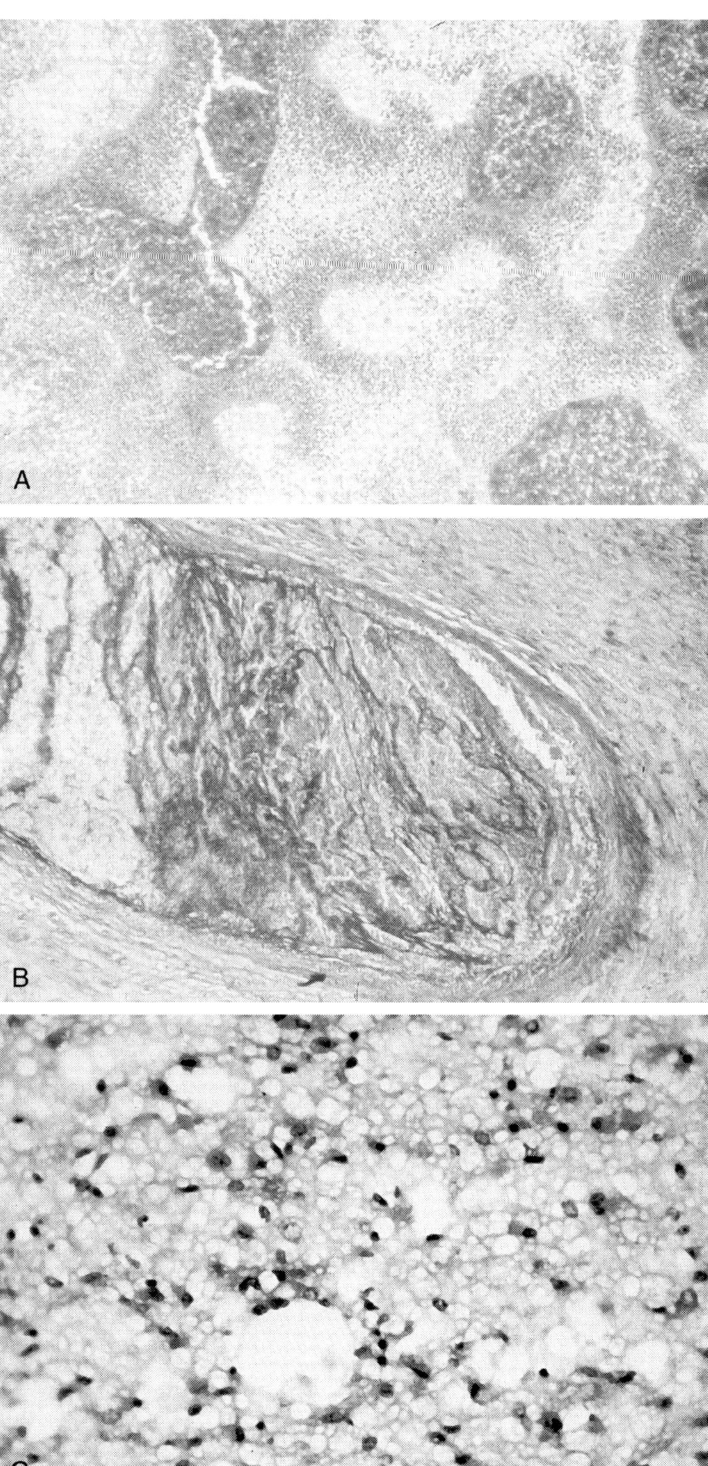

Figure 12–7. **A,** Densely cellular and highly vascular zone of fetal cerebral teratoma, predominantly ependymal and glial tissue. Whether the latter were part of the brain invaded by tumor or local tumor differentiation is not clear. Foci of immature cartilage and immature neuroblasts were also found. The mass was diagnosed by sonography at 33 weeks' gestation and was confirmed by repeat sonograms at 37 weeks. Two separate decompressions were performed 15 to 16 hours before delivery. Fetal autopsy revealed macrocrania rather than hydrocephaly (H&E, ×100). **B,** Striated thromboembolism in major ramar artery of the placenta in a case of decompression of a cerebral teratoma (see **A**) and macrocrania. The fibrinous lamellae are fairly regular near the center of the photograph; the fainter zones to the left are glial fibers (see **C**) (Phosphotungstic acid–hematoxylin, ×100). **C,** Details of embolic glial tissue from a decompressed intracranial teratoma (see **A** and **B**). A small number of cells were positive for glial fibrillary acid protein by special stain (H&E, ×250).

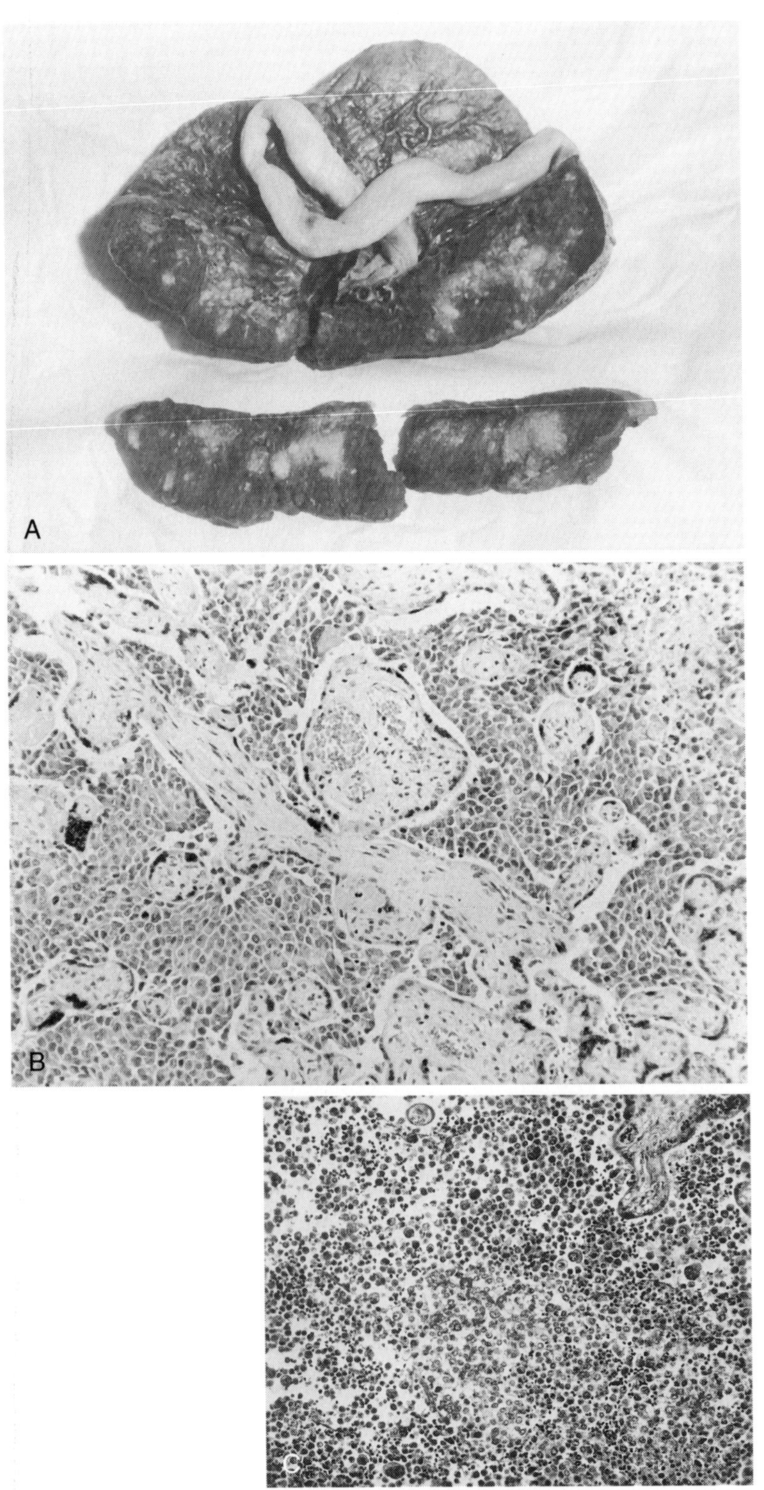

Figure 12–8. A, Sectioned surfaces of a 37-week placenta with multiple nodular metastases from poorly differentiated epidermoid carcinoma of the lung in the mother. She died 6 months after delivery; autopsy confirmed a primary lesion in the left upper pulmonary lobe. **B,** Extensive infiltration of intervillous space by poorly differentiated epidermoid carcinoma from lung (**A**). The tumor conforms to the villous outline. No sites of direct infiltration of villi are apparent in this field (H&E, ×100). **C,** Expansive growth of intervillous space metastasis from an ovarian carcinoma, late second trimester. The tumor cells are dissociated and do not form nodules or aggregates (H&E, ×160). (*A:* specimen courtesy JD Libre, MD, Jacksonville, Florida. *B* and *C* from Shanklin DR: Tumors of the placenta and umbilical cord. Philadelphia, 1990, BC Decker, pp 157 and 155.)

lous space growth pattern of metastatic disease.[98] Far too many assessments of malignant disease in pregnancy have overlooked the potential for placental and fetal involvement. The largest single study, that of Barber and Brunschwig,[99] exemplifies this omission. Significant numbers of colonic,[100] renal,[101] and ovarian[102] tumors occur in pregnant women. I identified a case of Ewing's sarcoma metastatic to the placenta at the Armed Forces Institute of Pathology in 1978. Another example of Ewing's sarcoma in the placenta was reported by Greenberg and colleagues.[103]

Occasionally the intervillous space is filled with enormous numbers of metastatic tumor cells (Fig. 12–8*C*).

Many mothers with cancer die soon after giving birth, whether vaginally or by section. This underscores the contribution to placental metastasis of tumor spread late in the course of disease. In some cases melanoma was found in fetal placental capillaries and not elsewhere in the fetus.[104,105]

Malignancies of the Lymphoreticular System

As neoplastic disorders occurring in a somewhat younger age group than most solid tumors, leukemia and lymphoma have been found during or diagnosed before pregnancy on many occasions.[106,107] Pelvic involvement of these disorders is uncommon.[108] Fetoplacental spread by Hodgkin's disease is rare, but at least one case with neonatal death has been reported.[109] A fairly high perinatal mortality is associated with maternal leukemia, mostly with chronic myelogenous leukemia and in about 10% with acute forms.[110] Miller,[110] in a large survey published in 1976, identified 259 mothers who died of leukemia, with a perinatal mortality just under 40%. Leukemia in both mother and infant is exceedingly rare.[111,112]

Recently, trophoblastic phagocytosis of atypical maternal cells, probably leukemic lymphoblasts, has been reported.[113] This unique finding suggests both an active role of placental epithelium in defense against the spread of malignant tumors and a possible mechanism of transfer. Further observational study and analysis are needed.

Collision (Incorporation) Tumors

The most common tumor of the reproductive system in women is the uterine leiomyoma. Many of these are submucous, and a few in that location are somewhat pedunculated. Nevertheless, the main interest in leiomyomas and pregnancy is the failure of the latter in face of the former. Occasionally, multiple myomectomy has permitted successful pregnancy in relatively infertile women. It seems remarkable that reports of placental incorporation of uterine leiomyomas are rare. Tapia and associates[114] reported such a case in 1985. The tumor measured 3.5 cm in maximum dimension and penetrated two thirds of the thickness of the discoid placenta. A large depression in the placenta filled with blood clot, which might have represented an adaptation to submucous leiomyoma without incorporation, was described by Shanklin and Scott.[115] So far no true placental leiomyoma has been reported; to establish such a case, one would have to show the vascular connection to the fetoplacental circuit and the presence of trophoblast on at least part of the perimeter.

SPECIAL STUDIES ON PLACENTAL TUMORS

Modern histochemistry has not fulfilled the broad early expectations for tumor diagnosis, largely because so many tumors have variable attributes. Nevertheless, when positive, certain tests are helpful in making a specific diagnosis. For example, Chen and associates [60] did find some α_1-antitrypsin staining in their case of hepatic adenoma. Differentiation of some lymphoreticular cases might come from use of muramidase staining.[116] Melanosomes can be stained histochemically or examined by electron microscopy. If tumor markers have been applied to neoplastic tissue from a pregnant woman, a comparison study of placental lesions might assist in identification. The extremely rare cases of joint maternal and fetal leukemia might be assessed with leukocyte alkaline phosphatase, but in one case in which this was done the information achieved was not useful.[117]

The dilemma for the front-line pathologist, with

a reasonable panel of histochemical and immunohistochemical methods available, is whether to use them as detectives in searching for data or as confirmation of a working hypothesis obtained by ordinary diagnostic study with hematoxylin and eosin and occasional connective tissue stains. There is no best answer at present, partly because these tumors are uncommon to rare and published comparative experience is lacking. Perhaps the most prudent rule, beyond the importance of describing the placenta in cases of maternal neoplasm, is to examine the tumor and apply to it the techniques that would be used on such a tumor elsewhere in the body. An underused technique is the periodic acid–Schiff and hematoxylin stain for vascular and trophoblastic basement membranes. This can demonstrate whether intervillous space tumor has penetrated the villi and ramuli chorii, and if so, to what degree and extent.

REFERENCES

1. Shanklin DR: Tumors of the placenta and umbilical cord. Philadelphia, 1990, BC Decker, p 102.
2. Benirschke K, Driscoll SG: The pathology of the human placenta. New York, 1967, Springer-Verlag, p. 381.
3. Fox H: Haemangiomata of the placenta. J Clin Pathol 19:133, 1966.
4. Fox H: Pathology of the placenta. Philadelphia, 1978, WB Saunders, pp 343 (chorangioma), 355 (placental teratoma), 362 (placental leukemia).
5. Hertig AT: On the development of the amnion and exocoelomic membrane in the pre-villous human ovum. Yale J Biol Med 18:107, 1945.
6. Hertig AT: Human trophoblast. Springfield, Ill., 1968, Charles C Thomas, p 77.
7. Marchetti AA: A consideration of certain types of benign tumors of the placenta. Surg Gynaecol Obstet 68:733, 1939.
8. Clarke J: Account of a tumour found in the substance of the human placenta. Philos Trans R Soc Lond 1:361, plates XIX-XX.
9. Shanklin DR: Tumors of the placenta and umbilical cord. Philadelphia, 1990, BC Decker, p 97.
10. Deugnier Y, Jouan H, Beurton D, et al: L'hemangiome placentaire. Arch Anat Cytol Pathol 31:154, 1983.
11. Siddall RS: Chorioangiofibroma (chorioangioma). Am J Obstet Gynecol 8:430, 1924.
12. Kuhnel P: Placental chorioangioma. Acta Obstet Gynecol Scand 13:143, 1933.
13. DeCosta EJ, Gerbie AB, Andresen RH, Gallanis TC: Placental tumors: hemangiomas. Obstet Gynecol 7:249, 1956.
14. Wallenburg HCS: Chorioangioma of the placenta. Obstet Gynecol Surv 26:411, 1971.
15. Jaffe R, Siegal A, Bernheim J, et al: Placental chorioangiomatosis—a high risk pregnancy. Postgrad Med J 61:453, 1985.
16. Wentworth P: The incidence and significance of haemangioma of the placenta. J Obstet Gynaecol Br Commonw 72:81, 1965.
17. Shaw-Dunn RI: Haemangioma of placenta (chorioangioma). J Obstet Gynaecol Br Empire 66:51, 1959.
18. Shanklin DR: Tumors of the placenta and umbilical cord. Philadelphia, 1990, BC Decker, p 103.
19. Javert CT: Spontaneous and habitual abortion. New York, 1957, McGraw-Hill.
20. Folkman J: What is the role of the endothelial cells in angiogenesis? Lab Invest 51:601, 1984.
21. Folkman J: Angiogenesis in cancer, vascular, rheumatoid and other disease. Nature Med 1:27, 1995.
22. Folkman J, Klagsbrun M: Angiogenic factors. Science 235:442, 1987.
23. Nahmanovici C, Pancrazi J, Philippe E: Chorioangiome placentaire: diagnostic echographique a la 19[e] semaine. J Gynecol Obstet Biol Reprod (Paris) 11:593, 1982.
24. Asadourian LA, Taylor HB: Clinical significance of placental hemangiomas. Obstet Gynecol 31:551, 1968.
25. Greene EE, Iams JD: Chorioangioma: a case presentation. Am J Obstet Gynecol 148:1146, 1984.
26. Hurwitz A, Milwidsky A, Yarkoni S, Palti Z: Severe fetal distress with hydramnios due to chorioangioma. Acta Obstet Gynecol Scand 62:633, 1983.
27. Mann L, Alroomi L, McNay M, Ferguson-Smith MA: Placental haemangioma: case report. Br J Obstet Gynaecol 90:983, 1983.
28. Willard DA, Moeschler JB: Placental chorioangioma: a rare cause of elevated amniotic fluid alpha-fetoprotein. J Ultrasound Med 5:221, 1986.
29. Shalev E, Weiner E, Feldman E, Zuckerman H: Prenatal diagnosis of placental hemangioma—clinical implication: a case report. Int J Gynaecol Obstet 22:291, 1984.
30. Shanklin DR: Tumors of the placenta and umbilical cord. Philadelphia, 1990, BC Decker, p 113.
31. Storch ED: Fälle von Sogenanntem partiellem Myxöm der placenta. Virchows Arch Pathol Anat 72:582, 1878.
32. Potter EL: Pathology of the fetus and the newborn. Chicago, 1952, Year Book, p. 26.

33. Hormann G: Zur Systematik einer pathologie der menschlichen placenta. Arch Gynecol Obstet 191:297, 1958.
34. Altshuler G: Chorangiosis: an important placental sign of neonatal morbidity and mortality. Arch Pathol Lab Med 108:71, 1984.
35. Shanklin DR: Tumors of the placenta and umbilical cord. Philadelphia, 1990, BC Decker, p 116.
36. Dupin and Chabaud: Gaz de Hop de Toulouse 3:73, 1889 (cited by Sidall RS: Chorioangiofibroma. Am J Obstet Gynecol 8:430, 1924).
37. Benson PF, Joseph MC: Cardiomegaly in a newborn due to placental chorioangioma. Br Med J 1:102, 1961.
38. Fisher JH: Chorioangioma of the placenta. Am J Obstet Gynecol 40:493, 1940.
39. Reiner L, Fries E: Chorangioma associated with arteriovenous aneurysm. Am J Obstet Gynecol 93:58, 1965.
40. Earn AA, Penner DW: Five cases of chorangioma. J Obstet Gynaecol Br Empire 57:442, 1950.
41. Yule R, O'Connor D: Haemangioma of placenta. Med J Aust 1:157, 1964.
42. Zarou GS, Carabba O Jr: Placental hemangioma. Am J Obstet Gynecol 83:1069, 1962.
43. Shanklin DR: Tumors of the placenta and umbilical cord. Philadelphia, 1990, BC Decker, p 120, plate IV.
44. Jones CEM, Rivers RPA, Taghizadeh A: Disseminated intravascular coagulation and fetal hydrops in a newborn infant in association with a chorangioma of placenta. Pediatrics 50:901, 1972.
45. Sweet L, Reid WD, Roberton NRC: Hydrops fetalis in association with chorioangioma of the placenta. J Pediatr 82:91, 1973.
46. Conway DF Jr, Barone R: Hemangioma of the placenta. Obstet Gynecol 19:505, 1962.
47. Sims DG, Barron SL, Wadehra V, Ellis HA: Massive chronic feto-maternal bleeding associated with placental chorioangiomas. Acta Paediatr Scand 65:271, 1976.
48. Leonidas JC, Beatty EC, Hall RT: Chorioangioma of the placenta. Am J Roentgenol Rad Ther Nucl Med 123:703, 1975.
49. Rodan BA, Bean WJ: Chorioangioma of the placenta causing intrauterine fetal demise. J Ultrasound Med 2:95, 1983.
50. Lopez-Herce Cid J, Escriba Polo R, Escudero Lou R: Corioangioma placentario y hemorragia intracraneal neonatal. An Esp Pediatr 19:405, 1983.
51. Shanklin DR: Tumors of the placenta and umbilical cord. Philadelphia, 1990, BC Decker, p 118.
52. Shanklin DR: The influence of placental lesions of the newborn infant. Pediatr Clin North Am 17:25, 1970.
53. Chan KW, Leung CY: Recurrent multiple chorioangiomas and intrauterine death. Pathology 20:77, 1988.
54. Wurster DH, Hoefnagel E, Benirschke K, Allen FH Jr: Placental chorioangiomata and mental deficiency in a child with 2/15 translocation: 46,XX,t(2q-;15q+). Cytogenetics 8:389, 1969.
55. Thom H, Campbell AG, Farr V, et al: The impact of maternal serum alpha fetoprotein screening on open neural tube defect births in north-east Scotland. Prenat Diagn 5:15, 1985.
56. Stiller AG, Skafish PR: Placental chorioangioma: a rare cause of fetomaternal transfusion with maternal hemolysis and fetal distress. Obstet Gynecol 67:296, 1986.
57. Shanklin DR: Tumors of the placenta and umbilical cord. Philadelphia, 1990, BC Decker, p 122.
58. Shanklin DR: Tumors of the placenta and umbilical cord. Philadelphia, 1990, BC Decker, p 125.
59. Jauniaux E, Zucker M, Meuris S, et al: Chorangiocarcinoma: an unusual tumor of the placenta; the missing link? Placenta 9:607, 1988.
60. Chen KTK, Ma CK, Kassel SH: Hepatocellular adenoma of the placenta. Am J Surg Pathol 10:436, 1986.
61. Cox JN, Chavrier F: Heterotopic adrenocortical tissue within a placenta. Placenta 1:131, 1980.
62. Labarrere CA, Caccamo D, Telenta M, et al: A nodule of adrenocortical tissue within a human placenta: light microscopic and immunocytochemical findings. Placenta 5:139, 1984.
63. Potter, EL: Pathology of the fetus and the newborn. Chicago, 1952, Year Book, pp. 144, 267.
64. Meyer AW: A congenital intra-cranial intra-dural adrenal. Anat Rec 12:43, 1917.
65. Wiener MF, Dallgaard SA: Intracranial adrenal gland. Proc NY State Assoc Pub Health Labs 38:8, 1958.
66. Barry FE, McCoy CP, Callahan WP: Hemangioma of the umbilical cord. Am J Obstet Gynecol 62:675, 1951.
67. Potter EL: Pathology of the fetus and the newborn. Chicago, 1952, Year Book, p 34.
68. Shanklin DR: Tumors of the placenta and umbilical cord. Philadelphia, 1990, BC Decker, p 135.
69. Shanklin DR: Tumors of the placenta and umbilical cord. Philadelphia, 1990, BC Decker, p 128.
70. Haendly P: Teratom der Nabelschnur. Arch Gynakol 116:578, 1923.
71. Browne FJ: On the abnormalities of the umbilical cord which may cause antenatal death. J Obstet Gynaecol Br Empire 32:17, 1925.
72. Shanklin DR: Tumors of the placenta and umbilical cord. Philadelphia, 1990, BC Decker, p 137.
73. Heckmann U, Cornelius HV, Freudenberg V: Das

Teratom der Nabelschnur. Geburtshilfe Frauenheilkd 32:605, 1972.
74. Gonzalez-Crussi F: Extragonadal teratomas. In Atlas of tumor pathology, 2nd series, Fascicle 18. Washington, D.C., 1982, Armed Forces Institute of Pathology, p 174.
75. Joseph TJ, Vogt PJ: Placental teratomas. Obstet Gynecol 41:574, 1973.
76. Smith LA, Pounder DJ: A teratoma-like lesion of the placenta. Pathology 14:86, 1982.
77. Kyriazis A, Arean VM, Shanklin DR: Placental-radiographic analysis of parasitic acardiac fetus: partially common umbilical circulation. J Reprod Med 12:74, 1974.
78. Harris LE, Wenzel JE: Heterotopic pancreatic tissue and intestinal mucosa in the umbilical cord. N Engl J Med 268:721, 1963.
79. Reed WB, Snyder W, Horowitz RE: A giant pigmented nevus with invasion into umbilical cord. Acta Derm Venereol (Stockh) 53:318, 1973.
80. Birner WF: Neuroblastoma as a cause of antenatal death. Am J Obstet Gynecol 82:1388, 1961.
81. Potter EL, Parrish JM: Neuroblastoma, ganglioneuroma and fibroneuroma in a stillborn fetus. Am J Pathol 18:141, 1942.
82. Shanklin DR: Tumors of the placenta and umbilical cord. Philadelphia, 1990, BC Decker, p 142.
83. Smith CR, Chan HSl, deSa DJ: Placental involvement in congenital neuroblastoma. J Clin Pathol 34:785, 1981.
84. Strauss L, Driscoll SG: Congenital neuroblastoma involving the placenta. Pediatrics 34:23, 1964.
85. Shanklin DR: Tumors of the placenta and umbilical cord. Philadelphia, 1990, BC Decker, p 145.
86. van der Slikke JW, Balk AG: Hydramnios with hydrops fetalis and disseminated fetal neuroblastoma. Obstet Gynecol 55:250, 1980.
87. Shanklin DR, Sotelo-Avila C: In situ tumors in fetuses, newborns and young infants. Biol Neonat 14:286, 1969.
88. Demian SEE, Donnelly WH, Frias JL, Monif GRG: Placental lesions in congenital giant pigmented nevi. Am J Clin Pathol 61:438, 1974.
89. Shanklin DR: Tumors of the placenta and umbilical cord. Philadelphia, 1990, BC Decker, p 151.
90. Perrin EV: Case of presumed fetal placental leukemia. Personal communication cited in Benirschke K, Kaufmann P: Pathology of the human placenta, 2nd ed. New York, 1990, Springer-Verlag, p 427.
91. Robinson HB, Bolande RP: Fetal hepatoblastoma with placental metastases. Pediatr Pathol 4:163, 1985.
92. Semchyshyn S, Mangurten H, Benawra R, et al: Fetal tumor: antenatal diagnosis and its implications. J Reprod Med 27:231, 1982.
93. Francois H, de Queiroz F, Kerisit J: Les metastases placentaires. Arch Anat Cytol Pathol 31:157, 1983.
94. Shanklin DR: Tumors of the placenta and umbilical cord. Philadelphia, 1990, BC Decker, p 154.
95. Eltorky M, Khare VK, Osborn P, Shanklin DR: Placental metastasis from maternal carcinoma; a report of three cases. J Reprod Med 40:399, 1995.
96. Shanklin DR: Tumors of the placenta and umbilical cord. Philadelphia, 1990, BC Decker, p 155.
97. Sedgely MG, Ostor AG, Fortune DW: Angiosarcoma of breast metastatic to the ovary and placenta. Aust NZ J Obstet Gynaecol 25:299, 1985.
98. Marsh R de W, Chu N-M: Placental metastasis from primary ocular melanoma: a case report. Am J Obstet Gynecol 174:1654, 1996.
99. Barber HRK, Brunschwig A: Gynecologic cancer complicating pregnancy. Am J Obstet Gynecol 85:156, 1963.
100. Green LK, Harris RE, Massey FM: Cancer of the colon during pregnancy. Obstet Gynecol 46:480, 1975.
101. Pelosi M, Hung CT, Langer A, et al: Renal carcinoma in pregnancy. Obstet Gynecol 45:461, 1975.
102. Novak ER, Lambrou CD, Woodruff JD: Ovarian tumors in pregnancy. Obstet Gynecol 46:401, 1975.
103. Greenberg P, Collins JD, Voet RL, Jariwala L: Ewing's sarcoma metastatic to placenta. Placenta 3:191, 1982.
104. Brodsky I, Baren M, Kahn SB, et al: Metastatic malignant melanoma from mother to fetus. Cancer 18:1048, 1965.
105. Gray J, Kenny M, Sharpey-Schafer EP: Metastasis of maternal tumour to products of gestation. J Obstet Gynaecol Br Empire 46:480, 1975.
106. Smith RBW, Sheehy TW, Rothberg H: Hodgkin's disease and pregnancy. Arch Intern Med 102:77, 1958.
107. Barry RM, Diamond HD, Craver LF: Influence of pregnancy on the course of Hodgkin's disease. Am J Obstet Gynecol 84:445, 1962.
108. Sweet DL: Malignant lymphoma: implications during the reproductive years and pregnancy. J Reprod Med 17:198, 1976.
109. Priesel A, Winkelbauer A: Placentare Ubertragung des Lympho-granuloms. Virchows Arch Pathol Anat 262:749, 1926.
110. Miller JB: Chronic myelocytic leukemia and the myeloproliferative diseases during the child-bearing years. J Reprod Med 17:217, 1976.
111. Bernard J, Jacquillat C, Chavelet F, et al:

Leucemie aigue de'une enfant de 5 mois nee d'une mere atteinte de leucemia aigue au moment de l'accouchement. Nouv Rev Fr Hematol 4:140, 1964.
112. Cramblett HG, Friedman JL, Najjar S: Leukemia in an infant born of a mother with leukemia. N Engl J Med 259:727, 1958.
113. Wang T, Hamann W, Hartge R: Structural aspects of a placenta from a case of maternal acute lymphatic leukemia. Placenta 4:185, 1983.
114. Tapia RW, White VA, Ruffolo EH: Leiomyoma of the placenta. South Med J 78:863, 1985.
115. Shanklin DR, Scott JS: Massive subchorial thrombohaematoma (Breus' mole). Br J Obstet Gynaecol 82:476, 1975.
116. Ree HJ, Song JY, Leone LA, et al: Occurrence and patterns of muramidase containing cells in Hodgkin's disease, non-Hodgkin's lymphomas, and reactive hyperplasia. Hum Pathol 12:49, 1981.
117. Rigby PG, Hanson TA, Smith RS: Passage of leukemic cells across the placenta. N Engl J Med 271:124, 1964.

13

Infectious Disorders of the Placenta

Scott R. Hyde and Geoffrey Altshuler

Many years ago Shakespeare eloquently wrote of seven ages of man. Regarding study of infectious diseases of the placenta in recent decades, we have encountered three perceptible ages. In the sixties a few obstetricians and pathologists wrote that chorioamnionitis causes prematurity and its complications. In the seventies and eighties clinicians doubted the importance of chorioamnionitis and were unaware of the high prevalence and implications of other placental inflammation. Now, at the dawn of a new century, emerging information from microbiologists, molecular biologists, pharmacologists, and epidemiologists is causing clinicians to reexamine the impact of infection and placental changes on the fetus and newborn. In reviewing these events traditional considerations of pathology and pathogenesis are a reasonable beginning.

BASIC PATTERNS OF INTRAUTERINE INFECTION

There are two basic patterns of intrauterine infection. Organisms that ascend to the amniotic cavity from the cervix and vagina produce clinically diagnosed amniotic infection syndrome. Chorioamnionitis is the histologic hallmark of ascending intrauterine infection. The second major pathway by which infectious agents reach the fetus is via a maternofetal bloodborne route. Maternal bloodborne infections are much less common than chorioamnionitis. These infections are manifested histologically by placental intervillositis and villitis. The pattern of placental inflammation provides useful information, occasionally including clues to the specific infectious cause. Other facts are noteworthy. Whereas chorioamnionitis is a major cause of premature labor, villitis is not. *Fusobacterium* and other anaerobic bacteria are common causes of chorioamnionitis, but they do not produce villitis.

The severity and type of placental inflammation provide clinically helpful information. Maternal genital tract infection by group A or B *Streptococcus, Streptococcus pneumoniae,* and herpes simplex may produce severe symptomatic infection of the fetus and newborn with relatively little inflammation of the placenta, the extraplacental membranes, and the umbilical cord. With most other organisms we have found a positive correlation between the severity of placental and umbilical cord inflammation and the risk of symptomatic or serious congenital infection.[1]

PATHOGENESIS OF INTRAAMNIOTIC INFECTIONS

Benirschke[2] clarified many considerations of chorioamnionitis, including its infectious cause and its causative relationship to prematurity. Often, however, no organisms are demonstrable by practical laboratory methods. Bacterial vaginosis, which occurs in approximately 20% of pregnant women, is the most frequent vaginal infection of sexually active women. This condition is probably initiated by hormone-induced changes in the environment of the vagina and cervix. Bacterial vaginosis is diagnosed when the pH of vaginal secretions is greater than 4.5 and when *Lactobacillus* is replaced by *Bacteroides, Gardnerella vaginalis, Mycoplasma hominis, Ureaplasma urealyticum,* and *Mobiluncus.*[3,4] The extent to which bacterial vaginosis is the primary cause of histopathologic chorioamnionitis is unknown, but definite relationships exist among bacterial vaginosis, premature rupture of membranes, and intraamniotic infections.[5]

Transgression of the cervical mucous plug by microbiologic organisms and their products is the initial phase of intraamniotic infection. The cervical mucous plug functions as a biologic filter,[6] protecting the uterus and fetal adnexa from potential pathogens that may ascend from the vagina. Enzymatic degradation of cervical mucus is one proposed mechanism whereby bacteria gain access to the endocervix and amniotic cavity. Proteolytic enzymes that may digest cervical mucus include collagenase, gelatinase, and elastinase. These proteins are produced locally by endocervical polymorphonuclear leukocytes and by bacteria commonly associated with chorioamnionitis.[7] McGregor and colleagues[8] have provided experimental evidence that these proteases are involved in degradation of the extraplacental membranes, as manifested by loss of tissue elasticity and tensile strength. Proteolytic digestion of subamniotic collagen and elastin is probably the fundamental antecedent of infection-related premature rupture of membranes.

Inflammation of the amniotic cavity is initiated by decidual inflammation adjacent to the internal cervical os. Proteases of bacterial and leukocytic origin facilitate bacterial penetration into the amniotic cavity, even in the absence of ruptured membranes. Bacterial products and inflammatory leukoattractants are subsequently elaborated into the amniotic fluid. This stimulates chemotaxis of both maternal and fetal leukocytes toward the amniotic cavity. Depending on the duration of the infection and the biologic properties of the causative microbe, severe or slight histopathologic chorioamnionitis develops.

The extraplacental membranes and much of the superficial chorionic plate lack fetal blood vessels. Therefore most of the inflammatory cells of chorioamnionitis would be expected to originate from the mother. Mothers with intact membranes and clinical features of chorioamnionitis are likely to have leukocytes in their amniotic fluid. When the fetus is male, DNA analysis provides an opportunity to determine whether the leukocytes originate from the mother or fetus. By fluorescence in situ hybridization, Sampson and co-workers[9] recently found that 90% of the inflammatory cells floating freely within amniotic fluid originate from the fetus. The investigators, however, did not study the associated placental pathology or document the extent to which fetal pneumonia may have produced many of the intraamniotic polymorphonuclear leukocytes.

HISTOLOGIC GRADING OF CHORIOAMNIONITIS

The most severe histopathologic manifestations of an intraamniotic infection include subchorionic microabscesses (Fig. 13–1*A*) and necrotizing chorioamnionitis (Fig. 13–1*B*). Although those features may occur in a single placenta, they often develop independent of each other. At least two staging systems for classification of chorioamnionitis have been published.[10,11] In our experience, however, no staging or grading system can be accurately used to document the duration of the inflammation or the risk of associated perinatal sepsis. Table 13–1 summarizes the method with which we record histopathologic details of chorioamnionitis. In the descriptive part of our pathology reports we often grade chorioamnionitis on a scale of 0 to 3. In our diagnosis and comment sections, however, we do not conclude that the amount of inflammation indicates the duration of the infection or firmly predicts the clinical outcome.

EFFECTS OF UMBILICAL CORD INFLAMMATION ON FETOPLACENTAL CIRCULATION

Because the vessels of the fetal-placental unit lack innervation, their contractility is influenced by vasoactive substances in the fetal circulation, the umbilical cord Wharton's jelly, and the fetal vascular endothelium and smooth muscle. Complex interactions of prostaglandins, amines, and proteins in the fetal vascular media determine the tone of these vessels.[12] Commensurate with the fetal need for abundant blood flow, mechanisms that promote vasodilatation of umbilical cord vasculature are predominant throughout gestation. After delivery, umbilical cord vasoconstriction becomes dominant. Activation of the umbilical cord's in-

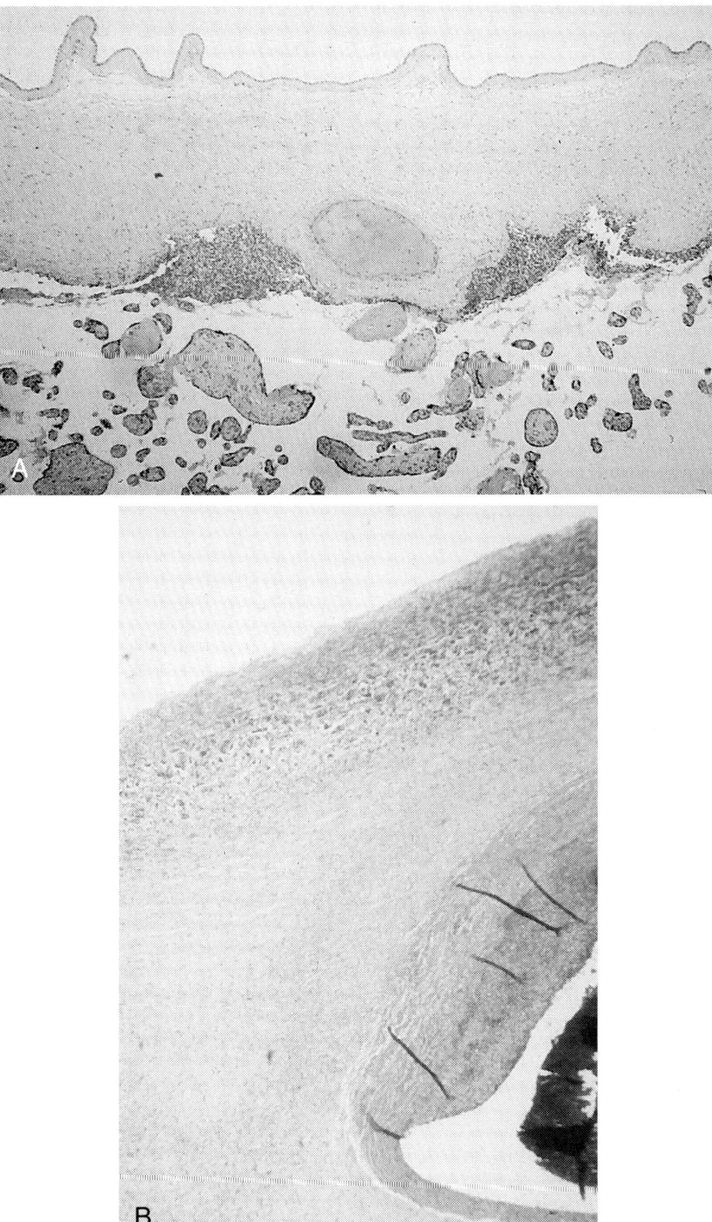

Figure 13–1. Placenta. **A,** Chorionic plate demonstrating two subchorionic microabscesses, one on either side of a fetal blood vessel. The inflammatory cells are of both fetal and maternal origin (H&E, ×25). **B,** Chorionic plate demonstrating severe necrotizing inflammation subjacent to the amniotic epithelium primarily involving the subamniotic connective tissue (H&E, ×100).

Table 13–1. Descriptive Scoring Method for Chorioamnionitis

Variable	Score
Extraplacental membranes or membranitis	
Polymorphs confined to the deep connective tissue next to the chorion	1
Polymorphs present in all of the chorion and amnion	2
Necrotizing inflammation or microabscesses, even if confined to the decidua	3
Fetal placental surface inflammation	
Polymorphs confined to the deep connective tissue above the chorionic plate	1
Polymorphs present in all of the chorion and amnion	2
Necrotizing chorioamnionitis or microabscesses	3
Placental fetal plate vasculitis	
Absent	0
Mild	1
Moderate	2
Severe	3
Umbilical cord vasculitis	
Each vessel involved	0.5
Each severely involved vessel	0.5
Umbilical cord funisitis	
Focally present	1
Diffusely present	2
Necrotizing (with or without calcification)	3

nate ability to constrict the blood vessels involves multiple stimuli. These mechanisms are initiated by exposure of the umbilical cord to air, which is colder than the intrauterine environment and has much higher oxygen content. Retraction of the umbilical cord during its delivery may cause perivascular mast cells to release histamine, a potent vasoconstrictor. Fetal platelets also participate in vasoconstriction by releasing serotonin and thromboxane A_2.[13]

Pathophysiologic effects of intraamniotic infections on the fetus include biochemical mechanisms that can cause fetal hypoxia. Hemodynamic abnormalities accompanying umbilical cord inflammation may affect fetal blood flow by prematurely activating innate vasoconstrictor mechanisms of the umbilical cord blood vessels.[14] Several lines of evidence support opinion that ascending infections produce fetal hypoxia through umbilical and placental vasospasm. Bodelsson and associates[15] determined that a binding site for the potent vasoactive peptide endothelin-1 is located in vascular smooth muscle of the umbilical cord. Ohno and co-workers showed increased umbilical vein endothelin-1 levels in infants who suffered variable decelerations and hypoxia.[16] Inflammatory mediators may be one endogenous source of vasoactive substances. Bacterial products may separately contribute vasoactive compounds. Group B *Streptococcus* infection is a common example. Affected fetuses and newborns sustain asphyxia, and some of them have periventricular leukomalacia and other ischemic brain damage.[17,18] This often occurs in the absence of severe placental inflammation. The mechanism of these asphyxial events involves the ability of a group B streptococcal polysaccharide exotoxin to provoke severe contraction of fetal vascular smooth muscle.[14] Bacterial toxins and noxious agents such as meconium may act alone or synergistically with inflammation to produce severe fetal hypoxic damage.[19]

DIAGNOSTIC PATTERNS OF UMBILICAL CORD INFLAMMATION

Subacute Necrotizing Funisitis

Subacute necrotizing funisitis is an uncommon form of chronic umbilical cord inflammation. Leukotoxins in the amniotic fluid diffuse into Wharton's jelly and destroy fetal neutrophils that are chemotactically migrating from umbilical vessels toward the amniotic cavity. This produces calcifying necrotic zones between the vessels of the umbilical cord and its amniotic surface (Fig. 13–2).

Navarro and Blanc[20] provided considerable information about necrotizing funisitis. This entity is caused by a multitude of organisms,[21] but in most instances the cause is unknown. Although it can be seen with congenital syphilis, a normal-appearing umbilical cord is the most common finding.[22] Necrotizing funisitis should never be considered pathognomonic of congenital syphilis.[23] Histopathologic placental findings are probably more specific.

Necrotizing funisitis is associated with substantial morbidity and mortality in newborns. Craver and Baldwin[24] reported 65 cases in which 28% of the newborns were growth retarded, 18% were stillborn, and 22% had necrotizing enterocolitis. These clinical findings support the opinion that noxious agents interact with umbilical cord blood vessels, producing vasoconstriction, placental blood flow reduction, and severe fetal hypoxic injury.[25]

Fungal Chorioamnionitis With Funisitis

Candida vaginitis is a common complication of pregnancy, reported to occur 10 to 20 times more frequently in pregnant women than in nonpregnant age-matched control subjects.[26] Although the incidence of *Candida* vaginitis is high during pregnancy, these fungi rarely cause chorioamnionitis. Factors such as premature rupture of membranes, retained intrauterine device, trauma, and coexistent infection are probably involved in the pathogenesis of *Candida* chorioamnionitis. The fungal agent that most commonly causes chorioamnionitis is *Candida albicans.* Occasional infections are produced by *Torulopsis glabrata, Candida parapsilosis,* and *Candida tropicalis.*

Fungal chorioamnionitis, particularly in term neonates, is often asymptomatic. The most common clinical consequence of fungal chorioamnionitis is superficial invasion of the skin and oral cavity.[27] Several cases of disseminated candidiasis have been reported.[28] Candidiasis can be life threatening, particularly in premature infants.

The umbilical cord of placentas with *Candida* infection often has grossly recognizable 0.1 cm diameter superficial microabscesses. The presence of umbilical cord microabscesses is almost pathognomonic for fungal chorioamnionitis. The diagnosis can be rapidly established if scrapings of the umbilical cord surface reveal clumps of neutrophils with fungal hyphae and yeast (Fig. 13–3). The membranes and fetal placental surface often have necrotizing inflammation and organisms.

Herpes Simplex Viral Chorioamnionitis with Plasmacytic Funisitis

In the United States herpes simplex virus annually affects more than 2000 infants and causes one of the most often fatal perinatal infections.[29] Herpes simplex infection is most commonly acquired

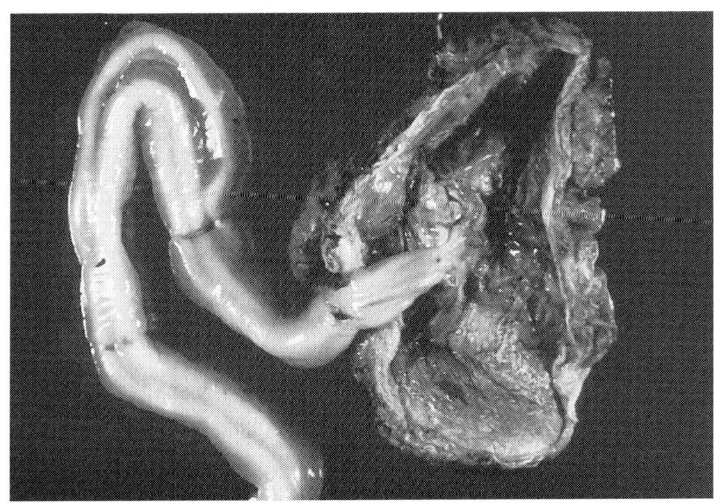

Figure 13–2. Necrotizing funisitis. Placenta with umbilical cord that manifests extensive edema and prominent blood vessels but not a so-called barber's pole appearance. On cut section the cord had chalky white linear streaks between the blood vessels and the amniotic surface of the umbilical cord.

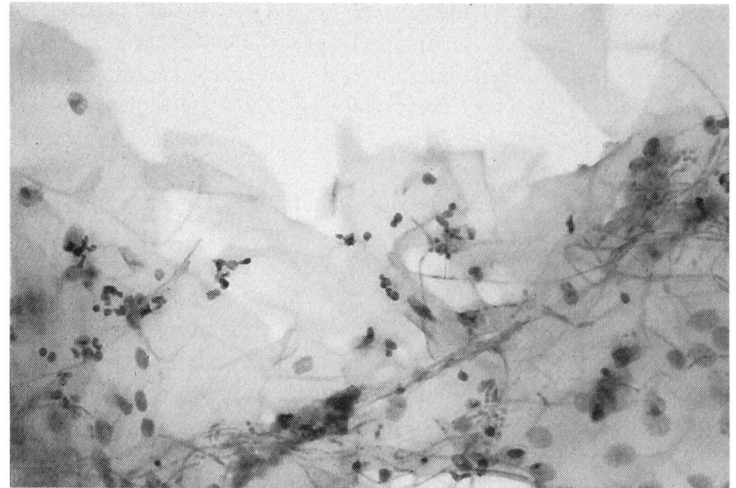

Figure 13–3. Scrapings from the amniotic surface of an umbilical cord with numerous punctate, 0.1 cm diameter areas of opacification. A number of fungal forms, including yeast and hyphae, can be seen along with many neutrophils. The presence of yeast and hyphae indicates *Candida* infection (H&E, ×250).

during delivery through an infected birth canal or after prolonged rupture of membranes. The associated placentas are often free of inflammation. With prolonged rupture of membranes, exudative inflammation from secondary bacterial infection may mask the bland necrosis that is typical of herpes viruses. Several cases of congenital herpes simplex infection have been described.[30–34] Witzleben and Driscoll[30] reported a probable case of congenital herpes infection acquired via a hematogenous route. They described multiple foci of bland villous necrosis associated with possible viral inclusions in necrotic syncytiotrophoblast. Other documented cases of congenital herpes infection have featured plasmacytic chorioamnionitis (Fig. 13–4).[31–34] In our opinion plasmacytic funisitis probably indicates herpes simplex infection, if not syphilis or other rare cause. Heifetz and Bauman[34] recently reported four cases of necrotizing funisitis, one of which was associated with congenital herpetic infection. In the remaining cases herpes antigen was demonstrable only in the decidua. Detection of viral protein or nucleic acid within decidua and other maternal tissues does not necessarily mean fetal infection.[35,36] An increased incidence of herpes viral antigens has been documented in fetal tissues associated with spontaneous abortion and stillbirth.[37] These findings may indicate that herpes simplex virus commonly causes pregnancy failure. Further investigation is warranted to establish the clinical significance of latent perinatal herpetic infections.

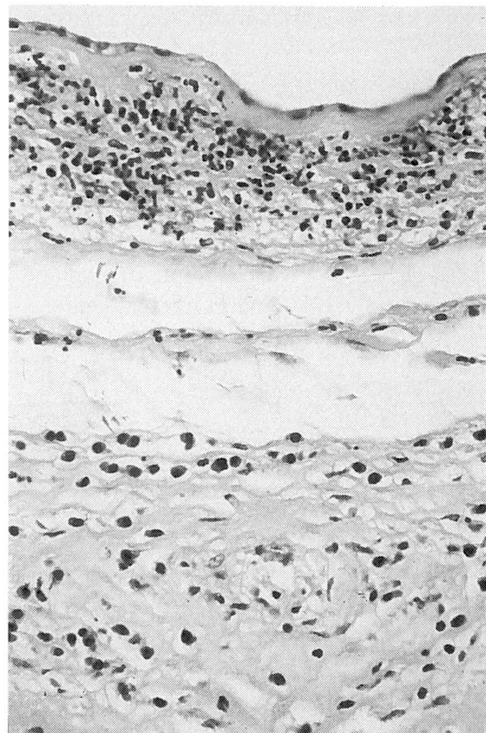

Figure 13–4. Congenital herpes simplex. Chorionic plate demonstrating necrotizing inflammation within the subamniotic connective tissue and lymphoplasmacytic infiltrates deep within the chorionic plate (H&E, ×100).

CLINICAL COMPLICATIONS ASSOCIATED WITH INTRAAMNIOTIC INFECTIONS

INTRAAMNIOTIC INFECTIONS AS A CAUSE OF PREMATURE LABOR

Intraamniotic infections are the single most common cause of perinatal morbidity and mortality. Whereas devastating fetal and maternal sepsis may accompany histopathologic chorioamnionitis, the major clinical impact of chorioamnionitis is prematurity and its complications.

Complex and incompletely delineated interactions are involved in the pathophysiology of preterm labor. The fundamental biochemical link between chorioamnionitis and premature labor is the generation of high levels of intraamniotic prostaglandin.[38] The various steps presented in Table 13–2 represent a logical progression of events that culminate in prostaglandin-induced uterine contraction and premature labor. These biochemical interactions should not be considered isolated events, nor are these suggested mechanistic details mutually exclusive.

MICROBIAL ACTIVATION OF THE UTERINE INNATE IMMUNE SYSTEM

Prostaglandins are derived from decidual and amniotic epithelial cells via a cascade of events initiated by the interaction of bacterial products with the host's immune system. Once liberated or elaborated into the amniotic fluid,[39–41] the bacterial products induce resident and subsequently recruited subamniotic and decidual macrophages to secrete cytokines. These agents act like inflammatory hormones that have a broad spectrum of biologic activities. The major proinflammatory cytokines involved in chorioamnionitis include tumor necrosis factor (TNF), interleukin-1 (IL-1), IL-6, and IL-8.[42]

YIELDING OF ARACHIDONIC ACID FROM PHOSPHOLIPASE FOR PROSTAGLANDIN SYNTHESIS

Prostaglandin synthesis depends on the availability of its metabolic precursor free arachidonic acid. Most cellular membranes contain endogenous phospholipases. TNF and IL-1 split arachidonic acid from the lipid bilayer through direct activation of endogenous cell membrane–associated phospholipase.[43,44] Monokine-induced secondary mediators may further promote endogenous phospholipase activity. Murray and colleagues[45] demonstrated that TNF, IL-1, and IL-6 induce amnion cells to produce endothelin. Endothelin, in turn, has been shown to stimulate phospholipase activity.[46,47] Neutrophils are involved in a third proposed pathway for the generation of free arachidonic acid. Both TNF- and IL-1-activated neutrophils synthesize and directly secrete phospholipase A_2.[48] Separate from endogenous sources of phospholipases, several bacterial species commonly associated with chorioamnionitis secrete

Table 13–2. Biochemical Mechanisms of Infection-Induced Premature Labor

Bacteria ascend the birth canal and enter the amnionic cavity
(protease digestion of cervical mucus with release of bacterial products)
↓
Microbial activation of the uterine innate immune system
(bacterial products cause leukocytes to secrete interleukin-1, 6, -8, and tumor necrosis factor)
↓
Cytokines activate endogenous cell membrane phospholipases
(amniotic neutrophils, endothelin, and bacterial phospholipases)
↓
Phospholipases yield arachidonic acid for prostaglandin synthesis
(arachidonic acids are split from cell membranes by phospholipase activity)
↓
Cyclooxygenase conversion of arachidonic acid into prostaglandin
(interleukin-1 stimulates inducible form of cyclooxygenase synthase)
↓
Intrauterine concentration of prostaglandin is greatly increased
(cervical ripening, uterine contractions, and premature labor)

high levels of phospholipase A_2. These include *Fusobacterium, Bacteroides,* and *Ureaplasma.*[49–51]

Conversion of Arachidonic Acid into Prostaglandin

Free arachidonic acid in the amniotic fluid is converted into prostaglandin H_2 by the enzyme cyclooxygenase. Prostaglandin H_2 is the metabolic precursor of the more stable prostaglandins E_2 and $F_{2\alpha}$. Cyclooxygenase is a cytokine-inducible enzyme. On induction, synthesis of cyclooxygenase is greatly increased over unstimulated conditions. One signal for cyclooxygenase induction is IL-1.[52] It is noteworthy that the onset of labor is associated with a concomitant increase in levels of both intraamniotic IL-1 and decidual and amnion cell cyclooxygenase mRNA.[53] These findings support the contention that IL-1-induced cyclooxygenase activity is a key step in the prostaglandin cascade and the onset of premature labor.

Biochemical Countermeasures to Prevent Premature Labor

Premature labor resulting from intraamniotic infections is refractory to current tocolytic therapy.[54] The biochemical complexity of the prostaglandin cascade may in part explain this. From a teleologic viewpoint it makes sense to prevent minor insults from resulting in premature delivery. Naturally occurring antiinflammatory mediators do occur. A pivotal point within the cascade is cyclooxygenase conversion of arachidonic acid to prostaglandin. IL-1 induction of this enzyme may provide a focus for intervention. Romero and colleagues[55] have investigated an intraamniotic IL-1 receptor antagonist. This protein has physical properties similar to IL-1. It reacts with the IL-1 receptor and prevents intracellular signal transduction in target tissues. In a murine model, IL-1 receptor antagonist blocks IL-1-induced labor in a dose-dependent manner.[56] Several lines of evidence support the hypothesis that this protein may be a useful adjunct to current tocolytic therapy. IL-1 receptor antagonist is a normal constituent of amniotic fluid. In vitro it blocks amnion cell prostaglandin synthesis in a dose-dependent manner. Because premature labor in mice is preventable in a dose-dependent manner, the molar ratio between IL-1 and its receptor antagonist may be important. The high levels of IL-1 generated during intraamniotic infections may overwhelm this naturally occurring blockade and subsequently initiate the prostaglandin cascade. Other cytokines may reduce the proinflammatory effects of IL-1. IL-4 and transforming growth factor–β_1 increase production of IL-1 receptor antagonist and inhibit prostaglandin production. IL-10 decreases synthesis of other proinflammatory cytokines.[57,58]

Intraamniotic Infections as a Cause of Placental Abruption

Abruptio placentae is a major cause of preterm labor. Infection-related exudative or necrotizing deciduitis is often present. Thrombosis of decidual vessels and hemorrhage into the surrounding soft tissues have been reported in association with abruptio placentae.[59] Decidual arteriopathy, maternal high blood pressure, preeclampsia, lupus anticoagulant, and diabetes are other etiologic factors of abruptio placentae and prematurity. Illicit drugs (e.g., cocaine) and abuse of cigarettes may also cause premature placental separation.

Intraamniotic Infections as a Cause of Fetal Pneumonia and Sepsis

Chorioamnionitis is caused by a diverse group of organisms that vary greatly in their pathogenic potential. Often it results from a mixed infection. Although intraamniotic meconium does not singly produce chorioamnionitis, severe inflammation occurs when there is accompanying infection, even when the causative microbe is relatively innocuous. Bacterial synergy has been well documented in other forms of infection, but it is rarely considered in clinical studies of chorioamnionitis. Epidemiologic investigations of clinically diagnosed chorioamnionitis have been incomplete, and some of them have not included placental examinations. These deficiencies explain why many clinicians have failed to recognize the importance of clinically inapparent histopathologic chorioamnionitis. Romero and his colleagues[60] found that only one of nine patients with preterm labor and positive amniotic fluid cultures had clinical features of chorioamnionitis.

Of cases of bacterial chorioamnionitis in the placenta, approximately half are caused by aerobic bacteria and the other half by anaerobic bacteria.[61] Diverse factors determine the fetal outcome of intraamniotic infections. These include host immune responses, gestational age, portal of entry, inoculum size, viability of organisms, bacterial growth requirements, adherence factors, and toxin production. Because of these numerous variables, histopathologic grades or features of chorioamnionitis provide only a limited amount of clinically useful information. The following generalizations are nevertheless reasonable.

1. If group B *Streptococcus* or herpes simplex viral infections are not present in the mother's genital tract, early or slight acute chorioamnionitis is unlikely to be accompanied by clinically demonstrable congenital sepsis. The same conclusion is applicable to group A *Streptococcus* and to *Streptococcus pneumoniae;* however, those organisms are only rarely to cause congenital infection.
2. When chorioamnionitis is severe, the risk of fetal congenital pneumonia, meningitis, and sepsis increases. Also, the combination of placental chorionic microabscesses with inflammation in all three umbilical cord vessels correlates with clinical features of neonatal sepsis.

SELECTED ORGANISMS THAT COMMONLY CAUSE INTRAAMNIOTIC INFECTIONS

Gram-Negative Bacteria

Fusobacterium

Fusobacterium is one of the most common causes of acute chorioamnionitis. We have detected *Fusobacterium* in as many as 18% of placentas with chorioamnionitis.[62,63] Other investigators have confirmed the importance of *Fusobacterium* as a common cause of premature labor and occult chorioamnionitis.[64] These bacteria have a remarkable ability to penetrate between amniotic epithelial cells (Fig. 13–5) and to extend deeply into Wharton's jelly of the umbilical cord. Virulence factors associated with the capacity of the organism to penetrate the cervical mucous plug and amniotic membranes are unknown. We suspect that bacterial proteolytic enzymes such as hyaluronidase and collagenase play a prominent role in the development of *Fusobacterium* chorioamnionitis.

Fusobacterium colonizes normal mucous membranes, including the mouth, intestines, and urogenital tract, and can be routinely cultured from fecal material.[65] Although *Fusobacterium* has the potential to cause severe fetal pneumonia and sep-

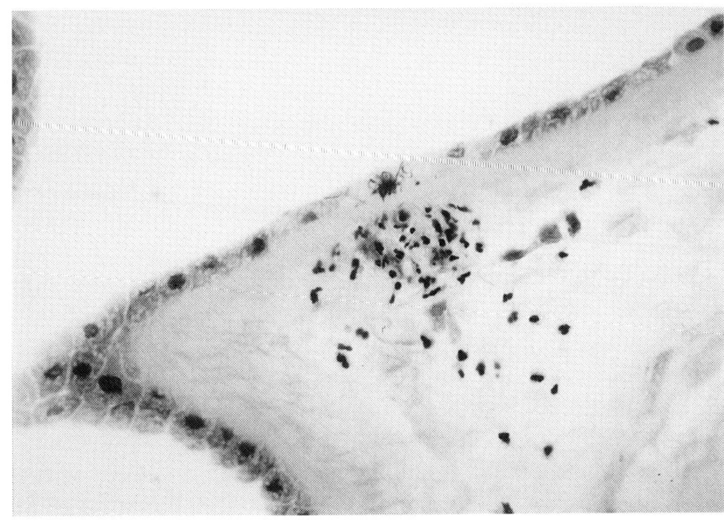

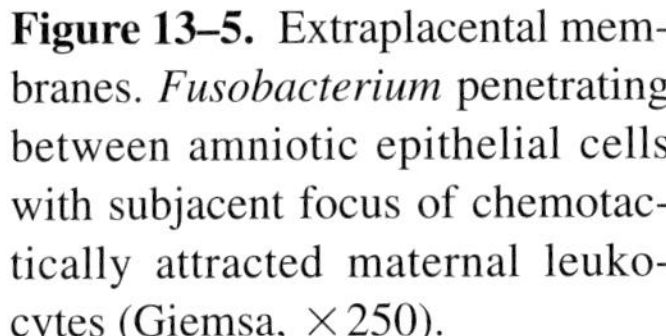

Figure 13–5. Extraplacental membranes. *Fusobacterium* penetrating between amniotic epithelial cells with subjacent focus of chemotactically attracted maternal leukocytes (Giemsa, ×250).

sis, the newborn is usually not thus affected. As is common in many anaerobic infections the bacterial population is frequently mixed. We have seen several cases of *Fusobacterium* chorioamnionitis associated with group B *Streptococcus*.

In routine hematoxylin and eosin–stained sections, *Fusobacterium* chorioamnionitis is characterized by long, slender (filamentous) bacteria in amorphous, necrotic amniotic epithelium. The organisms are most clearly delineated by Giemsa stain.

Nontypable *Haemophilus influenzae*

Haemophilus influenzae frequently causes chorioamnionitis and other perinatal infections. Rusin and co-workers[66] reported that over a 10-year period only group B *Streptococcus* and *Escherichia coli* were more frequently associated with early neonatal bacteremia. More than 80% of maternal and neonatal *Haemophilus* infections are produced by nontypable strains.[67,68] These infections may clinically mimic early-onset group B *Streptococcus* infections, since they are manifested as pneumonia, respiratory distress, and sepsis.

In tissue and smears of infected materials, nontypable *Haemophilus influenzae* appears as small, pleomorphic, coccobacillary gram-negative bacteria.[69] In contrast to placentas with group B streptococcal placentitis, those with *H. influenzae* often have severe acute chorioamnionitis with occasional monocytes and macrophages. This is occasionally accompanied by acute villitis. The best methods for diagnosis of nontypable *H. influenzae* are Gram's stain and culture of the tissue.

Escherichia coli

Escherichia coli is second only to group B *Streptococcus* as the cause of congenital pneumonia, meningitis, and sepsis.[70] Most infants are colonized during or shortly after delivery. Bacterial strains that possess the K1 antigen are associated with neonatal meningitis and other severe congenital infections.[71,72]

In tissue *E. coli* organisms are uniform, gram-negative bacilli approximately 3 to 4 μm in length. The typical pattern of inflammation is acute chorioamnionitis, which may be severe. Some cases of *E. coli* chorioamnionitis also manifest suppurative intervillositis and villitis (similar to the inflammation caused by *Listeria monocytogenes*). This inflammatory pattern facilitates the differential diagnosis.

Bacteroides Species

Bacteroides spp. are the most abundant organisms in human fecal flora and the most common clinical isolates of gram-negative anaerobic bacteria. *Bacteroides* is frequently isolated from placentas with chorioamnionitis. These organisms probably represent an underdiagnosed cause of fetal and neonatal infections.[73] *B. fragilis* has been documented to cause neonatal meningitis.[74]

Histologic study has shown that *Bacteroides* infections produce acute chorioamnionitis. We have never encountered *Bacteroides* villitis. Using immunofluorescence techniques, Evaldson and associates[75] found *B. fragilis* in 5 of 15 patients with chorioamnionitis and premature rupture of membranes (Fig. 13–6).[75] *B. fragilis* possesses a thick polysaccharide coat that causes a distinctive safety pin appearance on light microscopy. Histopathologic, culture, and immunofluorescence techniques are the best means of making specific diagnoses.[76]

Gram-positive Bacteria

Group B *Streptococcus*

Group B beta-hemolytic *Streptococcus* (GBS) is the most common cause of neonatal sepsis. It is present at term in up to 30% of women with normal pregnancies.[77] Although many infants are thus exposed to GBS, sepsis occurs in only a small percentage.[78] The size of the inoculum[79] and the capacity of the organism to produce a vasoactive polysaccharide "exotoxin" appear to be significant factors in determining perinatal outcome.[80]

GBS produces two distinct types of neonatal infection. Early GBS infections are characterized by sudden-onset hypotensive septic shock and respiratory distress. The late-onset form is strongly associated with neonatal meningitis. A less well-recognized form of GBS infection produces

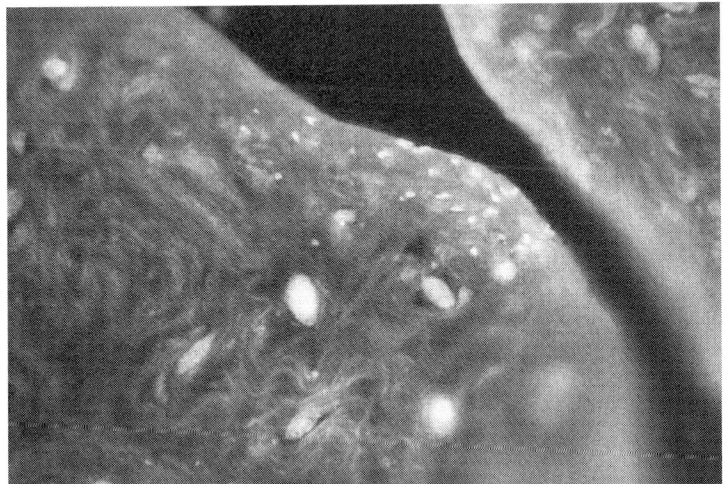

Figure 13–6. Extraplacental membranes. Immunofluorescence-labeled *Bacteroides fragilis*. The organisms have a rounded shape and have been described as resembling safety pins. (×250).

intrauterine asphyxia. Severe ischemic brain damage including periventricular leukomalacia may occur. Intrauterine infections caused by GBS typically exhibit minimal placental inflammation. Even in cases of neonatal death resulting from overwhelming GBS sepsis and pneumonia, the lungs and other organs typically lack purulent inflammation. These findings support the opinion that death results from a bacterial toxin.

Group B *Streptococcus* produces a 2 million molecular weight, heat-stable exotoxin composed of polysaccharide and protein. In sheep this extracellular bacterial product causes severe, sustained contractions of bronchial and vascular smooth muscle.[81] The polysaccharide is the vasoactive portion of the molecule. Because polysaccharide antigens are T cell independent, the antibody response may be exclusively of the IgM class.[82,83] Since IgM antibodies do not cross the placenta, maternal antibodies directed against the exotoxin would not protect the fetus. This may partially explain why pooled and hyperimmune serum vaccines have not been entirely successful in protecting newborns from GBS sepsis.[84–86]

In tissue, GBS organisms are small cocci that sometimes occur in small chains. Often GBS in infected placentas is not appreciable by light microscopy. When the organisms are seen, their morphologic features seldom assist light microscopic diagnosis. With group B streptococcal chorioamnionitis, however, we have seen a noteworthy presence of eosinophils accompanying very slight exudative chorionic plate vasculitis. In the clinical context of rapid-onset neonatal pneumonia and sepsis these placental findings warrant strong consideration of GBS. Although experienced placental pathologists can recognize these changes in frozen section slides, rapid immunologic tests are preferable methods for diagnosis.

Other Gram-positive Cocci

Enterococcus, Lancefield groups A, D, C, G, and F streptococci, *Pneumococcus,* and anaerobic *Peptostreptococcus* are common organisms causing chorioamnionitis. Unfortunately, however, they do not produce any particular or characteristic type of inflammation. Bacterial cultures are thus required for their diagnosis. *Staphylococcus aureus* typically produces severe acute chorioamnionitis that may be accompanied by suppurative villitis. Because of potent hemolytic enzymes, the fetal placental surface may have a yellow-green appearance. With declining numbers of illegal abortions in the United States, this kind of infection and inflammation is now rare.

Listeria Monocytogenes

Listeria organisms spread to humans through contaminated vegetables and animal products.[87] Pregnancy does not appear to change the rate of vaginal or gastrointestinal colonization[88]; it alters immune function and predisposes gravid carriers to infection.[89–91] If listeriosis occurs early in gestation, spontaneous or repeated abortions may result.[92] Listeriosis in the newborn resembles GBS infection. The early-onset form is characterized by pneumonia and disseminated disease. The late-onset form may develop up to 8 weeks after delivery. It is characterized by meningitis in 96% of cases.[93]

In tissue, *Listeria* elicits two types of inflammation. The initial inflammation is suppurative with granulocytes and occasional macrophages. Because *Listeria* is able to resist macrophage intracellular killing, a granulomatous reaction may ensue. The organisms multiply in the cytosol of the macrophage and are eliminated when macrophages become bactericidal after activation by T helper cell–derived γ-interferon. Infected cells may also be eliminated after direct lysis by cytotoxic T cells.[94] Neonates are predisposed to disseminated listeriosis because of age-related defects in macrophage intracellular killing,[95] reduced production of γ-interferon,[96] and reduced opsonization of bacteria by IgM.[97]

Listeria placentitis is characterized by suppurative chorioamnionitis, intervillositis, and villitis (Fig. 13–7). Areas of intervillositis may form grossly recognizable microabscesses resembling millet seeds. The chorioamnionitis may contain many eosinophils. The bacteria are difficult to detect in placental inflammatory cell infiltrates.[98] Because of cold enrichment at 4° C, they are often easier to detect in placentas that have been refrigerated before processing.

Fastidious Organisms that Cause Intraamniotic Infections

Chlamydia trachomatis

Cervical *Chlamydia* infections are a common complication of pregnancy. The organisms have been cultured from neonates with pneumonitis or ocular infections and from stillbirths. In our experience *Chlamydia* rarely produces chorioamnionitis. The histopathologic features of chlamydial placentitis in humans have not been described. *Chlamydia* injected into the amniotic cavity of rats, however, produces lesions that simulate human chorioamnionitis.[99] The organisms cannot be detected by routine light microscopy or culture. Immunofluorescence demonstration of the organisms and special culture studies are required to establish the diagnosis.

Ureaplasma urealyticum

Ureaplasma is reported to cause acute chorioamnionitis and recurrent abortions.[100,101] The organisms are commonly recovered from placentas and abortion and stillbirth materials.[102] A major

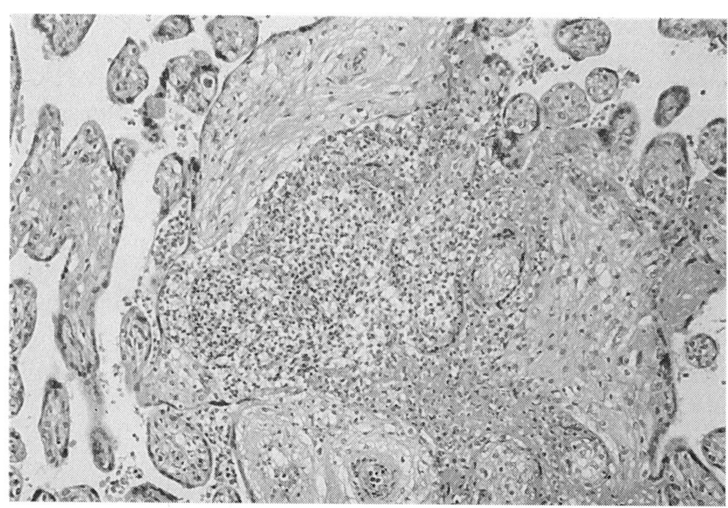

Figure 13–7. Placental tissue demonstrating focal intense acute intervillositis with perivillous fibrin deposition induced by congenital *Listeria* infection. There is also acute villitis (H&E, ×50).

Table 13–3. Empirical Reasons that Villitis of Unknown Etiology (VUE) is Primarily a Fetal Immune Response to an Infectious Agent

1. Lesions indistinguishable from VUE occur with diverse placental infections including cytomegalovirus, enteroviruses, *Mycoplasma,* and syphilis.
2. Placentas from immunologically immature fetuses and embryos do not have VUE.
3. VUE does not accompany chronic fetomaternal blood transfusion. This is particularly noteworthy because in that condition fetal cells with both class I and class II major histocompatibility complex antigens are released into the maternal circulation.
4. Diseases that involve fetomaternal immunologic aberrations do not manifest VUE. These include ABO and Rh blood group incompatibilities and isoimmune thrombocytopenia.
5. In the early phase of VUE, inflammatory cells migrate from the fetal villous capillaries to the villous trophoblastic surface. This indicates that the primary inflammatory response is fetal. Perhaps cytokines secondarily attract maternal cells.

problem in interpreting these data is that *Ureaplasma* organisms are ubiquitous in gravid populations.[103,104] Some serotypes of *Ureaplasma* exhibit high phospholipase A_2 activity.[105] It may be that strains possessing this enzyme are more often associated with chorioamnionitis and with mothers who have had recurrent reproductive failure.

Ureaplasma chorioamnionitis may cause severe mucopurulent inflammation. This is particularly true in placentas of immature fetuses. Because the inflammation evolves over many hours, *Ureaplasma* probably produces premature labor only after prolonged infection. Immunofluorescence studies would be helpful in delineating which serotypes are important pathogens.

INFECTIOUS AGENTS THAT CAUSE VILLITIS

Organisms that infect the placenta elicit a fetal immune response in stem, anchoring, and terminal villi. The route of infection may be of a maternofetal bloodborne type or involve direct extension from the uterus. This inflammation occurs in at least 10% of placentas associated with sick or at risk fetuses and newborns.[106–108] In at least 95% of placentas with chronic villous inflammatory cell infiltrates the causative agent is not identified. The term "villitis of unknown etiology" (VUE) is used to distinguish this entity from villitis of known cause. Some authors have emphasized the role of immunopathologic factors in the pathogenesis of villitis.[109,110] For various reasons we contend that although immunopathologic factors are important, in the vast majority of cases they are ancillary to infection (Table 13–3). VUE encompasses a broad spectrum of placental inflammatory cell infiltrates. These include lymphohistiocytic, lymphocytic, plasmacytic, granulomatous, suppurative, sclerotic, and evanescent inflammatory features (Fig. 13–8*A* to *C*). Whereas proliferative hypercellularity characterizes the developing phase of the infectious process (Fig. 13–8*D*), reparative features are represented by cicatricial changes and evanescent villitis (Fig. 13–8*E*). Several of these protean inflammatory patterns are often present within a single placenta, and close examination often reveals accompanying fetal villous vascular thrombosis or obliteration and focal or multifocal villous capillary hypervascularity (Fig. 13–8*F*).

The clinical consequences of VUE are diverse. Severe placental inflammation may develop in infants and mothers who have no overt abnormality, and conversely many newborns with severe clinical abnormalities have only subtle villitis. Because limited information is available from epidemiologic investigations of VUE, the risk of associated neurodevelopmental and other disorders has not been established. Depending on sociocultural, socioeconomic, and other population-based factors, there is a wide range in the prevalence of VUE. However, VUE is present in the placentas of at least 25% of small for gestational age newborns.[111–113] In specimens without coexistent histopathologic signs of low uteroplacental blood flow, the pathogenesis of VUE-related fetal growth retardation cannot be ascertained. Heyborne, Witkin, and McGregor[114] have provided evidence that activation of the cytokine network causes impaired fetal growth and that at midtrimester some growth-retarded fetuses have TNF in their amniotic fluid. These authors further demonstrated a dose-response relationship between TNF levels and birth weight percentiles. Because of the role of TNF in tissue wasting as-

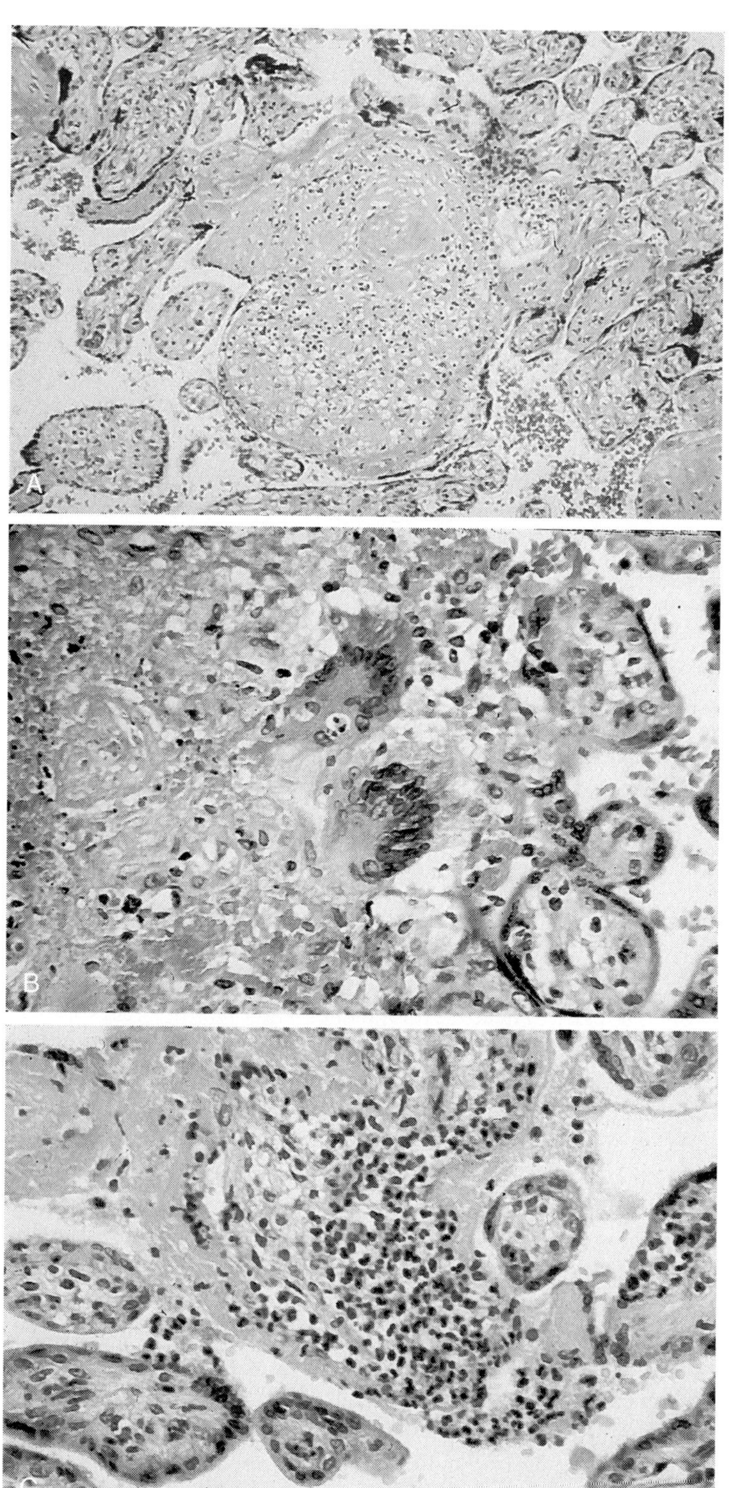

Figure 13–8. Placenta. **A,** Lymphohistiocytic villitis of unknown etiology. Note the disruption of the normal villous cytoarchitecture, including fetal vascular obliteration (H&E, ×50). **B,** Granulomatous villitis of unknown etiology. Two multinucleated giant cells are located within a villus admixed with histiocytic inflammation. No organisms were demonstrable by special stains (H&E, ×100). **C,** Suppurative villitis of unknown etiology. No organisms were demonstrable on special stains, and neonatal blood cultures were negative (H&E, ×100).

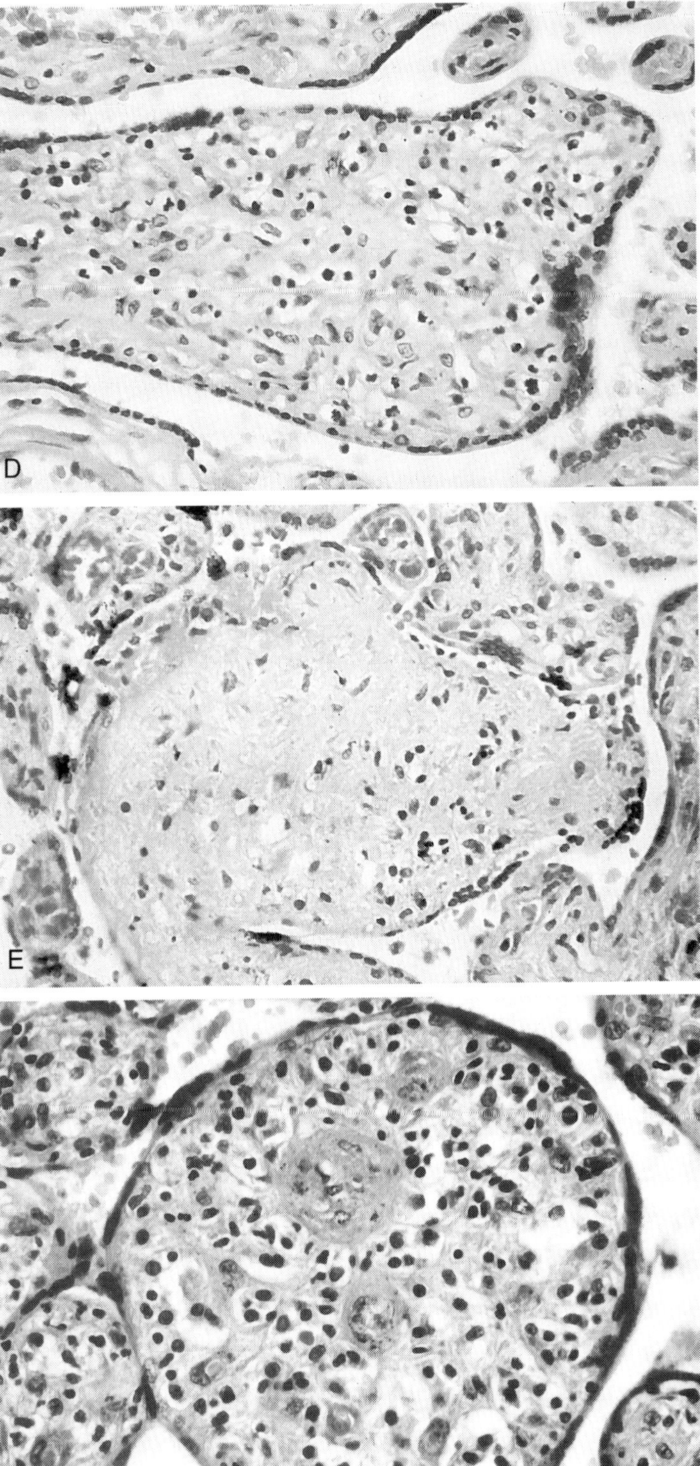

Figure 13–8 *Continued* **D,** Proliferative lymphohistiocytic villitis of unknown etiology. The villus is hypercellular with extensive disruption of the cytoarchitecture (H&E, ×100). **E,** Evanescent villitis of unknown etiology with accompanying villous stromal sclerosis (H&E, ×100). **F,** Proliferative lymphohistiocytic villitis with early vascular thrombosis of fetal capillaries (H&E, ×100).

sociated with chronic infections and cancer, it was originally known as cachectin. Catabolic actions of TNF involve the suppression of enzymes such as lipoprotein lipase.[115]

VUE has a remarkable tendency to recur in subsequent pregnancies. Russell[113] reported a recurrence rate of 27% and noted that the pattern of inflammation in the second placenta was indistinguishable from the inflammation in the previous pregnancy. This finding could indicate reactivation of a latent viral infection or sexually transmitted reinfection from a partner who is a chronic carrier. Alternatively, Redline and Abramowsky[116] have implied that immunologic aberrations have an important role in the pathogenesis of VUE and recurrent reproductive failure. They reported a 60% reproductive loss in patients with recurrent chronic villitis and a 37% loss accompanying nonrecurrent villitis.

VUE is probably caused by more than one infectious agent, and these organisms are not easily cultured or demonstrable by routine techniques. Recent use of molecular diagnostic methods has shown that echoviruses and an as yet unidentified nonsyphilitic spirochete produce some cases of VUE.[117,118] The polymerase chain reaction (PCR) method will probably elucidate several causes of VUE. In contrast to antibody techniques, PCR allows simultaneous detection of multiple related viruses, *Mycobacterium,* and other fastidious organisms. Conserved regions of DNA that occur in an entire genus of organisms can be detected by use of a single set of primers. Enteroviruses are one example.[119] Fragment length analysis of amplified PCR products or Southern blot can be used to identify the organism to the species level. Depending on the organism of interest, great care is required in selecting appropriate specimens for PCR analysis. Incorporation of viral DNA into the host cell genome and laboratory contamination of clinical samples are potential sources of false-positive results.

CLINICAL CONSIDERATIONS RELATIVE TO CHRONIC VILLITIS

The most common pattern of VUE consists of proliferative lymphohistiocytic infiltrates accompanied by disruption of villous architecture. Separate from immunopathologically mediated causes, these lesions warrant investigation for enteroviruses (including echoviruses and coxsackieviruses). Of 19 cases of confirmed maternal enteroviral infection, 17 had VUE in the placenta.[120] In the absence of ultrastructural study, coronavirus (a noncultivable virus) remains a possible cause of VUE, as do varicella, vaccinia, and nonviral organisms such as *Ureaplasma* and *Chlamydia.*

When villous inflammatory cell infiltrates are predominantly lymphocytic, diagnostic consideration of *Toxoplasma,* rubella virus, cytomegalovirus, herpes simplex virus, and syphilis is appropriate. These specific villitides have conspicuously more plasma cells. Such infiltrates occur only rarely in VUE. Histopathologic features of specific villitides include villous hemosiderin deposition, fetal vascular proliferative endovasculitis, villous dysmaturity, erythroblastosis, increased fetal nucleated red blood cells, viral inclusions, and pseudocysts of *Toxoplasma gondii* (Table 13–4). Clinical findings and serologic, culture, and molecular diagnostic tests are often necessary to substantiate placental light microscopic diagnosis.

Selected Organisms That Produce Chronic Villitis

Cytomegalovirus

Cytomegalovirus (CMV) is the most common of the so-called TORCHS infections. Approximately 1% of newborns have CMV viruria. Stagno and colleagues[121] estimate that 90% of these infants have clinically unrecognized disease. Only 5% have disseminated disease, and in the remaining 5% the most common long-term sequela is sensorineural deafness. Newborns with disseminated CMV infection often have hepatosplenomegaly, pneumonitis, microcephaly, periventricular calcifications, hydrops, and cutaneous extramedullary hematopoiesis or blueberry muffin spots. Like other herpesviruses, CMV often remains dormant after primary infection. Reactivation of latent maternal CMV infection is by far the most common source of congenital infection. It typically produces a mild or subclinical neonatal infection. Perhaps transplacentally acquired maternal antibody imparts protection. Hematopoietic

Table 13–4. Differential Diagnosis of Congenital TORCHS Infections

Toxoplasmosis	Lymphohistiocytic villitis with occasional plasma cells Pseudocysts in membranes and umbilical cord Features similar to erythroblastosis Granulomatous villitis also reported
Rubella	Lymphohistiocytic villitis, sometimes with plasma cells Extensive obliterative fetal vascular damage Intravillous hemosiderin deposition
Cytomegalovirus	Proliferative lymphoplasmacytic villitis Intravillous hemosiderin deposition Fetal endovascular sclerosis Viral inclusions in 20% of cases
Herpes simplex	Lymphoplasmacytic chorioamnionitis with funisitis Extensive subamniotic bland necrosis Viral cytopathic effect in amnion cells
Syphilis	Lymphoplasmacytic, acute, and granulomatous villitis Proliferative fetal endovasculitis Villous hypercellularity or dysmaturity Before antibiotics, Warthin-Starry-positive organisms

progenitor cells may be one site from which pregnancy-induced reactivation of a latent infection develops.[122]

CMV is excreted from the cervix during pregnancy in up to 10% of women at midtrimester and 29% at term.[123] Cervical excretion of the virus during pregnancy raises the possibility of an ascending infection. A recent case report by Weber and co-workers[124] documented intraamniotic CMV infection at 22 weeks' gestation by amniotic fluid culture, PCR, and shell vial techniques. No maternal antibody response to the virus was detected during pregnancy. The absence of an immune response argues against a systemic hematologic route of vertical transmission. Ohyama and her colleagues[125] have demonstrated, by similar diagnostic techniques including in situ hybridization, a second probable ascending congenital CMV infection. These considerations remind us of our observation of spermatozoa in placental subamniotic connective tissue and of literature of the 1970s.[126] CMV has been shown to persist in semen for many months, in the absence of clinical symptoms, and is considered a sexually transmitted disease. We suspect that ascending CMV infection is much more common than is realized. We have recently encountered a case of CMV villitis in which viral inclusions were identified in the subamniotic connective tissue of the extraplacental membranes.

The histopathologic features of CMV villitis typically include lymphoplasmacytic infiltrates associated with multifocal hemosiderin deposits, often within both avascular and nonavascular villi (Fig. 13–9*A*).[127] Hemosiderin deposition results from degeneration of microscopic stromal hemorrhages. Lymphocytic infiltrates of T cell lineage are also a consistent feature of CMV placentitis.[128] Placental cells susceptible to CMV replication are primarily fixed stromal cells, although viral proteins are also documented within endothelial cells, Hofbauer cells, and syncytiotrophoblast.[129] Other typical findings include increased fetal nucleated red blood cells, villous edema, stromal sclerosis, fetal villous endovascular sclerosis with thrombosis, and in approximately 20% of cases pathognomonic intranuclear viral inclusions (Fig. 13–9*B*).

Placental histopathologic findings occasionally raise the clinical suspicion of congenital CMV infection. Urine culture may require several days to manifest typical cytopathic effects. Shell vial techniques use monoclonal antibodies to detect early viral antigens in tissue culture cells.[130] This method is specific and greatly reduces the time needed for viral isolation. Tissue antibody stains or DNA diagnostic techniques are sometimes necessary to confirm light microscopic placental findings or clinical laboratory diagnosis.[131,132]

Syphilis

In the United States syphilis is now the second leading known cause of chronic intrauterine in-

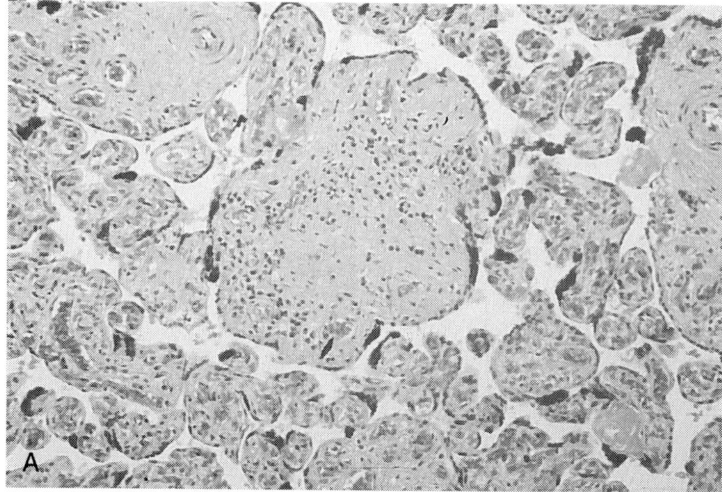

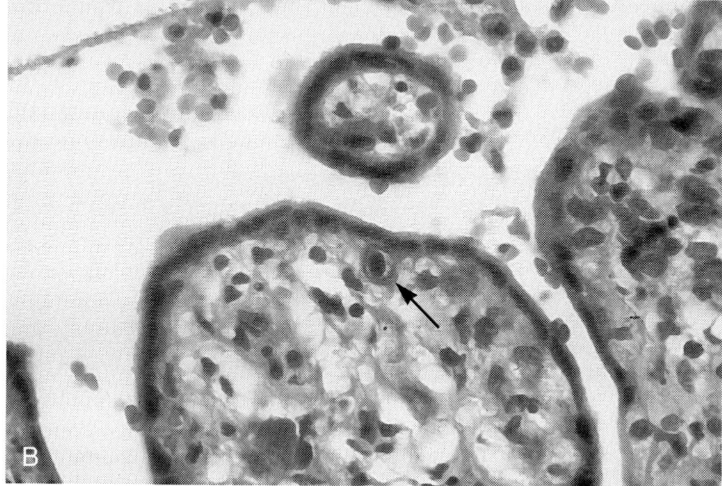

Figure 13–9. *Cytomegalovirus* placentitis. **A,** Lymphoplasmacytic villitis accompanied by focal intravillous hemosiderin deposits in a nonavascular villus (H&E, ×50). **B,** Villus containing pathognomonic intranuclear inclusions (H&E, ×50).

fection. The results of serologic tests for congenital syphilis are often inconclusive.[133] The diagnosis of syphilis should be strongly suspected on the basis of a triad of placental light microscopic findings: lymphohistiocytic villitis with focal plasma cells, proliferative endovasculitis with accompanying endovascular sclerosis, and placental stromal hypercellularity or dysmaturity.[134,135] Qureshi and his colleagues,[136] found these features in only seven of 25 congenital syphilis cases with diagnosis confirmed by PCR. Foci of acute or granulomatous villitis with multinucleated giant cells may also occur, and plasma cells are sometimes focally numerous. In our experience necrotizing funisitis and other inflammatory patterns have not been meaningful indicators of syphilis. Some of the observed placental lesions also occur with congenital CMV infection. Although both syphilis and CMV cause endovascular sclerosis (presumably via infection of endothelial cells), we cannot recall having seen proliferative endovasculitis with CMV (Fig. 13–10). In some placentas with congenital syphilis, lymphoplasmacytic chorioamnionitis occurs. We have never seen this entity with CMV placentitis. Greco and associates[137] found that villous stromal cells from CMV-infected placentas manifested a different pattern of macrophage cellular markers than syphilitic placentas.

If the mother has not received antibiotics before delivery, Warthin-Starry silver stains or immunofluorescence examination will readily stain spirochetes.[138] The organisms are then optimally seen in the umbilical cord, extraplacental membranes, and decidua basalis. PCR will probably become the test of choice for congenital syphilis. Because PCR amplifies DNA of the organisms, this test is more specific than methods measuring the immune response of the host.[139]

Toxoplasma gondii

Toxoplasmosis is caused by the protozoan *Toxoplasma gondii.* The organisms are ubiquitous in nature and readily infect many different types of animals. Felines, including domestic house cats, are the definitive host. In cats both a sexual and an asexual phase of reproduction occur within intestinal epithelium. The organism is commonly transmitted to humans by exposure to contaminated feline fecal material or ingestion of the undercooked meat of infected secondary hosts. Between 30% and 50% of infants whose mothers had a primary infection during pregnancy are affected. These infants can be asymptomatic or suffer severe damage. The triad of intracerebral calcifications, hydrocephalus, and chorioretinitis is considered the classic clinical presentation. Hydrops fetalis, hepatosplenomegaly, and erythroblastosis also occur.

The gross and light microscopic placental findings are similar to those of erythroblastosis fetalis. These include villous edema and numerous fetal nucleated red blood cells. In addition, however, foci of proliferative lymphohistiocytic, necrotizing, and plasma cell villitis are seen.[140–142] Popek[143] has described an 18-week fetus whose placenta manifested extensive granulomatous villous infiltrates and many organisms. The presence of pathognomonic pseudocysts, best seen in subamniotic connective tissue, establishes the diagnosis. Immunofluorescence delineation of tachyzoites in tissue sections or PCR detection of *Toxoplasma* DNA in tissue homogenates or amniotic fluid increases diagnostic sensitivity.[144]

Rubella

The teratogenic effects of rubella infection were first recognized by Sir Norman Gregg,[145] an Australian ophthalmologist who was investigating congenital cataracts. A triad of clinical findings, including congenital heart disease, cataracts, and deafness, characterizes the congenital rubella syndrome. In the 1960s an "expanded syndrome" with involvement of yet other organs was described. Since the introduction of extensive vaccination programs, congenital rubella infections have become rare in the United States. Even in major epidemics of rubella virus, however, reports of associated placentitis were remarkably few.[146,147] The placental inflammation consists of lymphocytic and lymphohistiocytic villitis with occasional plasma cells. As a result of attack of endothelial cells by rubella virus, acute endovasculitis of villous vessels, obliterative villous endovasculopathy, and intravillous deposits of hemo-

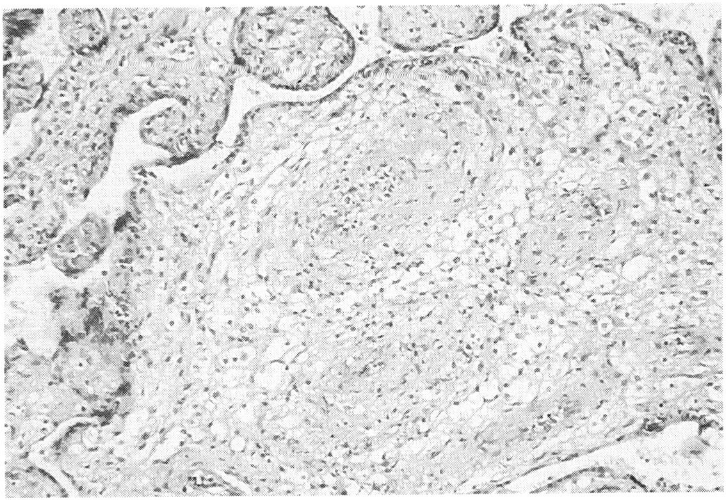

Figure 13–10. Placenta of congenital syphilis showing the triad of histopathologic findings including villous hypercellularity or dysmaturity, proliferative endovasculitis, and villitis (H&E, ×100).

siderin can be prominent features. Reverse transcriptase PCR is a sensitive and specific test that documents the virus in fetal placental tissues, amniotic fluid, and fetal blood.[148]

Varicella

In the United States each year approximately 9000 pregnancies may be complicated by maternal varicella infection.[149] Enders and colleagues[150] investigated 1373 cases of women who contracted varicella during the first 36 weeks of pregnancy. They found 9 cases of congenital varicella infection, each of which was contracted during the first 20 weeks of pregnancy. Although rare, congenital varicella can have devastating consequences for affected fetuses. These include cicatricial skin lesions, eye abnormalities, including microphthalmia and cataract, hypoplastic limbs, and central nervous system abnormalities. Placental findings include multifocal lymphohistiocytic and granulomatous infiltrates with occasional multinucleated giant cells.[151,152]

Chlamydia psittaci

In Europe *Chlamydia psittaci* is a relatively common cause of abortion in sheep and other mammals. If acquired during pregnancy, psittacosis may be a severe progressive febrile illness with headache, disseminated intravascular coagulation, liver enzyme abnormalities, and impaired renal function.[153] Recovery from this disease follows termination of pregnancy and appropriate antibiotic therapy. Direct exposure of gravid humans to infected products of conception is the most commonly reported mode of transmission. Diagnosis is suggested by the placental histopathologic findings, which consist of intense acute intervillositis, perivillous fibrin deposition with villous necrosis, and basophilic intracytoplasmic inclusions in the syncytiotrophoblast (Fig. 13–11).[154] Commercially available genus-specific monoclonal antichlamydial antibody facilitates the diagnosis.

Parvovirus B19

Parvovirus B19 infection is a common cause of acute transient aplastic anemia and aplastic crises in patients with sickle cell anemia and other chronic anemias.[155,156] It is also a relatively common cause of fetal anemia, nonimmune hydrops fetalis, spontaneous abortion, and stillbirth. Parvovirus is a single-stranded DNA virus that attacks rapidly dividing cells. Although the primary targets are erythroid precursor cells, heart muscle and other tissues are also susceptible.[157,158] Mothers contracting the disease during pregnancy appear to have a relatively low rate of vertical transmission. Affected fetuses typically manifest generalized edema, anemia, hepatomegaly, and hemo-

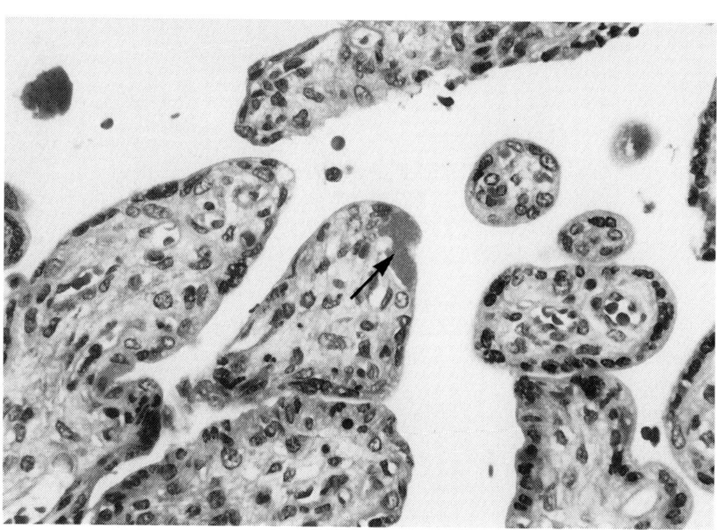

Figure 13–11. Placenta. Compared with *Chlamydia trachomatis,* this intracytoplasmic inclusion produced by *Chlamydia psittaci* has an irregular contour and does not distort the nucleus. It is basophilic in hematoxylin and eosin–stained sections and glycogen negative via periodic acid–Schiff reaction (×250).

siderin deposits in the spleen and liver. Circulating erythroblasts may be numerous. The placenta typically shows erythroblastosis and edema. On hematoxylin and eosin–stained slides, pink intranuclear inclusions can be seen in nucleated red blood cells, although sometimes with difficulty.[159,160] The diagnosis is established by in situ DNA hybridization. Formalin-fixed air-dried blood and bone marrow films stained with routine Wright's Giemsa stain are reported to provide the best view of intranuclear inclusions.[161]

Human Immunodeficiency Virus

Vertical transmission of human immunodeficiency virus (HIV) is well documented. Its transmission rate is estimated to be between 25% and 40%.[162] Jauniaux and colleagues[163] reported the histopathologic findings in 49 documented HIV-positive mothers, including placental or abortus specimens. Light microscopic findings were unremarkable and nonspecific. In 43% chorioamnionitis was present, and others manifested villous hypercellularity. Lewis and associates[164] found HIV antigen and nucleic acids in decidual leukocytes, trophoblasts, and Hofbauer cells of fetuses at 8 weeks' gestation. Therefore vertical transmission probably occurs early in gestation. In cases of high-risk or seropositive mothers, PCR optimally confirms neonatal infection.[165]

FUTURE OF THE HISTOLOGIC DIAGNOSIS OF INFECTIOUS DISEASE

Histopathologic examination of light microscopic placental slides continues to be essential for the diagnosis of intrauterine infection and the estimation of chronicity of infection. A few years from now techniques of molecular biology may become cost effective and reliable. Identification of DNA from an infectious agent does not establish the cause of a disease. PCR, for example, has misleadingly indicated CMV genome in about 50% of liver biopsies from patients with neonatal hepatitis.[166] Probably this results from laboratory contamination. The most fundamental questions of congenital infection should always be focused on the clinical facts, the pattern of placental inflammation, and immunologic and other microbiologic methods.

REFERENCES

1. Altshuler G: Placental pathology compared with clinical outcome: a retrospective blind review. Am J Dis Child 131:1224, 1977.
2. Benirschke K: Routes and types of infection in the fetus and newborn. Am J Dis Child 99:714, 1960.
3. Spiegel CA, Amsel R, Eschenbach DA, et al: Anaerobic bacteria in nonspecific vaginitis. N Engl J Med 303:601, 1980.
4. Westrom L, Evaldson G, Holmes KK, et al: Taxonomy of vaginosis: bacterial vaginosis, a definition. In Mardh PA, Taylor-Robinson D (eds): Bacterial vaginosis Stockholm, 1985, Almqvist & Wiksell, p 259.
5. Gravett MG, Nelson HP, DeRouen T, et al: Independent associations of bacterial vaginosis and *Chlamydia trachomatis* infection with adverse pregnancy outcome. JAMA 256:1899, 1986.
6. Confino E, Friberg J, Silverman S, et al: Penetration of bacteria and spermatozoa into bovine cervical mucus. Obstet Gynecol 70:134, 1987.
7. McGregor JA, Lawellin D, Franco-Buff A, et al: Protease production by microorganisms associated with reproductive tract infection. Am J Obstet Gynecol 154:109, 1986.
8. McGregor JA, French JI, Lawellin D, et al: Bacterial protease-induced reduction of chorioamniotic membrane strength and elasticity. Obstet Gynecol 69:167, 1987.
9. Sampson JE, Theve RP, Blatman RN, et al: Fetal origin of amniotic fluid polymorphonuclear leukocytes. Am J Obstet Gynecol 176:77, 1997.
10. Naeye RL: Acute chorioamnionitis, its origins and its clinical consequences. In Bellisario R, Mizejewski GJ (eds): Transplacental disorders: perinatal detection, treatment, and management (including pediatric AIDS). New York, 1990, Alan R Liss.
11. Salafia CM, Wiegl C, Silberman L: The prevalence and distribution of acute placental inflammation in uncomplicated term pregnancies. Obstet Gynecol 73:383, 1989.
12. Boura ALA, Walters WAW: Autacoids and the vascular tone in the human umbilical-placental circulation. Placenta 12:453, 1991.
13. White RP: Pharmacodynamic study of maturation and closure of human umbilical arteries. Obstet Gynecol 160:229, 1989.
14. Hyde SR, Smotherman J, Moore JI, Altshuler G: A model of bacterially induced umbilical vein spasm, relevant to fetal hypoperfusion. Obstet Gynecol 73:966, 1989.
15. Bodelsson G, Sjoberg NO, Stjernquist M: Contractile effect of endothelin in the human uterine

artery and autoradiographic localization of its binding sites. Am J Obstet Gynecol 167:745, 1992.

16. Ohno Y, Mizutani S, Kurauchi O, et al: Umbilical plasma concentration of endothelin-1 in intrapartum fetal stress: effect of fetal heart rate abnormalities. Obstet Gynecol 86:822, 1995.
17. Peevy KJ, Chalhub EG: Occult group B streptococcal infection: an important cause of intrauterine asphyxia. Am J Obstet Gynecol 146:989, 1983.
18. Faix RG, Donn SM: Association of septic shock caused by early-onset group B streptococcal sepsis and periventricular leukomalacia in the preterm infant. Pediatrics 76:415, 1985.
19. Altshuler G, Hyde S: Meconium-induced vasoconstriction: a potential cause of cerebral and other fetal hypoperfusion and of poor pregnancy outcome. J Child Neurol 4:137, 1989.
20. Navarro CN, Blanc WA: Subacute necrotizing funisitis: a variant of cord inflammation with a high rate of perinatal infection. Fetal Neonat Med 85:689, 1973.
21. Jacques SM, Qureshi F: Necrotizing funisitis: a study of 45 cases. Hum Pathol 23:1278, 1992.
22. Schwartz DA, Larsen SA, Beck-Sague C, et al: Pathology of the umbilical cord in congenital syphilis: analysis of 25 specimens using histochemistry and immunofluorescent antibody to *Treponema pallidum.* Hum Pathol 26:784, 1995.
23. Benirschke K: Congenital syphilis and necrotizing funisitis. JAMA 262:904, 1989.
24. Craver RD, Baldwin VJ: Necrotizing funisitis. Obstet Gynecol 79:64, 1992.
25. Altshuler G, Masayoshi A, Molnar-Nadasdy: Meconium-induced umbilical cord vascular necrosis and ulceration: a potential link between the placenta and poor pregnancy outcome. Obstet Gynecol 79:760, 1992.
26. Wallenburg HCS, Wladimiroff JW: Recurrence of vulvovaginal candidosis during pregnancy: comparison of miconazole vs nystatin treatment. Obstet Gynecol 48:491, 1976.
27. Delprado WJ, Baird PJ, Russell P: Placental candidiasis: report of three cases with a review of the literature. Pathology 14:191, 1982.
28. Keller MA, Sellers BB, Melish ME, et al: Systemic candidiasis in infants: a case presentation and literature review. Am J Dis Child 131:1260, 1977.
29. Whitley R, Arvin A, Prober C, et al: Predictors of morbidity and mortality in neonates with herpes simplex virus infections. N Engl J Med 324:450, 1991.
30. Witzleben CI, Driscoll SG: Possible transplacental transmission of herpes simplex infection. Pediatrics 36:192, 1965.
31. Altshuler G: Evidence of the pathogenesis of congenital herpesvirus infection: case report including description of the placenta. Am J Dis Child 127:427, 1974.
32. Hain J, Doshi N, Harger JH: Ascending transcervical herpes simplex infection with intact fetal membranes. Obstet Gynecol 56:106, 1980.
33. Hyde SR, Giacoia GP: Congenital herpes infection: placental and umbilical cord findings. Obstet Gynecol 81:852, 1993.
34. Heifetz SA, Bauman M: Necrotizing funisitis and herpes simplex infection of placental and decidual tissues: study of four cases. Hum Pathol 25:715, 1994.
35. Schwartz DA, Caldwell E: Herpes simplex virus infection of the placenta: the role of molecular pathology in the diagnosis of viral infection of placental-associated tissues. Arch Pathol Lab Med 115:1141, 1991.
36. Robb JA, Benirschke K, Mannino F, Voland J: Intrauterine latent herpes simplex virus infection. II. Latent neonatal infection. Hum Pathol 17:1210, 1986.
37. Robb JA, Benirschke K, Barmeyer R: Intrauterine latent herpes simplex virus infection. I. Spontaneous abortion. Hum Pathol 17:1196, 1986.
38. Romero R, Emamian M, Quintero R, et al: Amniotic fluid prostaglandin levels and intraamniotic infections. Lancet 1:1380, 1986.
39. Romero R, Roslansky P, Oyarzun E, et al: II. Bacterial endotoxin in amniotic fluid and its relationship to the onset of preterm labor. Am J Obstet Gynecol 158:1044, 1988.
40. Gravett MG, Eschenbach DA, Speigel-Brown, et al: Rapid diagnosis of amniotic fluid infection by gas-liquid chromatography. N Engl J Med 306: 725, 1982.
41. Cox SM, MacDonald PC, Casey ML: Assay of bacterial endotoxin (lipopolysaccharide) in human amniotic fluid: potential usefulness in diagnosis and management of preterm labor. Am J Obstet Gynecol 159:99, 1988.
42. Mitchell MD, Trautman MS, Dudly DJ: Cytokine networking in the placenta. Placenta 14:249, 1993.
43. Friers W, Beyaert R, Brouckaert P, et al: In vitro and in vivo action of tumor necrosis factor. In Bonavida B, Granger G (eds): Tumor necrosis factor: structure, mechanism of action, role in disease and therapy. Basel, 1990. Karger.
44. Chang J, Gilman SC, Lewis AJ: Interleukin-1 activates phospholipase A_2 in rabbit chondrocytes: a possible signal for IL-1 action. J Immunol 136:1283, 1986.

45. Murray MD, Phil D, Lundin-Schiller S, et al: Endothelin production by amnion and its regulation by cytokines. Obstet Gynecol 165:120, 1991.
46. Resink TJ, Scott-Burden T, Buhler FR: Activation of phospholipase A2 by endothelin in cultured vascular smooth muscle cells. Biochem Biophys Res Commun 158:279, 1989.
47. Resink TJ, Scott-Burden T, Buhler FR: Endothelin stimulates phospholipase C in cultured vascular smooth muscle cells. Biochem Biophys Res Commun 157:1360, 1988.
48. Movat HZ, Cybulsky MI, Golditz IG, et al: Acute inflammation in gram-negative infection: endotoxin, interleukin-1, tumor necrosis factor, and neutrophils. Fed Proc 46:97, 1987.
49. Bejar R, Curbelo V, Davis C, Gluck L: Premature labor. II. Bacterial sources of phospholipase. Obstet Gynecol 57:479, 1981.
50. Lamont RF, Anthony F, Myatt L, et al: Production of prostaglandin E_2 by human amnion in vitro in response to addition of media conditioned by microorganisms associated with chorioamnionitis and preterm labor. Am J Obstet Gynecol 162:819, 1990.
51. De Silva NS, Quinn PA: Endogenous activity of phospholipase A and C in *Ureaplasma urealyticum.* J Clin Microbiol 23:354, 1986.
52. Maier JAM, Hla T, Macraig T: Cyclo-oxygenase is an immediate early gene induced by interleukin-1 in human endothelial cells. J Biol Chem 265:10805, 1990.
53. Bennet PR, Henderson DJ, Moore GE: Changes in expression of the cyclo-oxygenase gene in human fetal membranes and placenta with labor. Am J Obstet Gynecol 167:212, 1992.
54. Romero R, Sirtori M, Oyarzun E, et al: Infection and labor. V. Prevalence, microbiology, and clinical significance of intra-amniotic infection in women with preterm labor and intact membranes. Am J Obstet Gynecol 161:817, 1989.
55. Romero R, Sepulveda W, Mazor M, et al: The natural interleukin-1 receptor antagonist in term and preterm parturition. Am J Obstet Gynecol 167:863, 1992.
56. Romero R, Tartakovsky B: The natural interleukin-1 receptor antagonist prevents interleukin-1-induced preterm delivery in mice. Am J Obstet Gynecol 167:1041, 1992.
57. Bry K, Lappalainen B: Interleukin-4 and transforming growth factor-β1 modulate the production of interleukin-1 receptor antagonist and of prostaglandin E_2 by decidual cells. Am J Obstet Gynecol 170:1194, 1994.
58. Lieles WC, Van Voorhis WC: Nomenclature and biological significance of cytokines involved in inflammation and the host immune response. J Infect Dis 172:1573, 1995.
59. Darby MJ, Caritis SN, Shen-Schwartz S: Placental abruption in the preterm gestation: an association with chorioamnionitis. Obstet Gynecol 74:88, 1989.
60. Romero R, Mazor M, Morrotti R, et al: Infection and labor. VII. Microbial invasion of the amniotic cavity in spontaneous rupture of membranes at term. Am J Obstet Gynecol 166:129, 1992.
61. Gibbs RS, Blanco JD, St. Clair PJ, Castaneda YS: Quantitative bacteriology of amniotic fluid from women with clinical intra-amniotic infection at term. J Infect Dis 145:1, 1982.
62. Altshuler G, Hyde S: Fusobacteria: an important cause of chorioamnionitis. Arch Pathol Lab Med 109:739, 1985.
63. Altshuler G, Hyde S: Clinicopathologic considerations of fusobacteria chorioamnionitis. Acta Obstet Gynecol Scand 67:513, 1988.
64. Easterling TR, Garite TJ: *Fusobacterium:* Anaerobic occult amnionitis and premature labor. Obstet Gynecol 66:825, 1985.
65. Ueno K, Sugihara PT, Bricknell KS, et al: Comparison of characteristics of gram negative anaerobic bacilli isolated from feces of individuals in Japan and the United States. In Balows A (ed): Anaerobic bacteria, role in disease. Springfield Ill., 1974, Charles C Thomas.
66. Rusin P, Adam R, Petersen E, et al: *Haemophilus influenzae:* an important cause of maternal and neonatal infections. Obstet Gynecol 77:92, 1991.
67. Campognone P, Singer DB: Neonatal sepsis due to nontypable *Haemophilus influenzae.* Am J Dis Child 140:117, 1986.
68. Wallace RJ, Baker CJ, Quinones FJ, et al: Nontypable *Haemophilus influenzae* (biotype 4) as a neonatal, maternal, and genital pathogen. Rev Infect Dis 5:123, 1983.
69. Berk SL, Holtsclaw SA, Wiener SL, Smith JK: Nontypable *Haemophilus influenzae* in the elderly. Arch Intern Med 142:537, 1982.
70. Marks MI, Welch DF: Diagnosis of bacterial infections of the newborn infant. Clin Perinatol 8:537, 1981.
71. Robbins JB, McCracken GH, Gotschurch EC, et al: *Escherichia coli* K1 capsular polysaccharide associated with neonatal meningitis. N Engl J Med 190:1216, 1974.
72. McCracken GH, Sarff LD, Glode MP, et al: Relation between *Escherichia coli* K1 capsular antigen and clinical outcome in neonatal meningitis. Lancet 2:246, 1974.

73. Chow AW, Leake RD, Yamauchi T, et al: The significance of anaerobes in neonatal bacteremia: analysis of 23 cases and review of the literature. Pediatrics 54:736, 1974.
74. Feder HM: *Bacteroides fragilis* meningitis. Rev Infect Dis 9:783, 1987.
75. Evaldson GR, Malmborg AS, Nord CE: Premature rupture of the membranes and ascending infection. Br J Obstet Gynaecol 89:793, 1982.
76. Kasper DL, Fiddian AP, Tabaqchali S: Rapid diagnosis of *Bacteroides* infections by indirect immunofluorescence assay of clinical specimens. Lancet 2:239, 1979.
77. Dillon HC, Gray E, Pass MA, Gray BM: Anorectal and vaginal carriage of group B streptococci during pregnancy. J Infect Dis 145:794, 1982.
78. Bascom AF: Carriage of group B streptococci during pregnancy: a puzzler. J Infect Dis 145:789, 1982.
79. Ancona RJ, Ferrieri P, Williams P: Maternal factors that enhance the acquisition of group B streptococci by newborn infants. J Med Microbiol 13:273, 1980.
80. Hellerqvist CG, Rojas J, Green RS, et al: Studies of group B beta-hemolytic streptococcus. I. Isolation and partial characterization of an extracellular toxin. Pediatr Res 15:892, 1981.
81. Sandberg K, Engelhardt B, Hellerqvist C, Sundell H: Pulmonary response to group B streptococcal toxin in young lambs. J Appl Physiol 2024, 1987.
82. Roitt I, Brostoff J, Male D: Immunology. St. Louis, 1985, Mosby.
83. Jann K, Westphal O: In Sela M (ed): The antigens. Vol III. New York, 1975, Academic Press.
84. Christensen RD, Rothstein G, Hill HR, Pincus SH: Treatment of experimental group B streptococcal infection with hybridoma antibody. Pediatr Res 18:1093, 1984.
85. Baker CJ, Rench MA, Edwards MS, et al: Immunization of pregnant women with a polysaccharide vaccine of group B *Streptococcus.* N Engl J Med 319:1180, 1988.
86. Santos JI, Shigeoka AO, Rote NS, Hill HR: Protective efficacy of a modified immune serum globulin in experimental group B streptococcal infection. J Pediatr 99:873, 1981.
87. Fleming DW, Cochi SL, MacDonald KL, et al: Pasteurized milk as a vehicle of infection in a outbreak of listeriosis. N Engl J Med 312, 1985.
88. Lamont RJ, Postlethwaite R: Carriage of *Listeria monocytogenes* and related species in pregnant and non-pregnant women in Aberdeen, Scotland. J Infect 13:187, 1986.
89. Hamada M, Kuroiwa A, Matsumoto T, et al: Modification of protective mechanisms against *Listeria monocytogenes* during pregnancy. J Clin Lab Immunol 6:169, 1981.
90. Luft BJ, Remington JS: Effect of pregnancy on resistance to *Listeria monocytogenes* and *Toxoplasma gondii* infections in mice. Infect Immunol 38:1164, 1982.
91. Bortolussi R, Campbell N, Krause V: Dynamics of *Listeria monocytogenes* type 4b infection in pregnant and infant rats. Clin Invest Med 7:273, 1984.
92. Gray ML: Genital listeriosis as a cause of repeated abortion. Lancet 2:296, 1960.
93. Visintine Am, Oleske JM, Nahmias AJ: *Listeria monocytogenes* infection in infants and children. Am J Dis Child 131:393, 1977.
94. McGregor D, Chen-Woan M: The cell response to *Listeria monocytogenes* is mediated by a heterogeneous population of immunospecific T cells. Clin Invest Med 7:243, 1984.
95. Speer CP, Amburso DR, Grimsley J, et al: Oxidative metabolism in cord blood monocytes and monocyte-derived macrophages. Infect Immun 50:919, 1985.
96. Wilson CB, Westall J, Johnson L, et al: Decreased production of gamma-interferon by human neonatal cells. J Clin Invest 77:860, 1986.
97. Bortolussi R, Issekutz A, Faulkner A: Opsonization of *Listeria monocytogenes* type 4b by human adult and newborn sera. Infect Immunol 52:493, 1986.
98. Kazuo Y, Price JT, Altshuler G: A placental view of the diagnosis and pathogenesis of congenital listerosis. Am J Obstet Gynecol 129:703, 1977.
99. Altshuler G, Rettig P: A rat model of *Chlamydia trachomatis* amniotic infection syndrome. Presented at the XIV International Congress of the International Academy of Pathology, Sydney, Australia, October 15, 1982.
100. Kundsin RB, Driscoll SG, Ming PML: Strain of *Mycoplasma* associated with human reproductive failure. Science 157:1573, 1967.
101. Madan E, Meyer MP, Amortegui AJ: Isolation of genital mycoplasmas and *Chlamydia trachomatis* in stillborn and neonatal autopsy material. Arch Pathol Lab Med 112:749, 1988.
102. Madan E, Meyer MP, Amortegui AJ: Histologic manifestations of perinatal mycoplasmal infection. Arch Pathol Lab Med 113:465, 1989.
103. Nugent RP: *Ureaplasma urealyticum* and pregnancy outcome: results of an observational study and clinical trial. Am J Epidemiol 128:929, 1988.
104. Romero R, Mazor M, Oyarzun E, et al: Is genital colonization with *Mycoplasma hominis* or *Ure-*

aplasma urealyticum associated with prematurity/low birth weight? Obstet Gynecol 73:532, 1989.
105. Hewish MJ, Birch DF, Fairly KF: *Ureaplasma urealyticum* serotypes in urinary tract disease. J Clin Microbiol 23:149, 1986.
106. Altshuler G: Placental villitis of unknown etiology: harbinger of serious disease? A four months' experience of nine cases. J Reprod Med 11:215, 1973.
107. Altshuler G, Russell P: The human placental villitides: a review of chronic intrauterine infection. In Grundman E, Kirsten WH (eds): Current topics in pathology. New York, 1975, Springer-Verlag.
108. Russell P: Inflammatory lesions of the human placenta. III. The histopathology of villitis of unknown etiology. Placenta 1:227, 1980.
109. Labarrere CA, McIntyre JA, Faulk WP: Immunohistological evidence that villitis in normal human term placentas is an immunologic lesion. Am J Obstet Gynecol 162:515, 1990.
110. Kliman HJ: Commentary: the placenta revealed. Am J Pathol 143:333, 1993.
111. Altshuler G, Russell P, Ermocilla R: The placental pathology of small for gestational age infants. Am J Obstet Gynecol 121:351, 1975.
112. Labarrere C, Althabe O, Telenta M: Chronic villitis of unknown aetiology in placentae of idiopathic small for gestational age infants. Placenta 3:309, 1982.
113. Russell P: Inflammatory lesions of the human placenta. II. Am J Diagn Gynecol Obstet 11:339, 1979.
114. Heyborne KD, Witkin SS, McGregor JA: Tumor necrosis factor in midtrimester amniotic fluid is associated with impaired intrauterine fetal growth. Am J Obstet Gynecol 167:920, 1992.
115. Evans RD, Argiles JM, Williamson D: Metabolic effects of tumor necrosis factor (cachectin) and interleukin-1. Clin Sci 77:257, 1989.
116. Redline RW, Abramowsky CR: Clinical and pathologic aspects of recurrent villitis. Hum Pathol 16:727, 1985.
117. Garcia AGP, Basso NGD, Fonseca MEF, Outanni HN: Congenital echovirus infection: morphologic and virological study of fetal and placental tissue. J Pathol 160:123, 1990.
118. Abramowsky C, Beyer-Patterson P, Cortinas E: Nonsyphilitic spirochetosis in second trimester fetuses. Pediatr Pathol 11:827, 1991.
119. Rotbart HA: PCR amplification of enteroviruses. In Innis MA, Gelfand DH, Sninsky JJ, White TJ (eds): PCR protocols: a guide to methods and applications. San Diego, 1990, Academic Press.
120. Garcia AGP, Basso NGD, Fonseca MEF, et al: Enterovirus associated placental morphology: a light, virological, electron microscopic and immunohistological study. Placenta 12:533, 1991.
121. Stagno S, Pass RF, Dworsky ME, Alford CA: Congenital and perinatal cytomegalovirus infections. Semin Perinatol 7:31, 1983.
122. Maciejewski JP, Bruening EE, Donahue RE, et al: Infection of hematopoietic progenitor cells by human cytomegalovirus. Blood 80:170, 1992.
123. Numazaki Y, Yano N, Morizuka T, et al: Primary infection with human cytomegalovirus: virus isolation from healthy infants and pregnant women. Am J Epidemiol 91:410, 1970.
124. Weber B, Opp M, Born HJ, et al: Laboratory diagnosis of congenital human cytomegalovirus infection using polymerase chain reaction and shell vial culture. Infection 20:155, 1992.
125. Ohyama M, Motegi Y, Goto A, et al: Ascending placentofetal infection caused by cytomegalovirus. Br J Obstet Gynaecol 99:770, 1992.
126. Lang DJ, Kummer JF, Hartly DP: Cytomegalovirus in semen: persistence and demonstration in extracellular fluids. N Engl J Med 291:121, 1974.
127. Benirschke K, Mendoza GR, Bazeley PL: Placental and fetal manifestations of cytomegalovirus infection. Virchows Arch B Cell Pathol 16:121, 1974.
128. Schwartz DA, Khan R, Stoll B: Characterization of the fetal inflammatory response to cytomegalovirus placentitis: an immunological study. Arch Pathol Lab Med 116:21, 1992.
129. Sinzger C, Muntefering H, Loning T, et al: Cell types infected in human cytomegalovirus placentitis identified by immunohistochemical double staining. Virchows Arch A Pathol Anat Histopathol 423:249, 1993.
130. Gleaves CA, Smith TF, Shuster EA, Pearson GR: Comparison of standard tube and shell vial culture techniques for detection of cytomegalovirus in clinical specimens. J Clin Microbiol 21:217, 1985.
131. Muhlemann K, Miller RK, Metlay L, Menegus MA: Cytomegalovirus infection of the human placenta: an immunocytochemical study. Hum Pathol 23:1234, 1992.
132. Nakamura Y, Sakuma S, Ohta Y, et al: Detection of human cytomegalovirus gene in placental chronic villitis by polymerase chain reaction. Hum Pathol 25:815, 1994.
133. Kaufman RE, Olansky DC, Wiesner PJ: The FTA-ABS (IgM) test for neonatal congenital syphilis: a critical review. J Am Vener Dis Assoc 1:79:1974.
134. Russell P, Altshuler G: Placental abnormalities of congenital syphilis: a neglected aid to diagnosis. Am J Dis Child 128:160, 1974.

135. Genest DR, Choi-Hong SR, Tate JE, et al: Diagnosis of congenital syphilis from placental examination: comparison of histopathology, Steiner stain, and polymerase chain reaction for *Treponema pallidum* DNA. Hum Pathol 27:366, 1996.
136. Qureshi F, Jacques SM, Reyes MP: Placental histopathology in syphilis. Hum Pathol 24:779, 1993.
137. Greco MA, Wieczorek R, Sachdev R, et al: Phenotype of villous stromal cells in placentas with cytomegalovirus, syphilis, and nonspecific villitis. Am J Pathol 141:835, 1992.
138. Hunter EF, Greer PW, Swisher BL, et al: Immunofluorescent staining of *Treponema* in tissues fixed with formalin. Arch Pathol Lab Med 108:878, 1984.
139. Wicher K, Noordhoek GT, Abbruscato F, Wicher V: Detection of *Treponema pallidum* in early syphilis by DNA amplification. J Clin Microbiol 30:497, 1992.
140. Desmonts G, Convreur J: Congenital toxoplasmosis. N Engl J Med 290:1110, 1974.
141. Benirschke K, Driscoll SG: Toxoplasmosis. In The pathology of the human placenta. New York, 1967, Springer-Verlag.
142. Altshuler G: Toxoplasmosis as a cause of hydranencephaly. Am J Dis Child 125:251, 1973.
143. Popek EJ: Granulomatous villitis due to *Toxoplasma gondii.* Pediatr Pathol 12:281, 1992.
144. Hohlfeld P, Daffos F, Costa JM, et al: Prenatal diagnosis of congenital toxoplasmosis with a polymerase chain reaction test on amniotic fluid. N Engl J Med 331:695, 1994.
145. Gregg NM: Congenital cataract following German measles in the mother. Trans Opthamol Soc Augt 3:35, 1941.
146. Driscoll SG: Histopathology of gestational rubella. Am J Dis Child 118:49, 1969.
147. Ornoy A, Segal S, Nishmi M, et al: Fetal and placental pathology in gestational rubella. Am J Obstet Gynecol 116:949, 1973.
148. Tanemura M, Suzumori K, Yagami Y, Katow S: Diagnosis of fetal rubella infection with reverse transcriptase and nested polymerase chain reaction: a study of 34 cases diagnosed in fetuses. Am J Obstet Gynecol 174:578, 1996.
149. Brunell PA: Varicella in pregnancy, the fetus, and the newborn: problems in management. J Infect Dis 166(suppl):S42, 1992.
150. Enders G, Miller E, Cradock-Watson J, et al: Consequences of varicella and herpes zoster in pregnancy: prospective study of 1739 cases. Lancet 343:1548-1551, 1994.
151. Qureshi F, Jacques SM: Maternal varicella during pregnancy: correlation of maternal history and fetal outcome with placental histopathology. Hum Pathol 27:191, 1996.
152. Robertson NJ, McKeever PA: Fetal and placental pathology in two cases of maternal varicella infection. Pediatr Pathol 12:545, 1992.
153. Hyde SR, Benirschke K: Gestational psittacosis: case report and literature review. Mod Pathol 10:602, 1997.
154. Wong SY, Gray ES, Buxton D, et al: Acute placentitis and spontaneous abortion caused by *Chlamydia psittaci* of sheep origin: a histological and ultrastructure study. J Clin Pathol 38:707, 1985.
155. Gray ES: Parvovirus B19 infection in the fetus, newborn, and child. Curr Opin Infect Dis 4:485, 1991.
156. Risks associated with human parvovirus B19 infection. MMWR 38:81, 1989.
157. Schwarz TF, Nerlich A, Hottentrager B, et al: Parvovirus B19 infection of the fetus: histology and in situ hybridization. Am J Clin Pathol 96:121, 1991.
158. Shmoys S, Kaplan C: Parvovirus and pregnancy. Clin Obstet Gynecol 33:268, 1990.
159. Berry PJ, Gray ES, Porter HJ, Burton PA: Parvovirus infection of the human fetus and newborn. Semin Diagn Pathol 9:4, 1992.
160. Caul EO, Usher J, Burton PA: Intrauterine infection with human parvovirus B19: a light and electron microscopy study. J Med Virol 24:55, 1988.
161. Krause JR, Penchansky L, Knisely AS: Morphological diagnosis of parvovirus B19 infection. Arch Pathol Lab Med 116:178, 1992.
162. MacDonald MG, Ginzburg HM, Bolan JC: HIV infection in pregnancy: epidemiology and clinical management. J Acquir Immune Defic Syndr 4:100, 1991.
163. Jauniaux E, Nessmann C, Imbert MC, et al: Morphological aspects of the placenta in HIV pregnancies. Placenta 9:633, 1988.
164. Lewis SH, Reynolds-Kohler C, Fox HE, et al: HIV-1 in trophoblastic and Hofbauer cells, and haematological precursors in eight week fetuses. Lancet 335:565, 1990.
165. Escaich S, Wallon M, Baginski I, et al: Comparison of HIV detection by virus isolation in lymphocyte cultures and molecular amplification of HIV DNA and DNA by PCR in offspring of seropositive mothers. J Acquir Immune Defic Syndr 4:130, 1991.
166. Chang M, Huang H, Huang E, et al: Polymerase chain reaction to detect human cytomegalovirus in livers of infants with neonatal hepatitis. Gastroenterology 103:1022, 1992.

14

Molecular Biology of the Placenta with Focus on Special Placental Studies of Infants with Intrauterine Growth Retardation

Dagmar K. Kalousek, Wendy Robinson, Brendan Harrington, and Valia S. Lestou

The placenta is probably the least studied of human organs, since for a long time it has been viewed as having a passive role, interposed between the maternal and fetal circulations and representing a physiologic sieve. In reality the placenta is anything but passive and would be better described as having a permissive role, regulating the growth of the fetus in utero and leaving a legacy for postnatal development.

The desired outcome of every pregnancy is a healthy mother with a healthy baby whose future well-being is secure. In the current technologically oriented world many parents feel angry and upset if the outcome of pregnancy is anything other than this, and physicians too are often at a loss to understand poor pregnancy outcomes. Considerable progress has been made in understanding of the pathogenesis of congenital abnormalities, intrauterine infection, and genetic defects, but much other pregnancy-related pathology remains unexplained.

Most studies of the placenta in pathologic situations focus on structural gross and microscopic features such as placental size, microscopic appearance of villi, blood vessel diameter, and presence of fibrinoid deposits. Such studies may supply the information on what has happened but not how or why. Until the how and why questions are answered, the possibility of preventive interventions is limited.

Molecular biology promises to be a powerful tool for the investigator who wishes to move beyond simply describing the changes in the placenta in embryopathologic states and to understand how those changes arose. The techniques of molecular biology have exploded into every area of investigation in the life sciences and revolutionized the knowledge of many fundamental processes. In view of the unglamorous position of placental research, it is perhaps not surprising that only recently has molecular biology been applied to the placenta. Yet it may be from the molecular biology of embryogenesis and placental function that we come to understand the most basic and important cellular mechanisms such as control of cellular differentiation.

Working on the genotypic characteristics of the placenta alone is also insufficient. Genes are transcribed in a controlled manner, and these transcripts are often modified and may or may not be immediately translated into a polypeptide product. This polypeptide product is usually subject to considerable modification before it acquires its final functional form and location. The functional activity of proteins determines an organism's phenotype, so additional studies should be directed to this area. Studying the activity of proteins in vitro and in vivo is conventionally the realm of the biochemist and the physiologist. Since abnormal proteins (in amount or structure) are the product of altered gene expression, complex molecular genetic techniques will play an increasing role in the elucidation of placental pathophysiology and cooperation among clinicians, pathologists, physiologists, and geneticists will be necessary to achieve advances.

FETAL AND PLACENTAL GROWTH

When the possible contribution of the placenta to adverse pregnancy outcome is studied, some characteristics of placental and fetal growth must be borne in mind. The progress of gestation is conventionally divided into development of the embryo and that of the fetus. (For a pictorial overview of mammalian embryogenesis, see Drews.[1] For a more comprehensive scientific review, see Pederson and Burdsal.[2]) The first 2 postconceptual weeks, termed the preembryonic period, include fertilization, preimplantation and implantation, and early differentiation of cell lineages in the blastocyst. In the embryonic period, from 2 to 8 weeks' gestation, the major differentiation and morphogenesis of organs occur. The remainder of gestation is called the fetal period and is the time of an accelerated fetal growth and increase in the size and maturation of organs. Some organs such as the brain and lung continue to differentiate even postnatally.

The above classification pays no attention to events in the placenta and its early progenitor cell lineages or the balance between placental and fetal growth. The preimplantation period is predominantly a phase of proliferation of cells that do not contribute to the fetal tissues. At the blastocyst stage most cells are committed to placental rather than embryonic development.[3] Specific cells of the inner cell mass, which eventually form the embryo, are few in number and less differentiated than trophectodermal cells as judged by the formation of gap junctions between cells.[4] The formation of gap junctions seems to be a marker for the terminal commitment and loss of totipotency during cell differentiation. During this period programmed cell death is already occurring[5] as a mechanism for morphogenesis.

Growth of the placenta greatly exceeds growth of the fetus gram for gram during the embryonic period. Not until well into the fetal period, around 14 weeks, does the fetus begin to grow faster than the placenta. At all stages of gestation, growth of the placenta and the embryo/fetus is discordant (Fig. 14–1). Investigators therefore should remember that the same event may affect the fetus and the placenta differently at different points in gestation depending on their growth phase. It is also possible that compromised functional development of the placenta at a given time will affect the fetus later in gestation; that is, a lag between the placental insult and fetal injury may be apparent. An example of this is intrauterine growth retardation (IUGR). Adverse effects on the placenta in the first or second trimester may not produce obvious fetal growth retardation (as measured by simple linear or circumferential ultrasound measures of fetal growth) until the second or third trimester. In this situation studies of the morphology and physiology of the placenta from the second or third trimester may miss the time of onset and the initial pathologic events.

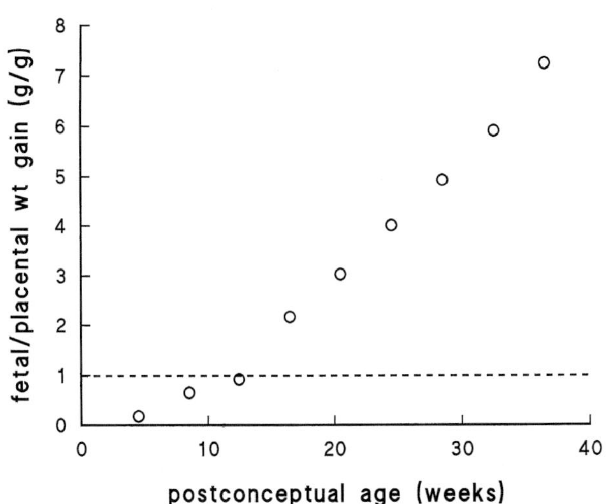

Figure 14–1. Relative weight gain of placenta and fetus. Values less than 1 indicate that the absolute growth of the placenta is faster than that of the fetus, that is, that the placenta grows by more than 1 g for every gram of fetal weight gain. Values greater than 1 indicate that the fetus has overtaken the placenta in absolute weight gain. The value of exactly 1 occurs at approximately 14 weeks' gestation. (Plotted from data in Kaufman.[145])

Table 14–1. Illustration of the Concept That Categorization of Birth Weight as Either Normal or Low and the Presence or Absence of Intrauterine Growth Retardation Are Not Concordant in All Cases

	Normal Birth Weight (appropriate for gestational age)	Low Birth Weight (small for gestational age)
Growth retarded in utero	Occult IUGR	True IUGR
Normal growth in utero	Normal	Small but normal

IUGR, Intrauterine growth retardation.

Fetal Intrauterine Growth Retardation

Many different problems in pregnancy can lead to the same endpoint: a smaller than expected baby as a result of IUGR. These small babies suffer a greater than expected amount of morbidity and mortality.[6]

Although extensive research is aimed at understanding IUGR, a widespread problem in studying IUGR is rarely acknowledged. Most studies adopt a stated lower percentile limit of birth weight, usually the 5th or 3rd percentile for birth weight on population charts. As with any population variable, the further from the mean a value lies, the greater the probability that a pathologic process is involved. However, even the 3rd percentile for birth weight (approximately 2 standard deviations below the mean) includes some healthy normal but small babies, especially if no allowance is made for ethnicity or maternal stature. These healthy but small babies have not had retarded growth in utero; they have achieved their full genetic growth potential. Including these babies in the study group diminishes the magnitude of any parameter of an active pathologic condition. Furthermore, the group with a birth weight above the given percentile, who will form the control population for normal data to be compared with the study group, will inevitably contain babies who have had their growth retarded in utero but not sufficiently to reduce birth weight below the 3rd percentile (see Table 14–1 for an illustration of this concept). These unsuspected cases in the control group will shift the mean of the control data closer to the mean of the study group and away from the true normal population mean. Such a shift makes statistically significant differences between study and control populations harder to detect. Data on birth weight are universally available, making retrospective data collection easy, but on their own they are a crude measure of fetal well-being. Other measurements, such as body length, head circumference, upper arm circumference, skinfold thickness, and placental weight, can add useful information on intrauterine fetal growth.[7,8]

Epidemiology of Fetal and Placental Growth

Although the role of the placenta ends with delivery, an expanding body of evidence from epidemiologic studies indicates that future health correlates strongly with fetal weight, placental weight, and the ratio between the two.[9] This is particularly so if groups are divided on the basis of weight gain in the first postnatal year, when weight gain no longer depends on the placenta. This effect of placental weight is seen in some of the most significant diseases causing morbidity and mortality in developed societies; non-insulin-dependent diabetes, coronary heart disease, and hypertension are among them. To explain these striking correlations Barker has proposed that postnatal metabolism may be programmed irreversibly in utero. Thus a fetus that suffers in utero starvation of essential nutrients such as amino acids or carbohydrate may be programmed to survive on a poor supply, and when it encounters adequate or excess supply in adult life, a greater proportion of any excess is diverted into lipid storage and hence atherosis. There is as yet no physiologic evidence to support this programming hypothesis, but the epidemiologic association is strong. If the hypothesis is true, altered gene expression must be programmed into a fetus in utero on the basis of its metabolic relationship with the placenta. Studies of the fetoplacental metabolism of glucose and certain amino acids and the transport of oxygen show that when supply is chronically compromised, the needs of the placenta are given priority at the expense of the fetus.[10] Studies on the birth weights of babies born to mothers who were themselves starved in utero have produced even more interesting possibilities. World War II produced severe deprivation in the Netherlands during the winter of 1944–1945. Nutritional and birth weight information was recorded, and the progress of children born during this "Dutch hunger winter" has been studied. The female children have had their own children, and an effect on birth weight appears to extend into the second generation; the grandchildren of women who were starved are smaller than expected by comparison with matched controls.[11] This may point to a programming of the ability of female fetuses to nourish their later offspring while they are still in utero.[9] It is said to represent a genetic memory of periodic famine (in the form of metabolic adaptation) passed from generation to generation. Evidence suggests that fetal insulin and insulin-like growth factors are the intermediary agents through which the availability of nutrition affects fetal growth.[12]

Although the significance of expression and imprinting of placental genes or confined placental mosaicism in the etiology of pathophysiologic states of pregnancy has not been established, genetic studies of these phenomena show great promise. Every person's start in life is determined by the activity of his or her placenta, and how far into adulthood the placental effect reaches only future studies will accurately document.

CONFINED PLACENTAL MOSAICISM

In most pregnancies the chromosomal complement detected in the fetus is also present in the placenta. The detection of an identical chromosomal complement in both the fetus and its placenta has always been expected, since both develop from the same zygote. However, in 1% to 2% of viable pregnancies studied by chorionic villous sampling (CVS) at 9 to 11 weeks of gestation, the cytogenetic abnormality, most often trisomy, is found to be confined to the placenta, a situation known as confined placental mosaicism (CPM).[13–16] CPM was first described in the placentas of term infants born with unexplained IUGR.[17] Contrary to generalized mosaicism, which is characterized by the presence of two or more karyotypically different cell lines within both the fetus and its placenta, CPM represents tissue-specific chromosomal mosaicism affecting the placenta only. CPM diagnosis is usually made when after the diagnosis of chromosomal trisomy incompatible with a liveborn infant (e.g., trisomy 16) in the CVS sample, the second prenatal testing (amniotic fluid culture or fetal blood culture analysis) shows a normal diploid karyotype (Table 14–2).

The three types of CPM are categorized according to the specific placental cell lineage(s) exhibiting the abnormal cell line (Fig. 14–2 and Table 14–2). Placental mosaicism can be confined to trophoblast (type I), chorionic stroma (type II), or both cell lineages (type III). CPM can arise either in a diploid conception (mitotic CPM) or in a viable chromosomally abnormal conceptus (meiotic CPM). CPM is the result of viable postzygotic mitotic mutation(s) occurring in either the progenitor cells of specific placental cell lineages (abnormal mitosis produces trisomy) or the true embryoblasts (abnormal mitosis results in the loss of one trisomic chromosome, restoring disomy). A diploid nonmosaic fetus with high levels of chromosomal trisomy confined to both cell lineages of the placenta (type III CPM) implies that the conceptus was originally trisomic (meiotic CPM). A

Table 14–2. Frequencies of Generalized and Confined Placental Mosaicism

Type of Mosaicism	Number of Pregnancies	Percent
Generalized	5:5612	0.19
Confined placental	51:5612	1.9
Type I: trophoblast	20:51	0.8
Type II: chorionic (villous) stroma	24:51	0.9
Type III: trophoblast and villous stroma	7:51	0.2

Data from Wang, Rubin, and Williams[146] and Kalousek and Vekemans.[147]

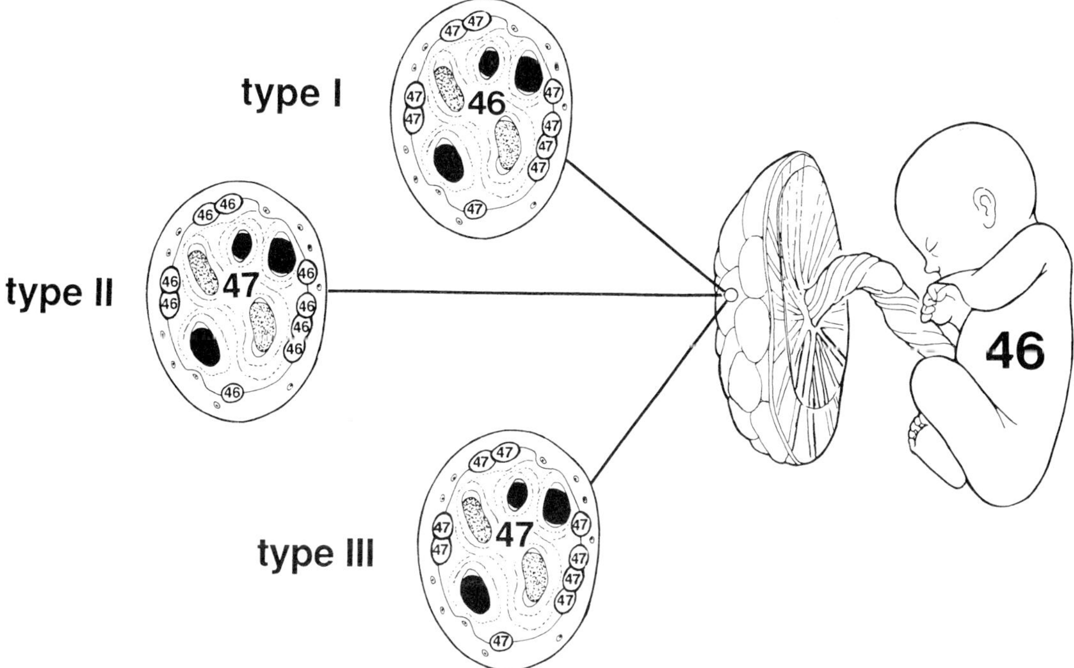

Figure 14–2. Three different types of confined placental mosaicism: I, trisomic trophoblast and diploid chorionic stroma; II, diploid trophoblast and trisomic chorionic stroma; and III, trisomic trophoblast and chorionic stroma. In all three types the mosaicism is confined to the placenta and the fetus is either nonmosaic diploid (in most cases) or nonmosaic aneuploid (in which case the cytotrophoblast is diploid).

CPM involving trisomy 16 is usually labeled as CPM 16. No nomenclature has been designated for the various types of CPM.

Development

Discrepancy in chromosomal constitution between the placental tissue and the embryonic/fetal tissues is the result of complex developmental events during early embryogenesis. The cell lineage involvement and the timing of the mitotic abnormality resulting in the second viable cell line are equally important in the final cell distribution.

In rodents, between the eight-cell stage and the blastocyst, the cells in the innermost layers contribute more frequently to the inner cell mass formation than do the peripheral cells.[18] The elegant experiments with manufactured hexaparental mice performed by Markert and Petters[3] have demonstrated that the wall of the blastocyst gives rise exclusively to the trophoblast. The complete embryo is derived from only three cells of the inner cell mass. The remaining cells of the inner cell mass contribute to the development of extraembryonic mesenchyme and extraembryonic structures such as the yolk sac and allantois.

The morphogenesis of human cleavage embryos has not been studied experimentally in as much detail as that of mouse embryos.[19] However, the histologic appearance of the inner cell mass and the pattern of formation of the embryo proper in the two species suggest great similarity in their early stages of embryogenesis.[20] The knowledge that only a few embryonic progenitor cells are selected from the inner cell mass at the blastocyst stage profoundly changed the understanding of the development of human mosaic morulas and blastocysts.[21]

The cell lineage involved in the chromosomal mutation and the time at which the second viable cell lines appears determine whether the mosaic morula develops into a conceptus characterized by generalized chromosomal mosaicism expressed in both the placenta and the fetus or by CPM recognized for its chromosomal dichotomy between placental chorionic and embryonic/fetal tissues (Fig. 14–2). When the second viable cell line arises at or shortly after the first postzygotic division, the distribution of the cells of both genotypes in the morula is more or less even. This increases the possibility of generalized chromosomal mosaicism expression in both the embryo and the placental trophoblast and chorion. When, however, the second viable cell line emerges at the morula/blastocyst stage, it is the position of a mutant cell in the morula/blastocyst that determines the impact of cell lineage on the formation of the embryo proper. An unequal distribution of both cell lines in the inner cell mass increases the probability that only one cell line will be involved in the formation of the embryo proper and that a mosaicism confined to the trophoblast or the chorion or both will result (Fig. 14–2). CPM can probably originate after the morula/blastocyst stage; however, no experimental data are available on the representation of the second cell line in term placentas.

Among several types of postzygotic mitotic errors that can result in CPM, the most significant is correction of aneuploidy. As illustrated in Figure 14–3, the outcome of the postzygotic loss of the extra chromosome depends mainly on the cell lineage involved but is also influenced by the timing of the correction and the nature and type of chromosome involved.

When the trisomic chromosome is lost in the trophoblast progenitors (epithelial lining of the placenta), a viable nonmosaic trisomic infant is delivered (Fig. 14–3*A*). For example, mosaicism involving diploidy in the cytotrophoblast appears to be required for the rescue of trisomy 13 and 18 conceptions.[22] If the correction of aneuploidy involves the loss of the extra chromosome in the embryoblast lineage, a diploid nonmosaic fetus/newborn develops supported by a trisomic placenta (Fig. 14–3*B*).

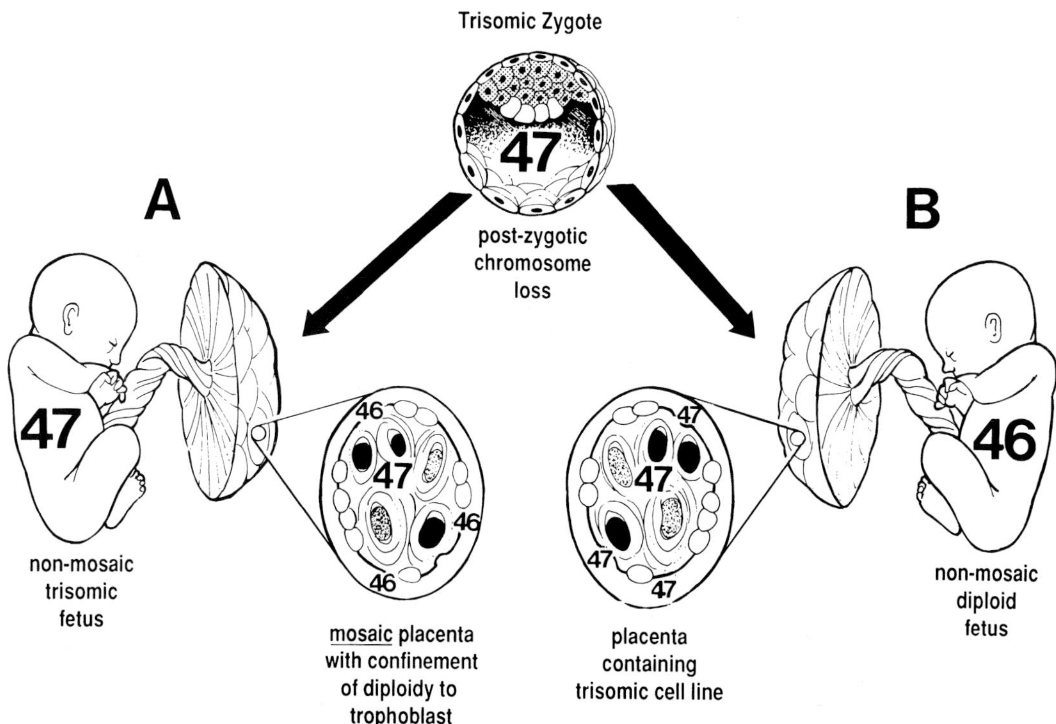

Figure 14–3. Trisomic zygote rescue. **A,** Intrauterine survival of a trisomic fetus correlates with the presence of a diploid cell line in the trophoblast resulting from early postzygotic mitotic loss of the trisomic chromosome. **B,** Mitotic mutation in the embryonic progenitor cells results in a diploid fetus and trisomic placenta.

Depending on the parental origin of the lost chromosome, the two remaining chromosomes in the fetus may be of both maternal and paternal origin (biparental disomy [BPD] or of only single-parent origin (uniparental disomy [UPD]). The concept of UPD in humans was introduced and later excellently reviewed by Eric Engel.[23] On average, one third of the aneuploidy correction would be expected to result in fetal UPD. Using this figure and assuming that all cases of CPM type III result from trisomic zygote rescue, one can estimate that the prevalence of UPD around 9 to 10 weeks' gestation is about 8:10,000.

Clinical and Genetic Consequences

CPM may be associated with a spectrum of fetal manifestations ranging from normal pregnancy outcome to intrauterine death of a chromosomally normal fetus, IUGR, or even unsuspected delivery of a larger than normal fetus.[24] It has been estimated that approximately 16% to 21% of pregnancies with CPM show prenatal or perinatal complications.[25,26] Other clinical reports have suggested that the effect of CPM is minimal or nonexistent.[27] When placental mosaicism detected by first-trimester CVS has been associated with poor prenatal or perinatal outcome (Table 14–3), it has been postulated that either chromosome-specific mosaicism is responsible for suboptimal placental function and associated pregnancy complications or the fetus had UPD (see below).

Recently it was shown that the effects of CPM on development depend on the origin of the extra chromosome in the placenta. Meiotic origin is highly correlated with type III CPM and elevated risk of pregnancy complications, whereas mitotic origin is found in types I and II and shows a specifically low risk of IUGR.[28]

The outcome of CPM appears to depend also on the nature of chromosome abnormality and the number and the viability of placental cells with an abnormal chromosomal complement. Trisomy 16 is the most common aneuploidy observed in CPM.[29] Other frequently reported aneuploidies are trisomies 2, 7, and 22. Interestingly, there is good correlation between trisomy 16 and 22 in chromosomally abnormal spontaneous abortions, the prominent involvement of trisomy 16 and 22 in CPM, and meiotic origin in CPM 16 and 22. On the other hand, for chromosome 7 it is the mitotic origin, since this chromosome is rare in spontaneous abortions.[30] Studies of pregnancies with CPM type II show both meiotic and mitotic origin.[31] CPM involving monosomy, except for sex chromosome monosomy, does not occur as frequently, presumably because chromosome loss is less likely to result in a viable placental cell progeny. However, other factors might also be involved.

Table 14–3. Outcome of Prenatally Diagnosed Confined Placental Mosaicism in 340 Pregnancies

Outcome	Number of Pregnancies
Normal birth weight	292
Intrauterine growth retardation and perinatal death	23
Pregnancy loss	25

Data from references 24, 25, 26, 146, 148, and 149.

The low predictive value of mosaicism diagnosed by CVS can be corrected by establishing the origin of the extra chromosome in the placenta (Table 14–4). Overall, CPM is confirmed at term in the majority of cases originally diagnosed with CVS. Among individual chromosomes there is heterogeneity, with meiotically derived extra chromosomes having the strongest tendency to persist to term in a form of high-trisomy/low-diploidy mosaic. Not all mitotically derived CPM persists to term, and mitotically derived CPM generally results in low-level mosaicism in the term placenta. Therefore the significance of correlation of pregnancy outcome with CVS diagnosis is limited unless the origin of trisomic chromosome is established or the term placenta is analyzed and the pregnancy course and outcome are correlated with the extent of aneuploid involvement in the term placenta.[32]

The genetic consequences of CPM can exert themselves on the fetus, the placenta, or both. The effect of CPM on the placenta remains unknown, but some information has been gathered concerning the genetic consequences of CPM for the fetus.

Fetal Uniparental Disomy and Chromosomal Imbalance in Placental Tissue

The effect of fetal UPD on prenatal and postnatal development in most pregnancies with CPM

Table 14–4. Correlation of Pregnancy Outcome, Birth Weight, Trisomic Chromosome Origin, and Level of Trisomy in 52 Pregnancies with Prenatally Diagnosed Confined Placental Mosaicism

Tissue Studied	Abnormal Outcome (%)	Normal Birth Weight (%)
Cultured chorionic villous sampling (stroma)	78	63
Term chorionic stroma	69	44
Term trophoblast	70	11

Adapted from Robinson WP, Barrett IJ, Bernard L, et al: Am J Hum Genet 60:917, 1997. © 1997 University of Chicago Press.

has not been well defined. Several reports in the literature document UPD in pregnancies with CPM for trisomies 7, 14, 15, and 16.[33–37] In these reports, however, the phenotypic consequences of fetal UPD may also depend on the specific chromosome involved in CPM and its effect on fetal and placental functions. For example, an association between CPM 16, fetal UPD 16, and IUGR was documented in one of the two cases reported by Bennett and associates[38] and in all four cases reported by Kalousek and co-workers.[39] Studies of CPM for chromosome 16 indicated that IUGR was related to the presence of a high percentage of placental trisomy 16 cells that caused placental malfunction rather than to fetal UPD 16. In cases of CPM with high levels of trisomy 16, IUGR is also found when the fetus has biparental origin of chromosome 16, and a normal birth weight has been recorded in an infant with UPD 16 and a low level of trisomy 16 in placental cells.[39]

Fetal Uniparental Disomy and Genomic Imprinting

One effect of UPD on prenatal and postnatal development depends on the presence of "imprinted" genes carried by the involved chromosomal pair. The term "genomic imprinting" refers to an epigenetic phenomenon that sets a parental signature on a specific DNA segment during gametogenesis or before fertilization so that it is modified and functions differently, depending on the parental original of the DNA segment. Among the first and most general indicators of the effect of genomic imprinting were observations that complete sets of both maternal and paternal chromosomes are essential for undisturbed embryonic and fetal development in mice.[40,41] Neither androgenic (diploid paternal) nor gynogenic (diploid maternal) embryos could complete normal intrauterine development. Gynogenic embryos constructed by replacement of a male pronucleus with a female pronucleus were found to grow normally only to early somite stages with unusually small extraembryonic placental tissue. An inverse situation was observed in androgenic embryos induced by transplantation of a male pronucleus into a zygote from which the female pronucleus had been removed. These gave rise to predominantly extraembryonic placental tissues with severely stunted embryos. From these experiments it was concluded that certain genes essential for growth of trophoblastic tissue are expressed preferentially from the paternally transmitted genome, whereas the maternally transmitted genome can provide all the genes needed for early development of the embryo proper. More specific evidence for the nonequivalence of maternal and paternal genome came from breeding experiments using strains of mice that carried various Robertsonian translocations. In appropriate crosses it was possible to produce UPD for particular chromosomes or chromosomal regions and to show an abnormal phenotype for certain UPD regions.[42] Clinical observations in humans correspond to those in experimental animals.[43,44] The expression and consequence of UPD and genomic imprinting in humans are probably best exemplified in two genetic syndromes, Prader-Willi syndrome (PWS) and Angelman's syndrome (AS).[45,46] Most often both syndromes result from chromosomal deletions in bands 15q11-13, with the deletion of paternal chromosome 15 in PWS and maternal chromosome 15 in AS. PWS also results from maternal UPD for chromosome 15, and AS is phenotypically expressed with paternal UPD for the same chromosome. Thus, in the cases of CPM 15 reported by Morichon-Delvallez,[35] Purvis-Smith,[47] and Cassidy,[48] and their associates, maternal UPD of chromosome 15 resulted, as expected, in a PWS phenotype. For chromosomes other than chromosome 15, phenotypic findings associated with UPD can include abnormal growth, mental retardation, nondistinctive minor anomalies, and less often congenital abnormalities as reviewed by Schinzel in 1993.[44]

Fetal Uniparental Disomy and Loss of Heterozygosity

A consequence of UPD is the expression of a recessively inherited mutation. For example, several autosomal recessive disorders have been found in association with UPD: methymalonic acidemia or transient neonatal diabetes mellitus and UPD 6,[49,50] cystic fibrosis or Silver-Russell syndrome and UPD 7,[51,52] rod monochromacy and UPD 14,[53] Bloom's syndrome and UPD 15,[54] and hemophilia and UPD X.[55] Knowing the frequency of isodisomy and of a recessively inherited mutation, one can estimate the frequency of an association of UPD and the expression of an autosomal recessive condition.[56] Interestingly, the lower the frequency of recessively inherited mutation, the higher the probability that UPD will be associated with this phenotype. Clearly, cystic fibrosis will be more common among carriers of UPD 7 than a rarer syndrome would be. However, a higher rate of UPD is expected among individuals with a rarer syndrome. This is somewhat equivalent to what has been observed for cousin marriages.

The clinical significance of fetal UPD for each specific chromosome needs careful study in a larger number of cases and correlation with findings in term mosaic placentas before any definite conclusions about CPM and UPD can be made and used for prenatal counseling.

GENE EXPRESSION IN THE PLACENTA

Studies of chromosome abnormalities indicate that a normal genetic constitution of both the placenta and fetus is critical for pregnancy outcome. In the case of trisomy there is no loss of genetic material, so the critical genes involved in intrauterine lethal or abnormal effects associated with any particular trisomy are probably limited to just a few dosage-sensitive genes that play important functions in placental development and function. For example, the fact that a fetus with trisomy 13 or trisomy 18 can survive to term only when some normal disomic cells are present in the trophoblast implies that the level of expression of a gene or genes on these chromosomes is highly regulated in this tissue. Trisomy 8 conceptuses are also normally aborted in the first trimester of pregnancy, yet mosaic liveborns with high levels of trisomy 8 and variable abnormalities have been reported. The trisomic cell line in liveborn mosaic cases has originated during development from a normal disomic fertilization, whereas a meiotic origin was always observed in spontaneous abortion trisomy 8.[28, 57–59] This implies that the lethal effects of trisomy 8 are associated with early differentiating lineages. As yet, however, virtually no data directly link a specific gene to the lethal effects caused by a specific chromosomal trisomy in the fetus or the placenta.

A wide variety of genes are expressed in placental tissues and play important roles in implantation and development of the placenta (see Cross, Werb and Fisher[19] for review. Mutations in most of these genes have been studied in mice, but few abnormal variants of the genes have been identified in humans. The proteins particularly important in placental development and function are cell adhesion molecules and other proteins involved in implantation of the blastocyst, proteins that code for a range of placental hormones that contribute to decidualization of the endometrium and invasion of the trophoblast, and placental and fetal growth factors. Table 14–5 lists some genes expressed in placental tissues that have been mapped to a specific human chromosome, a few of which are discussed in detail below. Mutations in many of these genes in mice result in developmental failure before the implantation stage. Nonetheless, null mutations in some other genes known to be highly expressed in the placenta do not cause failure of pregnancy,[19] indicating a redundancy in function of many of these genes.

Genes involved in implantation of the blastocyst include those encoding for various cytokines, adhesion molecules, and invasive proteinases (see for example Simón et al.[60]). Some of these are expressed in the maternal endometrium, such as colony-stimulating factor–1 and leukemia in-

Table 14–5. Some Localized Genes with Known Expression in Placenta

Gene	Chromosomal Location	Protein	Expression in Placental Tissue
IPP	1p32-p22	Intracisternal A partical promoted polypeptide	Trophoectoderm + endoderm linkage
CSF-1	1p21-p13	Colony-stimulating factor-1	Trophoblast
TSHB	1p13	Thyroid-stimulating hormone β chain	Syncytiotrophoblast
LAMB3	1q32	Laminin-β	Preimplantation
ACTH	2p25	Adrenocorticotropic hormone—corticotropin	Syncytiotrophoblast
IL1B	2q13-q21	Interleukin-1 β chain	Trophoblast
IL1A	2q13-q21	Interleukin-1 α chain	Trophoblast
ALPP	2q37	Placental alkaline phosphatase	Placenta
COL5A2	2q31	Collagen type V	Placenta
TRH	3p	Thyrotropin-releasing hormone	Cytotrophoblast
GHF1	3p11	Growth hormone factor 1 (Pit-1)	
GNRHR	4q21.1	Gonadotropin-releasing hormone receptor	Trophoblast
LIFR	5p13-p12	Leukemia inhibitory factor receptor	Blastocyst
CRHBP	5q11.2-13.3	Corticotropin-releasing hormone binding protein	
HLA-G	6	Human leukocyte antigen-G	Trophoblast
CGA	6q12-q21	Chorionic gonadotropin α chain	Syncytiotrophoblast
IGFBP1	7p14-p12	Insulin-like growth factor binding protein 1	Placenta
LAMB1	7q31.1-.3	Laminin-β 1	Preimplantation
GNRH	8p21-11.2	Gonadotropin-releasing hormone	Cytotrophoblast
CRH	8q13	Corticotropin-releasing hormone	Cytotrophoblast
TRHR	8q23	Thyrotropin-releasing hormone receptor	
INS4	9p24	Insulin-like peptide	Placenta (first trimester)
IGF2	11p15.5	Insulin-like growth factor 2	Placenta
MASH2	11p15.5	Mouse aschete-scute homolog-2	Trophoblast
IGF1	12q22-q24.1	Insulin-like growth factor 1	
PGF	14q24-q31	Placental growth factor (vascularization)	Placenta
CYP19	15q21.1	Cytochrome P450; placental aromatase	Placenta
CDH1	16q22.1	E-cadherin (Uvomorulin)	Preimplantation
CDH3	16q22.1	P-cadherin (placental type)	Preimplantation
CDH5	16q22.1	VE-cadherin, also H-cadherin located on 6q24	
CDH-11	16	OB-cadherin	Syncytiotrophoblast
CRHR	17q12-q22	Corticotropin-releasing hormone receptor	
CS-A	17q22-q24	Chorionic somatotropin-A	Syncytiotrophoblast
CS-B	17q22-q24	Chorionic somatotropin-B	Syncytiotrophoblast
GHN	17q22-q24	Growth hormone—normal	Syncytiotrophoblast
GHV	17q22-q24	Growth hormone variant	Syncytiotrophoblast
PL	17q22-q24	Placental lactogen	Syncytiotrophoblast
TIMP2	17q25	Tissue inhibitor of metalloproteinase-2	Placenta
LAMA3	18q22.1	Laminin-α 3	Preimplantation
PSG1	19q13.1-.3	Pregnancy-specific glycoprotein I	Syncytiotrophoblast
PSG12	19q13.1-.3	Pregnancy-specific glycoprotein 12	Syncytiotrophoblast
CEA	19q13.1-.3	Carcinoembryonic antigen	Syncytiotrophoblast
CGB	19q13.1-.3	Chorionic gonadotropin β chain	Syncytiotrophoblast
LHB	19q13.32	Luteinizing hormone β subunit	
PTP1B	20q13.1-.2	Protein-tyrosine phosphatase	Trophoblast
MMP-9	20q11.2-13.1	Metalloproteinase-9	Placenta
TIMP3	22	Tissue inhibitor of metalloproteinase-3	Placenta

Data from Online Mendelian inheritance in man, (OMIM); Center for Medical Genetics, Johns Hopkins University, Baltimore; and National Center for Biotechnology Information, National Library of Medicine, Bethesda Md., 1996.
World Wide Web URL: http://www3.ncbi.nlm.nih.gov/omim/

hibitory factor, whereas the receptors for these proteins are expressed in trophoblasts. Defects in such proteins could result in infertility through failure of embryonic development at or before the implantation stage. For example, human cadherin is thought to be an important component in cell adhesion at the implantation stage (Table 14–5). Riethmacher, Brinkmann, and Birchmeier[61] introduced a targeted mutation into the E-cadherin gene by homologous recombination in mouse embryonic stem cells, removing sequences essential for Ca^{2+} binding and adhesive function. Heterozygous mutant animals appeared normal and were fertile. However, the homozygous mutation was incompatible with life; the homozygous embryos showed severe abnormalities before implantation. Particularly, the adhesive cells of the morula dissociated shortly after compaction had occurred. Studies of such gene mutations in humans are difficult for obvious reasons. Possibly with the increasing use of in vitro fertilization techniques, carriers of mutations in such genes will be identified.

Many hormones are also produced in the trophoblast throughout pregnancy, and failure of pregnancy or inappropriate growth could be due to inappropriate dosage of such hormones. For example, epidermal growth factor is expressed in trophoblast and involved in human trophoblast invasion.[62] Mutations of this gene in mice result in embryonic death shortly after implantation.[19] Human chorionic gonadotropin (hCG) is a glycoprotein hormone produced by the trophoblastic cells of the placenta 10 to 12 days after conception. This hormone is important in maintaining pregnancy through the first trimester, and its rate of increase can be used to measure the viability of a pregnancy. Abnormal levels of hCG are associated with increased risks of trisomy 13, 16, 18, and 21.[63] This protein is coded for by chromosomes 6 and 19; conceptuses with trisomies for these chromosomes are lost early in pregnancy, and such trisomies are never observed in CPM.

Corticotropin-releasing hormone (CRH) maps to chromosome 8 and is expressed from cytotrophoblast. Human placenta produces large amounts of CRH, which appears to be part of a "placental clock" that determines length of gestation.[64] CRH levels increase exponentially near the end of pregnancy and trigger parturition and delivery. Deficiency of CRH has been associated with varying fetal manifestations, including hypoglycemia, hepatitis, facial dysmorphism, convulsions, and agenesis of the corpus callosum, as well as with frequent death in childhood.[65] Low maternal urinary levels of estriol were observed prenatally, and cortisol and adrenocorticotropic hormone (ACTH) were undetectable at birth. Because this gene is dosage sensitive, overexpression of CRH may contribute to in utero effects of trisomy 8, although presumably other placental genes also map to chromosome 8 and influence the viability of conceptions with trisomy 8.

Placental growth hormone is expressed from the syncytiotrophoblast of the placenta and appears in maternal serum from midpregnancy onward.[66] The chorionic somatotropin A and B genes are related and show similar expression patterns in development, suggesting a common regulatory element. A splice site mutation in this gene resulting in a longer than normal mRNA was found in one of 20 placentas examined, but there was no evidence of a significant adverse effect on pregnancy or fetal development.[67]

Estrogen production in the placenta depends on aromatization and desulfation of fetal adrenal androgens. Placental aromatase deficiency caused by defects in the CYP19 gene has been reported in association with maternal virilization during the second trimester of pregnancy and with pseudohermaphroditism of female fetuses.[68] Development in one affected male fetus was normal, but adult stature was very tall (greater than three standard deviations from normal) and macroorchidism and infertility were present. Laboratory findings include low levels of estrogen and high levels of androgens in maternal serum during pregnancy plus various abnormalities in the affected individuals.[68] Placental estrogen levels are also deficient in X-linked ichthyosis because of placental sulfatase deficiency, although no effect on in utero growth and development has been noted.

Defects in expression of a number of other genes expressed in the placenta have been observed in humans, including thyroid-stimulating hormone–β chain, thyrotropin-releasing hormone, and ACTH deficiencies. However, abnormalities in these cases appeared to be due to lack of expression in fetal or adult tissues, with no mention of placental defects or IUGR. Studies of genomic imprinting have shown greater evidence for the influence of specific genes on in utero growth in humans.

Imprinted Gene Expression

The evidence from gynogenetic or androgenetic zygotes and parent-of-origin effects in human triploids suggests particularly dramatic effects of genomic imprinting in the extraembryonic tissues. Many authors have proposed that imprinting may have evolved to control in utero growth in mammals.[69–71] Furthermore, placental UPD for some chromosomes may have greater adverse effects on in utero development than fetal UPD for that particular chromosome. Normal placental and fetal development clearly depend on inheritance of one normal chromosome complement from the mother and one from the father, and the imprinted genes active in placental development may be distinct from those acting in the fetus.

Two major regions in humans that contain a cluster of imprinted genes have been identified: 11p15.5 and 15q11.2-q13. The expression patterns of most of the identified imprinted genes (Table 14–6) have not yet been well characterized in human placentas. However, some genes in the mouse (e.g., *Ins1, Ins2, Mash2, Mas,* and *Xist*) show imprinted expression in specific extraembryonic tissues but show biallelic or random maternal-paternal expression in the embryo proper and adult tissues (Table 14–6 and below). Furthermore, the imprinting phenomenon possibly is not limited to on-off expression but may involve differential splicing of mRNA, RNA stability, or transportation of mRNA to the transcriptional machinery.[72]

Mouse embryos with two paternal copies of distal chromosome 7 (syntenic to 11p15.5 in humans) die at about 10 days' gestation, whereas those with two maternal copies die at later stages of development and show growth retardation.[73,74] Paternal UPD for chromosome 11p15.5 in humans is associated with Beckwith-Wiedemann syndrome (BWS), an overgrowth disorder.[75] All observed cases of UPD have apparently been due to somatic postmeiotic events, suggesting that nonmosaic paternal UPD for this region may be lethal early in development, as it is in mice. Chimeric uniparental-paternal inheritance of this region in mice is associated with somatic overgrowth similar to BWS.[74]

The 11p15.5 region includes at least five so far identified imprinted genes: *H19, IGF2, INS, KIP2 (p57 KIP2),* and *MASH2.*[76–82] The early embryonic lethality of paternal UPD of chromosome 7 in mice and possibly paternal UPD of chromosome 11 in humans is probably due to lack of the maternally expressed *Mash2* gene product, which is essential for development and differentiation of the trophoblast.[78,79] This gene encodes a transcription factor of the basic-helix-loop-helix class and is expressed at high levels in trophoblast progenitors and derivatives, oocytes, and preimplantation embryos. The *Mash2* paternal allele is expressed by trophoblastic cells at 6½ to 7½ days post coitum in mice but later is repressed, and only the maternal allele is expressed by 8½ days post coitum. *Mash2* −/− homozygous and pat+/mat− heterozygous mutant mouse embryos die at 10 days post coitum because of placental failure, specifically failure of the spongiotrophoblast to develop.

Table 14–6. Some Imprinted Genes in Mouse and Human

Mouse			Human		
Gene	Expression	Location	Gene	Expression	Location
Ins1	Paternal*	6 proximal	—	—	—
MEST/Peg-1	Paternal	6 proximal	?		
Ins2	Paternal*	7 distal	*INS*	n.d.	11p15.5
Igf2	Paternal	7 distal	*IGF2*	Paternal	11p15.5
H19	Maternal	7 distal	*H19*	Maternal	11p15.5
Mash2	Maternal*	7 distal	*MASH2*	nd.	11p15.5
KIP2(p57 *KIP2*)	Maternal	7 distal	*KIP2*	Maternal	11p15.5
?			*WT1*	Maternal*	11p13
Snrpn	Paternal	7 central	*SNRPN*	Paternal	15q11-q13
Znf127	Paternal	7 central	*ZNF127*	Paternal	15q11-q13
Ipw	Paternal	7 central	*IPW*	Paternal	15q11-q13
U2af1-rs1	Paternal	11 proximal	?		
Igf2r/M6P	Maternal	17 proximal	*IGF2R*	Possible maternal*	6q25-q27
Mas	Paternal*	17 proximal	*MAS*	n.d.	6q25-q27
Xist	Maternal*	X	*XIST*	n.d.	Xq13

n.d.,
*Uniparental inheritance observed in placenta or early embryonic development only.
Data from references 72, 150, and 151.

Growth restriction associated with maternal UPD of chromosome 7 in mice (11p15.5 in humans) could be due to lack of insulin-like growth factor 2 *(Igf2),* which is important in development and is expressed from the paternal allele in many tissues of both mouse and human. In humans paternal-only expression is observed in most embryonic tissues except those of the choroid plexus and leptomeninges, where *IGF2* is expressed from both alleles.[77,83] Biparental expression is also observed in kidney and postnatal liver after 12 weeks' gestation. The *H19* gene lies about 100 kilobases (kb) downstream of *IGF2* and shows a similar pattern of tissue-specific expression except that *H19* is usually maternally expressed in the tissues for which *IGF2* is paternally expressed. Neither *H19* nor *IGF2* is expressed from the maternal genome of gynogenetic gestations, and both are expressed from the paternal genome of androgenetic gestations.[84] Coexpression of *H19* and *IGF2* in androgenetic gestations was limited to trophoblast, the only placental tissue that is normally known to express these genes and that does not develop in gynogenotes in humans.[84] Biallelic expression of both genes appears to be a normal feature of trophoblast from placentas at less than 10 weeks' of gestation, whereas monoallelic (maternal) expression is observed after 10 weeks' gestation.[85] In situ hybridization results showed that expression of *H19* and *IGF2* was restricted to the cytotrophoblast and intermediate trophoblast cells and was not present in syncytiotrophoblast or stroma. "Leaky" or abnormal imprinting of *IGF2/H19* has been found in some patients with BWS and in some tumors.[86] It appears likely that abnormal imprinting of this gene in the placenta could also result in overgrowth or undergrowth in utero.

The insulin *(INS)* gene in humans is equivalent to the insulin2 gene of mice. Insulin2 is expressed in the pancreas, liver, and yolk sac during development of mice and rats.[87] Mutations in insulin affect embryonic development and growth, at times preceding the appearance of insulin effects on carbohydrate metabolism, which indicates a possible function for nonpancreatic insulin expression in early embryo development. Both parental copies of the insulin genes are expressed in mouse pancreas, whereas only paternal alleles are active in the yolk sac.[87] Expression of *INS* in human extraembryonic tissues has not been thoroughly investigated. However, inappropriate expression of this gene could also affect fetal growth.

Another cluster of imprinted genes lies within human chromosome 15q11.2-12. Lack of a paternal copy of this region through deletion or maternal uniparental disomy results in the Prader-Willi syndrome (PWS),[45,88–90] whereas a maternal deletion or paternal uniparental disomy results in the completely distinct phenotype of Angelman's syndrome (AS).[46,91] At least three genes *(SNRPN, IPW,* and *ZNF-127)* that are expressed only from the paternal chromosome have been identified in the PWS and AS deletion region.[92-95] *SNRPN* is a small nuclear ribosomal protein believed to be involved in splicing of mRNA and is expressed from a wide range of adult tissues, as well as in ovarian teratomas (gynogenetic) and hydatidiform moles (androgenetic).[96] *IPW* is widely expressed in adult and fetal tissues and in the placenta and apparently functions as an RNA, since there is no evidence that it is translated into protein.[95] Little has been reported about tissue-specific imprinted expression and function of these genes in extraembryonic tissues.

Paternal UPD of chromosome 6 is associated with intrauterine growth restriction and transient neonatal diabetes. The region responsible has been localized by linkage to 6q22.33-23.3.[97] Postnatal development in UPD6 cases appears normal except for problems related to those present at birth. Therefore chromosome 6–imprinted genes probably are functionally imprinted only during development. The insulin growth factor 2 receptor *(IGF2R)* maps to human chromosome 6q25-q27 and is biallelically expressed, although this gene is expressed from only the maternal chromosome in the mouse.[98] It remains possible that this gene is imprinted in humans in specific extraembryonic tissues or at a specific time of development. It could therefore be involved in the IUGR associated with paternal UPD6.

X CHROMOSOME INACTIVATION

Mammalian dosage compensation is achieved by the inactivation of one X chromosome in females during early embryogenesis.[99] The inactivation of the X chromosome(s) does not occur at a single time of development,[100] and not all genes are inactivated simultaneously.[101] At the morula stage both Xs are active, but during this or the next stage an X-counting mechanism occurs, resulting in only a single X remaining active in the epiblast and its derivatives in normal females, as well as in 47,XXY, 47,XXX, and 48,XXXX fertilizations. In the case of triploids with 69,XXX and 69,XXY chromosome constitution, two Xs remain active, indicating that the autosome/X ratio is important to this process.[102]

Cytogenetic studies of liveborns and aborted fetuses indicate that only approximately 0.3% of embryos with a 45,X constitution survive to birth.[102] Of liveborn patients, the majority have a mosaic 45,X constitution.[103] These findings suggest that biparental expression of both X chromosomes may be necessary for early stages of development in female conceptuses.

Although the paternal X chromosome is preferentially inactivated in the extraembryonic tissues of marsupials and rodents, results suggesting a parent-of-origin bias of X inactivation in extraembryonic tissues of normal human female fetuses are conflicting.[104–110] In the only study in which cytotrophoblast was enzymatically separated from the stroma cells of chorionic villi, most of the cytotrophoblast samples showed preferential inactivation of the paternally derived X chromosome whereas random X inactivation was seen in the stroma,[104] suggesting that nonrandom X inactivation might be restricted to the cytotrophoblast.

A gene that is proposed to have a role in the initiation of X inactivation is the X-inactive specific transcript *(XIST)* gene.[111] In addition to the imprinting phenomenon, primary nonrandom inactivation can be caused by mutations at the *XIST* locus.[112] Secondary nonrandom inactivation resulting from a selective advantage or disadvantage of cells caused by inactivation of one X chromosome has been observed in human females with X chromosome rearrangements and in carriers for certain X-linked diseases (reviewed in Belmont[113]).

Although no direct data have shown that skewed X inactivation may cause IUGR or other pregnancy problems, there are several reasons to think it may be indirectly associated. Skewed X inactivation can result in abnormalities because of preferential expression of the mutated copy in X-linked recessive conditions. In addition, skewed X inactivation is much more commonly associated with twin than nontwin births.[114] The presence of skewed X inactivation may also be associated with cases of vanishing twin or early implantation and developmental problems. In any situation in which the fetus develops from an unusually small number of progenitor cells, skewed X inactivation is likely to be more common. Furthermore, the possibility that inactivation of the paternal X chromosome preferentially occurs in some placental tissues implies that X chromosome mosaicism in these tissues may have particularly harmful effects.

Table 14–7. Studies of Randomness of X Chromosome Inactivation in Extraembryonic Tissues*

Study	Tissues Examined	Results Obtained
Ropers et al[110]	Placenta (tissue not specified)	Excess maternal expression
Migeon and Do[106]	Chorion, amnion, chorionic villi (newborn)	Maternal contamination (chorion); no activity (amnion); random inactivation (villi)
Migeon and Do[108]	Chorion, chorionic villi, fetal tissue (first trimester)	Skewing in all tissues toward allele B of *G6PD*
Migeon et al[107]	Chorionic villi (fetal and newborn)	Random inactivation
Mohandas et al[109]	Chorionic villi (cultured and uncultured, first trimester)	Random inactivation
Harrison and Warburton[105]	Amnion, chorion, chorionic villi (cultured and fresh, newborn)	Preferential paternal inactivation in all
Harrison[104]	Cytotrophoblast, stroma	Preferential paternal inactivation in cytotrophoblast; random inactivation in stroma

*All were based on expression of *G6PD* except Mohandas et al.,[109] which also looked at *HPRT*.

CURRENT TECHNOLOGY USED FOR GENETIC STUDIES

In Situ Hybridization

The field of molecular cytogenetics was revolutionized by reports of the detection of DNA sequences in cytologic preparations through the technique of in situ hybridization (ISH).[115] Today a wide variety of ISH approaches exist. The development of nonradioactive methods of labeling and detecting nucleic acid probes using haptens and fluorochromes improved the ISH protocols and reduced the use of autoradiography. The rapid development of fluorescence light microscopy in the 1990s has provided investigators with several fluorescence in situ hybridization (FISH) methodologies.[116] In general, FISH shows a high detection sensitivity, less than 1 kb (e.g., in highly extended DNA fibers), and a wide-range genomic resolution (e.g., from microdeletion detection to whole chromosome painting).[117,118] FISH allows visualization of chromosomes or of the number and rearrangement of chromosomal segment copies irrespective of cell cycle stage.[119] The use of interphase nuclei as targets for the examination of chromosome aneuploidy or rearrangement enables screening of large numbers of cells.[120] A major advantage is elimination of the need for metaphase chromosomes, thus reducing preparation time, eliminating tissue culture bias, and allowing a large number of interphase nuclei to be scored rapidly. The results obtained by FISH represent the in vivo status of the tissue being examined. The introduction of multicolor FISH and combinatorial labeling of a probe so that more than one hapten is detected with different fluorochromes or fluorochrome-conjugated nucleotides along with digital microscopy allows the visualization of at least 15 target sequences. This technique has tremendously increased FISH capacity.[121,122] As a consequence, FISH has already strongly affected many clinical and research fields, such as cytogenetics, pathology, hematology, molecular genetics, and cell biology (Fig. 14–4; see Color Plate).

At present FISH is used largely to detect known or suspected chromosomal abnormalities using specific probes. In a clinical setting FISH with commercially available DNA probes can be used for a variety of diagnostic purposes. When classic cytogenetic analysis reveals chromosomal aneuploidy, FISH using alpha satellite probes for a specific chromosomal centromere is the technique of choice for follow-up studies.[123] Phenotypically identified genetic syndromes (e.g., Miller-Dieker syndrome, PWS, AS) are confirmed by use of specific probes for the microdeletion in question. Use of FISH for confirming prenatally diagnosed chromosomal mosaicism in term placentas and infants has been developed into a rapid, accurate, and powerful method of analysis.[32,39] FISH has become a screening test for detection of specific chromosomal aneuploidies. With use of sophisticated multicolor FISH approaches it is possible to distinguish and to discriminate each human chromosome in a different color.[124]

To overcome the limitations in diagnostic and research cytogenetic analysis using FISH methodology, new techniques have been developed: primed in situ labeling (PRINS), comparative genomic hybridization (CGH), multiplex FISH (M-FISH), and multicolor spectral karyotyping. The choice of method depends on the nature of the sample and the clinical diagnosis. (For detailed methodology see Verma and Babu.[125])

Primed In Situ Labeling

PRINS is an alternative to traditional FISH methodology.[126] The PRINS method includes the annealing of unlabeled synthetic oligonucleotides or denatured double-stranded DNA fragments to complementary sequences on denatured metaphase chromosome preparations or interphase nuclei. This reaction is followed by a DNA polymerase–driven extension in the presence of labeled deoxynucleotides. The newly synthesized DNA can then be visualized by fluorescence detection.[127,128] Compared with traditional ISH methods, PRINS has the advantage of being fast and convenient, since detection of repeat sequences can be obtained in less than 1 hour and of unique DNA sequences in less than 3 hours. Multicolor PRINS enhances the potential for simultaneous visualization of multiple sequences in both metaphase and interphase nuclei. Moreover, a high-quality chromosome R banding using Alu-oligonucleotides can be produced, allowing simultaneous multiprobe analysis and mapping.[126,129] Because of the high efficiency of PRINS, structural abnormalities can be confirmed even in a small number of scorable metaphases. Numerical abnormalities can be detected in interphase nuclei. Because of the small size of the primer sequences, penetration of the nuclei is easily accomplished. PRINS has been extensively applied to analysis of sperm[130]; it can also be applied to uncultured blood samples.[131]

Comparative Genomic Hybridization

CGH is a new molecular cytogenetic approach based on two-color fluorescence in situ suppression hybridization.[132] CGH allows the comprehensive analysis of entire chromosome imbalances, as well as unbalanced copy numbers of chromosomal subregions. To date CGH has been used extensively to detect genetic changes in malignancies.[133] CGH has great potential as a rapid screening method for chromosomal aneuploidy in the evaluation of term placentas from abnormal pregnancies. The principle of CGH in brief is as follow: The genomic test DNA from the tissue sample of interest, such as a placenta, and a control DNA derived from cells with a normal karyotype (46,XX or 46,XY) are labeled differentially with different reporter molecules (e.g., biotin dUTP and digoxigenin dUTP). Equal amounts of the test and reference DNAs are mixed and hybridized on high-quality normal metaphase chromosomal preparations together with an excess of unlabeled Cot1 DNA fraction, which suppresses the repetitive human sequences along the genome.[134] Immunocytochemical methods are used to detect the hybridized control and test DNA. Usually fluorescein isothiocyanate (FITC) is used for labeling of the test DNA, and tetrarhodamine isothiocyanate (TRITC), for the reference DNA. The ratios of the fluorescence intensities along the chromosomes are measured. The normal state and the overrepresentation or underrepresentation of DNA from a given chromosome or chromosomal segment can be identified. Visualization occurs by epifluorescence microscopy with selective filters, and quantitation is performed by computer analysis, using a software program to calculate the ratio of red (TRITC) to green (FITC) fluorescence. Any deviation of the test sample from normal diploidy results in a shift in wavelength with abundance of red if the test sample is trisomic or an abundance of green if the test sample is monosomic (Fig. 14–5; see Color Plate). CGH reveals only the relative copy number changes. Ratios of signals for diploid and triploid cells cannot be distinguished from each other. This problem is easy to overcome using additional FISH analysis, with one specific chromosomal probe. Thus CGH combined with FISH provides a global view of the gains and losses that exist in the DNA of a test sample.[135]

In contrast to traditional cytogenetic analysis, CGH does not require preparation of metaphase chromosomes from the cell population studied. Like any other method, CGH has resolution and sensitivity limitations. The validity of a CGH experiment depends critically on the percentage of cells carrying chromosomal imbalances. For example, in placenta samples, maternal decidual cell contamination may cause false-negative results. Another limitation of the CGH method is its inability to detect balanced structural rearrangements, since only deviations from diploid complement can be visualized in the comparison by hybridization of control and test DNA (Fig. 14–6; see Color Plate).

Multiplex FISH and Spectral Karyotyping

The development of M-FISH and spectral karyotyping using a set of new epifluorescence filters and computer software allows the detection and discrimination of each human chromosome after FISH.[136,137] A pool of human chromosome painting probes, each labeled with a different fluor combination, is used for karyotyping analysis. Both simple and complex chromosomal rearrangements that could not be detected with conventional cytogenetic analysis can be rapidly defined. M-FISH fluorochrome discrimination is based on the measurement of a single intensity through fluorochrome-specific filters. In contrast, spectral karyotyping is based on the use of a triple-pass filter measurement of a discrete fluorochrome spectrum without image shift. Both techniques make a useful contribution to complex cytogenetic analysis but are not candidates for a simple screening method.

Molecular Genomic Analysis

Molecular DNA analysis is useful to complete the cytogenetic studies. After initial screening and definition of a chromosomal abnormality in the placenta, molecular studies of placental and parental DNA can determine the parental origin of the extra chromosome in the placenta or fetus. The origin of fetal disomy in cases of CPM can also be determined. At present the method of choice is the polymerase chain reaction (PCR) for amplification of polymorphic microsatellite loci.

PCR technology is an essential part of any molecular biology laboratory. PCR is used in many aspects of human genome analysis, including genetic and physical mapping of chromosomes (e.g., detection of small DNA polymorphisms) and the examination of gene expression using reverse transcription of mRNA into cDNA.

Collection and Storage of Samples

Studies evaluating the contribution of placental mosaicism to pregnancy outcome should begin with appropriate collection and storage of material. Before sampling, placentas to be analyzed should have detailed gross examination including measurement and weighing. Samples for histologic examination should be taken for analysis after routine pathology protocols. Both normal findings and abnormalities should be recorded. The results of cytogenetic prenatal diagnosis based on analysis of CVS, cultured amniotic fluid cells, or fetal blood cells should be noted if available.

For complete evaluation of the placental genome after delivery, multiple samples (about 10 per placenta) and both cell lineages (trophoblast and chorion) should be analyzed. The approximate location of these samples (each about 100 mg) should be recorded in a schematic map. Each sample should include chorionic villi and chorionic plate representing tissue of extraembryonic origin and amniotic membrane that is of fetal origin. If possible, blood from the umbilical cord should be collected in ethylenediamine tetraacetic acid (EDTA). The samples can be analyzed immediately or stored at $-70°$ C before processing. Separation of the two cell lineages forming placental villi (i.e., the trophoblast and villous stroma cells) using tissue digestion is important before analysis. This separation before cytogenetic and molecular analysis allows accurate diagnosis of three different types of CPM and prevents "dilution" of trisomic clone if found only in one of the placental cell lineages.[28,138] For any pregnancy with prenatally diagnosed CPM, fetal tissues, if available, should also be collected and stored at $-70°$ C to allow the exclusion of generalized mosaicism.

In a clinical setting, when placentas of infants with IUGR are being selected for FISH or CGH cytogenetic analysis, it is a good practice to exclude pregnancies in which IUGR is caused by maternal smoking, infection, essential maternal hypertension, or poor nutrition. One sample in the area of cord insertion should be taken from the fetal side of the placental and stored at $-70°$ C. This sample should include amnion, chorionic plate, and chorionic villi. Avoiding contamination with maternal decidua is important.

CONCLUSION

Extensive epidemiologic studies of poor pregnancy outcomes have been published, focusing on maternal health, nutrition, socioeconomic factors, gestational age, and race.[139,140] The problem has also been approached by comparing the histologic findings in the placenta with gestational age, placental and fetal karyotypes, and fetal development.[141,142] These studies have not been essentially helpful for clinicians, since in the epidemiologic studies the genetic component was excluded and since no correlation was found between placental histology and cytogenetics.

Studies of perinatal mortality show that although the factors contributing to fetal death are multiple and varied, the development and survival of humans depend largely on the quality and quantity of their genes. The outcome of pregnancies with a mosaic trisomic placenta and a diploid fetus shows the effect of the specific chromosome involved in the aneuploid placental mosaic cell line on the presence or absence of UPD in the fetus.[143,144] It is important to establish a karyotype-phenotype correlation for all aneuploidies leading to abnormal intrauterine growth development and consequently to intrauterine fetal death, abortion, growth retardation, or premature delivery. Long-term follow-up is imperative for children with IUGR at birth to evaluate their risk for specific diseases, such as diabetes and cardiovascular diseases. Close collaboration between clinicians, pathologists, and geneticists is required to accomplish this task.

ACKNOWLEDGMENTS

I gratefully acknowledge the financial support of the Medical Research Council of Canada grant No. MA-12152 and the March of Dimes Birth Defects Foundation grant No. 6-FY95-0131. The work of Dr. Brendan Harrington while visiting scientist at the British Columbia Research Institute for Child and Family Health was generously supported by the University of Manchester, U.K., and grants from the Central Manchester Healthcare Research & Development Initiative, the British Paediatric Association/Allen & Hanbury Research Award, and The British Council in Canada Young Research Workers Award.

REFERENCES

1. Drews U: Color atlas of embryology. Stuttgart, 1995, Georg Thieme Verlag.
2. Pederson RA, Burdsal CA: Mammalian embryogenesis. In Knobil E, & Neill JD (eds): The physiology of reproduction, 2nd ed. New York, 1994, Raven Press, p 319.
3. Markert CL, Petters RM: Manufactured hexaparental mice show that adults are derived from three embryonic cells. Science 202:56, 1978.
4. Ducibella T, Albertini DF, Andersen E, Biggers J: The preimplantation mammalian embryo: characterization of intracellular junctions and their appearance during development. Dev Biol 45:231, 1975.
5. Copp AJ: Interaction between inner cell mass and trophectoderm of the mouse blastocyst. I. A study of cellular proliferation. J Embryol Exp Morphol 48:109, 1978.
6. Jones RA, Roberton NR: Problems of the small-for-dates baby. Clin Obstet Gynaecol 11:499, 1984.
7. Georgieff M, Sasonow S, Mammel M, Pereira G: Mid-arm circumference to occipitofrontal circumference ratios for identification of symptomatic LGA, AGA and SGA infants. J Pediatr 109:316, 1986.
8. Excler J, Sann L, Lasne Y, Picard J: Anthropometric assessment of nutritional status in newborn infants: discriminative value of mid-arm circumference and skinfold thickness. Early Hum Dev 11:169, 1985.
9. Barker DJP: Mothers, babies, and disease in later life. London, 1994, BMJ Publishing Group.
10. Gu W, Jones CT, Parer JT: Metabolic and cardiovascular effects on fetal sheep of sustained reduction of uterine blood flow. J Physiol 368:109, 1985.
11. Lumey LH: Decreased birthweights in infants after maternal in utero exposure to the Dutch famine of 1944-45. Paediatr Perinat Epidemiol 6:240, 1992.
12. Fowden AL: The role of insulin in prenatal growth. J Dev Physiol 12:173, 1989.
13. Simoni G, Gimelli G, Cuoco C, et al: Discordance between prenatal cytogenetic diagnosis after chorionic villi sampling and chromosomal constitution of the fetus. In Fraccaro M, Simoni G, Brambati B (eds): First trimester fetal diagnosis. Berlin, 1985, Springer-Verlag, p 137.
14. Mikkelsen M: Cytogenetic findings in first trimester chorionic villi biopsies: a collaborative study. In Fraccaro M, Simoni G, Brambati B (eds): First trimester fetal diagnosis. Berlin, 1985, Springer-Verlag, p 109.
15. Ledbetter DH, Zachery JM, Simpson JL, et al: Cytogenetic results from the U.S. collaborative study on CVS. Prenat Diagn 2:317, 1992.
16. Teshima LE, Kalousek DK, Vekemans MJJ, et al: Chromosome mosaicism in CVS and amniocentesis samples. Prenat Diagn 12:443, 1992.
17. Kalousek DK, Dill FJ: Chromosomal mosaicism confined to the placenta in human conceptions. Science 221:665, 1983.
18. Graham CF, Deussen ZA: Features of cell lineage in preimplantation mouse development. J Embryol Exp Morphol 48:53, 1978.
19. Cross J, Werb Z, Fisher S: Implantation and the placenta: key pieces of the developmental puzzle. Science 262:1508, 1994.
20. Bianchi DW, Wilkins-Haug LE, Enders AC, Hay ED: Origin of extraembryonic mesoderm in experimental animals: relevance to chorionic mosaicism in humans. Am J Med Genet 46:542, 1993.

21. James RM, West JD: A chimeric animal model for confined placental mosaicism. Hum Genet 93:603, 1994.
22. Kalousek DK, Barrett IJ, McGillivray BC: Placental mosaicism and intrauterine survival of trisomies 13 and 18. Am J Hum Genet 44:338, 1989.
23. Engel E: A new genetic concept: uniparental disomy and its potential effect, isodisomy. Am J Med Genet 6:137, 1991.
24. Wolstenholme J, Rooney DE, Davison EV: Confined placental mosaicism, IUGR and adverse pregnancy outcome: a controlled retrospective U.K. collaborative survey. Prenat Diagn 14:345, 1994.
25. Johnson J, Wapner RJ, Davies GH, et al: Mosaicism in chorionic villus sampling: an association with poor perinatal outcome. Gynecology 75:573, 1990.
26. Breed ASPM, Mantingh A, Vosters R, et al: Follow-up and pregnancy outcome after a diagnosis of mosaicism in CVS. Prenat Diagn 11:577, 1991.
27. Schwinger E, Seidl E, Klink F, Rehder H: Chromosomal mosaicism of the placenta: a cause of developmental failure of the fetus. Prenat Diagn 9:639, 1989.
28. Robinson WP, Barrett IJ, Bernard L, et al: Meiotic origin of trisomy in CPM is correlated with presence of fetal uniparental disomy, high levels of trisomy in trophoblast and increased risk of fetal intrauterine growth restriction. Am J Hum Genet 60:917, 1997.
29. Wolstenholme J: An audit of trisomy 16 in man. Prenat Diagn 15:109, 1995.
30. Kalousek DK, Langlois S, Robinson WP, et al: Trisomy 7 CVS mosaicism: pregnancy outcome and DNA analysis in 14 cases. Am J Med Genet 65:348, 1996.
31. Shaffer LB, Langlois S, McCaskill C, et al: Analysis of nine pregnancies with confined placental mosaicism for trisomy 2. Prenat Diagn 16:899, 1996.
32. Henderson KG, Shaw TE, Barrett IJ, et al: Distribution of mosaicism in human placentae. Hum Genet 97:650, 1996.
33. Langlois S, Wilson RD, Yong SL, et al: Prenatal and postnatal growth failure associated with maternal heterodisomy for chromosome 7. J Med Genet 32:871, 1995.
34. Morichon-Delvallez N, Segues B, Pinson B, et al: Maternal uniparental disomy for chromosome 14 by secondary nondisjunction of an initial trisomy. In Zakut M (ed): Proceedings of 7th International Conference on Early Prenatal Diagnosis, Jerusalem, 1994. Bologna, Monduzzi Editore.
35. Morichon-Delvallez N, Mussat P, Dumez Y, et al: Trisomy 15 in chorionic villi and Prader Willi syndrome at birth. Prenat Diagn 12:S125, 1993.
36. Vaughan J, Ali Z, Bower S, et al: Human maternal uniparental disomy for chromosome 16 and fetal development. Prenat Diagn 14:751, 1994.
37. Dworniczak B, Koppers B, Kurlemann G, et al: Maternal origin of both chromosomes 16 in a phenotypically normal newborn. Am J Hum Genet 51:1, 1992.
38. Bennett, P, Vaughan J, Henderson D, et al: The association between confined placental trisomy, fetal uniparental disomy and early intrauterine growth retardation. Lancet 340:1284, 1992.
39. Kalousek DK, Langlois S, Barrett I, et al: Uniparental disomy for chromosome 16 in humans. Hum Genet 52:8, 1993.
40. Norris ML, Barton SC, Surani MAH: The differential roles of parental genomes in mammalian development. Oxf Rev Reprod Biol 12:225, 1990.
41. Surani MA, Reid W, Allen ND: Transgenes as molecular probes for genomic imprinting. Trends Genet 4:59, 1988.
42. Cattanach BM, Kirk M: Differential activity of maternally and paternally derived chromosome regions in mice. Nature 315:495, 1985.
43. Spence JE, Perciaccante RG, Greig CM, et al: Uniparental disomy as a mechanism for human genetic disease. Am J Hum Genet 42:217, 1988.
44. Schinzel A: Genomic imprinting: consequences of uniparental disomy for human disease. Am J Med Genet 46:683, 1993.
45. Nicholls RD, Knoll JHM, Butler MG, et al: Genetic imprinting suggested by maternal heterodisomy in non-deletion Prader-Willi syndrome. Nature 342:281, 1989.
46. Malcolm S, Clayton-Smith J, Nichols M, et al: Uniparental paternal disomy in Angelman's syndrome. Lancet 337:694, 1991.
47. Purvis-Smith SG, Saville T, Manass S, et al: Uniparental disomy 15 resulting from "correction" of an initial trisomy 15. Am J Hum Genet 50:1348, 1992.
48. Cassidy SB, Lai L, Erickson RP, et al: Trisomy 15 with loss of the paternal 15 as a cause of Prader-Willi syndrome due to maternal disomy. Am J Hum Genet 51:701, 1992.
49. Abramosicz MJ, Andrieu M, Dupont E, et al: Isodisomy of chromosome 6 in a newborn with methylmalonia cells causing diabetes mellitus. J Clin Invest 418, 1994.
50. Temple IK, James RS, Crolla JA, et al: An imprinted gene(s) for diabetes? Nature Genet 9:110, 1995.

51. Voss R, Ben Simon E, Avital A, et al: Isodisomy of chromosome 7 in a patient with cystic fibrosis: could uniparental disomy be common in humans? Am J Hum Genet 45:373, 1989.
52. Kotzot D, Schmitt S, Bernasconi F, et al: Uniparental disomy 7 in Silver-Russel syndrome and primordial growth retardation. Hum Mol Genet 4:583, 1995.
53. Pentao L, Lewis RA, Ledbetter DH, et al: Maternal uniparental isodisomy of chromosome 14: association with autosomal recessive rod monochromacy. Am J Hum Genet 50:690, 1992.
54. Woodage T, Prasad M, Dixon JW, et al: Bloom syndrome and maternal uniparental disomy for chromosome 15. Am J Hum Genet 55:74, 1994.
55. Vidaud D, Vidaud M, Plassa F, et al: Father to son transmission of hemophilia due to uniparental disomy. Am J Hum Genet 45:226, 1989.
56. Warburton D: Uniparental disomy: a rare consequence of the high rate of aneuploidy in human gametes. Am J Hum Genet 42:215, 1988.
57. Bernasconi F, Barrett I, Telenius A, et al: Survival of trisomy 8 correlates with somatic origin of the trisomy. Am J Hum Genet 58:A, 1996.
58. James RS, Jacobs PA: Molecular studies of the aetiology of trisomy 8 in spontaneous abortions and the liveborn population. Hum Genet 97:283, 1996.
59. Robinson WP, Binkert F, Bernasconi F, et al: Molecular studies of chromosomal mosaicism: relative frequency of chromosome gain or loss and possible role of cell selection. Am J Hum Genet 56:444, 1995.
60. Simón C, Gimeno MJ, Mercader A, et al: Cytokines–adhesion molecules–invasive proteinases: the missing paracrine/autocrine link in embryonic implantation? Mol Hum Reprod 2:405, 1996.
61. Riethmacher D, Brinkmann V, Birchmeier C: A targeted mutation in the mouse E-cadherin gene results in defective preimplantation development. Proc Natl Acad Sci USA 92:855, 1995.
62. Bass KE, Morrish D, Roth I, et al: Human cytotrophoblast invasion is up-regulated by epidermal growth factor: evidence that paracrine factors modify this process. Dev Biol 164:550, 1994.
63. Zimmerman R, Lauper U, Streicher A, et al: Elevated alpha-feto protein and human chorionic gonadotropin as a marker for placental trisomy 16 in the second trimester? Prenat Diagn 15:1121, 1995.
64. McLean M, Bisits A, Davies J, et al: A placental clock controlling the length of human pregnancy. Nature Med 1:460, 1995.
65. Mandel H, Berant M, Gotfried E, Hochberg Z: Autosomal recessive hypothalamic corticotropin deficiency: a new entity and its metabolic consequences. Am J Hum Genet 47(suppl):A66, 1990.
66. Liebhaber SA, Urbanek M, Ray J, et al: Characterization and histologic localization of human growth hormone–variant gene expression in the placenta. J Clin Invest 83:1985, 1989.
67. MacLeod JN, Worsley I, Ray J, et al: Human growth hormone variant is a biologically active somatogen and lactogen. Endocrinology 128: 1298, 1991.
68. Bulun SE: Clinical review: aromatase deficiency in women and men; would you have predicted the phenotypes? J Clin Endocr Metab 81:867, 1996.
69. Moore T, Haig D: Genomic imprinting in mammalian development: a parental tug-of-war. Trends Genet 7:45, 1991.
70. Pfeifer K, Tilghman SM: Allele-specific gene expression in mammals: the curious case of the imprinted RNAs. Genes Dev 8:1867, 1994.
71. Solter D: Differential imprinting and expression of the maternal and paternal genomes. Annu Rev Genet 22:127, 1988.
72. Franklin G, Adam G, Ohlsson R: Genomic imprinting and mammalian development. Placenta 17:3, 1996.
73. Beechey C: Further localization of the distal chromosome 7 imprinting region. Mouse Genome 91:310, 1993.
74. Ferguson-Smith A, Cattanach B, Barton SEA: Embryonic and molecular investigations of imprinting on mouse chromosome 7. Nature 351:667, 1991.
75. Henry I, Bonaiti-Pellie C, Chehensse V, et al: Uniparental paternal disomy in a genetic cancer-predisposing syndrome. Nature 351:665, 1991.
76. Bartolomei MS, Zemel S, Tighlman SM: Parental imprinting of the mouse H19 gene. Nature 351:153, 1991.
77. DeChiara TM, Robertson EJ, Efstratiadis A: Parental imprinting of the mouse insulin-like growth factor II gene. Cell 64:849, 1991.
78. Guillemot F, Nagy A, Auerbach A, et al: Essential role of Mash-2 in extraembryonic development. Nature 371:333, 1994.
79. Guillemot F: Genomic imprinting of Mash-2: a mouse gene required for trophoblast development. Nat Genet 9:235, 1995.
80. Hatada I, Inazawa J, Abe T, et al: Genomic imprinting of $p57^{kip2}$ and its reduced expression in Wilms tumors. Hum Mol Genet 5:783, 1996.
81. Hatada I, Mukai T: Genomic imprinting of a p57(kip2); acyclin inhibitor in mouse. Nat Genet 11:204, 1995.

82. Zemel S, Bartolomei M, Tilghman SM: Physical linkage of two mammalian imprinted genes, H19 and insulin-like growth factor 2. Nat Genet 2:61, 1992.
83. Ohlsson R, Hedborg F, Holmgren L, et al: Overlapping patterns of IGF2 and H19 expression during human development: biallelic IGF2 expression correlates with a lack of H19 expression. Development 120:361, 1994.
84. Mutter GL, Stewart CL, Chaponot ML, Pomponio RJ: Oppositely imprinted genes H19 and insulin-like growth factor 2 are coexpressed in human androgenetic trophoblast. Am J Hum Genet 53:1096, 1993.
85. Jinno Y, Ikeda Y, Yun K, et al: Establishment of functional imprinting of the H19 gene in human developing placentae. Nat Genet 10:318, 1995.
86. Reik W, Brown KW, Schneid H, et al: Imprinting mutations in the Beckwith-Wiedemann syndrome suggested by altered imprinting pattern in the IGF2-H19 domain. Hum Mol Genet 4:2379, 1995.
87. Giddings SJ, King CD, Harman KW, et al: Allele specific inactivation of insulin 1 and 2, in the mouse yolk sac, indicates imprinting. Nat Genet 6:310, 1994.
88. Mascari M, Gottlieb W, Rogan P, et al: The frequency of uniparental disomy in Prader-Willi syndrome: implications for molecular diagnosis. N Engl J Med 326:1599, 1992.
89. Robinson WP, Bottani A, Yagang X, et al: Molecular, cytogenetic, and clinical investigations of Prader-Willi syndrome patients. Am J Hum Genet 49:1219, 1991.
90. Zackowski J, Nicholls R, Gray B, et al: Cytogenetic and molecular analysis of Angelman syndrome. Am J Med Genet 46:7, 1993.
91. Knoll JHM, Nicholls RD, Magenis RE, et al: Angelman and Prader-Willi syndromes share a common chromosome 15 deletion but differ in parental origin of the deletion. Am J Med Genet 32:285, 1989.
92. Leff S, Brannan C, Reed M, et al: Maternal imprinting of the mouse Snrpn gene and conserved linkage homology with the human Prader-Willi syndrome region. Nat Genet 2:259, 1992.
93. Özçelik T, Leff S, Robinson W, et al: Small nuclear ribonucleoprotein polypeptide N (SNRPN), an expressed gene in the Prader-Willi syndrome critical region. Nat Genet 2:265, 1992.
94. Reed M, Leff S: Maternal imprinting of human SNRPN, a gene deleted in Prader-Willi syndrome. Nat Genet 6:163, 1994.
95. Wevrick R, Kerns J, Francke U: Identification of a novel paternally expressed gene in the Prader-Willi syndrome region. Hum Mol Genet 3:1877, 1994.
96. Glenn C, Saitoh S, Jong M, et al: Gene structure, DNA methylation, and imprinted expression of the human SNRPN gene. Am J Hum Genet 58:335, 1996.
97. Temple IK, Gardner RJ, Robinson DO, et al: Further evidence for an imprinted gene for neonatal diabetes localised to chromosome 6q22-q23. Hum Mol Genet 5:1117, 1996.
98. Kalscheuer V, Mariman E, Schepens M, et al: The insulin-like growth factor type-2 receptor gene is imprinted in mouse but not in humans. Nat Genet 5:74, 1993.
99. Lyon MF: Gene action in the X-chromosome of the mouse *(Mus musculus L.)*. Nature 190:372, 1961.
100. Tan S-S, Williams EA, Tam PPL: X-chromosome inactivation occurs at different times in different tissues of the post-implantation mouse embryo. Nat Genet 3:170, 1993.
101. Graves JAM, Dawson GW: The relationship between position and expression of genes on the kangaroo X chromosome suggests a tissue-specific spread of inactivation from a single control site. Genet Res 51:103, 1988.
102. Jacobs PA, Matsuyama AM, Buchanan IM, Wilson C: Late replicating X chromosomes in human triploidy. Am J Hum Genet 31:446, 1979.
103. Hassold T, Pettay D, Robinson A, Uchida I: Molecular studies of parental origin and mosaicism in 45,X conceptuses. Hum Genet 89:647, 1992.
104. Harrison KB: X-chromosome inactivation in the human cytotrophoblast. Cytogenet Cell Genet 52:37, 1989.
105. Harrison KB, Warburton D: Preferential X-chromosome activity in human female placental tissues. Cytogenet Cell Genet 41:163, 1986.
106. Migeon BD, Do TT: In search of non-random X-inactivation: studies of the placenta from newborns heterozygous for G6PD. In Russell LB (ed): Genetic mosaics and chimaeras in mammals. New York, 1978, Plenum Press, p 379.
107. Migeon BR, Wolf SF, Axelman J, et al: Incomplete X chromosome dosage compensation in chorionic villi of human placenta. Proc Natl Acad Sci USA 82:3390, 1985.
108. Migeon BD, Do TT: In search of non-random X inactivation: studies in the placenta from newborns heterozygous for G6PD. Am J Hum Genet 31:581, 1979.
109. Mohandas TK, Passage MB, Williams JW, et al:

X-chromosome inactivation in cultured cells from human chorionic villi. Somat Cell Mol Genet 15:131, 1989.

110. Ropers H, Wolff G, Hitseroth H: Preferential X inactivation in human placenta membranes: is the paternal X inactive in early embryonic development of female mammals? Hum Genet 42:265, 1978.
111. Brown CJ, Hendrich BD, Rupert JL, et al: The human XIST gene: analysis of a 17 kb inactive X-specific RNA that contains conserved repeats and is highly localized within the nucleus. Cell 71:527, 1992.
112. Plenge RM, Hendrich BD, Willard HF: A mutation in the XIST promoter in a family with nonrandom X chromosome inactivation. Am J Hum Genet 57(suppl):A30, 1995.
113. Belmont JW: Genetic control of X inactivation and processes leading to X-inactivation skewing. Am J Hum Genet 58:1101, 1996.
114. Goodship J, Carter J, Burn J: X-inactivation patterns in monozygotic and dizygotic female twins. Am J Med Genet 61:205, 1996.
115. Pardue ML, Gall JG: Molecular hybridization of radioactive DNA to the DNA of cytological preparations. Proc Natl Acad Sci USA 64:600, 1969.
116. Lichter P, Ward DC: Is non-isotopic in situ hybridization finally coming of age? Nature 345:93, 1990.
117. Lengauer C, Riethman H, Cremer T: Painting of human chromosomes generated from hybrid cell lines by PCR with Alu and L1 primers. Hum Genet 86:1, 1990.
118. Lestou VS, Strehl S, Lion T, et al: High resolution FISH of the entire integrated Epstein-Barr virus genome on extended human DNA. Cytogenet Cell Genet 74:211, 1996.
119. Lawrence JB, Singer RH, McNeil JA: Interphase and metaphase resolution of different distances within the human dystrophin gene. Science 249:928, 1990.
120. Philip J, Bryndorf T, Christensen B: Prenatal aneuploidy detection in interphase cells by fluorescence in situ hybridization (FISH). Prenat Diagn 14:1203, 1994.
121. Nederlof PM, Van Der Flier S, Wiegant J, et al: Multiple fluorescence in situ hybridization. Cytometry 11:126, 1990.
122. Ried T, Baldini A, Rand T, Ward DC: Simultaneous visualization of seven different probes by in situ hybridization using combinatorial fluorescence and digital imaging microscopy. Proc Natl Acad Sci USA 89:1388, 1992.
123. Emanuel BS: The use of fluorescence in situ hybridization to identify human chromosomal anomalies. Growth Genet Horm 9:6, 1993.
124. Le Beau M: One FISH, two FISH, red FISH, blue FISH. Nat Genet 12:341, 1996.
125. Verma RS, Babu A: Human chromosomes principles and techniques, 2 ed. New York, 1994, McGraw-Hill.
126. Baldini A, Ward DC: In situ hybridization banding of human chromosomes with Alu-PCR products: a simultaneous karyotype for gene mapping studies. Genomics 9:770, 1991.
127. Baldini A, Ross M, Nizetic D, et al: Chromosomal assignment of human YAC clones by fluorescence in situ hybridization: use of single-yeast colony PCR and multiple labeling. Genomics 14:181, 1992.
128. Gosden J, Lawson D: Instant PRINS: a rapid method for chromosome identification by detecting repeated sequences in situ. Cytogenet Cell Genet 68:57, 1995.
129. Volpi EV, Baldini A: MULTIPRINS: a method for multicolor primed in situ labeling. Chromosome Res 1:257, 1993.
130. Pellestor F, Girardet A, Coignet L, et al: Assessment of aneuploidy for chromosomes 8, 9, 13, 16 and 21 in human sperm by using primed in situ labeling technique. Am J Hum Genet 58:797, 1996.
131. Gosden J, Scopes G: Uncultured blood samples can be labeled by PRINS and ready for chromosome enumeration analysis 1 H after collection. Biotechniques 21:88, 1996.
132. Kallionemi A, Kallionemi OP, Sudar D, et al: Comparative genomic hybridization for molecular cytogenetic analysis of solid tumors. Science 258:818, 1992.
133. Schütz BR, Scheurlen W, Krauss J, et al: Mapping of chromosomal gains and losses in primitive neuroectodermal tumors by comparative genomic hybridization. Genes Chromosomes Cancer 16:196, 1996.
134. Du Manoir S, Schrock E, Bentz M, et al: Quantitative analysis of comparative genomic hybridization. Cytometry 19:27, 1995.
135. Raap T: Editorial: cytometry for CGH. Cytometry 19:1, 1995.
136. Speicher MR, Gwyn Ballard S, Ward DC: Karyotyping human chromosomes by combinatorial multi-fluor FISH. Nature Genet 12:368, 1996.
137. Schrock E, Du Manoir S, Veldman T, et al: Multicolor spectral karyotyping of human chromosomes. Science 273:494, 1996.

138. Kalousek DK: The effect of confined placental mosaicism on development of the human aneuploid conceptus. Birth Defects 29:39–51, 1993.
139. Berg CG, Zupan J, D'Almada PJ, et al: Gestational age and intrauterine growth retardation among white and black very low birthweight infants: a population-based cohort study. Paediatr Perinat Epidemiol 8:53, 1994.
140. Shoham-Vardi I, Leiberman JR, Kopernik G: The association of primiparity with intrauterine growth retardation. Eur J Obstet Gynecol Reprod Biol 53:95, 1994.
141. Salafia C, Maier D, Vogel C, et al: Placental and decidual histology in spontaneous abortion: detailed description and correlations with chromosome number. Obstet Gynecol 82:295, 1993.
142. Van Lijnschoten G, Arents JW, Thunissen FBJM, Geraedts JPM: A morphometric approach to the relation of karyotype, gestational age and histological features in early spontaneous abortion. Placenta 15:189, 1994.
143. Kalousek DK, Barrett I: Confined placental mosaicism and stillbirth. Pediatr Pathol 14:151, 1994.
144. Schubert R, Raff R, Schwanitz G: Molecular-cytogenetic investigations of the term placentae in cases of prenatally diagnosed mosaicism. Prenat Diagn 16:907, 1996.
145. Kaufman P: Entwicklung der Plazenta. In Becker V et al (eds): Die Plazenta des Menschen. Stuttgart, 1981, Georg Thieme Verlag, p 13.
146. Wang BB, Rubin CH, Williams J 3rd: Mosaicism in chronic villus sampling: an analysis of incidence and chromosomes involved in 2612 consecutive cases. Prenat Diagn 13:179, 1993.
147. Kalousek DK, Vekemans M: Confined placental mosaicism. review article. J Med Genet 33:529, 1996.
148. Leschot NJ, Wolf H: Is placental mosaicism associated with poor perinatal outcome? Prenat Diagn 11:403, 1991.
149. Wapner RJ, Simpson JL, Golbus MS, et al: Chorionic mosaicism: association with fetal loss but not with adverse perinatal outcome. Prenat Diagn 12:347, 1992.
150. Beechey C, Cattanach B: Genetic imprinting map. Mouse Genome 94:96, 1996.
151. Ledbetter DH, Engel E: Uniparental disomy in humans: development of an imprinting map and its implications for prenatal diagnosis. Hum Mol Genet 4:1757, 1995.

15

Clinical Ultrasound and Pathologic Correlation of the Placenta

Eric Jauniaux and John C.P. Kingdom

The development of a placental lesion is a dynamic process. The longer the interval between the discovery of a lesion in utero and delivery, the more marked the difference in the sonographic and the pathologic findings. Because little attempt has been made to compare ultrasound and pathologic findings in placental abnormalities, ultrasonographers continue to use inaccurate and misleading expressions to describe placental and cord lesions. Structural abnormalities of the placenta and the cord are discussed separately, since most placental lesions involve a vasculopathy of the umbilicoplacental or uteroplacental circulation whereas cord lesions are often a marker of a more complex fetal abnormality (Table 15–1).

STRUCTURAL ABNORMALITIES

PLACENTA

Placental Maturation

A sonographic classification system for grading placentas in utero according to maturational changes was developed by Grannum and associates.[1] The placentas were graded from 0 to III on the basis of compound B scan changes in the placental structures and the amount of calcification present, and the results were correlated with fetal pulmonary maturity evaluated by amniotic fluid lecithin-sphingomyelin (L/S) ratios. Mature L/S ratios were found in 68% of grade I, 88% of grade II, and 100% of grade III placentas, suggesting that invasive amniocentesis might be replaced by ultrasound placental grading as a standard test for fetal pulmonary maturity. However, subsequent reports did not support these findings, since they showed that a grade III placenta was associated with an immature L/S ratio in 8% to 42% of the cases. Therefore ultrasound was not accurate enough to replace amniocentesis in predicting fetal pulmonary maturity.[1] Factors such as chronic hypertension, preeclampsia, intrauterine growth restriction (IUGR), and maternal smoking are associated with accelerated placental maturation (see Fig. 7–12), whereas diabetes and fetomaternal immunization are associated with delayed placental maturation (see Fig. 7–11). A randomized controlled trial has demonstrated that pregnant women with mature placental appearance (grade III) on ultrasonography between 34 and 36 weeks' gestation have an increased risk of problems during labor, low-birth-weight infants, intrapartum distress, and perinatal death. Revealing this information to the clinician can reduce the risk of death.[2]

Placental Vascular Lesions

Large sonolucent intraplacental spaces (maternal lakes) can be found by ultrasound within the placental tissue from the second trimester until the end of pregnancy.[1] They contain turbulent blood flow on real-time imaging, and their shape can be modified by maternal position or uterine contractions (Fig. 15–1). Large sonolucent spaces are found in pregnancies with elevated maternal serum α-fetoprotein (MSAFP) levels if the spaces develop at the time of AFP screening.[3] Large spaces can also be observed in excessively thick

Table 15–1. Differential Diagnosis of the Principal Placental Sonographic Features

Location	Sonographic Features	Pathologic Classification
Fetal plate	Multiple sonolucent areas to placental periphery	Circumvallate placenta; circummarginate placenta
	Single sonolucent or hypoechoic area surrounded by thin membrane	Subamniotic cyst; old subamniotic; hematoma
	Single hyperechoic area surrounded by thin membrane	Recent subamniotic hematoma
	Heterogeneous mass protruding into amniotic cavity	Chorioangioma; teratoma
Placental tissue	Small sonolucent area in center of cotyledon	Centrocotyledonary cavity
	Hypoechoic round mass, well circumscribed	Chorioangioma; old infarct
	Large sonolucent area	Cavern; recent thrombosis; septal cyst
	Large hyperechoic area	Old thrombosis; recent infarct
	Multiple sonolucent areas of various sizes and shapes	Hydatidiform-like transformations
Maternal plate	Large hyperechoic area	Recent retroplacental hematoma
	Large hypoechoic area	Old retroplacental hematoma

Modified from Jauniaux E, Campbell S: Am J Obstet Gynecol 163:1650, 1990.

placentas (Fig. 15–2) and can be associated with fetal growth restriction and premature delivery.[4,5]

Katz and colleagues[6] found that large placental subchorionic lucencies are not associated with other placental or fetal anomalies and that these pregnancies are not at higher risk of perinatal complication. Our data agree with these findings for the large sonolucent space isolated in otherwise normal placental tissue. In contrast, in 16 cases we found an enlarged jellylike placenta with a patchy decrease in echogenicity, numerous sonolucent spaces throughout its substance, and a turbulent blood flow pattern on real-time imaging to be associated with abnormal fetal growth.[5] In particular, we found a jellylike placental appearance in 12 of 17 pregnancies complicated by both intrauterine growth retardation (IUGR) and preeclampsia. In ten of the cases with jellylike placentas there were also elevated MSAFP levels and abnormal Doppler features.

The combination of MSAFP elevations, abnormal placental morphology on ultrasound, and high resistance to flow in the uteroplacental circulation is more strongly associated with adverse fetal outcome than when these variables are present in isolation. A high incidence of placental vascular lesions such as large infarcts or thrombosis (Fig. 15–3) is found at delivery and fetal serum AFP levels are normal in pregnancies with elevated MSAFP levels and complicated by preeclampsia

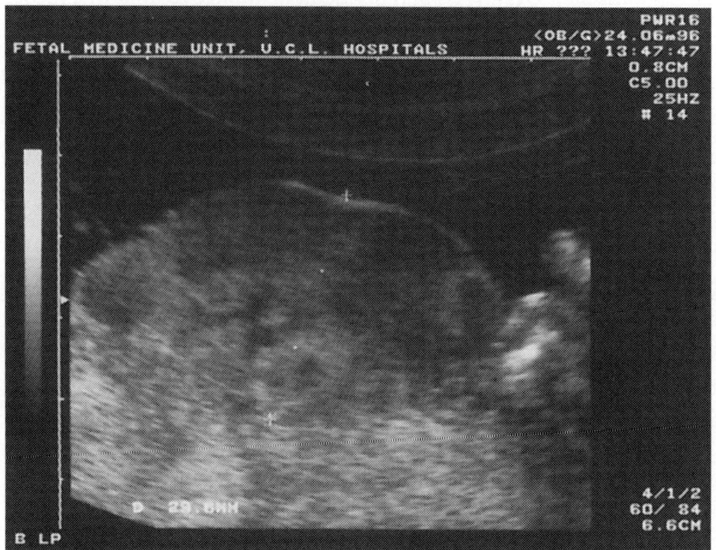

Figure 15–1. Sonogram of a large placental sonolucent space (maternal lake) at 20 weeks' gestation. The lake is under the chorionic plate and contains slow-moving turbulent flow.

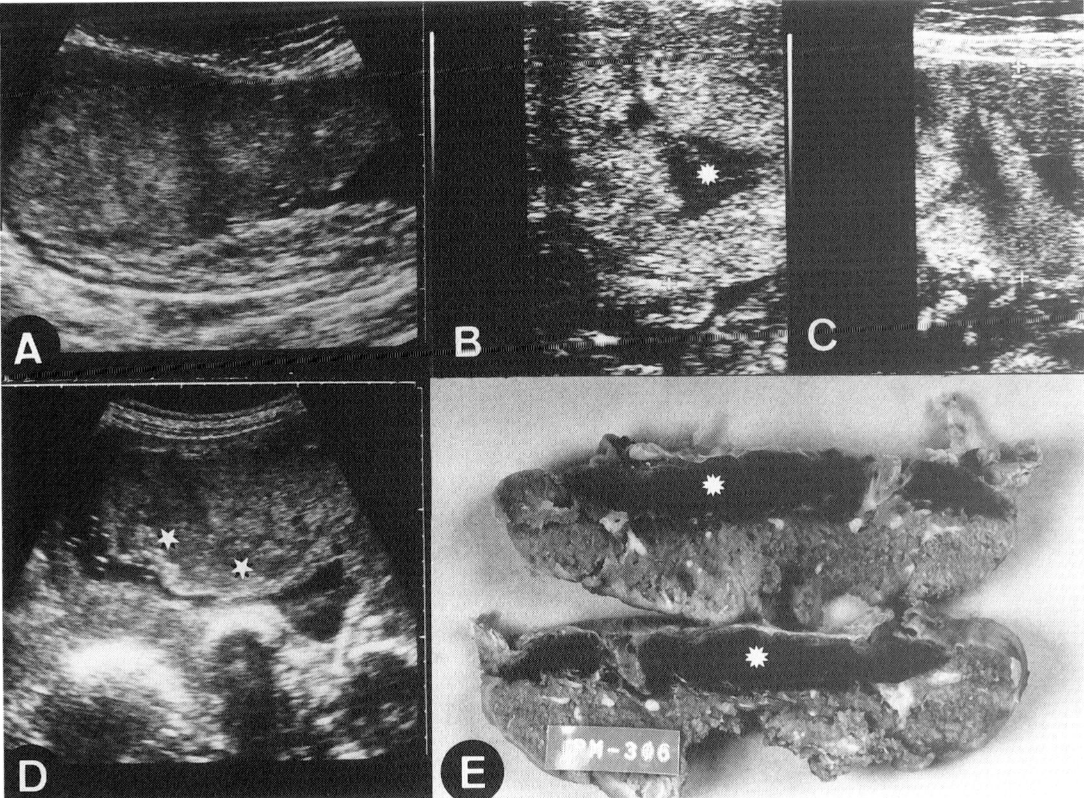

Figure 15–2. Sonograms at 20 weeks' gestation showing a large placenta (thickness > 4 cm) with patchy decreased echogenicity **(A)** and large sonolucent spaces **(B)** containing turbulent blood flow **(C** and **D)**. These placental sonographic features (jellylike placenta) were associated with elevated maternal serum α-fetoprotein. A large subchorial thrombosis *(stars)* was found at delivery in the early third trimester **(E).**

or IUGR. These findings support the concept of an increased AFP transfer through the placenta as the result of a breakdown of the trophoblastic barrier.[4] Joint assessment of uterine Doppler waveforms, placental ultrasound abnormalities, and MSAFP and maternal serum human chorionic gonadotropin (MShCG) levels around midgestation and uric acid levels after 24 weeks may refine the screening of pregnancies at risk of pregnancy-induced hypertension (PIH) and IUGR (Table 15–2).

Abnormal Placental Location and Abnormal Placentation

Placental localization by ultrasound was introduced by Donald in 1965, shortly after his first recording of an early gestational sac.[7,8] Placental visualization by sonography rapidly became standard practice, replacing older methods such as soft tissue radiography and radioisotope scanning. Respiratory distress syndrome associated with premature delivery and severe fetal anemia related to antepartum maternal hemorrhage are the major cause of neonatal morbidity and mortality associated with placenta previa. Placenta previa also produces high maternal morbidity because of massive intrapartum or postpartum hemorrhage, sometimes necessitating therapeutic hysterectomy.[9] The incidence of placenta previa varies from 0.3% to 0.5% of third-trimester pregnancies, probably reflecting differences in definition. The majority of the "low placentation" in early pregnancy has been shown not to be placenta previa at delivery, since 90% of low placentas appear subsequently to move into the upper portion of the uterus.

The prenatal ultrasound diagnosis of major placenta previa is usually easy because of the large

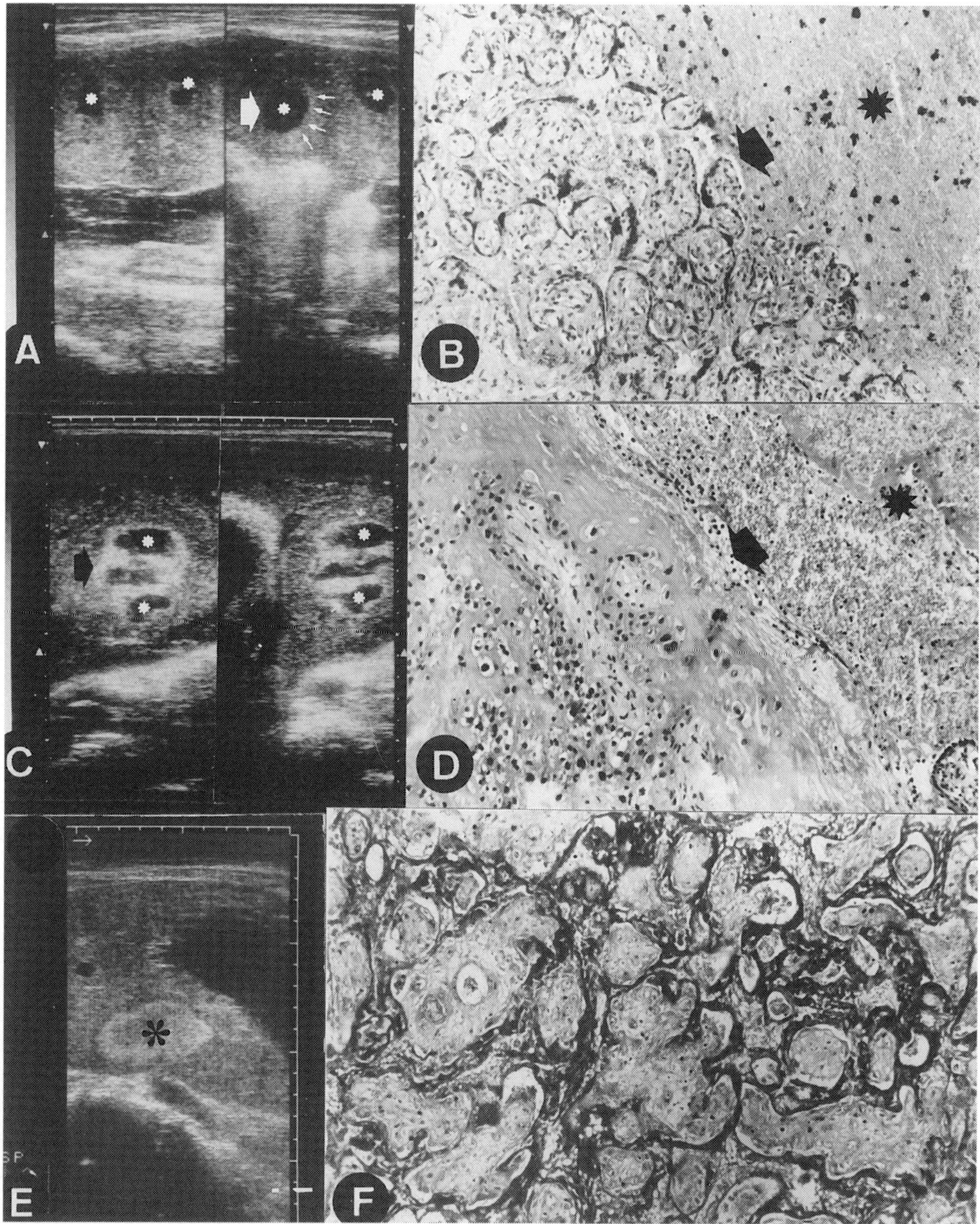

Figure 15–3. A, Sonograms at 35 weeks' gestation showing small and large placental sonolucent spaces *(stars)* containing turbulent blood flow. Note the increased echogenicity of the surrounding villi (*small arrows*). **B,** Histologic section (H&E, ×50) at the level of the large arrow showing a recent intervillous thrombosis *(star)* and normal villi (*arrow*). The villi surrounding the lesion at the level of the small arrows were compressed and infarcted. **C,** Sonograms at 39 weeks showing a large placental lesion *(stars)* corresponding to an organized intervillous thrombosis *(star)* **(D)** with extensive fibrin deposition *(large arrows)* in periphery (H&E, ×50). **E,** Large placental hyperechoic area *(star)* located near the basal plate at 32 weeks' gestation corresponding to a chronic infarct **(F)** (H&E, ×50). (From Jauniaux E, Campbell S: Am J Obstet Gynecol 163:1650, 1990.)

Table 15–2. Placental Ultrasound Features, Pregnancy Outcome, and Maternal Serum Biochemistry at 16 to 22 Weeks

USS Findings	Biochemistry	Doppler	Pathology	Outcome
Large sonolucent area (marginal-subchorionic)	Normal to high MSAFP; normal MShCG	Normal resistance to flow	Subchorionic thrombosis/ fibrin depot	Normal
Placenta thickness > 4 cm with diffuse sonolucent areas	High MSAFP; normal to high MShCG	High resistance in umbilical circulation	Diffuse fibrin depots/ thrombosis and microinfarcts	IUFD; IUGR
Diffuse dense areas (hypoechoic to hyperechoic)	High MSAFP; high MShCG	High resistance in both placental circulations	Large infarcts and fibrin depots	IUGR; PE
Large circumscribed hypoechoic area	High MSAFP; normal MShCG	Normal resistance to flow	Chorioangioma	Polyhydramnios

USS, Ultrasound study; *MSAFP,* maternal serum α-fetoprotein; *MShCG,* maternal serum human chorionic gonadotropin; *IUFD,* intrauterine fetal death; *IUGR,* intrauterine growth restriction; *PE,* preeclampsia.
Data from references 3, 4, and 5.

amount of placental tissue overlying the internal os. However, low-lying posterior placentas may not be distinguishable by sonography from marginal or partial placenta previa. Several conditions such as maternal obesity, posterior localization of the placenta, overdistended bladder, local myometrial thickening, and acoustic shadow of the fetal head can make accurate transabdominal ultrasound diagnosis of the different types of placenta previa difficult. These considerations have led recently to the proposal that transvaginal sonography is a more accurate method of diagnosing placenta previa. This new technique appears in comparative series to be as safe as and diagnostically superior to abdominal sonography.[10]

Decidua basalis deficiency with deep attachment of the placental villi inside the myometrium is considered the primary mechanism of the development of placenta accreta. In theory any endometrial trauma is a predisposing factor for the development of placenta accreta, and a previous cesarean section is most commonly found in the patient history.[11] Women with an anterior placenta previa and a previous cesarean section have a 20% to 30% risk of placenta accreta during a subsequent pregnancy. With the increasing rate of elective cesarean sections in some developed countries, the incidence of the various forms of placenta accreta is increasing. Since this condition is associated with a 25% maternal mortality, the potential for identifying placenta accreta before delivery holds considerable clinical interest. The absence of a decidual interface with a normal placental echogenicity is pathognomonic for placenta accreta.[12] Color Doppler sonography may highlight areas of increased vascularity with dilated blood vessels crossing the placenta and uterine wall (Fig. 15–4*A*).

The placenta extrachorialis (circummarginate and circumvallate placenta) is a common abnormality found in about 25% of placentas and characterized by a transition of membranous to villous chorion at a distance from the placental edge.[1] Insertion of the membranes within the placental margin results in placental tissue not covered by the chorionic plate (extrachorialis, accounting for antepartum bleeding in some cases) and in a smaller than normal amniotic cavity (Fig. 15–4*B*).

Nontrophoblastic Placental Tumors

Chorioangiomas are found in 0.5% to 1% of the placentas examined at term.[1] The microscopic appearance may be that of a capillary angioma (vascular), mesenchymal hyperplasia (cellular), or usually a mixture of the two. Most chorioangiomas are single, encapsulated, small, round, and intraplacental. Large chorioangiomas are well circumscribed, have a different echogenicity from the rest of the placental tissue (Fig. 15–5*A*), and are easily detectable by sonography early in pregnancy. Small intraplacental chorioangiomas have rarely been documented sonographically.[13] Chorioangiomas are associated with an increased incidence of polyhydramnios and IUGR. Large tumors (greater than 5 cm in diameter) can also be complicated by fetal cardiac failure with hydrops

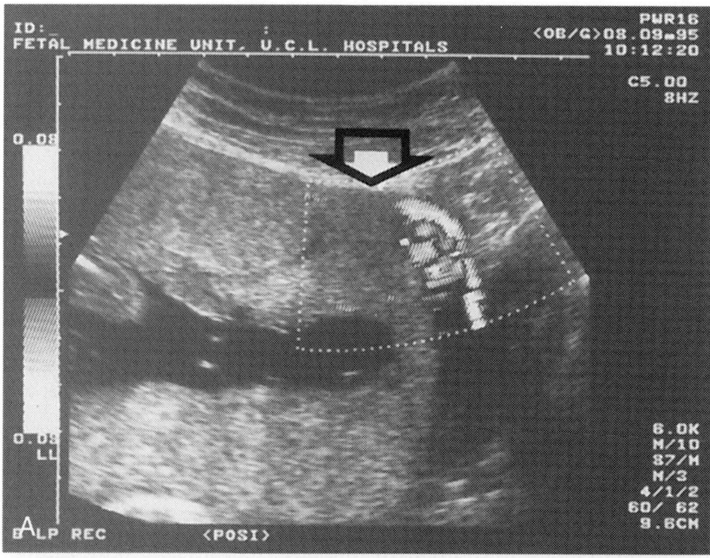

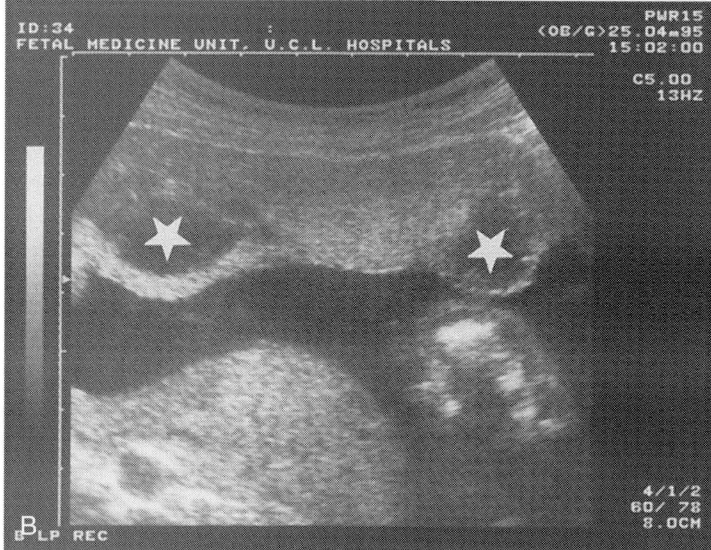

Figure 15–4. A, Longitudinal view of a complete placenta previa located partially under the scar of a previous cesarean section *(arrow).* Note the absence of decidual interface and an area of increased vascularity with dilated blood vessels. **B,** Hypoechoic spaces *(stars)* under the chorionic placental plate at 20 weeks' gestation. The lesions are all around the edge of the placenta and indicate the abnormal insertion of the membrane inside the placenta (circumvallate).

because of the shunting of blood through the tumor (Fig. 15–5*B*). Therefore, when a placental mass consistent with a chorioangioma is diagnosed antenatally, it is important to perform color Doppler mapping of the lesion.[14] Increase in echogenicity of the tumor with gestation has been related to fibrotic degeneration of the lesion, which may reduce the risk of high-output fetal cardiac failure. Placental chorioangiomas can be associated with elevated levels of AFP in the maternal serum and the amniotic fluid.[1] Associated fetal angiomas (cutaneous or hepatic) occur in 10% to 15% of cases of placental chorioangiomas, and a detailed examination of the neonate is recommended in these cases.

Umbilical Cord

Variations in the Placental Insertion

Marginal and markedly eccentric insertions of the umbilical cord have not been clearly distinguished in the literature. This may explain the wide variation of their incidence at term. By measuring the distance between the cord insertion and the closest placental margin, one can avoid classification problems. With this method, a significantly shorter distance was found in placentas from in vitro fertilization compared with control placentas.[15] This form of cord insertion may be caused by a malrotation of the blastocyst at implantation. Pregnancy complications can occur (see Chapter 5).

Velamentous insertion of the cord is a well-defined pathologic entity with a frequency of about 1% of all pregnancies.[1] The relation between this abnormal cord insertion and associated developmental defects is a matter of debate. Some authors have observed a high incidence of fetal malformations associated with extraplacental cord insertion, whereas others have found only an increase in the number of small for date neonates but not of malformations. From a clinical viewpoint, attachment of the cord to the extraplacental membranes is important because of the risk of severe fetal hemorrhage during labor,[1] as well as thrombosis (see Chapter 5).

Single Umbilical Artery Syndrome

The absence of one umbilical artery is among the most common congenital fetal malformations,

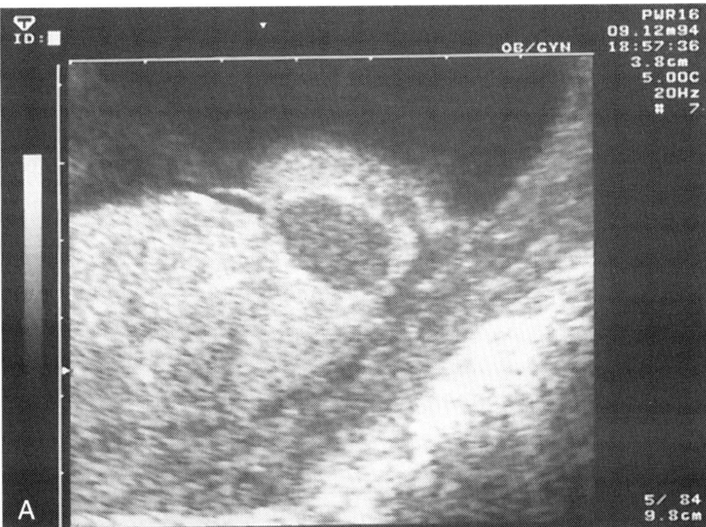

Figure 15–5. A, Longitudinal sonogram of the placenta at 20 weeks' gestation showing an hypoechoic mass corresponding to a chorioangioma. Polyhydramnios had been noted. **B,** Flow velocity waveforms obtained from the lesion shown in **A** indicating the vascularization of the tumor by fetal vessels (vascular chorioangioma).

with an incidence of approximately 1% of deliveries.[16] With the advent of ultrasound imaging the search for the cord with the missing vessel became part of the second-trimester ultrasonographic screening. Single umbilical artery syndrome (SUAS) occurs three to four times more frequently in twins and almost invariably accompanies the acardia malformation and sirenomelia or caudal regression syndrome.[16] There is also a six-fold increase in the incidence of velamentous insertion of the cord among SUAS infants. A single umbilical artery in the cord is in many cases the result of secondary atrophy of one of the arteries, and that vessel may disappear completely only after the second-trimester routine ultrasound examination. Thus two distant sonographic sections of the umbilical cord showing only two vessels are required for the antenatal diagnosis of single umbilical artery in the second or the third trimester of pregnancy. The examination of the fetal end of the cord including the lower pelvis is usually the easiest approach for the screening of a one-artery cord.[17] Color Doppler imaging (Fig. 15–6) is of particular clinical value in early pregnancy (less than 16 weeks), in monoamniotic twins, if gray-scale images are of poor quality, or to investigate the associated hemodynamic changes within the abdominopelvic fetal vasculature.[18]

Most cases of SUAS are discovered within the context of another fetal anatomic defect or obstetric problem. These complications are largely responsible for the high perinatal loss related to this disorder.[19] Associated fetal malformations are common in cases of single umbilical artery and can affect any organ system. In his comprehensive review of 237 autopsy cases of fetuses with a single umbilical artery, Heifetz[16] estimated that about 20% of malformed newborns have this anomaly. The comparison of sonographic and postnatal findings in cases of SUAS has shown that minor malformations of the musculoskeletal and cardiovascular systems or of the genitourinary tract are often misdiagnosed by ultrasonography, especially when they are isolated.[19] The discovery of a single umbilical artery in the perinatal period justifies a detailed ultrasound examination of the neonate to exclude minor anomalies of internal organs such as the kidney or heart, which may lead to deleterious sequelae if left untreated until late infancy. The incidence of IUGR is significantly elevated among fetuses with a single umbilical artery, and IUGR may be present without any other congenital anomalies in 15% to 20% of the cases.[19] A single umbilical artery is not a specific marker of chromosomal abnormalities, and the higher incidence of such artery in trisomies 13 and 18 is probably related only to the higher incidence in these cases of major fetal defects that are known to be associated with aplasia or atrophy of one of the umbilical arteries.[19]

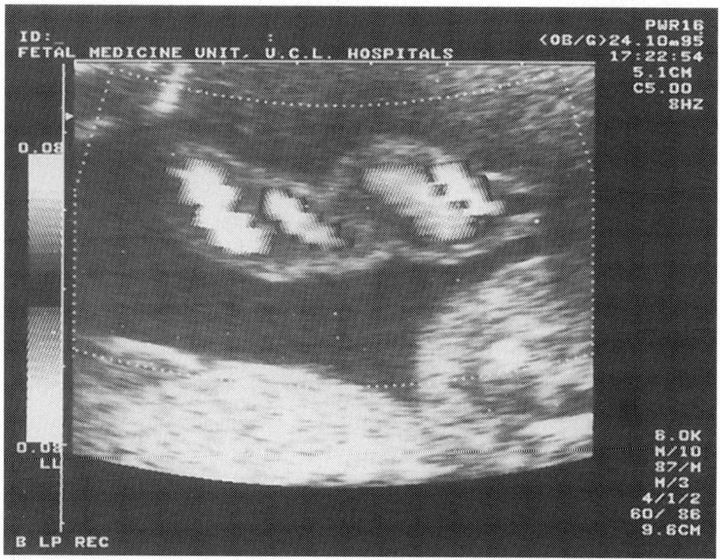

Figure 15–6. Color flow mapping at 22 weeks' gestation showing only one umbilical artery (*right*) next to the umbilical vein (*left*).

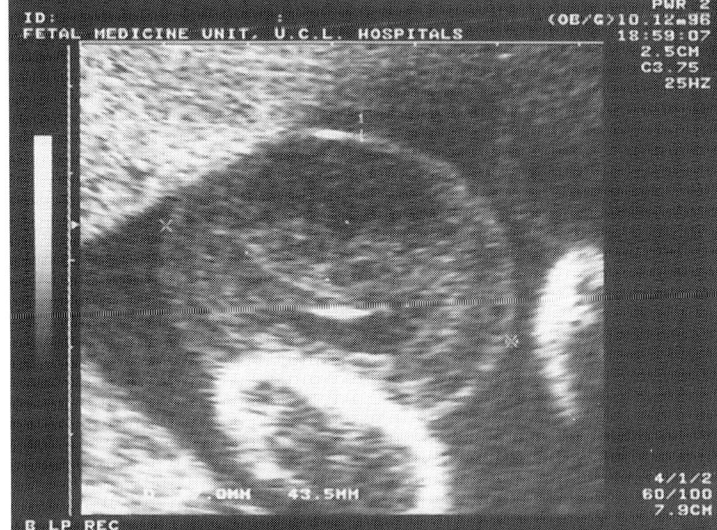

Figure 15–7. Sonogram of a large hypoechoic area (pseudocyst) at 32 weeks' gestation.

Umbilical Cord Masses

Umbilical cord remnants of the allantoic duct (urachus), omphalomesenteric duct (vitelline duct), or embryonic vessels are classic findings on microscopic examination of the cord.[20] Traces of the allantoic duct are found in 22.8% of cords examined histologically and have a similar incidence on both sides of the cord insertion. Allantoic cysts are rarely diagnosed in utero. They may coexist with an omphalocele or with patent urachus caused by a distal genitourinary tract obstruction.[21] Needle biopsy of cord masses can be performed under ultrasound guidance but should not be done without taking into consideration the risk of potential fetal hemorrhage, since some of these masses are vascularized. Serial ultrasound examinations to verify the evolution in size of the lesion must be performed regularly, combined with Doppler velocimetry to detect secondary effects on the cord circulation. Color flow Doppler imaging may also help the sonographer make a precise differential diagnosis without using invasive procedures.

Remnants of embryonic vessels are observed in 11% of the cords examined histologically.[20] They occur mainly at the fetal extremity of the cord and are often associated with allantoic remnants. The majority of cord angiomyxomas consist of nodules clearly attached to the cord.[22] Potential fetal complications of cord angiomyxomas include vascular compression of the main vessels with abnormal growth or possible intrauterine death and shortening of the cord length. These tumors appear sonographically as focal hyperechoic areas corresponding to myxoid tissue and vascular proliferation, with adjacent hypoechoic (pseudocystic) formation caused by focal edema (myxomatous degeneration) of Wharton's jelly. The abnormal vascular pattern of this type of cord tumor is well demonstrated by color Doppler imaging.[18]

Giant focal cord edema (myxomatous degeneration of Wharton's jelly) gives an ultrasound appearance of an anechoic fluid-filled multicystic mass (Fig. 15–7). These pseudocysts are presumably due to compression of umbilical cord vessels resulting from anterior fetal abdominal defects or from development of a cord angiomyxoma.[1] They can be easily diagnosed in utero from the end of the first trimester and could be an early marker of lethal aneuploidy or congenital anomalies.[23,24]

IATROGENIC LESIONS OF THE CORD AND PLACENTA

Growing use of invasive prenatal procedures has resulted in an increase in cord and placental damage with potential consequences for the fetus. Amniocentesis has been the most frequently used procedure but is being progressively replaced by chorionic villous sampling and percutaneous umbilical blood sampling (PUBS) or cordocentesis.

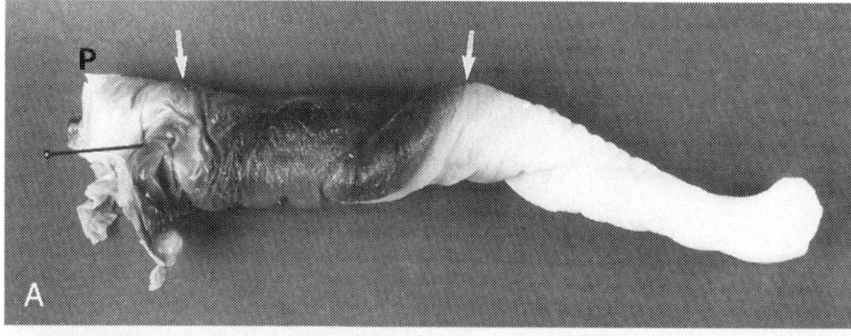

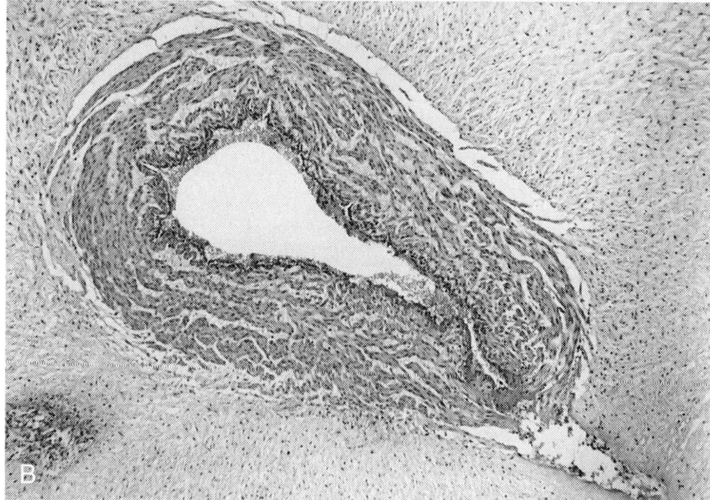

Figure 15–8. A, The cord near its placental *(P)* insertion showing a large hematoma (between arrows) that developed after fetal transfusion in utero. **B,** Umbilical cord at the site of needle puncture (bottom right) 1 week after percutaneous umbilical blood sampling (H&E, ×125).

Cord and placental trauma associated with severe fetal distress or fetal death was described during the early days of amniocentesis when no ultrasound guidance was used. Uncontrolled movements of the needle in PUBS are reduced by precise insertion of the needle in the cord under ultrasound guidance and by the increased experience of perinatal teams in these invasive procedures. Lacerations of superficial umbilical vessels may lead to substantial hemorrhage into the amniotic sac with severe adverse hemodynamic consequences.[25] A small hematoma usually does not compromise the fetal umbilical circulation because the blood can drain into the amniotic cavity via the needle entry. The extension of the hematoma is probably also limited by the tension created by Wharton's jelly and the amniotic cavity. The end result of a cord hematoma may range from complete occlusion of the cord vessels with inevitable fetal death to varying degrees of acute or chronic fetal distress.[26] Macroscopic examination of cords after delivery may elucidate how often procedure-related bradycardia is associated with specific cord damage (Fig. 15–8*A*). Microscopic examination of the cords of fetuses born after PUBS[25] demonstrates a rapid regeneration of the vessel wall within a week after the procedure (Fig. 15–8*B*).

ZYGOSITY IN MULTIPLE PREGNANCY

The ultrasound identification of more than one gestational sac and one embryo before 10 weeks' gestation does not ensure the continued survival of all fetuses. The vanishing twin phenomenon is the spontaneous abortion or resorption of one of the twins and occurs in about 20% of twins recognized in the first trimester, which is similar to the incidence of clinical loss in singleton pregnancies at the same gestational age. Vaginal bleeding is the main symptom but is reported in only 20% of the cases of vanishing twin.[27] The pregnancy outcome of the surviving twin is not otherwise affected, and a careful examination of the placenta after delivery often permits the identification of embryonic remnants.[27]

The prenatal outcome in twins is related primarily to chorionicity, which is the major factor in determining pregnancy outcome.[28] In monochorionic twins, perinatal morbidity and mortality are twice as high as in dichorionic twins. Conjoined twins or a shared placenta is the cause for twin-twin transfusion (TTT) syndrome and twin-reversed atrial perfusion (TRAP) syndrome. Furthermore, the death of a monochorionic twin jeopardizes the co-twin, putting it at high risk of sudden death or severe neurologic impairment.[29] Therefore accurate identification of monochorionic twins enables close monitoring of these very high risk fetuses. The traditional diagnostic scanning method of chorionicity has been visualization of two sacs before 10 weeks' gestation, different fetal sexes, and two complete separate placentas at 14 to 16 weeks' gestation. Examination of the intertwin membrane characteristics, such as width and number of layers (<2 mm for diamnionic/monochorionic twins; four layers and more echogenicity typically for dichorionic/diamniotic twins) is a more accurate diagnostic method.[30,31] The extension of placental tissue in a triangular projection at the base of the intertwin membrane is known as the twin peak or lambda sign in twins and the ipsilon sign in triplets.[32,33] Prospective studies using transabdominal first-trimester scanning have reported a high reliability for determining chorionicity in twin pregnancies based on an intertwin membrane assessment (Fig. 15–9).

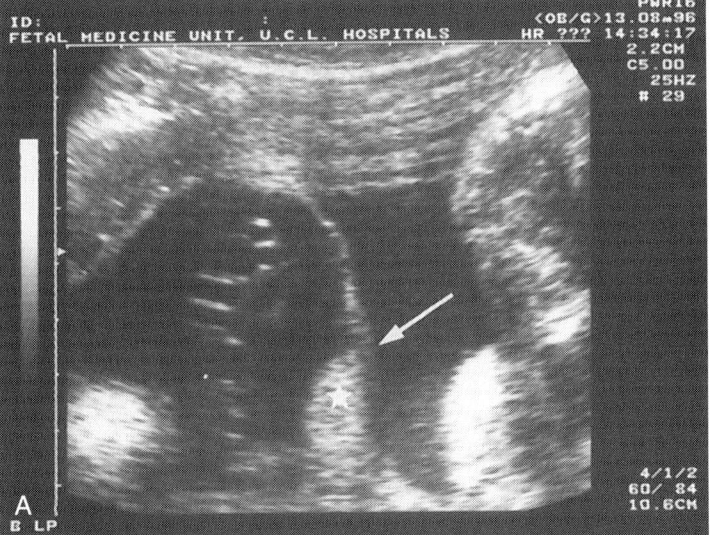

Figure 15–9. A, Dichorionic twin pregnancy at 14 weeks' gestation. Note the twin peak at the base of the membrane *(arrow).* **B,** Monochorionic monozygotic twin pregnancy at 13 weeks' gestation. Note the presence of one placenta *(arrow)* and a thin membrane *(arrows).*

Vascular connections between the two cord insertions are a frequent pathologic finding in monochorionic monozygotic twin placentas. Unusual flow velocity waveforms showing cyclic changes in systolic velocities with intermittent reversal of end-diastolic velocities can be demonstrated in utero in these cases.[35,36] A computer model has shown that these Doppler signals were the result of two opposing pulsatile blood flow waveforms with different velocities and frequencies.

ABNORMAL UMBILICAL ARTERY BLOOD FLOW

Clinical Utility of Umbilical Artery Doppler Ultrasound

Absence of or reversed end-diastolic flow (EDF) velocity in the umbilical arteries, detected by pulsed Doppler ultrasound, is a poor prognostic sign in the late second and early third trimesters, typically associated with severe IUGR.[37] Perinatal mortality in pregnancies with umbilical artery Doppler abnormalities is reduced by about one third as a result of fetal monitoring and planned delivery by cesarean section,[38] hence the current level of enthusiasm about this technique among clinicians. The lack of long-term neurodevelopmental outcome data among survivors remains an important concern.[39] Furthermore, absence of EDF velocity can be associated with aneuploidy and other intrauterine pathologic conditions,[40,41] necessitating careful sonographic examination of the fetus, amniotic fluid, umbilical cord, and placenta to evaluate the likely underlying cause.

Development of the Placental Villi

The first-trimester placenta is characterized by gradual capillarization of primitive villi, which impede blood flow, leading to "physiologic" absence of EDF velocity.[42] Intervillous blood flow is not demonstrable at this stage, resulting in "intraplacental" hypoxia,[43] which in turn favors trophoblast proliferation (thereby forming new primitive mesenchymal villi), capillary angiogenesis, and hence villous growth. Intervillous blood flow and EDF velocities in the umbilical arteries develop during the early second trimester and increase steadily thereafter toward term.[44] The growing part of the developing villous tree is the immature intermediate villi (IIV), and these are transformed proximally, through the formation of a muscularized media, into stem villi.[45] By about 20 to 24 weeks' gestation, the stem villi have largely formed, and further placental villous growth is directed toward the differentiation of IIV into their gas-exchanging mature counterparts, the mature intermediate villi (MIV) and their numerous terminal villi.[45] These structures are illustrated in Figure 15–10. By term the exponential increase in MIV and terminal villi caused by capillary angiogenesis results in an area of placenta available for gaseous exchange of more than 12 m^2 and a fetoplacental capillary volume of 80 ml.[46]

Pathology of Absence of EDF Velocity in the Umbilical Arteries

Confirmed absence of EDF velocity in the umbilical arteries generally persists or worsens until delivery,[47,48] which is the rationale for Doppler-based monitoring in severe IUGR.[49] The concept of a "fixed" lesion that often worsens is clinically important because the fetus is at increasing risk of hypoxia and acidosis until delivery,[50] indicating that absence of EDF is associated with a major impairment of transplacental gas exchange.

The macroscopic appearance of a placenta from a pregnancy complicated by severe IUGR is often abnormal, as the angiograms in Figure 15–11 illustrate. Vascular impedance is governed by the small stem arterioles or the distal capillaries within the peripheral villous tree. Figure 15–12 illustrates the normal structure of a typical stem villus containing several muscularized vessel profiles. The original proposal for absence of EDF velocities in the umbilical arteries was a reduction, caused by vessel obliteration, in the density of small-diameter (<90 μm) stem arterioles.[51] Subsequent publications supported this theory, but all suffered from lack of attention to tissue collection, processing, and analysis.[52] A newer approach, localization of muscularized stem vessel profiles by actin immunohistochemistry, failed to detect any selective loss of vessel profiles, even in the very smallest

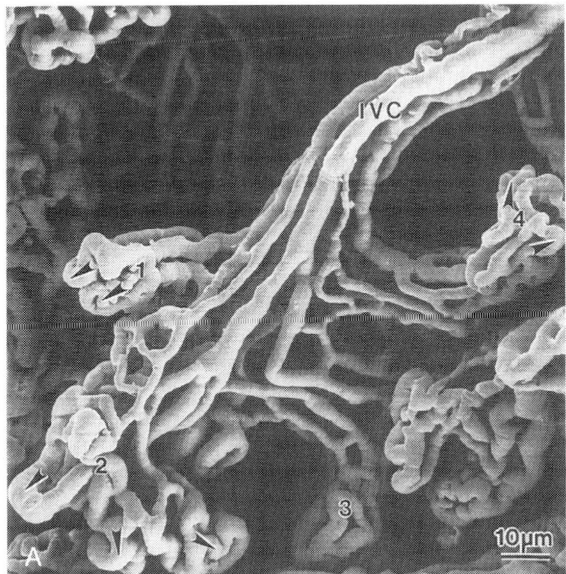

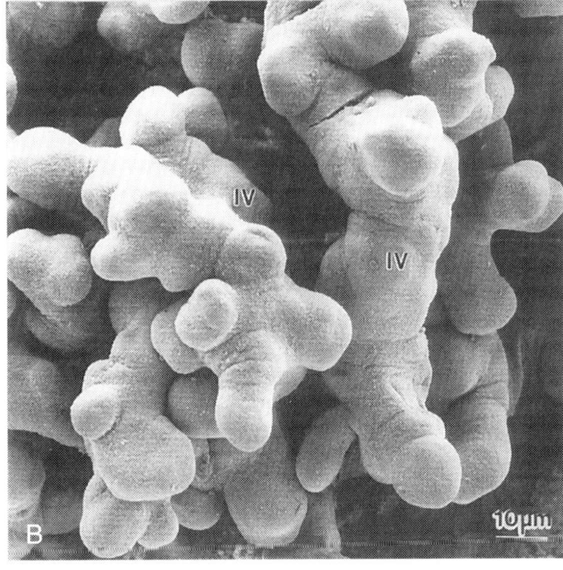

Figure 15–10. Scanning electron micrographs. **A,** Mature intermediate villous capillaries (IVC) and four terminal convolutes (*1* to *4, arrows*) from a normal placenta at 32 weeks' gestation. **B,** Corresponding mature intermediate villi *(IV)* with their microvillous surface. Terminal capillaries bulge out to form terminal villi. (From Krebs C, Macara LM, Leiser R, et al: Am J Obstet Gynecol 175:1534, 1996.)

(10 to 30 μm) postfixation diameter range, but did not use random block sampling.[53]

Even if the anatomy of the stem arterial tree is largely unaltered in IUGR pregnancies with absence of EDF, the vessels themselves may have significant pathologic damage. An elegant transmission electron microscopic study of stem muscularized vessels in preeclamptic placentas, often associated with IUGR and umbilical artery Doppler abnormalities, demonstrated occlusion of the vessel lumen by the endothelium.[54] These findings are reproduced in Figure 15–13. Caution is advised when assessing the findings because the tissues were not immediately perfusion fixed and postdelivery vasoconstriction could have produced artifacts at the electron microscopic level. However, a further study at the light microscopic level has suggested vascular hypertrophy of stem arteries in placentas from IUGR pregnancies, the extent of which correlated with the degree of umbilical artery Doppler abnormality.[55] Damage to either the media or endothelium of stem arteries could profoundly alter the local vasomotor control of these noninnervated vessels. At present the ev-

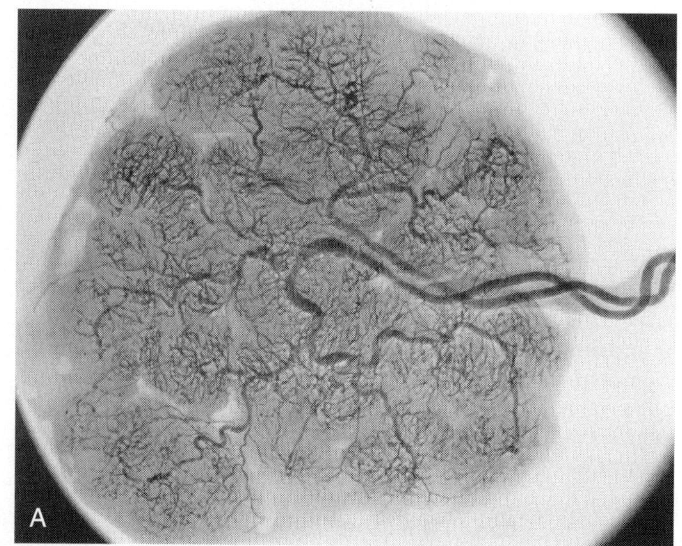

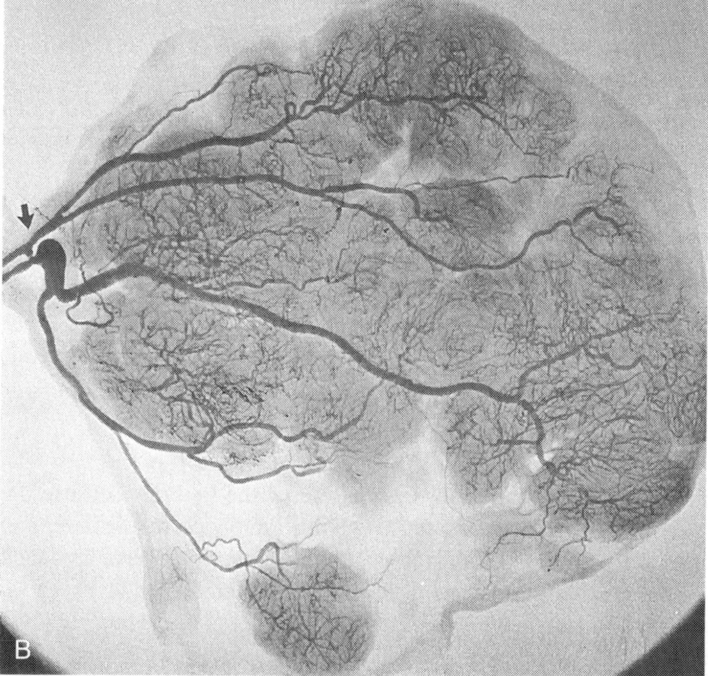

Figure 15–11. Angiogram of a normal term placenta **(A)** and a placenta from an IUGR pregnancy with umbilical artery Doppler abnormalities **(B)**. Note the normal dichotomous branching of the chorionic plate arteries, which is in contrast to the eccentric cord insertion and abnormal vascular arrangement in the IUGR case. (Reprinted from Nordenvall M, Ullberg I, Laurin J, et al: Placental morphology in relation to umbilical artery blood flow velocity waveforms. Eur J Obstet Gynaecol Reprod Biol 40:179–190, 1991, with kind permission from Elsevier Science Ireland Ltd., Bay 15K, Shannon Industrial Estate, County Clare, Ireland.)

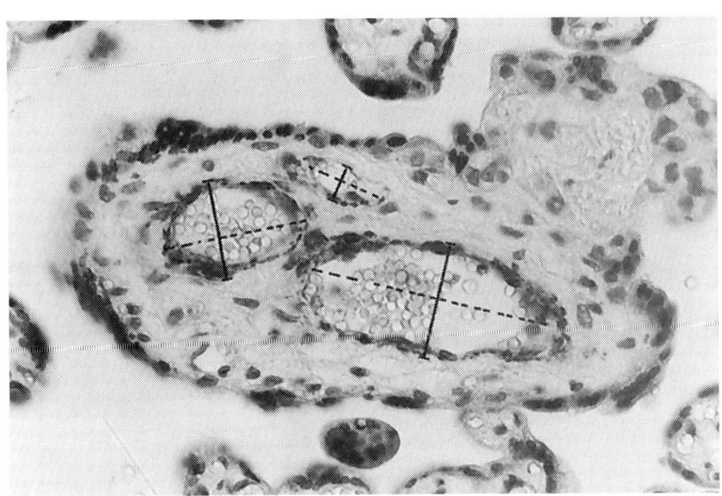

Figure 15–12. Immunohistochemical localization of muscularized stem vessel profiles using an antibody directed against α smooth muscle actin. Distinguishing arterioles from venules is not possible unless serial sections are taken and vessel reconstruction is performed. Similarly, adequate assessment of the vascular endothelium is not possible using light microscopy. (From Macara LM, Kingdom JCP, Kohnen G, et al: Br J Obstet Gynaecol 101:807, 1995.)

idence for a major vasomotor disorder, involving intense and sustained pathologic vasoconstriction, is lacking. The current literature is summarized in a recent review.[56]

Understanding of the developmental biology of the fetal villous tree has increased substantially over the past decade,[55,57] which has allowed various groups to focus their attention on the gas-exchanging villi. These are smaller and more numerous than stem villi, and precise microscopic methods are needed to assess differences in structure between study and control groups. Since these villi are responsible for gas exchange and at the same time their development parallels the physiologic decrease in fetoplacental vascular impedance, a failure of normal development of the gas-exchanging villi could account for most of the pathology of IUGR.[45] Two important light microscopy studies, in which the placenta was systematically sampled, concluded that the sectional area of placenta occupied by nonmuscularized villi was reduced when compared with gestational age–matched controls.[58,59] We recently used a three-dimensional approach, employing scanning electron microscopy of both villous tissue and plastic corrosion vascular casts to confirm the hypothesis of peripheral villous maldevelopment in severe preterm IUGR.[60] Severely maldeveloped villi are illustrated in Figure 15–14. Parallel two-dimensional structural analysis of terminal villi in these cases proved instructive as to the pathologic development of fetal hypoxia in this severe form of IUGR. Stromal fibrosis, reduced cytotrophoblast proliferation, and syncytiotrophoblast senescence or apoptosis were found, suggesting a local elevation of villous oxygen content before delivery.[61] The terminal capillaries were obstructed by fetal erythrocytes, suggesting that the "embolic process" does not primarily involve platelets in small arterioles, but rather aggregates of fetal erythrocytes within malformed peripheral capillaries and associated decidual vasculopathy (see Chapter 8).[60] Parallel maternal (intervillous) thrombosis occurs on the surface of the abnormal villi, a secondary pathway of placental failure, since transplacental gas exchange is worsened. This severe form of preterm IUGR and fetal hypoxia has been termed postplacental fetal hypoxia.[62] These anatomic studies are of clinical relevance because they reinforce the concept of a fixed and largely irreversible vascular lesion in the placenta. The clinical implication is that pregnancies with absence of EDF velocity in the umbilical arteries remain at high risk of fetal death until delivery by cesarean section.

A more precise understanding of the basis of absence of EDF in the umbilical arteries illustrates for the clinician the profound disorganization within the gas-exchanging villi in this condition, creating a greater awareness of the serious implications for the fetus and the need for intensive fetal monitoring until delivery. Fetal (capillary) or maternal (villous surface) thrombosis is demonstrable in these circumstances[59,60] (see Fig. 15–13*B*), and congenital or acquired thrombotic tendencies, such as the newly discovered factor V

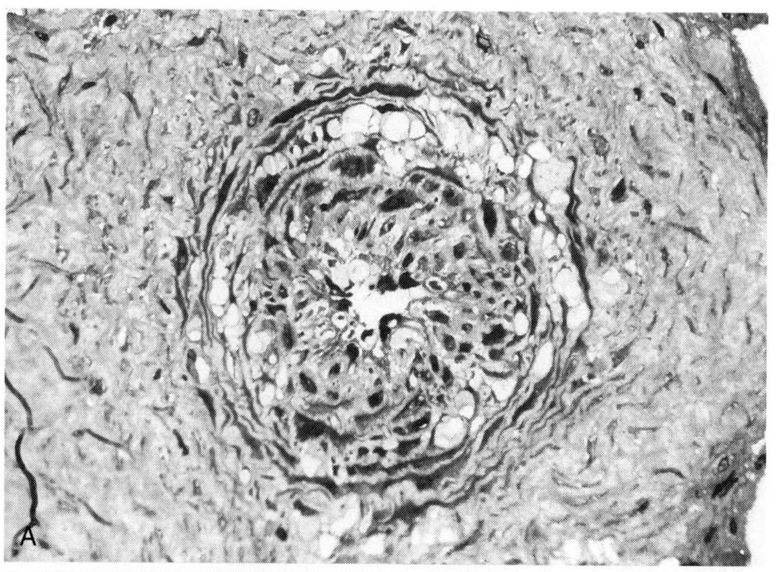

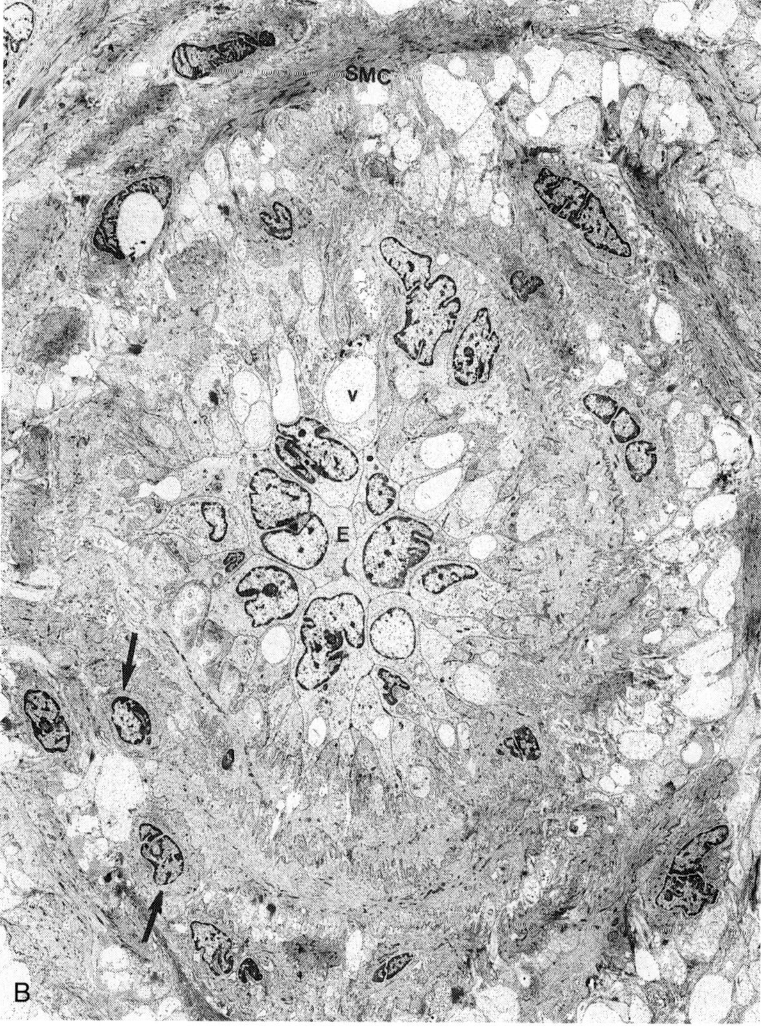

Figure 15–13. Light **(A)** and transmission electron **(B)** photomicrographs of muscularized stem vessels from the preeclamptic placenta. The vessel lumen is occluded by swollen endothelial cells, which is more obvious at the electron microscopic level. These features suggest pathologic activation of the normally flow-regulating arterial endothelial cells. (Permission was granted for use of the figures from work by Las Heras and Haust, Trophoblast Research 3:335, 1988.)

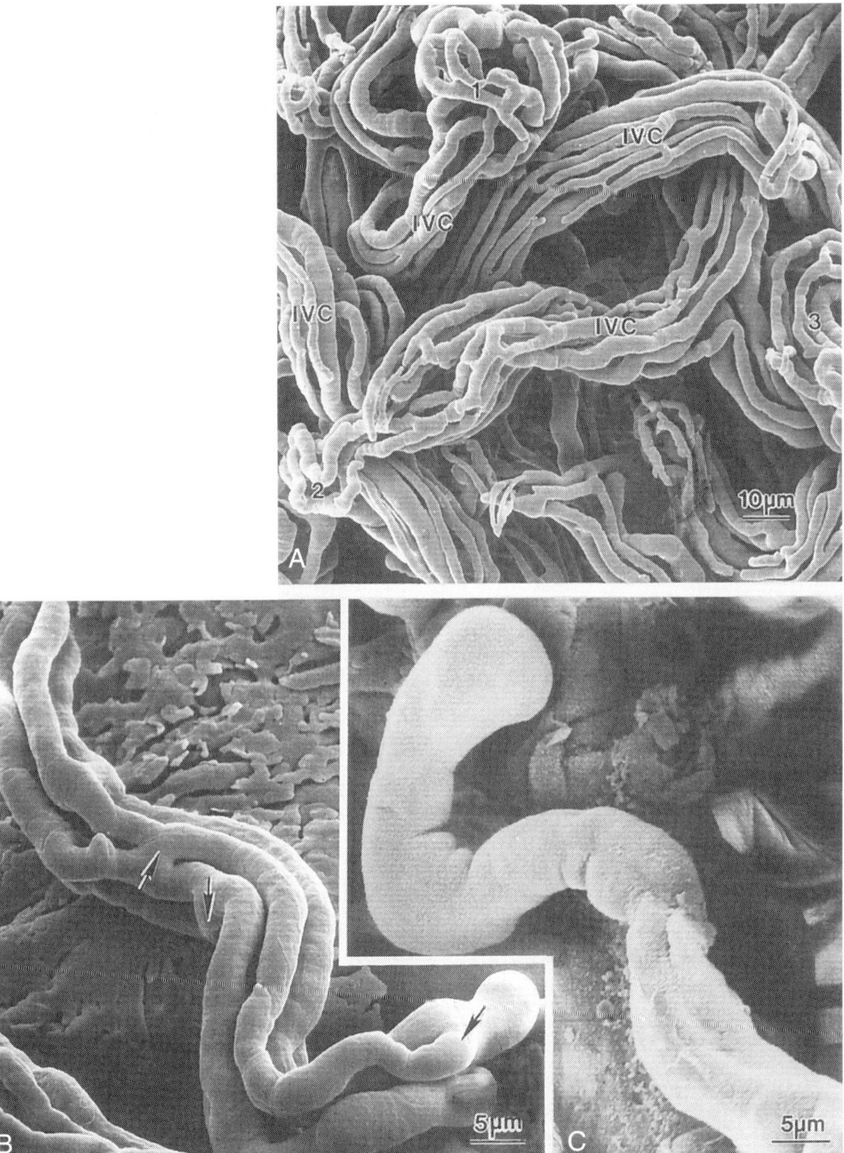

Figure 15–14. **A** to **C,** Maldeveloped, peripheral gas-exchanging villi, together with their capillaries, from a severe IUGR case with absence of EDF velocities detected in the umbilical arteries before delivery. **A,** Bundles of elongated intermediate villous capillaries (IVC) are seen with occasional terminal convolutes *(1,2,3).* **B** and **C,** Higher views show an extremely elongated villous ending with no coiling and few branches *(arrows)* (**B,** Cast; **C,** corresponding villus).

Illustration continued on following page

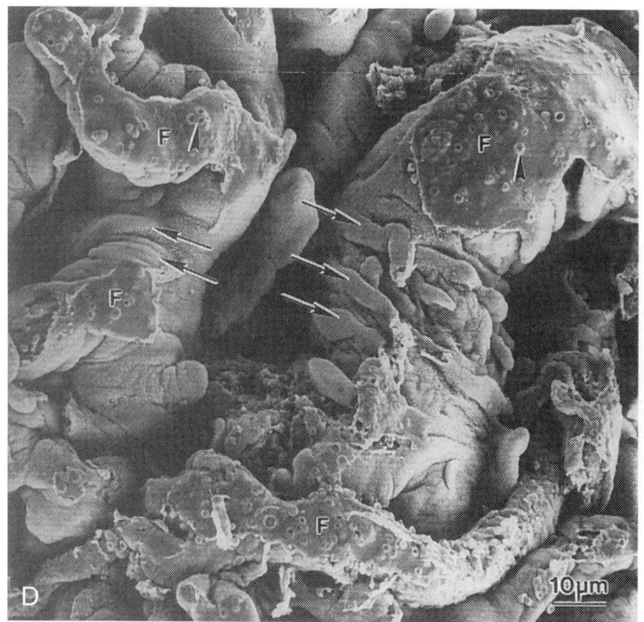

Figure 15–14 *Continued* **D,** Abnormal villous surface in severe preterm IUGR demonstrating plaques of fibrin *(F)* engulfing maternal erythrocytes. The syncytiotrophoblast was often found to be wrinkled, which is due to arrest of trophoblast turnover.[60] Apoptosis is probably responsible for these appearances. (From Krebs C, Macara LM, Leiser R, et al: Am J Obstet Gynecol 175:1534, 1996.)

Leiden mutation in protein C, are found in up to 30% of cases of severe preterm preeclampsia, which is often associated with IUGR and umbilical artery Doppler abnormalities.[63,64] Clearly a number of factors contribute to disordered placental angiogenesis, and in the most severe forms of preterm IUGR, oxygen "accumulation" within the villous placenta may prevent normal branching angiogenesis.[61] Further pathologic studies, concentrating on uteroplacental ischemia and on the factors controlling villous angiogenesis, are awaited with interest.

REFERENCES

1. Jauniaux E, Campbell S: Sonographic assessment of placental abnormalities. Am J Obstet Gynecol 163:1650, 1990.
2. Proud J, Grant AM: Third trimester placental grading by ultrasonography as a test of fetal wellbeing. Br Med J 294:1641, 1987.
3. Jauniaux E, Moscoso G, Campbell S, et al: Correlation of ultrasound and pathologic findings of placental anomalies in pregnancies with elevated maternal serum alpha-fetoprotein. Eur J Obstet Gynecol 37:219, 1990.
4. Jauniaux E, Ramsay B, Campbell S: Ultrasonographic investigation of placental morphology and size during the second trimester of pregnancy. Am J Obstet Gynecol 170:130, 1994.
5. Jauniaux E, Gulbis B, Tunkel S, et al: Maternal serum testing for alpha-fetoprotein and human chorionic gonadotropin in high risk pregnancies. Prenat Diagn 16:1129, 1996.
6. Katz VL, Blanchard GF, Watson WJ, et al: The clinical implications of subchorionic placental lucencies. Am J Obstet Gynecol 164:99, 1991.
7. Donald I: On launching a new diagnostic science. Am J Obstet Gynecol 103:609, 1968.
8. Gottesfeld KR, Thompson HE, Holmes JH, Taylor D: Ultrasonic placentography—a new method for placental localization. Am J Obstet Gynecol 96: 538, 1967.
9. McShane PM, Heyl PS, Epstein MF: Maternal and perinatal morbidity resulting from placenta praevia. Obstet Gynecol 65:176, 1985.
10. Lauria MR, Smith RS, Treadwell MC, et al: The use of second-trimester transvaginal sonography to predict placenta previa. Ultrasound Obstet Gynecol 8:337, 1996.
11. Weckstein LN, Masserman JSH, Garite TJ: Placenta accreta: a problem of increasing clinical significance. Obstet Gynecol 69:480, 1986.
12. Jauniaux E, Toplis PJ, Nicolaides KH: Sonographic diagnosis of a non-praevia placenta accreta. Ultrasound Obstet Gynecol 7:58, 1996.
13. Jauniaux E, Kadri R, Donner C, Rodesch F: Not all chorioangiomas are associated with elevated ma-

ternal serum alpha-fetoprotein. Prenat Diagn 12:73, 1992.

14. Jauniaux E, Jurkovic D, Campbell S, et al: Investigation of placental circulations by color Doppler ultrasound. Am J Obstet Gynecol 164:486, 1991.
15. Jauniaux E, Englert Y, Vanesse M, et al: Pathologic features of placentas from singleton pregnancies obtained by in vitro fertilization and embryo transfer. Obstet Gynecol 76:61, 1990.
16. Heifetz SA: Single umbilical artery: a statistical analysis of 37 autopsy cases and review of the literature. Perspect Pediatr Pathol 8:345, 1984.
17. Jauniaux E: Screening for the single umbilical artery cord: is it worth screening for antenatally? Ultrasound Obstet Gynecol 5:75 1995.
18. Jauniaux E, Campbell S, Vyas S: The use of color Doppler imaging for prenatal diagnosis of umbilical cord anomalies: report of three cases. Am J Obstet Gynecol 161:1195, 1989.
19. Jauniaux E, De Munter C, Pardou A, et al: Evaluation echographique du sydrome de l'artere ombilicale unique: une serie de 80 cas. J Gynecol Obstet Biol Reprod 18:341, 1989.
20. Jauniaux E, De Munter C, Vanesse M, et al: Embryonic remnants of the umbilical cord: morphological and clinical aspects. Hum Pathol 20:458, 1989.
21. Jauniaux E, Jurkovic D, Campbell S: Prenatal features of an umbilical cord pseudocyst associated with a small omphalocele. Eur J Obstet Gynecol Reprod Biol 40:245, 1991.
22. Jauniaux E, Moscoso G, Chitty L, et al: An angiomyxoma involving the whole length of the umbilical cord: prenatal diagnosis by ultrasonography. J Ultrasound Med 9:419, 1990.
23. Smith GN, Walker M, Johston S, Ash K: The sonographic findings of persistent umbilical cord cystic mass is associated with lethal aneuploidy and/or congenital anomalies. Prenat Diagn 16:1141, 1996.
24. Ross JA, Jurkovic D, Zosmer N, et al: Umbilical cord cysts in early pregnancy. Obstet Gynecol 89:442, 1997.
25. Jauniaux E, Donner C, Simon P, et al: Pathologic aspects of the umbilical cord after percutaneous umbilical blood sampling. Obstet Gynecol 73:215, 1989.
26. Jauniaux E, Nicolaides KH, Campbell S, Hustin J: Hematoma of the umbilical cord secondary to cordocentesis for intrauterine fetal transfusion. Prenat Diagn 10:477, 1990.
27. Jauniaux E, Elkhazen N, Leroy F, et al: Clinical and morphologic aspects of the vanishing twin phenomenon. Obstet Gynecol 72:577, 1988.
28. Bejar R, Vigliocco K, Gramajo H, et al: Antenatal origin of neurologic damage in newborn babies. II. Multiple gestation. Am J Obstet Gynecol 162:1230, 1990.
29. Bajoria R, Kingdom J: The case for routine determination of chronicity and zygosity in multiple pregnancy. Prenat Diagn 17(13):1207, 1997.
30. D'Alton ME, Dudley DK: The ultrasound prediction of chorionicity in twin gestation. Am J Obstet Gynecol 160:557, 1989.
31. Winn HN, Gabrielli S, Reece EA, et al: Ultrasonographic criteria for the prenatal diagnosis of placental chorionicity in twin gestations. Am J Obstet Gynecol 161:1540, 1989.
32. Fineberg J: The twin peak sign: reliable evidence of dichorionic twinning. J Ultrasound Med 11:571, 1992.
33. Sepulveda W, Sebire NJ, Odibo A, et al: Prenatal determination of chorionicity in triplet pregnancy by ultrasonographic examination of the ipsilon zone. Obstet Gynecol 88:855, 1996.
34. Wood SL, Onge RST, Connors G, Elliot PD: Evaluation of the twin peak or lambda sign in determining chorionicity in multiple pregnancy. Obstet Gynecol 88:6, 1996.
35. Sepulveda W, Sebire NJ, Hughes A, et al: The lambda sign at 10-14 weeks of gestation as a predictor of chorionicity in twin pregnancies. Ultrasound Obstet Gynecol 7:421, 1996.
36. Hecher K, Jauniaux E, Campbell S, et al: Artery to artery anastomosis in monochorionic twins. Am J Obstet Gynecol 171:570, 1994.
37. Pattinson RC, Norman K, Odendaal HJ: The role of Doppler velocimetry in the management of high risk pregnancies. Br J Obstet Gynaecol 101:114, 1994.
38. Alfirevic Z, Neilson JP: Doppler ultrasonography in high-risk pregnancies: systematic review with meta-analysis. Am J Obstet Gynecol 172:1379, 1995.
39. Kingdom JCP, Rodeck CH, Kaufmann P: Umbilical artery Doppler—more harm than good? Br J Obstet Gynaecol 104(4):393, 1997.
40. Rizzo G, Pietropolli A, Capponi A, Arduini D, Romanini C: Chromosomal abnormalities in fetuses with absent end-diastolic velocity in umbilical artery: analysis of risk factors for an abnormal karyotype. Am J Obstet Gynecol 171:827, 1994.
41. Snijders RJM, Sherrod C, Gosden CM, Nicolaides KH: Fetal growth retardation: associated malformations and chromosomal abnormalities. Am J Obstet Gynecol 168:547, 1993.
42. Jauniaux E, Jurkovic D, Campbell S, Hustin J: Doppler ultrasonographic features of the developing placental circulation: correlation with anatomic findings. Am J Obstet Gynecol 166:585, 1992.

43. Rodesch F, Simon P, Donner C, Jauniaux E: Oxygen measurements in endometrial and trophoblastic tissues during early pregnancy. Obstet Gynecol 80:283, 1992.
44. Hendricks S, Sorensen TK, Wang KY, et al: Doppler umbilical artery waveform indices—normal values from fourteen to forty-two weeks. Am J Obstet Gynecol 161:761, 1989.
45. Benirschke K, Kaufmann B: Pathology of the human placenta, 3rd ed. New York, 1995, Springer-Verlag.
46. Luckhardt M, Leiser R, Kingdom J, et al: Effect of physiologic perfusion-fixation on the morphometrically evaluated dimensions of the term placental cotyledon. J Soc Gynecol Invest 3:166, 1996.
47. Johanson R, Lindow SW, van der Elst C, et al: A prospective randomised comparison of the effect of continuous O_2 therapy and bedrest on fetuses with absent end-diastolic flow on umbilical artery Doppler waveform analysis. Br J Obstet Gynaecol 102:662, 1995.
48. Arduini D, Rizzo G, Romanini C: The development of abnormal heart rate patterns after absent end-diastolic velocity in umbilical artery: analysis of risk factors. Am J Obstet Gynecol 169:43, 1993.
49. Alstrom H, Axelsson O, Cnattingius S, et al: Comparison of umbilical artery velocimetry and cardiotocography for surveillance of small-for-gestational age fetuses. Lancet 340:936, 1992.
50. Nicolaides KH, Bilardo CM, Soothill PW, Campbell S: Absence of end-diastolic frequencies in the umbilical artery: a sign of fetal hypoxia and acidosis. Br Med J 297:1026, 1988.
51. Giles WB, Trudinger BJ, Baird P: Fetal umbilical artery flow velocity waveforms and placental resistance: pathological correlation. Br J Obstet Gynaecol 92:31, 1985.
52. Jauniaux E, Burton GJ: Correlation of umbilical Doppler features and placental morphometry: the need for uniform methodology. Ultrasound Obstet Gynecol 3:233, 1993.
53. Macara LM, Kingdom JCP, Kohnen G, et al: Elaboration of stem villous vessels in growth-restricted pregnancies with abnormal umbilical artery Doppler waveforms. Br J Obstet Gynaecol 101: 807, 1995.
54. Las Heras J, Haust MD: Ultrastructure of fetal stem arteries of human placenta in hypertensive disorders (toxemia) of pregnancy. Troph Res 3:335, 1988.
55. Fok RY, Pavlova Z, Benirschke K, et al: The correlation of arterial lesions with umbilical artery Doppler velocimetry in the placentas of small-for-dates pregnancies. Obstet Gynecol 75:578, 1990.
56. Kingdom JCP, Burrell SJ, Kaufmann P: Pathology and clinical implications of abnormal umbilical artery Doppler waveforms. Ultrasound Obstet Gynecol 9(4):271, 1997.
57. Castellucci M, Scheper M, Scheffen I, et al: The development of the human placental villous tree. Anat Embryol 181:117, 1990.
58. Hitschold T, Weiss E, Beck T, et al: Low target birthweight or growth retardation? Umbilical Doppler velocity waveforms and histometric analysis of fetoplacental vascular tree. Am J Obstet Gynecol 168:1260, 1993.
59. Jackson MR, Walsh AJ, Morrow RJ, et al: Reduced placental villous tree elaboration in small-for-gestational age pregnancies: relationship with umbilical artery Doppler waveforms. Am J Obstet Gynecol 172:518, 1995.
60. Krebs C, Macara LM, Leiser R, et al: Intrauterine growth restriction with absent end-diastolic flow velocity in the umbilical artery is associated with maldevelopment of the terminal placental villous tree. Am J Obstet Gynecol 175:1534, 1996.
61. Macara LM, Kingdom JCP, Kaufmann P, et al: Structural analysis of placental terminal villi in growth-restricted pregnancies with abnormal umbilical artery Doppler waveforms. Placenta 17:37, 1996.
62. Kingdom JCP, Kaufmann P: Oxygen and placental villous development: origins of fetal hypoxia. Placenta 18(8):613, 1997.
63. Dekker GA, de Vries JIP, Doelitzsch PM, et al: Underlying disorders associated with severe early-onset preeclampsia. Am J Obstet Gynecol 173: 1042, 1995.
64. Dizon-Townson DS, Nelson LM, Easton K, Ward K: The factor V Leiden mutation may predispose women to severe preeclampsia. Am J Obstet Gynecol 175:902, 1996.

16

The Placenta: Medicolegal Considerations

Richard L. Naeye

When claims are made that malpractice in the health care system was responsible for a stillbirth, a neonatal death, or a child's cerebral palsy, pathologists are often asked whether placental findings can clarify what took place. Providing such help can sometimes be difficult. First, the placenta probably was initially examined and the findings reported several years earlier without the pathologist having much clinical information about the case. Second, the information needed often requires integrating placental findings with many clinical, laboratory, and sometimes brain-imaging findings. Accumulating, organizing, and integrating all of this information can take many hours and require consultations with obstetricians, neonatalogists, and neuroradiologists. This chapter explains some of what the pathologist may need to know and how to use it in the investigation. The roots and timing of injury are emphasized because health care personnel cannot be held responsible for death or disability if the damage took place or was inevitable before they were in a position to intervene.

STILLBIRTHS AND NEONATAL DEATHS

The pathologist can determine the cause of most stillbirths and neonatal deaths if the results of a placental examination are integrated with clinical, laboratory, and autopsy findings. Autopsy findings often can answer questions about the results of therapy and the nature of terminal events, whereas identifying the initiating disorder commonly requires a placental examination. The most frequent of such initiating disorders is acute bacterial chorioamnionitis (Table 16–1).[1,2] It has a rather innocuous reputation because it most often arises too close to delivery for most of its untoward clinical consequences to develop before the child is born. That it is seldom recognized before death or brain damage has taken place is one key to understanding its role in wrongful death claims. If untreated it starts the prostaglandin cascade that leads to cervical dilatation, labor, and delivery. If this sequence occurs during the first or second trimester of pregnancy, the immaturity of the fetus and neonate in conjunction with the direct effects of the infection often determine the outcome, which includes brain damage and death. To indicate how helpless health care personnel usually are to control these events, the rates of preterm birth have changed little in recent decades in the industrial nations. The most frequent initiator of these premature births is acute chorioamnionitis.[2] It arises outside the control of the health care system and with rare exceptions proceeds to early delivery unaffected by any currently available therapy.[3] It is almost never identified as the cause of preterm birth without a placental examination because only about 1:20 of these infections produces signs or symptoms of their presence in gravidas.[2]

Understanding the major features of *acute chorioamnionitis* explains why the health care system can rarely prevent it and its consequences. It is a disorder in which bacteria or mycoplasms from the vagina and cervix invade the fetal membranes and enter the amniotic fluid.[2,4] The diagnosis of acute chorioamnionitis is made when acute inflammatory cells are found within the fetal (chorionic) plate of the placenta or in the blood clot just beneath the chorionic plate. Acute inflammatory cells are attracted to these sites by the presence of bacteria or mycoplasmas in the amniotic fluid. The role of amnionitis in fetal and neonatal deaths is more often indirect than direct. It can be direct

Table 16–1. Initiating Disorders That Led to Stillbirth, Neonatal Death, or Neurologic Abnormalities at 7 Years of Age

	Relative Risk Values		
Disorder	Stillbirth	Neonatal Death	Neurologic Abnormalities at 7 Years of Age
Placental disorders			
Mild acute chorioamnionitis	**2.0**	**2.0**	0.9
Moderate to severe chorioamnionitis	**5.2**	**5.0**	1.2
Low uteroplacental blood flow	**1.6**	**1.3**	1.4
Abruptio placentae	**4.1**	**1.9**	1.2
Maternal floor infarction	**21.2**	1.0	1.6
Severe villous edema	**3.1**	**5.3**	**1.7**
Umbilical cord disorders			
Abnormally short	**1.2**	**1.2**	**1.3**
Tight knot in cord	**19.1**	0.8	0.7
Tight nuchal cord	1.1	**0.6**	1.1
Cord prolapse	**2.9**	**1.9**	0.7
Cord grossly edematous	**2.4**	1.4	1.0
Blood vessel thrombus	**2.8**	**2.8**	1.0
Hematoma at delivery	**7.4**	0.9	0.6

The relative risk values are derived from multiple logistic analyses in which many independent risk factors were included in each analysis. Figures in boldface print are statistically significant.

Data from the Collaborative Perinatal Study. In Naeye R: Disorders of the placenta, fetus, and newborn: diagnosis and clinical significance. St. Louis, 1992, Mosby.

when virulent bacteria enter and propagate in the blood of the fetus or neonate. Hypotension and other evidence of shock are characteristically present in such cases. Evidence of a direct lethal effect by the infection includes virulent organisms in cultures of a neonate's blood, large numbers of neutrophils in the spleen and the hematopoietic centers of the liver, and severe pneumonia or meningitis at autopsy. Inflammatory cytokines have been postulated to be the agents that damage fetal tissues and cause death in such cases.[5,6]

Acute chorioamnionitis has an indirect role in many deaths by initiating preterm birth, placental villous edema, premature rupture of the fetal membranes, fetal defecation into the amniotic fluid with resultant toxic consequences of meconium in the amniotic fluid, placental abruptions, and umbilical vein thrombosis.[2] In 19 of 20 cases acute chorioamnionitis does not produce a fever or any other easily recognized clinical evidence of its presence in gravidas. The only means of identifying gravidas at risk of these infections has been serial cervicovaginal tests for fetal fibronectin, starting at 24 weeks' gestation, which is the age at which fetuses reach extrauterine viability.[7] Acute chorioamnionitis is by far the most frequent cause of *preterm birth* in every population in which it has been studied in both the industrial and developing nations.[1,2] The first sign of the infection is most often unanticipated preterm labor, unexpected painless dilatation of the cervix, or premature rupture of the fetal membranes. Since all efforts to stop such labors have failed, health care personnel can rarely be held responsible for preterm births that are initiated by these infections.[3]

A fatal consequence of acute chorioamnionitis before 28 weeks' gestation is *placental villous edema* (Table 16–1). It can develop within hours after acute chorioamnionitis begins.[2,8] It characteristically peaks several hours after it starts and recedes the next day. Placental villous edema almost never produces signs or symptoms in gravidas, so obstetric personnel can almost never be held responsible for its presence or its hypoxic-ischemic effects on fetuses. If delivery takes place while the edema is at its peak, its presence is most easily recognized by the abnormally large weight of the placenta, its characteristic appearance in the villi, and the hypoxemic, acidotic state of the neonate (Fig. 16–1). When edema is severe and diffuse, the resulting fetal hypoxemia often damages the lungs and other organs of the fetus. The lung damage, after birth, predisposes to hyaline membrane disease and the respiratory distress syndrome, which cause many neonatal deaths and serious brain damage.[2]

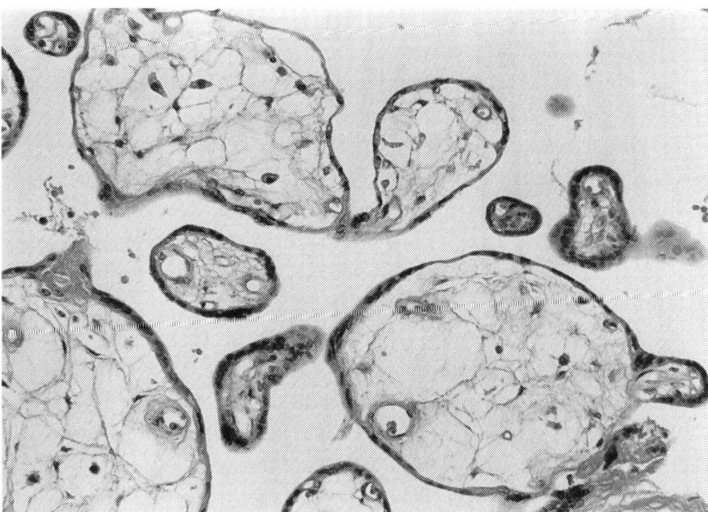

Figure 16–1. Severe edema in placental villi (H&E, ×200).

Many studies have shown that acute bacterial chorioamnionitis is the most frequent cause of *premature membrane rupture* through the damage it produces in the fetal membranes.[2] Analyses of data from the Collaborative Perinatal Study, which include information from the examinations of more than 35,000 placentas, determined that approximately half of the premature membrane ruptures were the consequence of acute chorioamnionitis.[2] Premature delivery most often occurs within a week of the rupture.[9]

Starting at about 30 weeks' gestation the fetal stress produced by acute chorioamnionitis can lead the fetus to defecate meconium into the amniotic fluid. The *meconium* often contains toxic bile acids.[10] When meconium is transported into the chorionic plate of the placenta and umbilical cord by macrophages, it sometimes causes veins at these sites to constrict, markedly reducing blood flow from the placenta to the fetus (Fig. 16–2).[11] Altshuler and Hyde[12] were the first to recognize that meconium sometimes has these vasoconstrictive properties. Evidence has appeared that the fetal hypoxemia induced by the vasoconstriction often lasts 10 to 14 hours.[11] Multiple logistic analyses of data from the Collaborative Perinatal Study have confirmed that meconium in the amniotic fluid is a major risk factor for stillbirth,

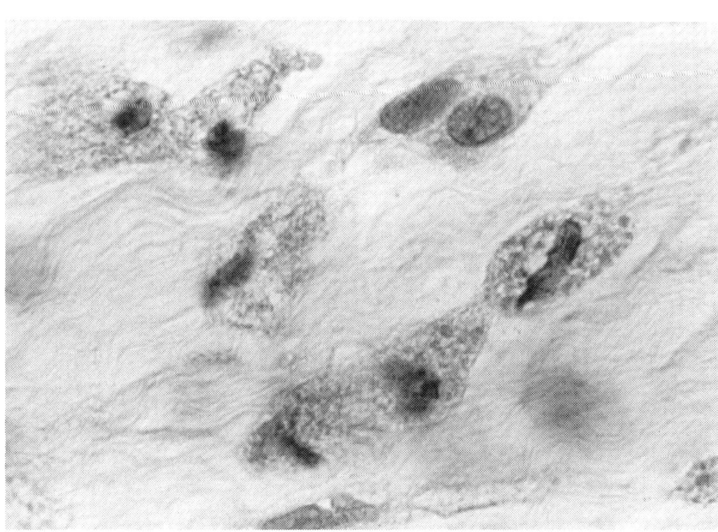

Figure 16–2. Macrophages in the chorionic plate of the placenta are filled with small and larger clumps of meconium (H&E, ×1000).

neonatal death, and hypoxic-ischemic cerebral palsy, independent of many other risk factors for these outcomes.[2] Meconium-initiated stillbirth almost always occurs without prior signs or symptoms, so medical system personnel almost never have an opportunity to prevent it.

Fetuses and neonates die in half or more of the cases in which a *placental abruption* suddenly occurs (Table 16–1).[2] Multiple logistic analysis found that 8% of the placental abruptions in the Collaborative Perinatal Study could be attributed to acute chorioamnionitis.[2] In these cases the infection had invaded the decidua basalis beneath the placenta. Decidual blood vessels that are engulfed by the infection usually thrombose. When instead the vessels rupture, the resulting hemorrhage can lead to an abruption.[2] The apparent ages of the blood clot within the decidua basalis and the infarcted tissue above the abruption often indicate if the abruption was hours, days, or weeks old.

Low uteroplacental blood flow is the third most frequent cause of fetal and neonatal death and the second most frequent cause of preterm birth (Table 16–1).[2] Its most frequent underlying disorders are preeclampsia-eclampsia, chronic maternal hypertension, and certain autoimmune disorders in the gravida. In preeclampsia-eclampsia not all blood vessels in the wall of the uterus are normally remodeled in early gestation.[2,4] The resulting low blood flow into the placenta produces an increase in the number and size of syncytial knots, a thinning of the syncytiotrophoblastic cell layer that covers the villi, and sometimes infarcts.[2,4] These findings are characteristically uneven from one microscopic field to another in the placenta because blood flow is normal through some uterine spiral arteries that pass blood into the placenta and low or absent through others. Whether health care personnel could have recognized the risks and prevented fetal or neonatal death is the central issue in many malpractice claims. If the fetal or neonatal death took place in the first or second trimester of pregnancy, there may have been no prior clinical manifestations of the low uteroplacental blood flow. The low blood flow is often not identified as the cause of death in such cases unless a pathologist recognizes its characteristic gross and microscopic features in the placenta. Since uteroplacental blood flow sometimes decreases rapidly and unexpectedly during the course of preeclampsia-eclampsia, even the most experienced obstetricians may find no prior clues that could have predicted the death.

Umbilical cord accidents are associated with a high rate of fetal and lesser neonatal mortality (Table 16–1).[2] They fall into five main categories: umbilical blood vessel thrombosis, umbilical cord prolapse, a tight knot in the umbilical cord, severe umbilical cord edema, and a hematoma in the cord. The major antecedents of umbilical vein and artery thrombosis in the Collaborative Perinatal Study were acute chorioamnionitis and physical trauma to the cord by vigorous fetal movements, neither of which can usually be anticipated or predicted.[2] The role of trauma was discovered by the association of thromboses with markers of vigorous fetal motor activity, such as very long umbilical cords, tight knots in the cord, and a greater than normal amount of fibrin beneath the chorionic plate of the placenta.[2,13]

Umbilical vein thrombosis has a high mortality for fetuses and neonates (Table 16–1).[2] The only clinical indicator of it has been the realization by gravidas that the fetus had stopped moving.

Umbilical cord prolapse, a tight cord knot, and a tight nuchal cord all kill by stopping blood flow in one or more umbilical blood vessels, particularly in the umbilical vein where blood pressure is lower than it is in the umbilical arteries (Table 16–1). Whether interventions by health system personnel can ever save infants with these conditions depends on whether blood flow is completely or only partially stopped and the duration of the flow reduction. If blood flow is completely stopped, severe irreversible brain damage may occur within 15 minutes.

It is important to distinguish the umbilical cord edema produced by clamping the cord at delivery from that which preceded birth. When edema is of very short duration, the tissue that constitutes its borders has a ragged appearance on microscopic examination. Edematous areas of much longer duration usually have a consolidated border. Edema that develops before delivery is associated with substantial fetal mortality (Table 16–1).

A *hematoma in the umbilical cord* at delivery is associated with a high fetal mortality rate, particularly when it was the result of a blood vessel rupture (Table 16–1).[2] Pathologists are accustomed to ignoring hematomas that have been produced by cord clamping at delivery, so they may need to be specifically notified when such a hemorrhage was present before the cord was clamped. In this latter circumstance the pathologist should examine multiple sections through the hemorrhagic segment to determine whether a blood vessel ruptured before delivery. A predelivery rupture can sometimes be identified by the relative paucity of lymphocytes and normoblasts in the dissecting blood in Wharton's jelly, whereas these cells are often present in large numbers in the child's blood at birth if the vessel rupture led to severe fetal hypoxemia.[2] The significance of this lymphocytosis and normoblastemia is discussed later in the chapter.

Placental maternal floor infarction is a poorly understood disorder characterized by the progressive heavy deposition of fibrin between individual villi.[2] It usually advances as pregnancy progresses, with fetal mortality increasing as more and more villi become nonfunctional (Table 16–1). The pathologist has a special responsibility to recognize and diagnose placental maternal floor infarction even if the child is stillborn because this disorder has a high risk of repeating in subsequent pregnancies.[2,14] The rate at which it destroys placental function in an individual pregnancy cannot be predicted. One fetus may survive whereas the fetus in the next pregnancy dies. Diagnosing the disorder in one pregnancy should be the signal for frequent monitoring of the fetus in the next pregnancy so that it might be saved by a quick delivery.

A single umbilical artery has a well-known association with *congenital anomalies* in other organs, some of which are fatal. A very short umbilical cord and absence of fibrin beneath the chorionic plate of the placenta in late gestation are evidence of weak or infrequent fetal movements, often because of fetal brain dysfunction, weak muscles, or some physical restraint that limited movement of the fetus (Fig. 16–3).[2,13] These findings increase the risk of both fetal and neonatal death.[2] A markedly undergrown placenta with seemingly normal villi for gestational age can be the manifestation of a serious, sometimes fatal developmental disorder.[2]

Fetal Deaths Between 14 and 20 Weeks' Gestation

Most deaths between 14 and 20 weeks' gestation result from acute chorioamnionitis, chronically low uteroplacental blood flow, or developmental disorders. The placental findings associated with each can pose special problems for diagnosis. Recognizing that a death was due to a bacterial infection is simple when acute chorioamnionitis is severe and the interval between death and birth was a day or less. Fetal neutrophils will have invaded the walls of umbilical blood vessels or blood vessels on the surface of the placenta. Acute chorioamnionitis can also develop after fetal death

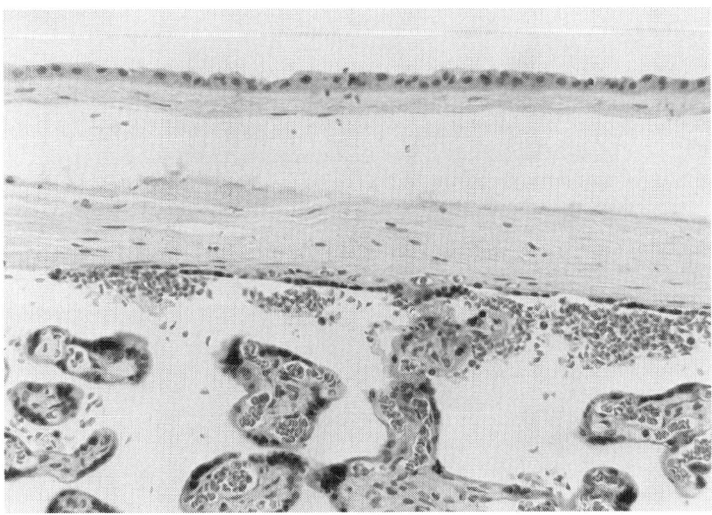

Figure 16–3. Note the absence of blood clot beneath the chorionic plate of the placenta in this full-term child born with a severe developmental disorder that was responsible for quadriplegic cerebral palsy (H&E, ×100).

and thus have no role in the fetal demise. In that case fetal neutrophils will not have reacted to the infection by invading the walls of umbilical or placental blood vessels.

Recognizing that *low uteroplacental blood flow* killed a fetus can be difficult if more than 2 or 3 days elapsed between death and birth because accelerated villous maturation, identical to that produced by chronic low uteroplacental blood flow, can develop rapidly after a fetus dies.[2,4] The pathologist can determine that this acceleration antedated death when it affected most but not all areas of the placenta.[2] Finding a few areas where villi are normally mature for gestational age indicates that uterine blood flow into the intervillous space of these areas was normal before death, whereas in all other areas uteroplacental blood flow was subnormal.

A *developmental disorder* can be suspected as the cause of death in the presence of multiple malformations in the fetus, a placenta that is markedly growth retarded for fetal size and microscopically normal for gestational age, or very dysmorphic placental villi that indicate the existence of a chromosomal disorder.[2]

Fetal and Neonatal Deaths After 42 Weeks' Gestation

Perinatal deaths that occur after 42 weeks' gestation are called postterm and are often attributed to placental senescence. Earlier delivery would no doubt have saved the lives of some of these children, but clinical indications for such a delivery may not have been present. In the Collaborative Perinatal Study most of the perinatal mortality increase after 42 weeks' gestation was due to the increasing frequencies of acute chorioamnionitis and developmental disorders.[2,15] A postterm fetal or neonatal death should be attributed to whatever fatal disorder is revealed from placental and autopsy findings and never to placental insufficiency unless conclusive evidence for such insufficiency is present in the placenta. Furthermore, most women have a predetermined pregnancy length that does not vary by more than 1 or 2 days in successive gestations unless disorders intervene to lead to an earlier delivery.[16] Some women have a predetermined pregnancy length that is 42 weeks or longer.

Estimating the Time of Fetal Death

David Genest and his collaborators[17–19] have identified progressive *time-predictable tissue changes* that take place in the placenta and fetal organs as the interval between death and birth increases (Table 16–2). In my experience the time of death they suggest almost always coincides with the time that gravidas reported their fetus had stopped moving or monitors documented that cardiac arrest had taken place. Genest's tissue timers

Table 16–2. Organ and Body Findings That Best Correlate with the Timing of Fetal Death

Finding	Time
Histologic features in fetal organs	
Loss of nuclear basophilia in individual renal cortical tubular cells	4 hours
Loss of such basophilia in hepatic cell nuclei	24 hours
Loss of nuclear basophilia in cells in the inner half of the myocardium	24 hours
Loss of nuclear basophilia in cells in the outer half of the myocardium	48 hours
Loss of nuclear basophilia in cells in the bronchial epithelium	96 hours
Loss of nuclear basophilia in tracheal cartilage, gastrointestinal tract, and adrenal gland	1 week
Histologic features in the placenta	
Villous intravascular karyorrhexis	6 or more hours
Fibroblast septation in the vascular lumina of stem villi	2 or more days
Extensive fibrosis of terminal villi	2 or more weeks
External fetal examination	
Desquamation of cells on the surface of the umbilical cord of at least 1 cm	6 hours or more
Brown-red discoloration of the umbilical cord stump	6 hours or more
Desquamation on the face, abdomen, or back	12 hours or more
Desquamation involving 5% or more of the body surface	18 hours or more
Brown skin discoloration	24 hours or more
Mummification	2 weeks or more

From Genest DR, Williams MA, Greene MF: Obstet Gynecol 80:575, 1992. Reprinted with permission from the American College of Obstetricians and Gynecologists.

Table 16–3. Risk Factors for Quadriplegic Cerebral Palsy at 7 Years of Age in Children Who Were Born at Full Term

Risk Factor	Attributable Risks (95% confidence intervals)
Genetic, developmental	**.59**
Major fetal malformations	.33 (.15, .50)
Minor fetal malformations	.08 (.05, .10)
Motor disorders in siblings	.05 (.02, .11)
Congenital syndromes	.04 (.00, .08)
Chronically low motor activity before birth	
Absence of subchorionic fibrin	.05 (0.1, .09)
A very short umbilical cord	.04 (.02, .06)
Hypoxemic-ischemic disorders	**.18**
Widely recognized asphyxial disorders	.04 (.00, .09)
Meconium in the amniotic fluid	.14 (.09, .19)
Other identified disorders	**.10**
TOTAL	**.86** (.77, .95)

Adapted from Naeye R: Disorders of the placenta, fetus, and newborn: diagnosis and clinical significance. St. Louis, 1992, Mosby.

are reliable only when the tissue being evaluated underwent quick fixation after delivery. For example, kidney fixation is commonly slow. As a result, often only the cortical tubular cells just beneath the renal capsule are fixed rapidly enough that the status of their nuclei can be used to estimate the time of fetal death.[17]

The *duration of acute chorioamnionitis* is sometimes an important issue in litigation. During the early course of the infection maternal neutrophils invade the blood clot beneath the chorionic (fetal) plate of the placenta. This is termed stage 1. Subsequently these neutrophils migrate through the clot and into the chorionic plate (stage 2). When they reach the glassy basement membrane just below the amnion cells, the infection is at stage 3. We plotted these stages against the time since fetal membranes had ruptured according to the database of the Collaborative Perinatal Study. When only a small or moderate number of neutrophils were involved in the inflammatory process, it was classified as mild. In the Collaborative Study mild acute chorioamnionitis usually remained at stage 1 for 3 days after the fetal membranes ruptured.[2] Between 4 and 6 days the infection reached stage 2, and after 7 days more than half reached stage 3.[2] If large number of neutrophils were present, the acute chorioamnionitis was classified as severe. Severe acute chorioamnionitis sometimes reached stage 3 within 24 hours after the membranes had ruptured. Thus the duration of acute chorioamnionitis before birth can be judged only when the inflammatory process is mild.

CEREBRAL PALSY AND OTHER CENTRAL NERVOUS SYSTEM DISORDERS

Claims that cerebral malfunction, particularly cerebral palsy, was the result of misdiagnosis or mismanagement by medical system personnel usually assume the damage took place during the last hours of labor and delivery and was hypoxic-ischemic or traumatic in origin. If true it is difficult to explain why the frequency of cerebral palsy has remained unchanged for many years in the general population despite the introduction and widespread use of fetal stress testing, fetal biophysical profiles, quick deliveries when fetal stress has been detected, improved methods of resuscitation, and sophisticated management of sick newborns.[20–22] Could most cerebral palsy be nonhypoxic in origin and that which is hypoxic usually be taking place outside the control of health care personnel? More than half the cases of cerebral palsy in the general population appear to be developmental in origin (Table 16–3). Such cases are rarely litigated once the true nature of the brain abnormalities is understood. The circumstances and timing of traumatic damage are usually well known from the obstetric history and brain imaging findings. Only 18% of cerebral palsy in children born at term had a hypoxic-ischemic origin in the Collaborative Study (Table 16–3).[2,23] The timing of this latter damage is a critical issue in many malpractice claims because it can show whether the gravida and her fetus were in a setting where obstetric interventions might have prevented the brain damage. Establishing the time and cause of brain damage usually requires the integration of clinical, laboratory, and sometimes brain imaging findings with placental findings.

In some cases placental findings can readily identify the cause of brain damage when a disorder has rendered most of the placenta dysfunctional. Such cases include widespread, destructive chronic villitis, very dysmorphic villi that suggest a chromosomal disorder was probably present, findings indicating that a complete or nearly complete placental abruption had taken place, a maternal floor infarction that had destroyed most of the villi in the placenta, or an umbilical cord accident that had blocked blood flow in the umbilical vein or arteries. Placental abruptions and cord accidents are usually recognized at birth, so the pathologist's confirming report is only rarely a surprise. When the pathologist's initial placental examination does not indicate an obvious cause and timing of brain damage, other possible abnormalities in the placenta should not be assumed present. Such overinterpretation has led to many diagnostic errors in the past and sometimes great confusion during trial testimony when the placental findings did not seem to relate to other findings in the case. Such mistakes will be rare if care is taken that the interpretation of placental findings is compatible with the other findings and conclusions in the case.

In beginning the process of gathering and integrating all of the information needed to establish the cause and timing of brain damage in a child, the first effort should be to determine whether the damage is developmental, infectious, traumatic, thromboembolic, or hypoxic-ischemic in origin. The development of abnormalities in images of the child's brain from birth onward usually provides this information. Abnormalities attributable to *developmental disorders* are described in detail in the textbooks by A. James Barkovich,[24] Harvey Sarnat,[25] and others.

The pathologist can sometimes identify the origin of a child's *hemiparesis.* The hemiparesis is usually due to an embolus, thrombus, or vasospasm in a cerebral artery, a developmental disorder, or a cerebral hemorrhage. If brain images and clinical findings disclose that the damage is in the distribution of a cerebral artery, particularly the middle cerebral artery, the pathologist should search for the origin of an embolus by looking for a predelivery thrombus in the umbilical vein or in the veins on the surface of the placenta. An embolus originating from a thrombus at one of these sites has an open pathway to a cerebral artery because before birth no capillary beds separate these veins from the cerebral arteries. The thrombi from which emboli sometimes arise can result from traumatic damage to these veins by vigorous fetal movements.[2] A thrombus sometimes also forms as the result of damage caused by acute funisitis, which is a common feature of acute bacterial chorioamnionitis.[2] Embolic infarction of the brain that originates after birth is most often the consequence of congenital cyanotic heart disease in which emboli from peripheral veins are shunted from the right to the left side of the heart without being stopped by passing through the pulmonary capillary bed.[26]

The most frequently litigated brain damage cases are those attributed to *hypoxia-ischemia.* The specific damage pattern in such cases depends on the maturity of various parts of the brain, including their blood supply; their metabolic rate; and the severity and duration of the hypoxia-ischemia. Various combinations of these factors produce distinctive injury patterns that can be recognized in brain images. When one of these patterns is identified and correlated with the psychomotor and sensory abnormalities in the child, conclusions can usually be drawn about the nature and timing of the injury. Detailed analyses of the clinical, laboratory, and placental findings in the case can then go forward to determine the more exact time and circumstances in which the damage took place. Quite different patterns of brain injury develop with very short episodes of severe hypoxia-ischemia and longer episodes of somewhat less severe hypoxia-ischemia. Irreversible brain damage can occur after only 12 to 15 minutes of very severe hypoxemia-ischemia.[26] If it lasts for 25 minutes or longer, most or all of the brain usually is severely damaged. Short periods of very severe hypoxemia-hypotension characteristically produce damage in the lateral thalami in 26 to 32 weeks' gestation and the lentiform nucleus, primarily the posterior putamen, the hippocampus, and sometimes the precentral and postcentral gyri, closer to term.[24] Before 34 weeks' gestation moderately severe fetal hypoxemia-ischemia that persists an hour or more damages the periventricular white matter.[24] Closer to term most of the damage is in marginally perfused regions between the distributions of the major cerebral arteries. These latter areas include the periventricular white matter, the cerebral cortex, and the subcortical white matter. Deep gray matter structures in the basal ganglia are usually spared.[24] Primate studies have shown that such brain damage often occurs during the second hour after the hypoxemia begins.[27-29] During the first hour of hypoxemia the autoregulation that normally matches blood flow to local tissue needs in the brain is usually lost. Brain damage during this first hour is often prevented by an increase in cardiac output, which increases blood flow through most areas of the brain.[30] Brain damage is then likely to occur during the second hour as hypoxic damage to the myocardium reduces cardiac output with resultant decreases in cerebral blood flow.[30–32]

Three types of imaging are widely employed to visualize hypoxic-ischemic brain injury in neonates and older children. Ultrasound is the most commonly used. It most easily detects hemorrhages and demonstrates the size and the shape of the cerebral ventricles. Reductions in ventricular size are sometimes manifestations of cerebral edema. Very experienced pediatric neuroradiologists can sometimes detect cerebral edema in the form of parenchymal hyperechogenicity on ultrasound images. Computed tomographic (CT) images are claimed to be the most reliable detectors of hypoxic-ischemic brain injury during the first week of life. An indication of such injury is low attenuation in the basal ganglia and sometimes in the cerebral cortex. As the child grows older, magnetic resonance images become progressively more sensitive and accurate than CT images in identifying the specific findings of hypoxic-ischemic brain injury.[24]

Once imaging has revealed a characteristic pattern of hypoxic-ischemic injury in a brain, tentative conclusions are often possible about the severity and duration of the hypoxia-ischemia and the time during gestation when the damage probably occurred. More information is of course needed to identify the disorder that initiated the hypoxia-ischemia, how and why it developed, its antecedents, and the exact time of injury.

Estimating the Time of Brain Injury

During the course of litigation expert witnesses are routinely asked about the opportunities that may or may not have existed to prevent the brain damage. Credible answers require reliable knowledge about the sequence of disorders that led to the damage, the time the damage occurred, and options that were available to prevent the damage at each stage before it took place. Knowing when severe hypoxemia began and the damage took place will automatically include or exclude many disorders that can cause hypoxic-ischemic brain damage. For example, if the damage took place a day or more before delivery and the child was no longer hypoxemic or acidotic at birth, placental disorders that keep a fetus hypoxemic and acidotic until delivery are implausible explanations for the damage. Such disorders include placental abruptions, maternal floor infarctions, rupture of an umbilical vein, and many other such irreversible conditions. If the child is no longer severely hypoxemic or acidotic at birth, the damage was presumably produced by a disorder that caused a transient period of hypoxia-ischemia. The evidence for these disorders can often be found in the placenta. Two such findings are residual foci of villous edema in the placenta and large amounts of meconium in the chorionic plate of the placenta.

The next step is to determine when the hypoxemia-ischemia began and when during its course the brain damage took place. The search for reliable ways to obtain this information has been long and frustrating. In practice fetal heart rate abnormalities have been widely used for this purpose. Unfortunately, such monitoring can rarely if ever meet this need. A recent large prospective study found that such heart rate abnormalities had a 99.8% false-positive rate for predicting long-term psychomotor impairments.[33] Metaanalyses have produced similar disappointing results.[34] Almost all the children with hypoxic-ischemic cerebral palsy in our studies have had fetal heart rate abnormalities during labor and delivery. Except for intractable fetal bradycardia, these abnormalities appear to have been first observed after the child's brain damage had taken place. This does not negate research that has linked some abnormal fetal heart rate patterns to fetal hypoxemia, but it does make implausible claims that these patterns are a valuable tool for determining when brain damage is taking place or about to occur.

With some exceptions low Apgar scores and severe acidosis in an infant at birth also do not reliably indicate when severe hypoxemia-ischemia began, its duration, or when during its course brain damage took place.[11] The presence or absence of acidosis in the cord blood of neonates at birth can be particularly misleading because in many cases it is mild or absent when severe hypoxic-ischemic brain damage had taken place hours or days earlier.[11] On the other hand, severe hypoxemia and acidosis can be present at birth without accompanying brain damage because the previously mentioned mechanisms that protect the fetal brain from hypoxic-ischemic damage for a time can still be in operation and effective at delivery.

Currently the most reliable methods for establishing when damaging hypoxemia-ischemia began in a fetus appear to be serial lymphocyte, normoblast, and platelet counts in a neonate's blood starting immediately after birth and continuing until these counts return to normal levels,[35] the interval between birth and the child's first observed seizure and the time before birth when a gravida noted that her fetus had stopped moving. In 1995 we monitored from birth the changing numbers of lymphocytes and normoblasts in the blood of 16 neonates who subsequently were found to have hypoxic-ischemic cerebral palsy of the type produced by cortical and subcortical damage in the brain.[35] Lymphocyte counts increased to greater than 10,000/mm^3 and normoblast counts to greater than 2000/mm^3 within an hour after brain-damaging ischemia and hypoxemia began (Fig. 16–4). These lymphocyte counts rapidly returned to normal or subnormal levels 24 hours after the hypoxemia-ischemia began, even when the hypoxemia persisted after birth. The beginning of hypoxemia could therefore be calculated by counting back 24 hours from the time blood lymphocyte counts rapidly decreased from abnormally high to normal or subnormal numbers.

Normoblasts also appeared in the blood of the 16 neonates with hypoxic-ischemic cerebral palsy within an hour after severe hypoxemia-ischemia began and disappeared or decreased to low numbers 24 to 30 hours later.[35] The only exception was counts in neonates whose hypoxemia persisted after birth. In these children the normoblastemia often continued beyond 30 hours.

Our initial findings raised many questions that must be answered before lymphocyte and normoblast counts can be accepted as reliable timers of when severe hypoxemia begins. Are the findings in this small study also present in a larger population of children with hypoxic-ischemic cerebral palsy? In a study of 28 additional children with hypoxic-ischemic cerebral palsy, blood lymphocyte and normoblast counts had time cycles of lymphocyte and normoblast counts that were identical to those reported in the original study.

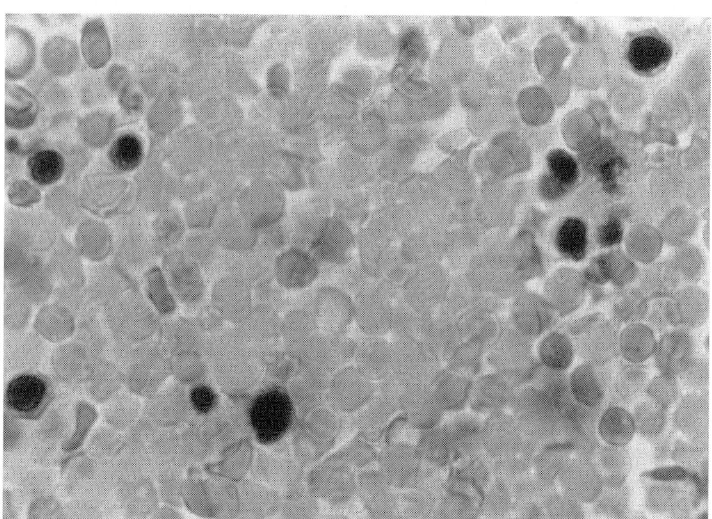

Figure 16–4. Most of the nucleated cells of the fetal blood in this placenta are lymphocytes and normoblasts. This child had severe hypoxic-ischemic cerebral palsy (H&E, ×1000).

How specific for acute hypoxemia-ischemia are lymphocyte and normoblast cycles? To date we found no other type of stress that can produce these cycles. Recent claims that acute chorioamnionitis can increase normoblast counts in the blood of neonates[36] require further study because as previously discussed acute chorioamnionitis often initiates processes that lead to hypoxemia.

What is the time interval between the beginning of severe hypoxemia-ischemia and the first seizures in neonates? This interval was determined from serial lymphocyte counts in 33 neonates whose hypoxic-ischemic cerebral palsy originated within 2 days of birth. The intervals between the start of their severe hypoxemia-ischemia as determined by lymphocyte counts and their first recognized seizure ranged from 16 to 101 hours. In most infants the interval was between 18 and 30 hours.

Can platelet counts in the blood of neonates be used to identify the time that ischemia and hypoxemia damaged their brains? We included 28 children with hypoxic-ischemic cerebral palsy in our study. Platelet counts were normal for the 20 to 26 hours after severe hypoxemia began and then progressively decreased for 2 to 4 days thereafter. This cycle was most predictable when brain damage was severe.

In almost all children with hypoxic-ischemic cerebral palsy severe or moderately severe hematuria is present for 2 and sometimes 3 days after the start of severe hypoxemia. This is presumably a reflection of damage to the lower nephron in the kidneys. When hematuria was present on the day of birth and absent the next day in a child, lymphocyte counts revealed that brain-damaging hypoxemia had begun 1 to 2 days before delivery.

Disorders Initiating Brain Injury

The next step in determining how and when hypoxic-ischemic brain damage took place in a child is to identify the initiating disorder. An earlier section of this chapter details the most frequent initiating disorders for stillbirth and neonatal death. Most of those disorders at least occasionally cause hypoxic-ischemic cerebral palsy as well (Table 16–1). Only one of those initiating disorders needs additional elaboration, in part because its role in initiating cerebral palsy appears to be very large. Eighteen percent of the quadriplegic cerebral palsy in children born at term in the Collaborative Perinatal Study was attributable to hypoxic-ischemic disorders.[2,24] Only 4% was attributable to the commonly recognized antenatal hypoxic-ischemic disorders such as placental abruptions, umbilical cord compression, umbilical vein ruptures, large fetomaternal hemorrhages, placental maternal floor infarctions, and fetal or maternal shock.[2,23] The rest (14%) was attributable to the presence of meconium in the amniotic fluid (Table 16–3). This result was derived from multiple logistic analyses that included many other potential risk factors for cerebral palsy. The Collaborative Perinatal Study data on which these analyses are based are old but presumably still valid because the health care system has not been able to reduce the incidence of cerebral palsy since the study was completed.[20–22]

To further determine what role meconium might have in the genesis of cerebral palsy, we studied in detail 42 children with hypoxic-ischemic cerebral palsy who had no recognized cause of their brain damage other than meconium in their amniotic fluid.[11] Based on this and several other lines of evidence, meconium, when present in the amniotic fluid for a day or more, can induce veins on the surface of the placenta and in the umbilical cord to constrict. As previously mentioned, indirect evidence exists that this constriction can persist for up to 14 hours and that the resulting fetal hypoxemia-ischemia can produce widespread hypoxic-ischemic cortical brain necrosis.[11] In the study in which vasoconstriction appeared to end after 10 to 14 hours, the affected fetuses with the longest interval between this time and birth had at least partially recovered from their earlier severe hypoxemia and acidosis at the time of delivery. This period in which oxygenated blood again flowed to the fetus before birth would not be expected to reverse brain damage that had already taken place, and this indeed was the finding in our study. Special circumstances must be present for meconium in the amniotic fluid to cause such damage. Most meconium in the amniotic fluid arrives during the second stage of labor when not enough time remains before delivery for it to be transported by macrophages into the placenta where it could induce vasoconstriction. Thus meconium in the amniotic fluid should not be considered a possible cause of fetal brain damage unless large quantities are in the chorionic plate of the placenta, a site in which it can presumably induce nearby veins and perhaps arteries to constrict.

CONCLUSION

Most claims of malpractice that relate to stillbirth, neonatal death, and antenatal brain damage require that information from many different sources be gathered, weighed, and integrated. Placental findings often have a key role in these analyses.

REFERENCES

1. Naeye RL, Tafari N: Risk factors in pregnancy and diseases of the fetus and newborn. Baltimore, 1983, Williams & Wilkins.
2. Naeye R: Disorders of the placenta, fetus, and newborn: diagnosis and clinical significance. St. Louis, 1992, Mosby.
3. Romero R, Sirtori M, Oyarzun E, et al: Prevalence, microbiology and clinical significance of intraamniotic infection in women with preterm labor and intact membranes. Am J Obstet Gynecol 161:817, 1989.
4. Benirschke K, Kaufman P: Pathology of the human placenta, 3rd ed. New York, 1995, Springer-Verlag.
5. Yoon BH, Jun JK, Roberto R, et al: Amniotic fluid inflammatory cytokines, neonatal brain white matter lesions and cerebral palsy. Am J Obstet Gynecol 177:19, 1997.
6. Hitti JH, Krohn MA, Patton DL, et al: Amniotic fluid tumor necrosis factor and the risk of respiratory distress syndrome among preterm infants. Am J Obstet Gynecol 177:50, 1997.
7. Goldenberg RL, Mercer BM, Iams JD, et al: The preterm prediction study: patterns of cervicovaginal fetal fibronectin as predictors of spontaneous preterm delivery. Am J Obstet Gynecol 177:8, 1997.
8. Naeye RL, Maisels MJ, Lorenz RP, Botti JJ: The clinical significance of placental villous edema. Pediatrics 71:588,1983.
9. Taylor J, Garite TJ: Premature rupture of the membranes before fetal viability. Obstet Gynecol 64:615, 1984.
10. Sepulveda WH, Gonzalez C, Cruz MA, Rudolph MI: Vasoconstrictive effect of bile acids on isolated human chorionic veins. Eur J Obstet Gynecol Reprod Biol 42:211, 1991.
11. Naeye RL: Can meconium in the amniotic fluid injure the fetal brain? Obstet Gynecol 86:720, 1995.
12. Altshuler G, Hyde S: Meconium-induced vasoconstriction: a potential cause of cerebral palsy, fetal hypoperfusion and poor pregnancy outcome. J Child Neurol 4:137, 1989.
13. Naeye RL: Umbilical cord length. J Pediatr 107:278, 1985.
14. Naeye RL: Maternal floor infarction. Hum Pathol 16:823, 1985.
15. Naeye RL: Causes of perinatal mortality excess in prolonged gestations. Am J Epidemiol 108:429, 1978.
16. Naeye RL: Reliability factors of delivery due dates. J Reprod Med 22:148, 1979.
17. Genest DR, Williams MA, Greene MF: Estimating the time of death in stillborn fetuses. I. Histologic evaluation of fetal organs, an autopsy study of 150 stillborns. Obstet Gynecol 80:575, 1992.
18. Genest DR: Estimating the time of death in stillborn fetuses. II. Histologic evaluation of the placenta: a study of 71 stillborns. Obstet Gynecol 80:585, 1992.
19. Genest DR: Estimating the time of death in stillborn fetuses. III. External fetal examination: a study of 86 stillborns. Obstet Gynecol 80:593, 1992.
20. Hagberg G, Hagberg G, Olow L, et al: The changing panorama of cerebral palsy in Sweden. V. The first year period 1979-82. Acta Paediatr Scand 78:283, 1989.
21. Stanley F, Watson L: Trends in perinatal mortality and cerebral palsy in Western Australia, 1967 to 1985. Br Med J 304:1658, 1992.
22. MacGillivray I, Campbell DM: The changing pattern of cerebral palsy in Avon. Paediatr Perinat Epidemiol 9:146, 1995.
23. Naeye RL, Peters EC, Bartholomew M, Landis JR: Origins of cerebral palsy. Am J Dis Child 143:1154, 1989.
24. Barkovich AJ: Pediatric neuroimaging, 2nd ed. New York, 1995, Raven Press.
25. Sarnat HB: Cerebral dysgenesis, embryology and clinical expression. New York, 1992, Oxford University Press.
26. Volpe J: Neurology of the newborn. Philadelphia, 1995, WB Saunders.
27. Meyers RS: Two patterns of perinatal brain damage and their conditions of occurrence. Am J Obstet Gynecol 112:246, 1972.
28. Low JA, Galbraith RS, Muir DW, et al: Factors associated with motor and cognitive deficits in children after intrapartum fetal hypoxia. Am J Obstet Gynecol 148:533, 1984.

29. Low JA: Fetal acid-base status and outcome. In Hill A, Volpe JJ (eds): Fetal neurology. New York, 1989, Raven Press.
30. Lou HC, Lassen NA, Tweed WA, et al: Pressure passive cerebral blood flow and breakdown of the blood-brain barrier in experimental fetal asphyxia. Acta Paediatr Scand 68:57, 1979.
31. Reivich M, Brann AW Jr, Shapiro HM, et al: Regional cerebral blood flow during prolonged partial asphyxia. In Meyer JS, Reivich M, Lechner H, et al (eds): Research on the cerebral circulation. Springfield, Ill., 1972, Charles C Thomas, p 217.
32. Dawes GS: Foetal and neonatal physiology. Chicago, 1968, Year Book, p 143.
33. Nelson KB, Dambrosia JM, Ting TY, Grether JK: Uncertain value of electronic fetal monitoring in predicting cerebral palsy. N Engl J Med 334:613, 1996.
34. MacDonald D: Cerebral palsy and intrapartum fetal monitoring. N Engl J Med 334:659, 1996.
35. Naeye RL, Localio AR: Determining the time before birth when ischemia and hypoxemia initiated cerebral palsy. Obstet Gynecol 86:713, 1995.
36. Salafia CM, Minior VK, Pezzulo JC, et al: Premature rupture of the membranes and preterm labor: neonatal nucleated erythrocyte numbers are related to histologic acute inflammation and not to placental markers of hypoxia. Am J Obstet Gynecol 174:318, 1996.

Index

Note: Page numbers in *italics* refer to illustrations; page numbers followed by t refer to tables.

M

ISBN 0-443-07586-7